THE
REHABILITATION
SPECIALIST'S
HANDBOOK

FOURTH EDITION

THE REHABILITATION SPECIALIST'S
HANDBOOK

Serge H. Roy, ScD, PT
Research Professor
NeuroMuscular Research Center, and
Sargent College of Health and Rehabilitation Sciences
Boston University
Boston, Massachusetts

Steven L. Wolf, PhD, PT, FAPTA, FAHA
Associate Professor, Department of Cell Biology
Emory University School of Medicine Center for Rehabilitation Medicine
Atlanta, Georgia

Professor, Health and Elder Care
Nell Hodgson Woodruff School of Nursing at Emory University
Senior Research Scientist, Atlanta VA Rehab R&D Center

David A. Scalzitti, PhD, PT, OCS
Associate Editor, Evidence-Based Resources
American Physical Therapy Association
Alexandria, Virginia

F.A. Davis Company • Philadelphia

F. A. Davis Company
1915 Arch Street
Philadelphia, PA 19103
www.fadavis.com

Printed in the United States of America
Last digit indicates print number: 10 9 8 7 6 5 4 3 2

Library of Congress Cataloging-in-Publication Data
Roy, Serge H., 1949-
  The rehabilitation specialist's handbook / Serge H. Roy, Steven L. Wolf, David A. Scalzitti.—4th ed.
    p. ; cm.
  Rev. ed. of: The rehabilitation specialist's handbook / Jonathan M. Rothstein ... [et al.]. 3rd ed. c2005.
  Includes bibliographical references and index.
  ISBN 978-0-8036-3906-5—ISBN 0-8036-3906-6
  I. Wolf, Steven L. II. Scalzitti, David A. III. Rehabilitation specialist's handbook. IV. Title.
  [DNLM: 1. Rehabilitation—Handbooks. 2. Physical Therapy Modalities—Handbooks. WB 39]

  617.03—dc23

                    2012041574

Editor-in-Chief: Margaret M. Biblis
Acquisitions Editor: Melissa A. Duffield
Senior Developmental Editor: Jennifer A. Pine
Manager of Content Development: George W. Lang
Art and Design Manager: Carolyn O'Brien

Preface

This *Fourth Edition of the Rehabilitation Specialist's Handbook* is a testament to the fact that information, and the technology for communicating it, has expanded at an exponential rate. While many of the early attributes designed for easy access in the *Handbook* have been retained, this one edition has undergone more extensive modifications than all previous editions combined. We may have even reached the point at which the term "revision" is outdated, because the new content in Edition 4 has surpassed that retained from previous editions.

If this is your first exposure to the *Handbook*, then these changes are inconsequential . . . just enjoy the book, and make full use of our efforts to keep pace with the times. To those of you who have consulted previous *Handbook* editions, we hope you will continue to appreciate the fact that we have not compromised our goal of providing you with information that is easily retrievable, substantive, and relevant to rehabilitation practice.

When first opening this book, you will notice that the content has been completely reorganized into sections that emphasize its relationship to rehabilitation practices, such as "Tools and Essentials for Practice," "Specialty Areas of Practice," and "Resources for Practice." More generalized information for the different body systems is now listed in a separate section. Each of the components within these sections has been expanded significantly—not only by updating the material from the third edition, but also by adding new sections that reflect either the growing importance of specific sub-specialties in rehabilitation (Women's Health, Oncology, Genetics, and Geriatrics), and new technological advancements that provide resources for practice (Prosthetics, Orthotics, Wheelchairs and Seating). The specialty areas and resources for practice have been particularly strengthened by recruiting experts in the field to co-author sections, or components within them, that have been revised, or in some cases originated, so that the content truly reflects contemporary, clinical expertise. These individuals, to whom we are greatly indebted, are listed prominently immediately following the Preface.

You may then notice that this edition offers a full-color re-design of the pages including easier-to-read tables and over 400 completely new illustrations. For the first time, photographs and digital imaging combine with full-color anatomical illustrations and other line drawings to more effectively convey information. The re-design also integrates a color-coded organizational structure (colored section tabs, outlines, etc.) making it simpler to find information.

We acknowledge with profound appreciation that past editions of the *Handbook* have been used widely by students while acquiring their clinical experiences and to prepare for licensure examinations. Although not specifically designed for examination preparation, students have recognized over the years that the *Handbook* has the depth and breadth of information to provide a valuable and unique resource for retrieving information that will make them better prepared for successfully completing this important milestone in their professional lives. Feedback from students over the years on Handbook content has been an extremely valuable resource. We are thankful for your input and welcome future generations of students to these pages to continue this important dialogue.

One of the most important changes, in terms of "keeping contemporary," may be the least recognizable. *Handbook 4* has been prepared so that it can be made available in contemporary digital format to support its use on a variety of portable devices that have become a mainstay of our professional and personal lives.

The Greek philosopher Aristotle is credited with the pensive and insightful statement that "change in all things is sweet." While certainly true in reflecting on the new developments in *Handbook 4*, one change, the loss of our dear co-founding author Jules Rothstein, is a profound exception that leaves a void in this evolving process, as well as in our personal and professional lives. We miss his friendship and brilliance in co-authoring the original text, and guiding us on past revisions. It is fitting that Dr. David Scalzitti, who was mentored by Jules, should now assume the role of co-author on *Handbook 4*, joining co-founding authors Drs. Serge Roy and Steven Wolf. David has made invaluable contributions to past editions, and has earned this advancement from hard work and insightful contributions. He has also earned our respect and appreciation.

S.H. Roy
Boston, 2011

S.L. Wolf
Atlanta, 2011

Contributors

Hilmir Agustsson, MHSc, DPT, MTC, CFC
University of St. Augustine
St. Augustine, Florida

Doris Armour, MD
Department of Rehabilitation Medicine
Emory University
Atlanta, Georgia

Diane Beckwith, PT, ATP
Center for Rehabilitation Medicine
Emory University
Atlanta, Georgia

Sarah Blanton, DPT, NCS
Division of Physical Therapy
Department of Rehabilitation Medicine
Emory University School of Medicine
Atlanta, Georgia

Charles D. Ciccone, PhD, PT,
Department of Physical Therapy
School of Health Sciences and Human Performance
Ithaca College
Ithaca, New York

Catherine L. Curtis, EdD, PT
Department of Physical Therapy
School of Health Sciences & Practice
Institute of Public Health
New York Medical College
Valhalla, New York

Edelle Field-Fote, PhD, PT
Department of Physical Therapy
University of Miami Miller School of Medicine
Miami, Florida

Wendy Gilleard, BAppSc, MSc, PhD
School of Health and Human Sciences
Southern Cross University
Lismore, NSW AUSTRALIA

Allon Goldberg, PhD, PT
Department of Physical Therapy
Wayne State University
Detroit, Michigan

Courtney Hall, PhD, PT
Auditory and Vestibular Dysfunction REAP
James H. Quillen VA Medical Center
Mountain Home, Tennessee

Susan Herdman, PhD, PT, FAPTA
Division of Physical Therapy
Department of Rehabilitation Medicine
Emory University School of Medicine
Atlanta, Georgia

Jeffrey Hoder, PhD, PT, DPT, NCS
Department of Neurology
Virginia Commonwealth University
Richmond, Virginia

Christopher Hovorka, MS, CPO, LPO, FAAOP
Prosthetics and Orthotics Program
School of Applied Physiology
Georgia Institute of Technology
Atlanta, Georgia

Zoher Kapasi, PhD, PT, MBA
Division of Physical Therapy
Department of Rehabilitation Medicine
Emory University School of Medicine
Atlanta, Georgia

Robert Kistenberg, MPH, CP, LP, FAAOP
Prosthetics and Orthotics Program
School of Applied Physiology
Georgia Institute of Technology
Atlanta, Georgia

Aimee B. Klein, DPT, DSc, OCS
Department of Physical Therapy
School of Health and Rehabilitation Sciences
MGH Institute of Health Professions
Boston, Massachusetts

Geza Kogler, PhD, CO
Prosthetics and Orthotics Program
School of Applied Physiology
Georgia Institute of Technology
Atlanta, Georgia

Andréa Leiserowitz, MPT, CLT
Oncology Physical Therapy
Eugene, Oregon

Edward Mahoney, MSPT, DPT, CWS
Department of Rehabilitation Sciences
School of Allied Health Professions
LSU Health Sciences Center
Shreveport, Louisiana

Irene McEwen, PT, DPT, PhD, FAPTA
The Department of Rehabilitation Sciences
College of Allied Health
University of Oklahoma HSC
Oklahoma City, Oklahoma

David Pleva, PT, Dip.MDT
Community Physical Therapy
Addison, Illinois

Chris Rorden, PhD
Center for Advanced Brain Imaging
Medical University of South Carolina
Charleston, South Carolina

Elizabeth Benson Smith
Habersham Medical Center
Demorest, Georgia

Anthony Y. Stringer, PhD, ABPP/CN, CPCRT
Department of Rehabilitation Medicine (Neuropsychology)
Emory University School of Medicine
Atlanta, Georgia

Anne Swisher, PT, PhD, CCS
Department of Physical Therapy
School of Medicine-Human Performance
West Virginia University
Morgantown, West Virginia

Elise Townsend, DPT, PhD, PCS
Department of Physical Therapy
School of Health and Rehabilitation Sciences
MGH Institute of Health Professions
Boston, Massachusetts

Michael T. Wexler, BS
Department of Biomedical Engineering
College of Engineering
Boston University
Boston, Massachusetts

Heather Wilsey, PT, DPT, NCS, CSCS
Habersham Medical Center
Demorest, Georgia

Joshua H. Wolf, MD
Piedmont Transplant Institute
Piedmont Hospital
Atlanta, Georgia

Laura Zajac-Cox, PT, NCS
Division of Physical Therapy
Department of Rehabilitation Medicine
Emory University School of Medicine
Atlanta, Georgia

Brief Contents

Contents

APPENDIX Reference Tables, Conversion Charts, and First Aid 1215

About the Authors

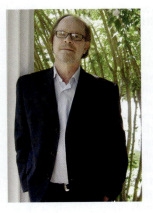

Serge H. Roy, ScD, PT, is a Research Professor at both the NeuroMuscular Research Center and the Sargent College of Health and Rehabilitation Sciences at Boston University. Dr. Roy received his entry-level degree in Physical Therapy from New York University, an MS degree in Physical Therapy and an ScD degree in Applied Anatomy and Kinesiology from Boston University Sargent College of Health and Rehabilitation Sciences. Dr. Roy is the recipient of the Elizabeth C. Adams Award from N.Y.U. and two group achievement awards from NASA. He was elected a Fellow of the American Institute for Medical and Biological Engineering (AIMBE) and the International Society of Electrophysiology and Kinesiology (ISEK), where he also served as past President of ISEK. Dr. Roy is a co-founding author of *The Rehabilitation Specialist's Handbook.* His research activities are focused on developing EMG systems for assessing muscle impairments; automated monitoring of movement disorders; and studying the effects of aging, bedrest, and microgravity on motor unit function.

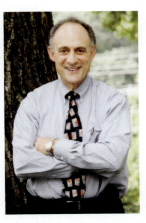

Steven L. Wolf, PhD, PT, FAPTA, FAHA, received his AB in Biology from Clark University, his physical therapy certificate from Columbia University, MS in Physical Therapy from Boston University, and his PhD in Neurophysiology from Emory University. He has defined the selection criteria for the application of EMG biofeedback to restore upper extremity function among chronic patients with stroke. These findings became the inclusion criteria for most constraint induced movement therapy stroke studies. He has served in multiple administrative and leadership capacities for the American Physical Therapy Association and for groups associated with the promotion of research and clinical service within neurorehabilitation. He is the recipient of the Marian Williams Award for Research Golden Pen Award, Georgia Merit Award, Physical Therapy Association of Georgia; Catherine Worthingham Fellowship; Robert C. Bartlett Recognition Award, Foundation for Physical Therapy; Distinguished Service Award, Section on Clinical Electrophysiology;

Helen J. Hislop Award for Excellence in Contributions to Professional Literature; Lucy Blair Service Award; Section on Geriatrics outstanding published paper award; Neurology Section, Outstanding Researcher Award; Mary McMillan Lecturer. He has been a keynote speaker for many organizations, a commencement speaker for several institutions, and has served on several study sections and advisory boards for the NIH and other foundations.

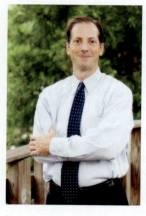

David A. Scalzitti, PhD, PT, OCS received his entry-level degree in Physical Therapy from the University of Illinois at Chicago (UIC) and after several years of clinical practice returned to the UIC for a Master of Science degree in Kinesiology and a PhD in Disability Studies. Dr. Scalzitti has overseen the growth of the American Physical Therapy Association's Hooked on Evidence database and has contributed to a number of other initiatives related to evidence-based physical therapy practice. David is an adjunct faculty member at George Washington University and is a frequent invited speaker at a number of physical therapy education programs and national meetings. He has been a contributing author to two previous editions of the *Rehabilitation Specialist's Handbook*.

Acknowledgments

The allocated page space would not afford us ample opportunity to properly acknowledge all of the generous contributions from the FA Davis team, colleagues, students, family, and friends who have provided valuable support throughout the creation of this 4th Edition. Special thanks are directed to Teresa Prince (photographer) and the Emory DPT student models (Mathew Ayers and Kelsey Gilman) for the photographs that appear for the first time in this edition. Thank you one and all!

SHR, SLW, DAS

Tools and Essentials for Practice

I

CONCEPTS AND CONSTRUCTS

International Classification of Functioning, Disability, and Health (ICF)

In 2001, the World Health Assembly endorsed the International Classification of Functioning, Disability, and Health (ICF), which represents a revision of the International Classification of Impairment, Disability and Health (ICIDH). The ICF has moved from being a "consequence of disease" classification to become a "components of health" classification. The ICF does not model the process of functioning and disability; instead, it provides a multi-perspective approach to classification as an interactive and evolutionary process. Terms used in the ICF are designed to be neutral in terms of etiology and are designed to include both positive and negative aspects.

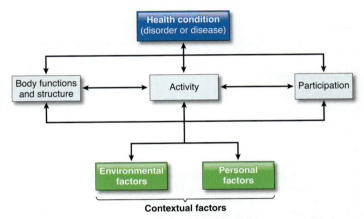

The components of the ICF model and the interactions between components. **From:** World Health Organization. *ICF: International Classification of Functioning, Disability, and Health.* World Health Organization, Geneva, Switzerland, 2002:18; with permission.

Definition of Terms in the ICF

body functions: The physiological functions of body systems (including psychological functions).

body structures: Anatomical parts of the body such as organs, limbs, and their components.

impairments: Problems in body function or structure, such as a significant deviation or loss.

activity: The execution of a task or action by an individual.

participation: The involvement in a life situation.

activity limitations: Difficulties that an individual may have in executing activities.

participation restrictions: Problems an individual may experience in involvement in life situations.

environmental factors: The physical, social, and attitudinal environment in which people live and conduct their lives.

personal factors: The particular background of an individual's life and living; these make up features of the individual that are not part of the health condition or health states. These factors may include gender, race, age, other health conditions, fitness, lifestyle, habits, upbringing, coping styles, social background, education, profession, past and current experiences, overall behavior pattern and character style, individual psychological assets, and other characteristics, all of which may play a role in disability at any level. Personal factors are not classified in the ICF; however, their contribution is recognized.

functioning: An umbrella term encompassing all body functions, activities, and participation.

disability: An umbrella term for impairments, activity limitations, or participation restrictions.

From:

World Health Organization. ICF: International Classification of Functioning, Disability and Health. World Health Organization, Geneva, Switzerland, 2002.

ICF Classification

Body Functions
1. Mental functions
2. Sensory functions and pain
3. Voice and speech functions
4. Functions of the cardiovascular, haematological, immunological, and respiratory systems
5. Functions of the digestive, metabolic, and endocrine systems
6. Genitourinary and reproductive functions
7. Neuromusculoskeletal and movement-related functions
8. Functions of the skin and related structures

Body Structures
1. Structures of the nervous system
2. The eye, ear, and related structures
3. Structures involved in voice and speech
4. Structures of the cardiovascular, immunological, and respiratory systems
5. Structures related to the digestive, metabolic, and endocrine systems
6. Structures related to the genitourinary and reproductive systems
7. Structures related to movement
8. Skin and related structures

Activities and Participation
1. Learning and applying knowledge
2. General tasks and demands
3. Communication
4. Mobility
5. Self-care
6. Domestic life
7. Interpersonal interactions and relationships

8. Major life areas
9. Community, social, and civic life

Environmental Factors
1. Products and technology
2. Natural environment and human-made changes to environment
3. Support and relationships
4. Attitudes
5. Service, systems, and policies

Guide to Physical Therapist Practice

Definitions of the Elements of Patient/Client Management

examination: A comprehensive screening and specific testing process leading to diagnostic classification or, as appropriate, to a referral to another practitioner. Includes the following:
- **history:** A systematic gathering of data related to the reason(s) the patient/client is seeking services.
- **systems review:** A brief or limited examination of (1) the anatomical and physiological status of the cardiovascular/pulmonary, integumentary, musculoskeletal, and neuromuscular systems; and (2) the communication ability, affect, cognition, language, and learning style of the patient.
- **tests and measures:** Specific standardized methods and techniques used to gather data about the patient/client.

evaluation: A dynamic process in which the physical therapist makes clinical judgments based on data gathered during the examination.

diagnosis: The process of integrating and evaluating the data that are obtained during the examination to describe the patient/client condition in terms that will guide the prognosis, the plan of care, and intervention strategies.

prognosis: The determination of the predicted optimal level of improvement in function and the amount of time needed to reach that level.

intervention: The purposeful interaction of the physical therapist with the patient/client, and, when appropriate, with other individuals involved in patient/client care, using various physical therapy procedures and techniques to produce changes in the condition.

outcomes: The intended results of patient/client management, which the changes in impairments, functional limitations, and disabilities and the changes in health, wellness, and fitness needs that are expected as the result of implementing the plan of care. The expected outcomes in the plan should be measurable and time limited.

Based on:

Guide to Physical Therapist Practice, ed. 2. Phys Ther 81:9–744, 2001.

Tests and Measures

- Aerobic capacity/endurance
- Anthropometric characteristics

- Arousal, attention, and cognition
- Assistive and adaptive devices
- Circulation (arterial, venous, lymphatic)
- Cranial and peripheral nerve integrity
- Environmental, home, and work (job/school/play) barriers
- Ergonomics and body mechanics
- Gait, locomotion, and balance
- Integumentary integrity
- Joint integrity and mobility
- Motor function (motor control and motor learning)
- Muscle performance (including strength, power, and endurance)
- Neuromotor development and sensory integration
- Orthotic, protective, and supportive devices
- Pain
- Posture
- Prosthetic requirements
- Range of motion (including muscle length)
- Reflex integrity
- Self-care and home management (including activities of daily living and instrumental activities of daily living)
- Sensory integrity
- Ventilation, respiration (gas exchange), and circulation
- Work (job/school/play), community, and leisure integration or reintegration (including instrumental activities of daily living)

Types of Interventions

- Coordination, communication, and documentation
- Patient/client-related instruction
- Procedural interventions
  - Therapeutic exercise (including aerobic conditioning)
  - Functional training in self-care and home management (including activities of daily living and instrumental activities of daily living)
  - Functional training in community and work (job/school/play) integration or reintegration (including instrumental activities of daily living, work hardening, and work conditioning)
  - Manual therapy techniques (including mobilization and manipulation)
  - Prescription, application, and, as appropriate, fabrication of devices and equipment
  - Airway clearance techniques
  - Integumentary repair and protection
  - Electrotherapeutic modalities
  - Physical agents and mechanical modalities

Preferred Practice Patterns

Musculoskeletal

Pattern A: Primary prevention/risk reduction for skeletal demineralization
Pattern B: Impaired posture

Pattern C: Impaired muscle performance

Pattern D: Impaired joint mobility, motor function, muscle performance, and range of motion associated with connective tissue dysfunction

Pattern E: Impaired joint mobility, motor function, muscle performance, and range of motion associated with localized inflammation

Pattern F: Impaired joint mobility, motor function, muscle performance, range of motion, and reflex integrity associated with spinal disorders

Pattern G: Impaired joint mobility, muscle performance, and range of motion associated with fracture

Pattern H: Impaired joint mobility, motor function, muscle performance, and range of motion associated with joint arthroplasty

Pattern I: Impaired joint mobility, motor function, muscle performance, and range of motion associated with bony or soft tissue surgery

Pattern J: Impaired motor function, muscle performance, range of motion, gait, locomotion, and balance associated with amputation

Neuromuscular

Pattern A: Primary prevention/risk reduction for loss of balance and falling

Pattern B: Impaired neuromotor development

Pattern C: Impaired motor function and sensory integrity associated with non-progressive disorders of the central nervous system—congenital origin or acquired in infancy or childhood

Pattern D: Impaired motor function and sensory integrity associated with nonprogressive disorders of the central nervous system— acquired in adolescence or adulthood

Pattern E: Impaired motor function and sensory integrity associated with progressive disorders of the central nervous system

Pattern F: Impaired peripheral nerve integrity and muscle performance associated with peripheral nerve injury

Pattern G: Impaired motor function and sensory integrity associated with acute or chronic polyneuropathies

Pattern H: Impaired motor function, peripheral nerve integrity, and sensory integrity associated with nonprogressive disorders of the spinal cord

Pattern I: Impaired arousal, range of motion, and motor control associated with coma, near coma, or vegetative state

Cardiovascular/Pulmonary

Pattern A: Primary prevention/risk reduction for cardiovascular/pulmonary disorders

Pattern B: Impaired aerobic capacity/endurance associated with deconditioning

Pattern C: Impaired ventilation, respiration/gas exchange, and aerobic capacity/endurance associated with airway clearance dysfunction

Pattern D: Impaired aerobic capacity/endurance associated with cardiovascular pump dysfunction or failure

Pattern E: Impaired ventilation and respiration/gas exchange associated with ventilatory pump dysfunction or failure

Pattern F: Impaired ventilation and respiration/gas exchange associated with respiratory failure

Pattern G: Impaired ventilation, respiration/gas exchange, and aerobic capacity/endurance associated with respiratory failure in the neonate

Pattern H: Impaired circulation and anthropometric dimensions associated with lymphatic system disorders

Integumentary

Pattern A: Primary prevention/risk reduction for integumentary disorders

Pattern B: Impaired integumentary integrity associated with superficial skin involvement

Pattern C: Impaired integumentary integrity associated with partial-thickness skin involvement and scar formation

Pattern D: Impaired integumentary integrity associated with full-thickness skin involvement and scar formation

Pattern E: Impaired integumentary integrity associated with skin involvement extending into fascia, muscle, or bone and scar formation

Evidence-Based Practice

Overview

Evidence-based practice is the integration of best research evidence with clinical expertise and the patient's unique values and circumstances.

Steps

- Develop an answerable clinical question.
- Search the literature for relevant clinical articles.
- Critically appraise the evidence for its validity and its usefulness.
- Implement useful findings in clinical practice.
- Evaluate performance.

PICO Clinical Questions

- The Patient or problem being addressed
- The Intervention
- A Comparison intervention
- The clinical Outcome or outcome of interest

Glossary of Terms Related to Evidence-Based Practice

absolute mean difference (AMD): A measure of effect size; simply the difference between the means of a treatment group and a comparison group.

absolute risk: The probability or chance that a person will have a medical event. Absolute risk is expressed as a percentage. It is the ratio of the number of people who have a medical event divided by all of the people who could have the event because of their medical condition.

cohort study: A clinical research study in which people who have a certain condition or receive a particular treatment are followed over time and compared with another group of people who are not affected by the condition. In a cohort study (also known as a prospective observational study), measurements of the people who belong to a cohort are obtained at several points in time.

comparative effectiveness: The conduct and synthesis of systematic research comparing different interventions and strategies to prevent, diagnose, treat, and monitor health conditions.

confidence interval (CI): The range in which a particular result is likely to occur for everyone who has a disease. For example, a 95% CI is the range of values within which we can be 95% sure that the true value for the whole population lies. A CI is defined by two numbers, one lower than the result found in the study and the other higher than the study's result. The size of the confidence interval is the difference between these two numbers.

cost-benefit analysis: A type of analysis that compares the financial costs with the benefits of two or more health-care treatments or programs. Health-care interventions that have the same or better benefit at a lower cost are better values than treatments or programs that are more expensive.

cost-effectiveness analysis: A type of analysis that is similar to a cost-benefit analysis but is used when the benefits cannot be measured in financial terms. It would be hard to put a price tag on living an extra year of life.

diagnostic test: A procedure to provide information about a person's condition that helps health-care providers to make a diagnosis. Diagnostic tests provide information about whether a person does or does not have a particular disease.

effect size: The amount of change in a condition or symptom as a result of a treatment (compared to not receiving the treatment). It is commonly expressed as a risk ratio (relative risk), odds ratio, difference in risk, number needed to treat, absolute mean difference, or standardized mean difference.

effectiveness: Whether a treatment works in real life. Effectiveness studies of drugs look at whether they work when they are used the way that most people take them. Effectiveness means that most people who have the disease would improve if they used the treatment.

efficacy: Whether a treatment works under the best possible conditions. In a research study about efficacy, the study participants are carefully selected, and the researchers can make sure the treatment is administered consistently. A treatment that has efficacy under the best conditions may not work as well in a different group of people with the same disease.

likelihood ratio (LR): A measure of the accuracy of a diagnostic test. It is used to determine how likely it is that a person has a specific disease based on test results. When the test result is positive, the likelihood ratio is known as a positive likelihood ratio (LR+). When the test result is negative, the likelihood ratio is known as a negative likelihood ratio (LR−). The likelihood ratio is a way of comparing the probability that the test result would occur in people with the disease as opposed to occurring in people without the disease. A positive likelihood ratio greater than 10 or a negative likelihood ratio less than 0.1 would be considered clinically useful in helping guide health-care decision making.

meta-analysis: A way of combining data from many different research studies. A meta-analysis is a statistical process that combines the findings from individual studies.

minimal clinically important difference (MCID): The smallest change in measurement that signifies an important improvement according to the patient/client's perspective. Also known as the minimal clinically important change (MCIC).

minimal detectable change (MDC): The amount of change in a variable that must be achieved to reflect a true difference. Also known as the minimal detectable difference (MDD).

negative predictive value (NPV): Indicates the likelihood that people with a negative test result would not have a condition. The higher the value of the negative predictive value (e.g., 99% is usually considered a high value), the more useful the test is for predicting that people do not have the condition.

number needed to harm (NNH): The number of people who would need to be treated over a specific period of time before one bad outcome of the treatment will occur.

number needed to treat (NNT): The number of people who need to be treated over a specific period of time to promote one additional good outcome (or prevent one additional bad outcome).

odds ratio (OR): The chance of an event occurring in one group compared to the chance of it occurring in another group. The OR is a measure of effect size and is commonly used to compare results in clinical trials. An OR of 1 indicates no difference between the treatment and comparison groups.

positive predictive value (PPV): Indicates the likelihood that a person with a positive test result would actually have the condition for which the test is used. The higher the value of the positive predictive value (e.g., 90% is considered a high value), the more useful the test is for predicting that the person has the condition.

prevalence: How often or how frequently a disease or condition occurs in a group of people. Prevalence is calculated by dividing the number of people who have the disease or condition by the total number of people in the group.

probability: The likelihood (or chance) that an event will occur. In a clinical research study, it is the number of times a condition or event occurs in a study group divided by the number of people being studied.

randomized controlled trial: A controlled clinical trial that randomly (by chance) assigns participants to two or more groups. There are various methods to randomize study participants to their groups.

relative risk (RR): A comparison of the risk of a particular event for different groups of people. Relative risk (RR) is usually used to estimate exposure to something that could affect health. In a clinical research study, the experimental group is exposed to a particular drug or treatment. The control group is not. The number of events in each group is compared to determine relative risk. An RR of 1 indicates no difference between the treatment and comparison group.

reliability: The consistency or repeatability of measurements; the degree to which measurements are error free and the degree to which repeated measurements will agree.

- **internal consistency:** The extent to which items or elements that contribute to a measurement reflect one basic phenomenon or dimension.
- **intertester reliability:** The consistency or equivalence of measurements when more than one person takes the measurements; indicates agreement of measurements taken by different examiners.
- **intratester reliability:** The consistency or equivalence of measurements when one person takes repeated measurements separated in time; indicates agreement in measurements over time.
- **parallel-forms (alternate-forms) reliability:** The consistency or agreement of measurements obtained with different (alternative) forms of a test;

indicates whether measurements obtained with different forms of a test can be used interchangeably.

- **test-retest reliability:** The consistency or repeated measurements separated in time; indicates stability (reliability) over time.

sensitivity: The ability of a test to identify correctly people with a condition. A test with high sensitivity will nearly always be positive for people who have the condition (the test has a low rate of false-negative results). Sensitivity is also known as the true-positive rate.

specificity: The ability of a test to identify correctly people without a condition. A test with high specificity will rarely be wrong about who does *not* have the condition (the test has a low rate of false-positive results). Specificity is also known as the true-negative rate.

standardized mean difference (SMD): The SMD is a measure of treatment effect size and is the ratio of the difference between the means of a treatment and comparison group and the pooled standard deviation of the means. An SMD of 0 indicates no difference between the treatment group and the comparison group.

systematic review: A summary of the clinical literature. A systematic review is a critical assessment and evaluation of all research studies that address a particular clinical issue. The researchers use an organized method of locating, assembling, and evaluating a body of literature on a particular topic using a set of specific criteria. A systematic review typically includes a description of the findings of the collection of research studies. The systematic review may also include a quantitative pooling of data, called a meta-analysis. A comparative effectiveness review is a type of systematic review in which all the available evidence about particular treatments for a disease is reviewed and compared.

validity: The degree to which a useful (meaningful) interpretation can be inferred from a measurement.

- **concurrent validity:** A form of criterion-based validity in which an inferred interpretation is justified by comparing a measurement with supporting evidence that was obtained at approximately the same time as the measurement being validated.
- **construct validity:** The conceptual (theoretical) basis for using a measurement to make an inferred interpretation; evidence for construct validity is through logical argumentation based on theoretical and research evidence.
- **content validity:** A form of validity that deals with the extent to which a measurement is judged to reflect the meaningful elements of a construct and not any extraneous elements.
- **criterion-based (criterion-related) validity:** Three forms of criterion-based validity exist: concurrent validity, predictive validity, and prescriptive validity; the common element is that with each of these forms of validity the correctness of an inferred interpretation can be tested by comparing a measurement with either a different measurement or data obtained by other forms of testing.
- **predictive validity:** A form of criterion-based validity in which an inferred interpretation is justified by comparing a measurement with supporting evidence that is obtained at a later point in time; examines the justification of using a measurement to say something about future events or conditions.

- **prescriptive validity:** A form of criterion-based validity in which the inferred interpretation of a measurement is the determination of the form of treatment a person is to receive; prescriptive validity is justified based on the successful outcome of the chosen treatment.

Definitions based on:
http://effectivehealthcare.ahrq.gov/tools.cfm?tooltype=glossary. *Accessed January 13, 2012.*
Rothstein, JM, and Echternach, JL: Primer on Measurement: An Introductory Guide to Measurement Issues. APTA, Alexandria, VA, 1993.
Straus, SE, et al: Evidence-Based Medicine: How to Practice and Teach EBM, ed. 4. Elsevier Churchill Livingstone, Edinburgh, Scotland, 2011.

Statistics for Evidence-Based Practice

🟠 TABLE 1.1 Studies of Diagnosis

	Target Condition Present	Target Condition Absent	Total
Diagnostic test positive	a (true positives)	b (false positives)	a + b
Diagnostic test negative	c (false negatives)	d (true negatives)	c + d
Total	a + c	b + d	a + b + c + d

Sensitivity = $a/(a + c)$
Specificity = $d/(b + d)$
Likelihood ratio for a positive test result = LR+ = sensitivity/(1 − specificity)
Likelihood ratio for a negative test result = LR− = (1 − sensitivity)/specificity
Positive predictive value = $a/(a + b)$
Negative predictive value = $d/(c + d)$
Pre-test probability (prevalence) = $(a + c)/(a + b + c + d)$
Pre-test odds = prevalence/(1 − prevalence)
Post-test odds = pre-test odds × likelihood ratio
Post-test probability = post-test odds/(post-test odds + 1)

Studies of Reliability

Minimal detectable change at the 95% confidence intervals (MDC_{95}) = 1.96 × $\sqrt{2}$ × standard error of the measurement, where the standard error of the measurement = standard deviation × $\sqrt{1-r}$ and r is the correlation coefficient

🟠 TABLE 1.2 Studies of Interventions With Dichotomous Outcomes

	Outcome Present	Outcome Absent	Totals
Treatment group	a	b	a + b
Comparison group	c	d	c + d
Totals	a + c	b + d	a + b + c + d

Odds ratio = $(a × d)/(b × c)$
Relative risk = $[a/(a + b)]/[c/(c + d)]$
Absolute risk reduction = $[a/(a + b)] − [c/(c + d)]$
Number needed to treat = $1/[a/(a + b)] − [c/(c + d)]$

Studies of Interventions With Continuous Outcomes

Standardized mean difference = (mean$_1$ – mean$_2$)/pooled standard deviation
where the pooled standard deviation =

$$\sqrt{\frac{[SD_1^2 \cdot (n_1 - 1)] + [SD_2^2 \cdot (n_2 - 1)]}{n_1 + n_2 - 2}}$$

PEDro Scale for Rating the Quality of Randomized Clinical Trials

The PEDro scale uses the following criteria to score randomized clinical trials based on the number of items present (0–10). A higher score represents higher quality in the information reported in the article regarding the validity of the trial.

- Random allocation
- Concealed allocation
- Groups similar at baseline
- Blinding of subjects
- Blinding of clinicians
- Blinding of assessors
- Adequate follow-up of outcomes (obtained from at least 85% of the participants randomized to groups)
- Intention to treat analysis
- Between group statistical comparisons reported
- Point estimates and measure of variability reported

Hypothesis-Oriented Algorithm for Clinical Decision Making

The purpose of the Hypothesis-Oriented Algorithm for Clinicians (HOAC-II) is to provide rehabilitation practitioners with a framework for clinical decision making, self-evaluation, and documentation. A central feature of the algorithm is the idea that all treatments must be based on a conceptual theme, that is, hypotheses as to why patients have problems or may anticipate developing problems.

The algorithm has two parts. Part One leads clinicians through the process of evaluation, hypothesis generation, and development of treatment strategies (overall purposes) and tactics (specific treatments). Part Two takes the clinician through the processes of reevaluation, with concrete items being considered (i.e., implementation of tactics and formulation of strategies) before theoretical issues (i.e., is the hypothesis correct?).

Hypothesis-Oriented Algorithm for Clinicians II
(HOAC II - PART 1)

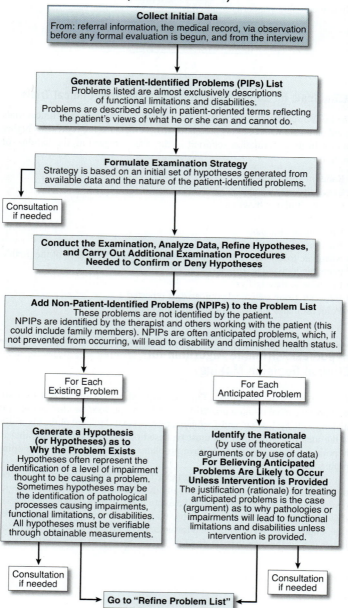

Collect Initial Data
From: referral information, the medical record, via observation before any formal evaluation is begun, and from the interview

Generate Patient-Identified Problems (PIPs) List
Problems listed are almost exclusively descriptions of functional limitations and disabilities.
Problems are described solely in patient-oriented terms reflecting the patient's views of what he or she can and cannot do.

Formulate Examination Strategy
Strategy is based on an initial set of hypotheses generated from available data and the nature of the patient-identified problems.

Consultation if needed

Conduct the Examination, Analyze Data, Refine Hypotheses, and Carry Out Additional Examination Procedures Needed to Confirm or Deny Hypotheses

Add Non-Patient-Identified Problems (NPIPs) to the Problem List
These problems are not identified by the patient.
NPIPs are identified by the therapist and others working with the patient (this could include family members). NPIPs are often anticipated problems, which, if not prevented from occurring, will lead to disability and diminished health status.

For Each Existing Problem

For Each Anticipated Problem

Generate a Hypothesis (or Hypotheses) as to Why the Problem Exists
Hypotheses often represent the identification of a level of impairment thought to be causing a problem. Sometimes hypotheses may be the identification of pathological processes causing impairments, functional limitations, or disabilities. All hypotheses must be verifiable through obtainable measurements.

Identify the Rationale
(by use of theoretical arguments or by use of data)
For Believing Anticipated Problems Are Likely to Occur Unless Intervention is Provided
The justification (rationale) for treating anticipated problems is the case (argument) as to why pathologies or impairments will lead to functional limitations and disabilities unless intervention is provided.

Consultation if needed

Consultation if needed

Go to "Refine Problem List"

Hypothesis-Oriented Algorithm for Clinicians II
(HOAC II - PART 1 continued)

Refine Problem List
Most problems will be maintained without modification.
Identify problems that should be treated by other
health-care workers (eliminate these problems from
the list), refer patient, and document the need for referral.
The problem statement should be annotated so that those
problems not amenable to full resolution are identified
and a modified problem statement needs to be generated.
Changes in the PIPs should only be done after discussion
with the patient and with proper documentation.

Referral
if needed

For Each Problem: Establish One or More Goals
Goals for existing problems usually represent measurable target levels of
function (disability) that a patient will achieve as a result of the intervention.
There must be a temporal element for each goal (an expectation as to when
the goal will be met). Goals for anticipated problems essentially consist of
statements as to what problems will be avoided as a result of intervention.
Goals are always patient centered and always represent outcomes that have
value to the patient's current quality of life or future quality of life.

For Each Existing Problem

For Each Anticipated Problem

Establish Testing Criteria
Testing criteria are used to examine
the correctness of the hypotheses.
Testing criteria usually represent
specified levels (measurements)
of achievements (often at the
impairment level) that if obtained
will result in the resolution of the
problem (attainment of the goal),
but only if the hypothesis is correct.

Establish Predictive Criteria
Predictive criteria are target levels
of measurements or behavioral
alterations that need to be obtained
to preclude the occurence of
anticipated problems. Because
anticipated problems and recurrence
are prevented, true testing of
hypotheses related to anticipated
problems is not possible.

Consultation if needed

Consultation if needed

Establish a Plan to Reassess Testing and Predictive Criteria
Establish a Plan to Assess the Status of Problems and Goals
The time interval between assessment of changes in the status of both
types of criterion measures (testing and predictive) should be based
on expected changes in those measurements, and those expectations in
turn should be based on theoretical arguements and data. Goals that
can be expected to be obtained sooner may be termed "short-term goals."
Short- and long-term goals, therefore, are not different in nature but only
in the time period expected before they are achieved.

Plan Intervention Strategy Based on
Hypotheses and Anticipated Problems
Indicate why the strategy should lead
to changes in the criterion measures.

Plan Tactics
Indicate how tactics are expected to alter criterion measures
(relate each tactic to a criterion measure). Indicate who
will implement tactics (eg, therapists, assistants, aides,
family members, teachers, and the patient).

Consultation
if needed

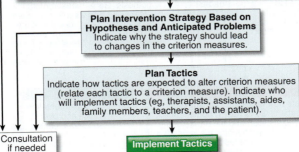

Implement Tactics

HOAC II - PART 2 (Existing Problems)

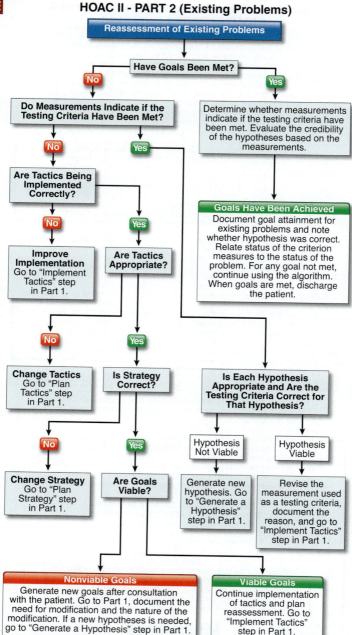

Reassessment of Existing Problems

Have Goals Been Met?

No — **Do Measurements Indicate if the Testing Criteria Have Been Met?**

Yes — Determine whether measurements indicate if the testing criteria have been met. Evaluate the credibility of the hypotheses based on the measurements.

No — **Are Tactics Being Implemented Correctly?**

Yes —

Goals Have Been Achieved
Document goal attainment for existing problems and note whether hypothesis was correct. Relate status of the criterion measures to the status of the problem. For any goal not met, continue using the algorithm. When goals are met, discharge the patient.

No — **Improve Implementation** Go to "Implement Tactics" step in Part 1.

Yes — **Are Tactics Appropriate?**

No — **Change Tactics** Go to "Plan Tactics" step in Part 1.

Yes — **Is Strategy Correct?**

Is Each Hypothesis Appropriate and Are the Testing Criteria Correct for That Hypothesis?

No — **Change Strategy** Go to "Plan Strategy" step in Part 1.

Yes — **Are Goals Viable?**

Hypothesis Not Viable — Generate new hypothesis. Go to "Generate a Hypothesis" step in Part 1.

Hypothesis Viable — Revise the measurement used as a testing criteria, document the reason, and go to "Implement Tactics" step in Part 1.

Nonviable Goals
Generate new goals after consultation with the patient. Go to Part 1, document the need for modification and the nature of the modification. If a new hypotheses is needed, go to "Generate a Hypothesis" step in Part 1.

Viable Goals
Continue implementation of tactics and plan reassessment. Go to "Implement Tactics" step in Part 1.

HOAC II – PART 2 (Anticipated Problems)

Reassessment of Anticipated Problems

↓

Have Problems Occurred?

No → / Yes →

No:

Have Predictive Criteria Been Met?

No → / Yes →

Yes:

Add problem to merged problem list in Part 1. Determine whether predictive criteria were met. Determine whether predictive criteria were appropriate.

Are Predictive Criteria Appropriate?

Appropriate Criteria | Inappropriate Criteria | Eliminate problem from the list.

Are Tactics Being Implemented Correctly?

Revise Criteria
Go to "Establish Predictive Criteria" step in Part 1.

No ↓

Improve Implementation
Go to "Implement Tactics" step in Part 1.

Goals Have Been Achieved
Document goal attainment. For anticipated problems, document the status of predictive criteria. For any goal not met, continue using the algorithm. When goals are met, discharge the patient.

Yes ↓

Are Tactics Appropriate?

No ↓

Change Tactics
Go to "Plan Tactics" step in Part 1.

Yes ↓

Is Strategy Correct?

No ↓

Change Strategy
Go to "Plan Strategy" step in Part 1.

Yes ↓

Are Goals Viable?

Nonviable Goals
Generate new goals after consultation with the patient. Go to Part 1, document the need for modification and the nature of the modification. If a new rationale is needed, go to "Refine Problem List" step in Part 1.

Viable Goals
Continue implementation of tactics and plan reassessment. Go to "Implement Tactics" step in Part 1.

AMERICANS WITH DISABILITIES ACT

Description of the Americans With Disabilities Act (ADA)*

The Americans with Disabilities Act of 1990 (ADA; Pub L. No. 101-336) is a federal anti-discrimination statute designed to prohibit discrimination on the basis of disability. The ADA gives civil rights protections to individuals with disabilities similar to those protections provided to individuals on the basis of race, color, sex, national origin, age, and religion. It guarantees equal opportunity for individuals with disabilities in employment (Title I), state and local government services (Title II), public accommodations (Title III), telecommunications (Title IV), and transportation (Title V). The ADA was later amended (effective January 1, 2009) by the ADA Amendments Act of 2008. Revised ADA regulations implementing Titles II and III are earmarked to take effect on March 15, 2011, including revisions to the ADA Standards for Accessibility Designs. They can be accessed via the ADA Home Page listed below.

Conditions of Applicability

- To be protected by the ADA, one must have a disability or have a relationship or association with an individual with a disability.
- An individual with a disability is defined by the ADA as a person who has a physical or mental impairment that substantially limits one or more major life activities, a person who has a history or record of such an impairment, or a person who is perceived by others as having such an impairment.
- The ADA does not specifically name all of the impairments that are covered.

Summary Description of the ADA

TABLE 2.1 Overview of the Americans With Disabilities Act (ADA)

Sections	Overview of Regulations
Title I: Employment	Applies to private employers, state and local governments, employment agencies, and labor organizations. Prohibits employers from discriminating against "a qualified individual with a disability" for application, hiring, advancements, and discharge. Employers are required to make "reasonable accommodations" to the known physical or mental limitation of an otherwise qualified individual with a disability, unless to do so would impose an "undue hardship."

(table continues on page 20)

ADA

■ TABLE 2.1 Overview of the Americans With Disabilities Act (ADA) (continued)

Sections	Overview of Regulations
Title II: Public Services	Prohibits discrimination against or excluding qualified individuals with disabilities from participating in services, programs, or activities of a "public entity" (any state or local government department, agency, and transportation authority).
Title III: Public Accommodations and Services Operated by Private Entities	Prohibits discrimination against individuals with disabilities in full and equal enjoyment of the goods, services, facilities, privileges, advantages, or accommodations of any place of public accommodation requiring that these be offered "in the most integrated setting appropriate to the needs of the individual," except when the individual poses a direct threat to the health or safety of others.
Title IV: Telecommunications	Requires that telephone companies provide services enabling hearing-impaired individuals to communicate with hearing individuals through the use of telecommunications devices for the deaf (TDD) or other nonvoice terminal devices.
Title V: Miscellaneous Provisions	Authorizes reimbursement of fees and actions if the plaintiff prevails as well as alternative methods of resolving disputes. Addresses access to wilderness areas. Lists sexual and other behaviors precluded from being a disability under the act.

From: *The Americans with Disabilities Act Handbook.* U.S. Equal Employment Opportunity Commission and the U.S. Department of Justice, Washington, DC, 1992.

ADA Amendment Act of 2008

The Americans with Disabilities Act of 1990 (ADA) was amended by the ADA Amendments Act of 2008 (Pub L. No. 110-325), which became effective on January 1, 2009. A copy of the amended ADA (ADAAA) can be downloaded at http://www.ada.gov/pubs/adastatute08.htm. Table 2.2 summarizes the major changes enacted by this amendment.

TABLE 2.2 Comparison of the ADA (as construed by the courts) and the ADA, as Amended

Issue	ADA (as construed by the courts)	ADA, as Amended by the ADA Amendments Act (ADAAA)
Scope of the Definition of "Disability": In General	Defines a "disability," in part, as a physical or mental impairment that substantially limits a major life activity of an individual. The Supreme Court has narrowly construed this definition in a way that has led lower courts to exclude a range of individuals from coverage, including individuals with diabetes, epilepsy, cancer, and artificial limbs.	Defines a "disability," in part, as a physical or mental impairment that substantially limits a major life activity of an individual. Rejects the Supreme Court's interpretation of "substantially limits" and reinterprets it as consistent with the ADAAA. Definition of "disability" construed in favor of broad coverage of individuals, to the maximum extent permitted by the terms of the ADA.
Mitigating Measures	Mitigating measures (such as medication or devices) are to be taken into account in determining whether a person was substantially limited in a major life activity. If medication or devices enabled a person with an impairment to function well, that person was often held by a court not to have a disability under the ADA.	The ameliorative effects of mitigating measures should not be considered in determining whether an individual has an impairment that substantially limits a major life activity. An exception is made for "ordinary eyeglasses or contact lenses," which may be taken into account.
"Substantially Limits"	The Supreme Court held that an impairment "substantially limits" a "major life activity" if it "prevents or severely restricts the individual" from performing the activity.	Requires that the term "substantially limits" be interpreted consistently with the findings and purposes of the act. When considering whether a person is substantially limited, the beneficial effects of any mitigating measures the person uses must be ignored.

(table continues on page 22)

TABLE 2.2 Comparison of the ADA (as construed by the courts) and the ADA, as Amended (continued)

Issue	ADA (as construed by the courts)	ADA, as Amended by the ADA Amendments Act (ADAAA)
The "Major Life Activity" Requirement	The Supreme Court ruled that a "major life activity" must be an activity that is "of central importance to most people's daily lives."	Includes a nonexhaustive list of major life activities, such as seeing, hearing, breathing, eating, sleeping, walking, learning, concentrating, caring for oneself, performing manual tasks, thinking, communicating, and working. Major life activities also include the operation of "major bodily functions."
Episodic or in Remission Conditions and Multiple Major Life Activities	In the past, a person whose condition was in remission or whose limitations are transient or only include one major life activity might not be covered by the ADA.	Makes clear that an impairment that substantially limits a major life activity need not also limit other major life activities to be considered a disability. Impairments that are episodic or in remission are considered disabilities if the impairment substantially limits a major life activity.
Regarded as Having a Disability	The Supreme Court established stringent requirements for an individual to show that he or she is substantially limited in working.	Transitory and minor impairments are excluded from this coverage, and employers and other covered entities under the ADA have no duty to provide a reasonable accommodation or modification.
Academic Requirements in Higher Education	Higher education institutions are subject to the ADA's requirements.	This provision thus restates current law to clarify that the changes in the definition of disability do not change the "fundamental alteration" provision of the ADA.

Source: Office of Disability Employment Policy (ODEP) Job Accommodation Network homepage (http://www.jan.wvu.edu) and the ADA homepage (http://www.ada.gov/).

ADA Accessibility Guidelines*

Refer to Table 2.3 for typographic conventions used in accessibility guidelines (see figures on pp. 23–32)

TABLE 2.3 Graphic Conventions Used to Describe Accessibility Requirements

Convention	Description
36" max **915 mm**	Typical dimension line showing U.S. customary units (in inches) above the line and SI units (in millimeters) below
12" **305 mm**	Dimension for short distances
(green arrow)	Direction of approach
max	Maximum
min	Minimum
– – – – – – – – – –	Boundary of clear floor area
————————— ₵	Centerline

From: *The Americans with Disabilities Act Handbook.* U.S. Equal Employment Opportunity Commission and the U.S. Department of Justice, Washington, DC, 1992.

Space for Wheelchairs

Minimum Clearance Width for Single Wheelchair

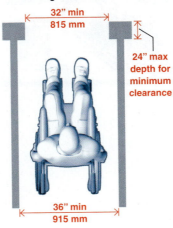

32" min **815 mm**

24" max depth for minimum clearance

36" min **915 mm**

Turning Space for Wheelchairs

Space Needed for Smooth U-Turn in a Wheelchair

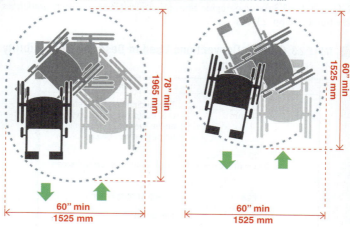

78" min
1965 mm

60" min
1525 mm

60" min
1525 mm

60" min
1525 mm

T – Shaped Space for 180° Turns

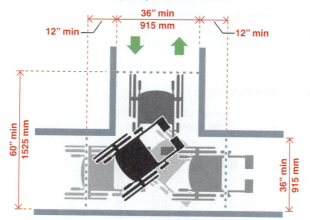

36" min
915 mm

12" min

12" min

60" min
1525 mm

36" min
915 mm

ADA

Forward Reach From Wheelchair

Maximum High and Minimum Low Forward Reach Limits

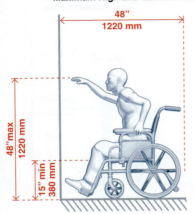

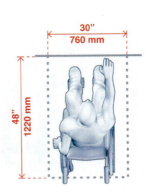

48"
1220 mm

48"max
1220 mm

15" min
380 mm

30"
760 mm

48"
1220 mm

Maximum Forward Reach over an Obstruction

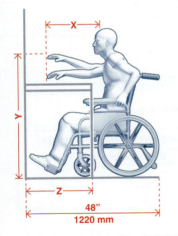

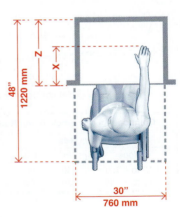

X

Y

Z

48"
1220 mm

48"
1220 mm

Z

X

30"
760 mm

Note: X shall be ≤ 25 in (635 mm); Z shall be ≥ X.
When X < 20 in (510 mm), then Y shall be 48 in (1220 mm) maximum.
When X is 20 to 25 in (510 to 635 mm), then Y shall be 44 in (1120 mm) maximum.

Side Reach From Wheelchair

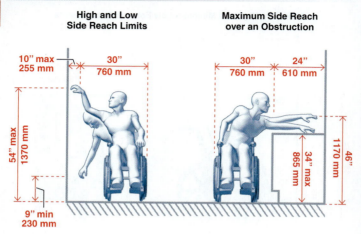

High and Low Side Reach Limits

10" max / 255 mm
30" / 760 mm
54" max / 1370 mm
9" min / 230 mm

Maximum Side Reach over an Obstruction

30" / 760 mm
24" / 610 mm
34" max / 865 mm
46" / 1170 mm

Ramp Dimensions

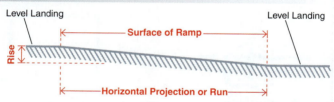

Level Landing

Level Landing

Rise

Surface of Ramp

Horizontal Projection or Run

Components of a Single Ramp Run and Sample Ramp Dimensions				
Maximum Rise			Maximum Horizontal Projection	
Slope	in	mm	ft	m
1:12 to < 1:16	30	760	30	9
1:16 to < 1:20	30	760	40	12

Shower Stall

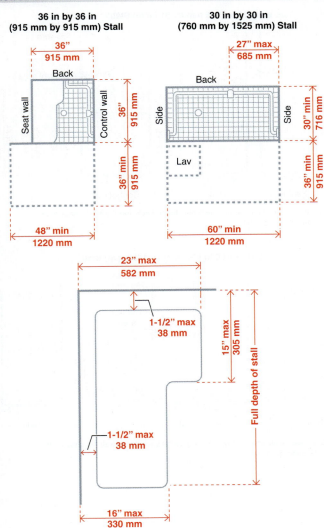

**36 in by 36 in
(915 mm by 915 mm) Stall**

36"
915 mm

Back

Seat wall

Control wall

36"
915 mm

36" min
915 mm

48" min
1220 mm

**30 in by 30 in
(760 mm by 1525 mm) Stall**

27" max
685 mm

Back

Side

Side

30" min
716 mm

36" min
915 mm

Lav

60" min
1220 mm

23" max
582 mm

1-1/2" max
38 mm

15" max
305 mm

Full depth of stall

1-1/2" max
38 mm

16" max
330 mm

Shower Seat Design

36 in by 36 in (915 mm by 915 mm) Stall

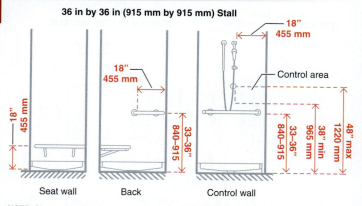

Seat wall   Back   Control wall

NOTE: Shower head and control area may be on back (long) wall (as shown) or on either side wall.

30 in by 60 in (760 mm by 1525 mm) Stall

Side   Back (long)   Side

NOTE: Shower head and control area may be on back (long) wall (as shown) or on either side wall.

Bathtubs

With Seat in Tub

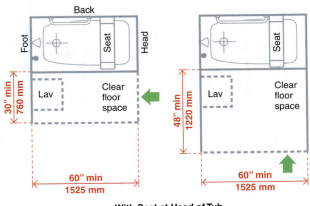

With Seat at Head of Tub

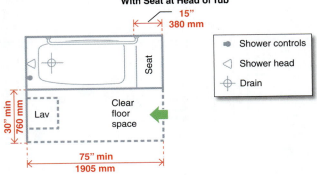

Shower controls
Shower head
Drain

With Seat in Tub

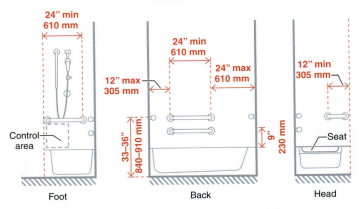

Foot

Back

Head

With Seat at Head of Tub (Grab Bars at Bathtubs)

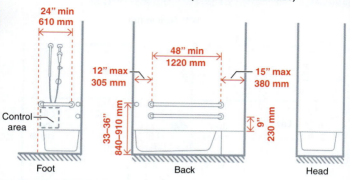

Control area

Foot

48" min 1220 mm

12" max 305 mm

15" max 380 mm

33–36" 840–910 mm

9" 230 mm

Back

Head

24" min 610 mm

Lavatories

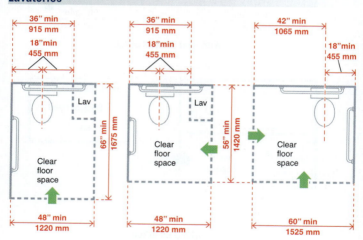

36" min 915 mm

18" min 455 mm

Lav

66" min 1675 mm

Clear floor space

48" min 1220 mm

36" min 915 mm

18" min 455 mm

Lav

56" min 1420 mm

Clear floor space

48" min 1220 mm

42" min 1065 mm

18" min 455 mm

Clear floor space

60" min 1525 mm

Grab Bars at Water Closets

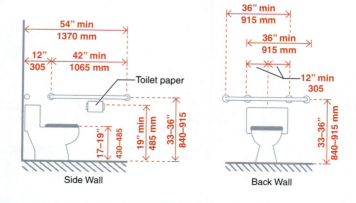

54" min 1370 mm

12" 305

42" min 1065 mm

Toilet paper

19" min 485 mm

17–19" 430–485

33–36" 840–915 mm

Side Wall

36" min 915 mm

36" min 915 mm

12" min 305

33–36" 840–915 mm

Back Wall

ADA

Sinks

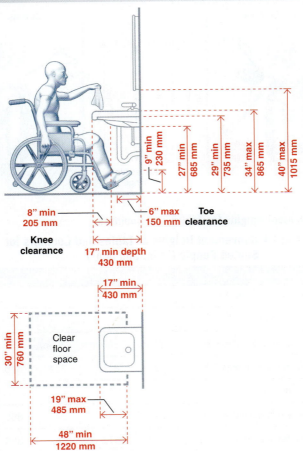

9" min 230 mm

27" min 685 mm

29" min 735 mm

34" max 865 mm

40" max 1015 mm

8" min 205 mm

6" max 150 mm

Toe clearance

Knee clearance

17" min depth 430 mm

17" min 430 mm

Clear floor space

30" min 760 mm

19" max 485 mm

48" min 1220 mm

Storage Shelves and Closets

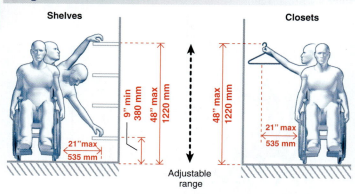

Convenient Heights for Tables and Counters

TABLE 2.4 Convenient Heights of Tables and Counters for Seated People (in in. and mm[1])

Conditions of Use	Short Women		Tall Men	
Seated in a wheelchair:				
Manual work:				
Desk or removable armrests	26 in.	660 mm	30 in.	760 mm
Fixed, full-size armrests[2]	32[3]	815	32[3]	815
Light, detailed work:				
Desk or removable armrests	29	735	34	865
Fixed, full-size armrests[2]	32[3]	815	34	865
Seated in a 16 in. (405 mm) high chair:				
Manual work	26	660	27	685
Light, detailed work	28	710	31	785

From: *The Americans with Disabilities Act Handbook.* U.S. Equal Employment Opportunity Commission and the U.S. Department of Justice, Washington, DC, 2002.

[1] All dimensions are based on a work-surface thickness of 1.5 in. (38 mm) and a clearance of 1.5 in. (38 mm) between legs and the underside of a work surface.

[2] This type of wheelchair arm does not interfere with the positioning of a wheelchair under a work surface.

[3] This dimension is limited by the height of the armrests: a lower height is preferable. Some people in this group prefer lower work surfaces, which require positioning the wheelchair back from the edge of the counter.

International Symbols

International symbol
of accessibility

International symbol
of TTY

Volume control
telephone

International symbol
of accessing for
hearing loss

Information Services

ADA Homepage
http://www.ada.gov/

ADA Hotline
800-514-0301 (voice)
800-514-0383 (TTY)
Monday, Tuesday, Wednesday, and Friday from 10:30 a.m. until 4:30 p.m.;
Thursday from 12:30 p.m. until 4:30 p.m. (Eastern time).

ADA Technical Assistance: Free CD-ROM
http://www.ada.gov/cdorderform/adatacd1.htm

U.S. Equal Employment Opportunity Commission (EEOC)
For information and instructions on reaching your local office, contact the
EEOC at
800-669-4000 (voice)
800-669-6820 (TDD)
In the Washington, DC, area, call 202-663-4900 (voice) or 202-663-4494 (TDD).

Job Accommodation Network
http://www.jan.wvu.edu
800-526-7234 (voice/TTY)
E-mail
http://www.jan.wvu.edu/JANonDemand.htm

Body Systems

MUSCULOSKELETAL

Skeletal Anatomy

The Skull

Anterior (Frontal) View

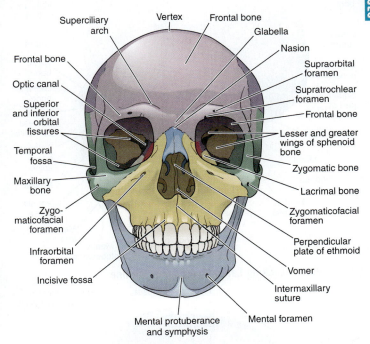

- Superciliary arch
- Vertex
- Frontal bone
- Glabella
- Nasion
- Supraorbital foramen
- Frontal bone
- Optic canal
- Supratrochlear foramen
- Superior and inferior orbital fissures
- Frontal bone
- Lesser and greater wings of sphenoid bone
- Temporal fossa
- Zygomatic bone
- Maxillary bone
- Lacrimal bone
- Zygomaticofacial foramen
- Zygomaticofacial foramen
- Perpendicular plate of ethmoid
- Infraorbital foramen
- Vomer
- Incisive fossa
- Intermaxillary suture
- Mental protuberance and symphysis
- Mental foramen

Lateral View

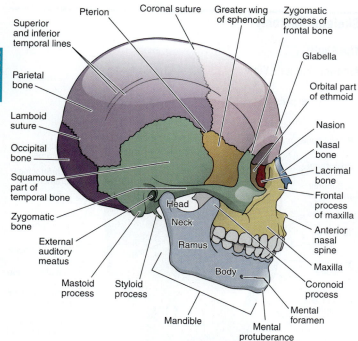

Pterion

Coronal suture

Greater wing of sphenoid

Zygomatic process of frontal bone

Superior and inferior temporal lines

Glabella

Parietal bone

Orbital part of ethmoid

Lamboid suture

Nasion

Occipital bone

Nasal bone

Lacrimal bone

Squamous part of temporal bone

Frontal process of maxilla

Zygomatic bone

Anterior nasal spine

External auditory meatus

Maxilla

Mastoid process

Styloid process

Coronoid process

Mandible

Mental foramen

Mental protuberance

Head

Neck

Ramus

Body

Interior View—Looking Laterally From the Midline

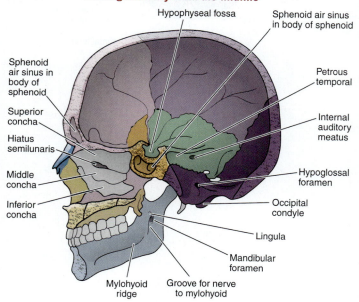

Hypophyseal fossa

Sphenoid air sinus in body of sphenoid

Sphenoid air sinus in body of sphenoid

Petrous temporal

Superior concha

Internal auditory meatus

Hiatus semilunaris

Middle concha

Hypoglossal foramen

Inferior concha

Occipital condyle

Lingula

Mandibular foramen

Mylohyoid ridge

Groove for nerve to mylohyoid

MUSCULO

Interior View—Inferior Surface

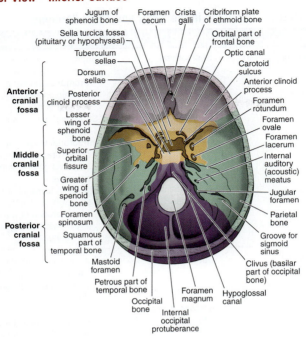

Jugum of sphenoid bone

Foramen cecum

Crista galli

Cribriform plate of ethmoid bone

Sella turcica fossa (pituitary or hypophyseal)

Orbital part of frontal bone

Tuberculum sellae

Optic canal

Dorsum sellae

Carotoid sulcus

Posterior clinoid process

Anterior clinoid process

Lesser wing of sphenoid bone

Foramen rotundum

Superior orbital fissure

Foramen ovale

Greater wing of spenoid bone

Foramen lacerum

Foramen spinosum

Internal auditory (acoustic) meatus

Squamous part of temporal bone

Jugular foramen

Mastoid foramen

Parietal bone

Petrous part of temporal bone

Groove for sigmoid sinus

Occipital bone

Clivus (basilar part of occipital bone)

Internal occipital protuberance

Foramen magnum

Hypoglossal canal

Anterior cranial fossa

Middle cranial fossa

Posterior cranial fossa

Inferior View

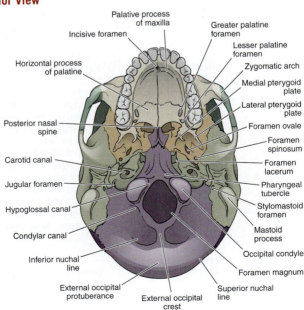

Palative process of maxilla

Incisive foramen

Greater palatine foramen

Horizontal process of palatine

Lesser palatine foramen

Zygomatic arch

Posterior nasal spine

Medial pterygoid plate

Lateral pterygoid plate

Carotid canal

Foramen ovale

Foramen spinosum

Jugular foramen

Foramen lacerum

Hypoglossal canal

Pharyngeal tubercle

Condylar canal

Stylomastoid foramen

Inferior nuchal line

Mastoid process

External occipital protuberance

Occipital condyle

External occipital crest

Foramen magnum

Superior nuchal line

TABLE 3.1 Openings in the Skull and Their Contents

View	Structure	Contents
Anterior (frontal)	Supraorbital foramen	Supraorbital vessels, supraorbital nerve (frontal branch of ophthalmic division of trigeminal nerve)
	Supratrochlear foramen	Supratrochlear vessels and nerve
	Infraorbital foramen	Infraorbital vessels and nerve (branch of maxillary division of trigeminal nerve)
	Zygomaticofacial foramen	Branch of lacrimal artery and zygomaticofacial nerve (branch of maxillary division of trigeminal nerve)
Orbital	Optic canal	Optic nerve, ophthalmic artery, meninges, ophthalmic plexus of sympathetic nerves
	Anterior ethmoidal foramen	Anterior ethmoidal vessels and nerve (nasociliary branch of ophthalmic division of trigeminal nerve)
	Posterior ethmoidal foramen	Posterior vessels and nerve (nasociliary branch of ophthalmic division of trigeminal nerve)
	Nasolacrimal canal	Nasolacrimal duct
	Infraorbital foramen	Infraorbital nerve and vessels
	Superior orbital fissure (lateral to origin of the lateral rectus muscle)	Lacrimal nerve, frontal nerve, trochlear nerve, meningeal branch of lacrimal artery, orbital branch of middle meningeal artery, sympathetic branches from the carotid plexus
	Superior orbital fissure (between the heads of the lateral rectus muscle)	Superior and inferior ophthalmic veins, oculomotor nerve, nasociliary nerve, abducens nerve
Posterior	Mastoid foramen	Emissary vein connecting sigmoid sinus to the posterior auricular vein

MUSCULO

View	Structure	Contents
Lateral	External auditory meatus	Air
	Tympanomastoid fissure	Auricular branch of vagus nerve
	Alveolar canals	Posterior superior alveolar nerves
	Infraorbital fissure	Infraorbital nerve and vessels
	Zygomaticofacial foramen	Branch of lacrimal artery and zygomaticofacial nerve (branch of maxillary division of trigeminal nerve)
	Zygomaticotemporal foramen	Zygomaticotemporal nerve of the mandibular division of the trigeminal nerve
Inferolateral	Pterygomaxillary fissure	Maxillary artery to infratemporal fossa artery
Anterior wall	Inferior orbital fissure	Structure that connects with orbit
Inferior wall	Greater palatine canal	Structure that extends to posterior surface of hard palate
	Foramen rotundum	Structure that connects with middle cranial fossa and allows for passage of maxillary division of the trigeminal nerve
Superior wall	Pterygoid canal	Structure that connects foramen lacerum via root of pterygoid process (vessel and nerve of pterygoid canal)
	Pharyngeal canal (palatinovaginal)	Structure that connects with posterior opening of nose
Medial wall	Sphenopalatine foramen	Structure that connects with superior meatus of nose
Inferior	Incisive foramen	Greater palatine artery, nasopalatine nerve
	Greater palatine foramen	Greater palatine artery and nerve

(table continues on page 42)

TABLE 3.1 **Openings in the Skull and Their Contents** (continued)

MUSCULO

View	Structure	Contents
	Palatinovaginal canal	Pharyngeal branches of pterygopalatine (pharyngeal canal) ganglion and third portion of maxillary artery
	Foramen spinosum	Middle meningeal artery
	Foramen ovale	Mandibular division of trigeminal nerve, motor root of mandibular nerve, accessory meningeal artery, lesser superficial petrosal nerve, emissary veins connecting cavernous sinus to pterygoid venous plexus
	Foramen magnum	Spinal roots of accessory nerve, two vertebral arteries, medulla oblongata, two posterior spinal arteries, one anterior spinal artery, sympathetic plexuses about vertebral arteries, tonsil of cerebellum
	Posterior condylar canal	Emissary vein connecting sigmoid sinus to suboccipital venous plexus
	Anterior condylar canal	Hypoglossal nerve, emissary veins connecting meningeal veins to pharyngeal venous plexus
	Stylomastoid foramen	Facial nerve
	Jugular foramen	
	Anterior compartment	Inferior petrosal sinus
	Middle compartment	Glossopharyngeal, vagus, and accessory nerves
	Posterior compartment	Sigmoid sinus to internal jugular vein
	Tympanic canaliculus	Tympanic branch of glossopharyngeal nerve
	Carotid canal	Internal carotid artery, sympathetic carotid plexus, emissary vein connecting cavernous sinus to pharyngeal plexus

MUSCULO

View	Structure	Contents
	Caroticotympanic canaliculi	Branches of carotid sympathetic plexus, tympanic branches of internal carotid artery
	Foramen lacerum	Meningeal branch of ascending pharyngeal artery, emissary vein connecting cavernous sinus to pharyngeal plexus, internal carotid artery, sympathetic plexus, deep petrosal nerve (from otic sympathetic plexus), greater petrosal nerve (parasympathetic from facial nerve)
	Canal for auditory tube (eustachian tube)	Temporal bone between tympanic plate and petrosal portion of temporal bone
	Petrotympanic fissure	Chorda tympani nerve of facial nerve
Internal		
Anterior cranial fossa	Foramen cecum	Emissary vein connecting superior sagittal sinus to veins of nose
	Cribriform plate of ethmoid bone	Filaments of olfactory nerve
Middle cranial fossa	Optic canal	Optic nerve, ophthalmic artery, meninges, ophthalmic plexus of sympathetic nerves
	Superior orbital fissure (lateral to origin of the lateral rectus muscle)	Lacrimal nerve, frontal nerve, trochlear nerve, meningeal branch of lacrimal artery, orbital branch of middle meningeal artery, sympathetic branches from the carotid plexus
	Superior orbital fissure (between the heads of the lateral rectus muscle)	Superior and inferior ophthalmic veins, oculomotor nerve, nasociliary nerve, abducens nerve

(table continues on page 44)

MUSCULO

◖ TABLE 3.1 Openings in the Skull and Their Contents (continued)

View	Structure	Contents
	Foramen rotundum	Structure that connects with middle cranial fossa and allows for passage of maxillary division of the trigeminal nerve
	Foramen ovale	Mandibular nerve of trigeminal nerve, motor root of mandibular division, accessory meningeal artery, lesser superficial petrosal nerve, emissary veins connecting cavernous sinus to pterygoid venous plexus
	Foramen spinosum	Middle meningeal artery
	Foramen lacerum	Meningeal branch of ascending pharyngeal artery, emissary vein connecting cavernous sinus to pharyngeal plexus, internal carotid artery, sympathetic plexus, deep petrosal nerve (from otic sympathetic plexus), greater petrosal nerve (parasympathetic from facial nerve)
	Pterygoid canal	Nerve of pterygoid canal (formed by greater and deep petrosal nerves), artery of pterygoid canal (branch of maxillary artery)
Posterior cranial fossa	Foramen magnum	Spinal roots of accessory nerve, two vertebral arteries, medulla oblongata, two posterior spinal arteries, one anterior spinal artery, sympathetic plexuses about vertebral arteries, tonsil of cerebellum

View	Structure	Contents
	Anterior condylar canal	Hypoglossal nerve, emissary veins connecting meningeal veins to pharyngeal venous plexus
	Posterior condylar canal	Emissary vein connecting sigmoid sinus to suboccipital venous plexus
	Mastoid foramen	Emissary vein connecting sigmoid sinus to the posterior auricular vein
	Jugular foramen Anterior compartment	Inferior petrosal sinus
	Middle compartment	Glossopharyngeal, vagus, and accessory nerves
	Internal auditory meatus	Motor and sensory roots of facial nerve, vestibulocochlear nerve
	Opening of aqueduct of vestibule	Endolymphatic duct
Mandible	Mandibular foramen	Inferior alveolar vessels and nerve (mandibular division of trigeminal)
	Mental foramen	Mental vessels and nerve (mandibular division of trigeminal)
	Mylohyoid groove	Mylohyoid vessels and mylohyoid nerve (mandibular division of trigeminal)
	Mandibular notch	Vessels to masseter muscle and nerve to masseter (mandibular division of trigeminal)

MUSCULO

The Vertebral Column

Lateral and Anterior Views

MUSCULO

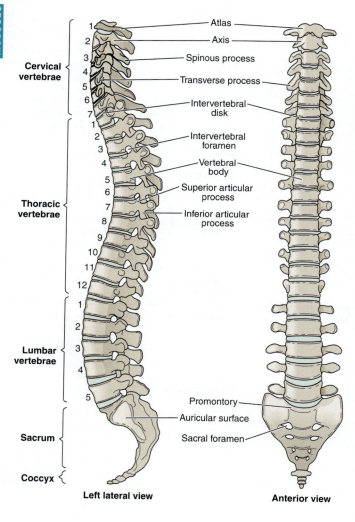

Atlas

Axis

Spinous process

Transverse process

Intervertebral disk

Intervertebral foramen

Vertebral body

Superior articular process

Inferior articular process

Cervical vertebrae
1 2 3 4 5 6 7

Thoracic vertebrae
1 2 3 4 5 6 7 8 9 10 11 12

Lumbar vertebrae
1 2 3 4 5

Sacrum

Coccyx

Promontory

Auricular surface

Sacral foramen

Left lateral view

Anterior view

Cervical Vertebrae
Superior Views

Atlas (C1)
(viewed from above)

Posterior
tubercle

Posterior arch

Vertebral
foramen

Groove for vertebral artery

Lateral mass

Facet for
dens of axis

Foramen transversarium

Transverse process

Superior
articular facet

Anterior
tubercle

Anterior arch

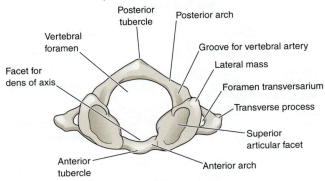

Axis (C2)

Bifid spinous process

Vertebral
foramen

Lamina

Pedicle

Inferior
articular process

Foramen
transversarium

Transverse
process

Superior
articular surface

Dens

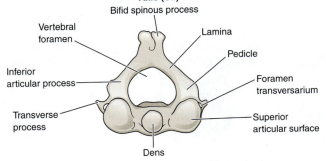

Typical cervical vertebra (fifth)

Bifid spinous process

Lamina

Vertebral foramen

Inferior articular process

Superior articular process

Foramen
transversarium

Pedicle

Posterior tubercle

Anterior tubercle

Sulcus for
spinal nerve

Body of vertebra

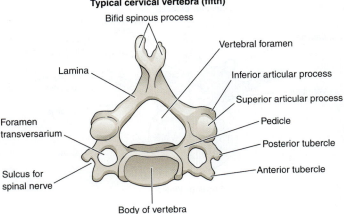

Vertebrae
Superior Views

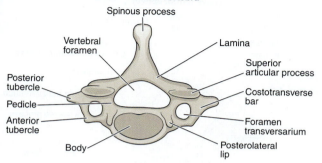

Seventh cervical vertebra

Spinous process

Vertebral foramen

Lamina

Superior articular process

Posterior tubercle

Costotransverse bar

Pedicle

Anterior tubercle

Foramen transversarium

Body

Posterolateral lip

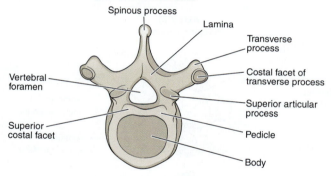

Sixth thoracic vertebra

Spinous process

Lamina

Transverse process

Costal facet of transverse process

Vertebral foramen

Superior articular process

Superior costal facet

Pedicle

Body

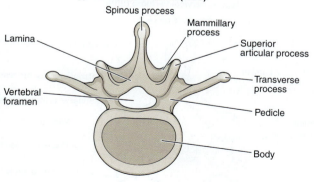

Typical lumbar vertebra (third)

Spinous process

Mammillary process

Lamina

Superior articular process

Vertebral foramen

Transverse process

Pedicle

Body

Superior Views

The Sacrum and Coccyx
Anterior and Posterior Views

Anterior

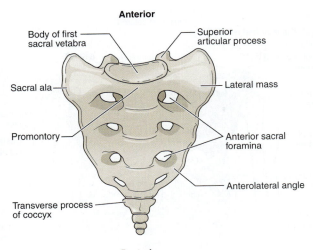

Body of first sacral vetabra

Sacral ala

Promontory

Transverse process of coccyx

Superior articular process

Lateral mass

Anterior sacral foramina

Anterolateral angle

Posterior

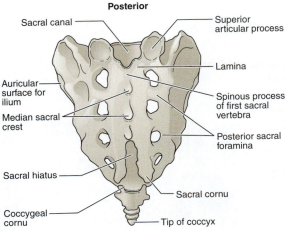

Sacral canal

Auricular surface for ilium

Median sacral crest

Sacral hiatus

Coccygeal cornu

Superior articular process

Lamina

Spinous process of first sacral vertebra

Posterior sacral foramina

Sacral cornu

Tip of coccyx

MUSCULO

Thorax

Anterior View

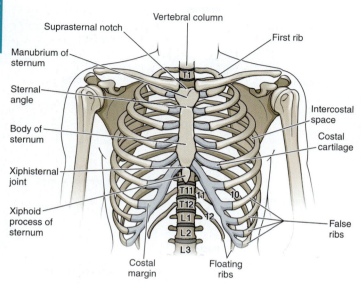

Vertebral column

Suprasternal notch

First rib

Manubrium of sternum

T1

Sternal angle

Intercostal space

Body of sternum

Costal cartilage

Xiphisternal joint

T11
T12
11
10

L1
12

Xiphoid process of sternum

L2

L3

False ribs

Costal margin

Floating ribs

Costovertebral and Costosternal Articulations

Lateral View

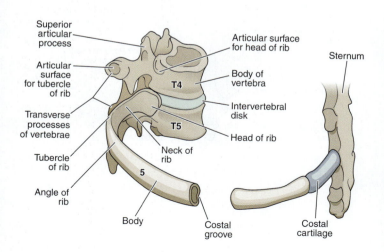

Superior articular process

Articular surface for head of rib

Sternum

Articular surface for tubercle of rib

Body of vertebra

T4

Transverse processes of vertebrae

Intervertebral disk

T5

Tubercle of rib

Head of rib

Neck of rib

Angle of rib

5

Body

Costal groove

Costal cartilage

Upper Extremity

The Clavicle

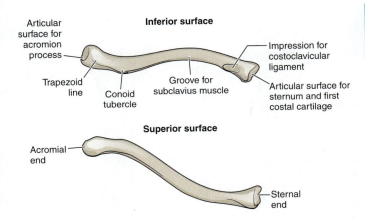

Inferior surface

Articular surface for acromion process

Trapezoid line

Conoid tubercle

Groove for subclavius muscle

Impression for costoclavicular ligament

Articular surface for sternum and first costal cartilage

Superior surface

Acromial end

Sternal end

The Scapula
Costal and Posterior Surfaces

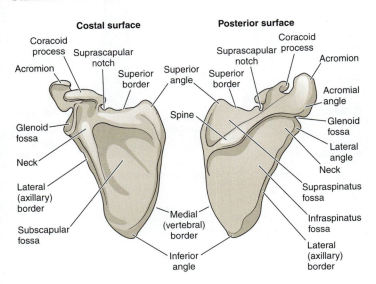

Costal surface

Coracoid process

Acromion

Suprascapular notch

Superior border

Superior angle

Glenoid fossa

Neck

Lateral (axillary) border

Subscapular fossa

Medial (vertebral) border

Inferior angle

Posterior surface

Suprascapular notch

Coracoid process

Acromion

Superior border

Superior angle

Acromial angle

Spine

Glenoid fossa

Lateral angle

Neck

Supraspinatus fossa

Infraspinatus fossa

Lateral (axillary) border

The Humerus
Anterior and Posterior Surfaces

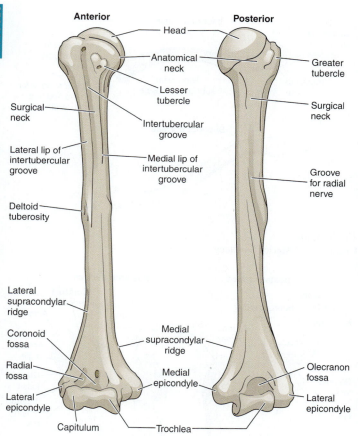

Anterior | **Posterior**

Head
Anatomical neck
Lesser tubercle
Intertubercular groove
Surgical neck
Lateral lip of intertubercular groove
Medial lip of intertubercular groove
Deltoid tuberosity
Lateral supracondylar ridge
Medial supracondylar ridge
Coronoid fossa
Radial fossa
Lateral epicondyle
Medial epicondyle
Capitulum
Trochlea

Greater tubercle
Surgical neck
Groove for radial nerve
Olecranon fossa
Lateral epicondyle

The Radius and Ulna
Anterior and Posterior Surfaces

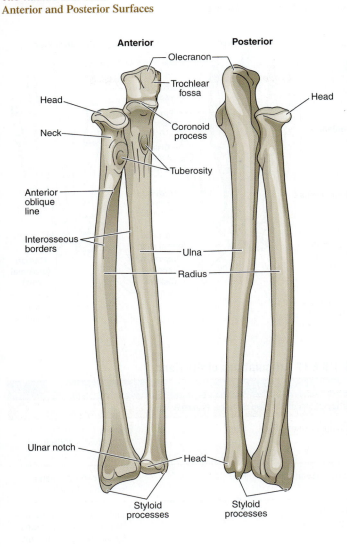

Anterior

Posterior

Olecranon

Trochlear fossa

Head

Head

Neck

Coronoid process

Tuberosity

Anterior oblique line

Interosseous borders

Ulna

Radius

Ulnar notch

Head

Styloid processes

Styloid processes

MUSCULO

The Hand
Anterior and Posterior Surfaces

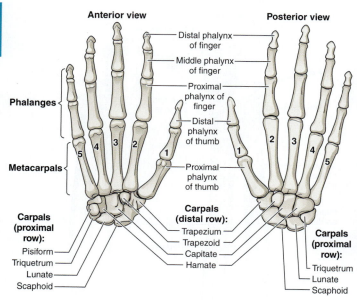

Anterior view

Posterior view

Distal phalynx of finger

Middle phalynx of finger

Proximal phalynx of finger

Distal phalynx of thumb

Proximal phalynx of thumb

Phalanges

Metacarpals

Carpals (proximal row):
Pisiform
Triquetrum
Lunate
Scaphoid

Carpals (distal row):
Trapezium
Trapezoid
Capitate
Hamate

Carpals (proximal row):
Triquetrum
Lunate
Scaphoid

TABLE 3.2 Articulations of the Hand

Bone	Number of Articulations	Articulates With
Articulations of the Carpal Bones: Proximal Row		
Scaphoid (navicular)	Five	Radius, trapezium, trapezoid, capitate, lunate
Lunate (semilunar)	Five	Radius, capitate, hamate, scaphoid, trapezium
Triquetrum (triangularis)	Three	Lunate, pisiform, hamate (separated from the ulna by the triangular articular disk)
Pisiform	One	Triquetrum
Articulations of the Carpal Bones: Distal Row		
Trapezium	Four	Scaphoid, first and second metacarpals, trapezoid

Bone	Number of Articulations	Articulates With
Articulations of the Carpal Bones: Distal Row		
Trapezoid	Four	Scaphoid, second metacarpal, capitate, trapezium
Capitate	Seven	Scaphoid; lunate; second, third, and fourth metacarpals; trapezoid; hamate
Hamate	Five	Lunate, fourth and fifth metacarpals, triquetrum, capitate
Articulations of the Metacarpal Bones		

First: trapezium, proximal phalanx
Second: trapezium trapezoid, capitate, third metacarpal, proximal phalanx
Third: capitate, second and fourth metacarpals, proximal phalanx
Fourth: capitate, hamate, third and fifth metacarpals, proximal phalanx
Fifth: hamate, fourth metacarpal, proximal phalanx

MUSCULO

The Pelvic Girdle

Anterior and Posterior Views

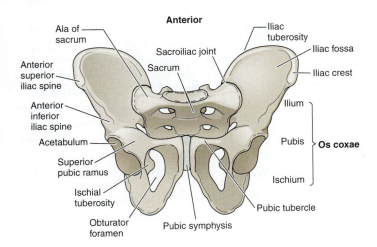

MUSCULO

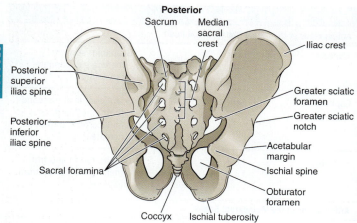

Posterior

Sacrum

Median sacral crest

Iliac crest

Posterior superior iliac spine

Greater sciatic foramen

Greater sciatic notch

Posterior inferior iliac spine

Acetabular margin

Sacral foramina

Ischial spine

Obturator foramen

Coccyx   Ischial tuberosity

Lateral and Medial Views

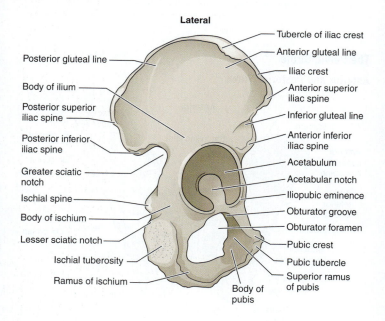

Lateral

Posterior gluteal line

Tubercle of iliac crest

Anterior gluteal line

Iliac crest

Body of ilium

Anterior superior iliac spine

Posterior superior iliac spine

Inferior gluteal line

Posterior inferior iliac spine

Anterior inferior iliac spine

Acetabulum

Greater sciatic notch

Acetabular notch

Ischial spine

Iliopubic eminence

Body of ischium

Obturator groove

Lesser sciatic notch

Obturator foramen

Ischial tuberosity

Pubic crest

Ramus of ischium

Pubic tubercle

Body of pubis

Superior ramus of pubis

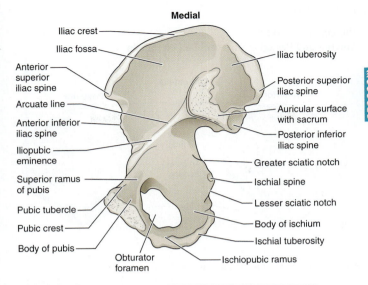

Medial

- Iliac crest
- Iliac fossa
- Anterior superior iliac spine
- Arcuate line
- Anterior inferior iliac spine
- Iliopubic eminence
- Superior ramus of pubis
- Pubic tubercle
- Pubic crest
- Body of pubis
- Obturator foramen
- Iliac tuberosity
- Posterior superior iliac spine
- Auricular surface with sacrum
- Posterior inferior iliac spine
- Greater sciatic notch
- Ischial spine
- Lesser sciatic notch
- Body of ischium
- Ischial tuberosity
- Ischiopubic ramus

Lower Extremity

The Femur
Anterior and Posterior Surfaces

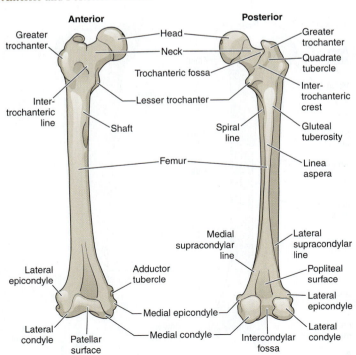

Anterior

- Greater trochanter
- Inter-trochanteric line
- Shaft
- Lateral epicondyle
- Lateral condyle
- Patellar surface

Posterior

- Greater trochanter
- Quadrate tubercle
- Inter-trochanteric crest
- Gluteal tuberosity
- Linea aspera
- Lateral supracondylar line
- Popliteal surface
- Lateral epicondyle
- Lateral condyle
- Intercondylar fossa

- Head
- Neck
- Trochanteric fossa
- Lesser trochanter
- Spiral line
- Femur
- Medial supracondylar line
- Adductor tubercle
- Medial epicondyle
- Medial condyle

MUSCULO

The Leg and Patella
Anterior and Posterior Surfaces of a Left Patella

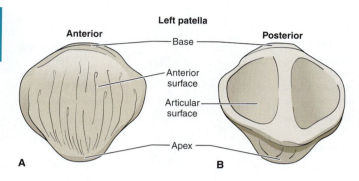

Left patella

Anterior · Base · Posterior

Anterior surface

Articular surface

Apex

A · B

Anterior and Posterior Surfaces of the Tibia and Fibula

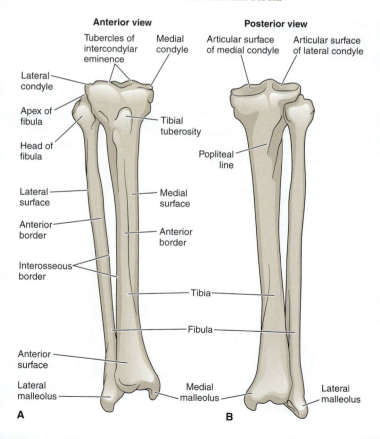

Anterior view

Tubercles of intercondylar eminence
Medial condyle
Lateral condyle
Apex of fibula
Head of fibula
Lateral surface
Anterior border
Interosseous border
Tibial tuberosity
Medial surface
Anterior border
Tibia
Fibula
Anterior surface
Lateral malleolus
Medial malleolus

Posterior view

Articular surface of medial condyle
Articular surface of lateral condyle
Popliteal line
Lateral malleolus

A · B

The Foot
Lateral and Medial Views

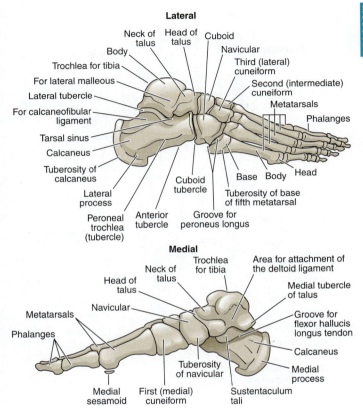

Lateral

Neck of talus
Head of talus
Cuboid
Body
Navicular
Trochlea for tibia
Third (lateral) cuneiform
For lateral malleous
Second (intermediate) cuneiform
Lateral tubercle
Metatarsals
For calcaneofibular ligament
Phalanges
Tarsal sinus
Calcaneus
Tuberosity of calcaneus
Base Body Head
Lateral process
Cuboid tubercle
Tuberosity of base of fifth metatarsal
Peroneal trochlea (tubercle)
Anterior tubercle
Groove for peroneus longus

Medial

Trochlea for tibia
Area for attachment of the deltoid ligament
Neck of talus
Head of talus
Medial tubercle of talus
Navicular
Groove for flexor hallucis longus tendon
Metatarsals
Phalanges
Calcaneus
Tuberosity of navicular
Medial process
Medial sesamoid
First (medial) cuneiform
Sustentaculum tali

See Table 3.3, Articulations of the Foot (pages 61–62).

Superior and Inferior Views

MUSCULO

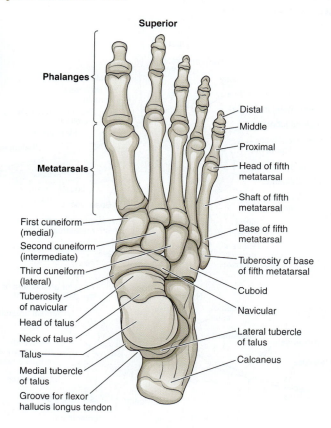

Superior

Phalanges

Metatarsals

Distal
Middle
Proximal
Head of fifth metatarsal
Shaft of fifth metatarsal
Base of fifth metatarsal
Tuberosity of base of fifth metatarsal
Cuboid
Navicular
Lateral tubercle of talus
Calcaneus

First cuneiform (medial)
Second cuneiform (intermediate)
Third cuneiform (lateral)
Tuberosity of navicular
Head of talus
Neck of talus
Talus
Medial tubercle of talus
Groove for flexor hallucis longus tendon

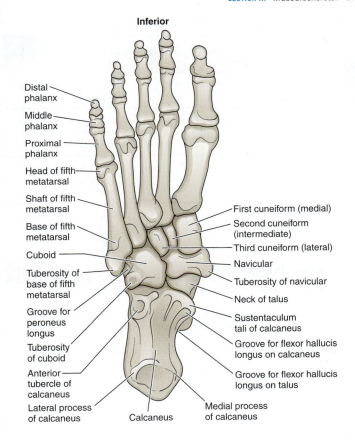

Inferior

Distal phalanx
Middle phalanx
Proximal phalanx
Head of fifth metatarsal
Shaft of fifth metatarsal
Base of fifth metatarsal
Cuboid
Tuberosity of base of fifth metatarsal
Groove for peroneus longus
Tuberosity of cuboid
Anterior tubercle of calcaneus
Lateral process of calcaneus
Calcaneus

First cuneiform (medial)
Second cuneiform (intermediate)
Third cuneiform (lateral)
Navicular
Tuberosity of navicular
Neck of talus
Sustentaculum tali of calcaneus
Groove for flexor hallucis longus on calcaneus
Groove for flexor hallucis longus on talus
Medial process of calcaneus

See Table 3.3, Articulations of the Foot.

TABLE 3.3 Articulations of the Foot

Bone	Number of Articulations	Articulates With
Articulations of the Tarsal Bones		
Calcaneus	Two	Talus, cuboid
Talus	Four	Tibia, fibula, calcaneus, navicular
Cuboid	Four (sometimes five)	Calcaneus, lateral cuneiform, fourth and fifth metatarsal, sometimes navicular

(table continues on page 62)

MUSCULO

TABLE 3.3 **Articulations of the Foot** (continued)

Bone	Number of Articulations	Articulates With
Articulations of the Tarsal Bones		
Navicular	Four (sometimes five)	Talus, three cuneiforms, sometimes cuboid
Medial cuneiform (first cuneiform)	Four	Navicular, intermediate cuneiform, first and second metatarsals
Intermediate cuneiform (second cuneiform)	Four	Navicular, medial and lateral cuneiforms, second metatarsal
Lateral cuneiform (third cuneiform)	Six	Navicular; intermediate cuneiform; cuboid; second, third, and fourth metatarsals
Articulations of the Metatarsal Bones		

First: second metatarsal, grooves for two sesamoids, medial cuneiform, proximal phalanx
Second: first and third metatarsals, three cuneiforms, proximal phalanx
Third: second and fourth metatarsals, lateral cuneiform, cuboid, proximal phalanx
Fourth: third and fourth metatarsals, lateral cuneiform, cuboid, proximal phalanx
Fifth: fourth metatarsal, cuboid, proximal phalanx

Radiology

ABCS of Radiographic Analysis
A: Alignment
General skeletal architecture
General contour of bone
Alignment of bones relative to adjacent bones

B: Bone Density
General bone density
Texture abnormalities
Local bone density

C: Cartilage Spaces
Joint space width
Subchondral bone
Epiphyseal plates

S: Soft Tissues
Muscles
Fat pads and fat lines

Joint capsules
Periosteum
Miscellaneous soft tissue findings

Based on:

McKinnis, LN: Fundamentals of Orthopedic Radiology, ed. 3. FA Davis, Philadelphia, 2010, pp 40–51.
Scheurger, SR: Introduction to critical review of roentgenograms. Phys Ther 68:1114, 1988.

MUSCULO

Images

Anteroposterior Open-Mouth Cervical Spine Radiograph

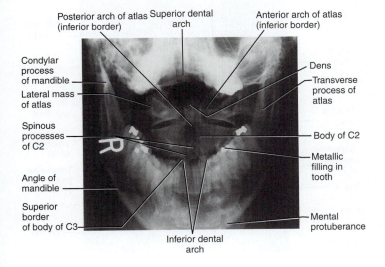

Posterior arch of atlas (inferior border) Superior dental arch Anterior arch of atlas (inferior border)

Condylar process of mandible Dens Transverse process of atlas

Lateral mass of atlas

Spinous processes of C2 Body of C2

Metallic filling in tooth

Angle of mandible

Superior border of body of C3 Mental protuberance

Inferior dental arch

MUSCULO

Anteroposterior Lower Cervical Spine Radiograph

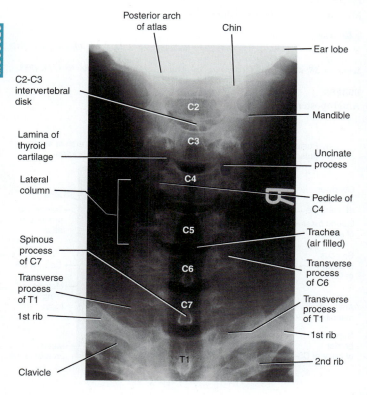

Posterior arch of atlas

Chin

Ear lobe

C2-C3 intervertebral disk

C2

C3

Mandible

Lamina of thyroid cartilage

C4

Uncinate process

Lateral column

C5

Pedicle of C4

Trachea (air filled)

Spinous process of C7

C6

Transverse process of C6

Transverse process of T1

C7

Transverse process of T1

1st rib

1st rib

Clavicle

T1

2nd rib

Lateral Cervical Spine Radiograph

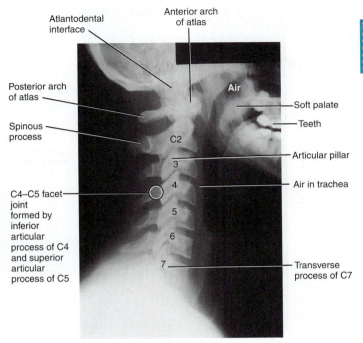

Atlantodental interface

Anterior arch of atlas

Posterior arch of atlas

Spinous process

Air

Soft palate

Teeth

C2

Articular pillar

3

4

Air in trachea

C4–C5 facet joint formed by inferior articular process of C4 and superior articular process of C5

5

6

7

Transverse process of C7

Anteroposterior Radiograph of the Lumbar Spine

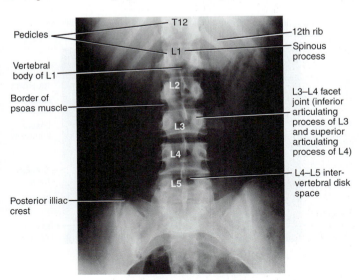

Pedicles

T12

12th rib

L1

Spinous process

Vertebral body of L1

L2

Border of psoas muscle

L3

L3–L4 facet joint (inferior articulating process of L3 and superior articulating process of L4)

L4

L5

L4–L5 inter-vertebral disk space

Posterior illiac crest

MUSCULO

Lateral Radiograph of the Lumbar Spine

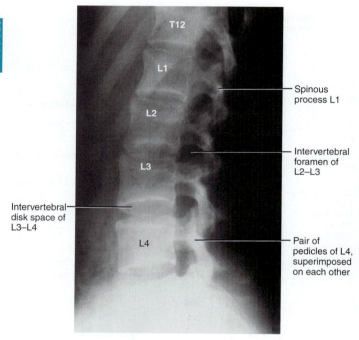

T12
L1 — Spinous process L1
L2
— Intervertebral foramen of L2–L3
L3
Intervertebral disk space of L3–L4
L4 — Pair of pedicles of L4, superimposed on each other

Anteroposterior External Rotation Radiograph of the Shoulder

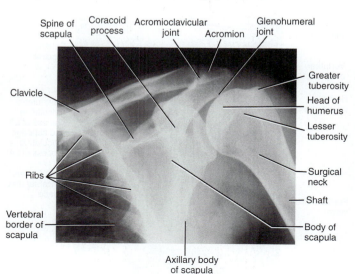

Spine of scapula
Coracoid process
Acromioclavicular joint
Acromion
Glenohumeral joint
Clavicle
Greater tuberosity
Head of humerus
Lesser tuberosity
Ribs
Surgical neck
Shaft
Vertebral border of scapula
Body of scapula
Axillary body of scapula

Anteroposterior Radiograph of the Right Elbow

MUSCULO

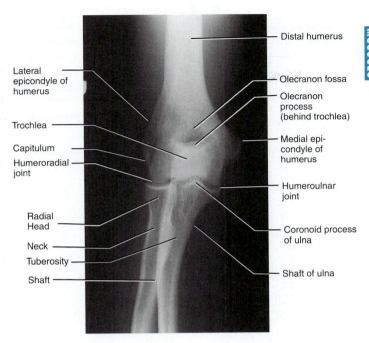

Distal humerus

Lateral epicondyle of humerus

Olecranon fossa

Olecranon process (behind trochlea)

Trochlea

Medial epi-condyle of humerus

Capitulum

Humeroradial joint

Humeroulnar joint

Radial Head

Coronoid process of ulna

Neck

Tuberosity

Shaft

Shaft of ulna

Anteroposterior Radiograph of the Pelvis

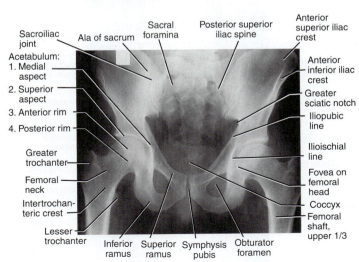

Sacroiliac joint

Ala of sacrum

Sacral foramina

Posterior superior iliac spine

Anterior superior iliac crest

Acetabulum:
1. Medial aspect
2. Superior aspect
3. Anterior rim
4. Posterior rim

Anterior inferior iliac crest

Greater sciatic notch

Iliopubic line

Ilioischial line

Greater trochanter

Fovea on femoral head

Femoral neck

Coccyx

Intertrochan-teric crest

Femoral shaft, upper 1/3

Lesser trochanter

Inferior ramus

Superior ramus

Symphysis pubis

Obturator foramen

Anteroposterior Radiograph of the Left Hip

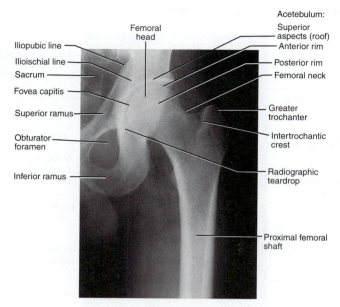

Femoral head

Iliopubic line

Ilioischial line

Sacrum

Fovea capitis

Superior ramus

Obturator foramen

Inferior ramus

Acetebulum:

Superior aspects (roof)

Anterior rim

Posterior rim

Femoral neck

Greater trochanter

Intertrochantic crest

Radiographic teardrop

Proximal femoral shaft

Anteroposterior Radiograph of the Right Knee

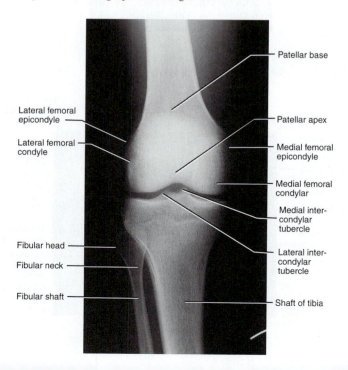

Patellar base

Lateral femoral epicondyle

Lateral femoral condyle

Patellar apex

Medial femoral epicondyle

Medial femoral condylar

Medial inter-condylar tubercle

Fibular head

Fibular neck

Fibular shaft

Lateral inter-condylar tubercle

Shaft of tibia

Lateral Radiograph of the Left Knee

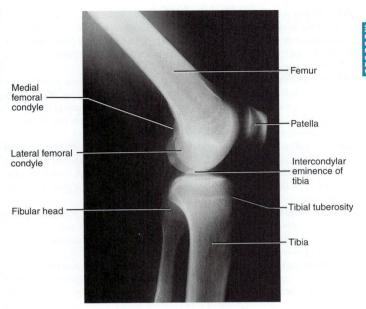

MUSCULO

Femur

Medial femoral condyle

Patella

Lateral femoral condyle

Intercondylar eminence of tibia

Tibial tuberosity

Fibular head

Tibia

Musculoskeletal Anatomy

Muscles Listed Alphabetically

The muscles of the body are listed in alphabetical order. The functions, secondary functions, origins, insertions, and innervations are listed for the major muscles.

abdominals: See *obliquus externus abdominis, obliquus internus abdominis, rectus abdominis,* and *transversus abdominis.*

abductor digiti minimi of the foot: *Function*—abducts the small toe; *origin*—medial and lateral processes of the calcaneal tuberosity, the plantar aponeurosis, and the intermuscular septum; *insertion*—the lateral side of the proximal phalanx of the fifth toe; *innervation*—lateral plantar nerve, S2–S3.

abductor digiti minimi of the hand: *Function*—abducts the fifth finger; *secondary function*—flexes the fifth finger; *origin*—the pisiform bone, the tendon of flexor carpi ulnaris; *insertion*—the ulnar side of the base of the proximal phalanx of the little finger; *innervation*—ulnar nerve, C8–T1.

abductor hallucis: *Function*—abducts and flexes the great toe; *origin*—the flexor retinaculum, the calcaneal tuberosity, the plantar aponeurosis, and the intermuscular septum; *insertion*—the medial side of the base of the proximal phalanx of the great toe; *innervation*—medial plantar nerve, L5–S1.

abductor pollicis brevis: *Function*—abducts the thumb; *origin*—the flexor retinaculum, the scaphoid, and the trapezium; *insertion*—the radial side of the proximal phalanx at the base of the thumb; *innervation*—median nerve, C8–T1.

abductor pollicis longus: *Function*—abducts and extends the thumb; *secondary function*—abducts the wrist; *origin*—the middle third of the posterior surface of the radius, the posterior surface of the ulna, and the interosseous membrane; *insertion*—the radial side of the base of the first metacarpal bone; *innervation*—radial nerve, C6–C7.

adductor brevis: *Function*—adducts and flexes the thigh; *secondary function*—rotates the thigh medially; *origin*—the external aspect of the body and inferior ramus of the pubis; *insertion*—by an aponeurosis to the line from the greater trochanter to the linea aspera of the femur; *innervation*—obturator nerve, L2–L4.

adductor hallucis: *Function*—adducts the great toe; *origin*—the oblique head arises from the second, third, and fourth metatarsal bones, and the transverse head arises from the plantar ligaments of the third, fourth, and fifth toes; *insertion*—the lateral sesamoid bone and base of the first phalanx of the large toe; *innervation*—lateral plantar nerve, S2–S3.

adductor longus: *Function*—adducts and flexes the thigh; *secondary function*—rotates the thigh medially; *origin*—the pubic crest and symphysis; *insertion*—by an aponeurosis to the middle third of the linea aspera of the femur; *innervation*—obturator nerve, L2–L4.

adductor magnus: *Function*—adducts the thigh; *secondary function*—upper fibers flex and rotate the thigh medially, and lower fibers extend and rotate the thigh laterally; *origin*—the inferior ramus of the pubis, the ramus of ischium, and the inferolateral aspect of the ischial tuberosity; *insertion*—by an aponeurosis to the linea aspera and adductor tubercle of the femur; *innervation*—obturator nerve, L2–L4, and tibial portion of the sciatic nerve, L2–L4.

adductor pollicis: *Function*—adducts the thumb; *origin*—the oblique head arises from the capitate, bases of the second and third metacarpals, and the palmar carpal ligaments, and the transverse head arises from the distal two-thirds of the palmar surface of the third metacarpal; *insertion*—fibers converge into a tendon containing a sesamoid bone that attaches to the ulnar side of the base of the proximal phalanx of the thumb; *innervation*—ulnar nerve, C8–T1.

anal sphincter (external): *Function*—closes the anal canal and orifice; *innervation*—S4 and inferior rectal branch of the pudendal nerve.

anal sphincter (internal): *Function*—assists external sphincter in an involuntary manner; *innervation*—sympathetic and sacral parasympathetic fibers by way of inferior mesenteric and hypogastric plexuses.

anconeus: *Function*—extends the forearm; *origin*—the posterior surface of the lateral epicondyle of the humerus; *insertion*—the lateral side of the olecranon and the proximal fourth of the posterior shaft of the ulna; *innervation*—radial nerve, C7–C8.

anterior deltoid: See *deltoid.*

articularis genus: *Function*—retracts the synovial membrane of the knee joint proximally (cephalad); *origin*—the anterior surface of the distal shaft of the femur; *insertion*—the upper part of the synovial membrane of the knee joint; *innervation*—femoral nerve, L3–L4.

aryepiglotticus: *Function*—closes the glottal opening; *innervation*—recurrent laryngeal branches of the vagus nerve.

arytenoid (arytenoideus): *Function*—closes glottal opening; *innervation*—recurrent branches of the vagus nerve.

auricularis anterior: *Function*—draws auricula forward and upward; *innervation*—temporal branches of the facial nerve.

auricularis posterior: *Function*—draws auricula backward; *innervation*—posterior auricular branches of the facial nerve.

auricularis superior: *Function*—draws auricula upward: *innervation*—temporal branches of the facial nerve.

biceps brachii: *Function*—flexes the arm (the long head), flexes the forearm (both heads), and supinates the forearm; *origin*—the short head arises from the coracoid process, and the long head arises from the supraglenoid tubercle at the apex of the glenoid cavity; *insertion*—the radial tuberosity of the radius; *innervation*—musculocutaneous nerve, C5–C6.

biceps femoris (long head): *Function*—flexes and laterally rotates the leg and extends and laterally rotates the thigh; *origin*—the ischial tuberosity and the sacrotuberous ligament; *insertion*—the head of the fibula and lateral condyle of the tibia; *innervation*—tibial portion of the sciatic nerve, S1–S3.

biceps femoris (short head): *Function*—flexes and laterally rotates the leg; *origin*—the lateral tip of the linea aspera of the femur; *insertion*—the head of the fibula and the lateral condyle of the tibia; *innervation*—peroneal portion of the sciatic nerve, L5–S2.

brachialis: *Function*—flexes the forearm; *origin*—the distal half of the anterior surface of the humerus; *insertion*—the tuberosity of the ulna and the coronoid process; *innervation*—musculocutaneous, C5–C6, and radial nerve (for sensory only).

brachioradialis: *Function*—flexes the forearm; *origin*—the proximal two-thirds of the lateral supracondylar ridge of the humerus; *insertion*—the styloid process of the radius; *innervation*—radial nerve, C5–C6.

buccinator: *Function*—compresses the cheek (assists in mastication); *origin*—the alveolar process of the maxillary bone, the pterygomandibular raphe, and the buccinator ridge of the mandible; *insertion*—the orbicularis oris; *innervation*—buccal branches of the facial nerve.

bulbospongiosus (bulbocavernosus): *Function*—empties the canal of the urethra and in the female reduces the orifice of the vagina; *innervation*—perineal branch of pudendal nerve, S2–S4.

chondroglossus: See *hyoglossus.*

ciliaris: *Function*—draws the ciliary process centrally and relaxes the suspensory ligaments of the lens, changing the convexity of the lens; *innervation*—short ciliary nerves.

coccygeus: *Function*—brings the coccyx ventrally; *innervation*—pudendal plexus including S4–S5.

constrictor inferior: See *inferior constrictor.*

constrictor medius: See *middle constrictor.*

constrictor superior: See *superior constrictor.*

coracobrachialis: *Function*—flexes and adducts the arm; *origin*—the coracoid process of the scapula; *insertion*—the middle of the medial surface of the humerus; *innervation*—musculocutaneous nerve, C6–C7.

corrugator supercilii: *Function*—draws the eyebrow down and medially; *origin*—the superciliary arch of the frontal bone; *insertion*—the skin over the middle third of the supraorbital margins; *innervation*—temporal and zygomatic branches of the facial nerve.

cremaster: *Function*—in the male draws testes up, and in the female draws labial folds up toward the superficial inguinal ring; *innervation*—genital branch of the genitofemoral nerve.

cricoarytenoideus lateralis: See *lateral cricoarytenoid.*

cricoarytenoideus posterior: See *posterior cricoarytenoid.*

cricothyroid (cricothyroideus): *Function*—tightens the vocal cords; *innervation*—internal laryngeal nerve of the vagus nerve.

deltoid: (see individual listings for anterior, middle, and posterior): *Function*—abducts the arm; *secondary function*—ventral fibers rotate the arm medially, and dorsal fibers rotate the arm laterally; *innervation*—axillary nerve, C5–C6.

deltoid (anterior): *Function*—flexes the arm; *origin*—the lateral third of the clavicle; *insertion*—the deltoid tuberosity of the lateral aspect of the humerus; *innervation*—axillary nerve, C5–C6.

deltoid (middle): *Function*—abducts the arm; *origin*—the superior surface of the acromion; *insertion*—the deltoid tuberosity of the lateral aspect of the humerus; *innervation*—axillary nerve, C5–C6.

deltoid (posterior): *Function*—extends the arm; *origin*—the spine of the scapula; *insertion*—the deltoid tuberosity of the lateral aspect of the humerus; *innervation*—axillary nerve, C5–C6.

depressor anguli oris: *Function*—Depresses the angle of mouth; *origin*—the oblique line of the mandible; *insertion*—the skin at the angle of the mouth; *innervation*—mandibular and buccal branches of the facial nerve.

depressor labii inferioris: *Function*—draws the lower lip down and back; *origin*—the oblique line of the mandible; *insertion*—the skin of the lower lip; *innervation*—mandibular and buccal branches of the facial nerve.

depressor septi: *Function*—draws the ala of the nose downward; *innervation*—buccal branches of the facial nerve.

diaphragm: *Function*—draws the central tendon downward and forward during inspiration to increase the volume and decrease the pressure within the thoracic cavity and also decreases the volume and increases the pressure within abdominal cavity; *origin*—the xiphoid process, the costal cartilages of the lower six ribs, and the lumbar vertebrae; *insertion*—the central tendon; *innervation*—phrenic nerve, C3–C5.

digastricus (anterior belly): *Function*—brings hyoid bone forward; *innervation*—mylohyoid nerve from the inferior alveolar branch of the mandibular division of the trigeminal nerve.

digastricus (posterior belly): *Function*—Brings hyoid bone backward; *innervation*—facial nerve.

dilator pupillae: *Function*—dilates the pupil; *innervation*—sympathetic efferents from the superior cervical ganglion.

dorsal interossei of the foot: See *interossei.*

dorsal interossei of the hand: See *interossei.*

extensor carpi radialis brevis: *Function*—extends the wrist; *secondary function*—abducts the wrist; *origin*—the lateral epicondyle of the humerus, the radial collateral ligament of the elbow and its covering aponeurosis;

insertion—the dorsal surface of the base of the third metacarpal; *innervation*—radial nerve, C6–C7.

extensor carpi radialis longus: *Function*—extends and abducts the wrist; *origin*—the distal one third of the lateral supracondylar ridge of the humerus; *insertion*—the radial side of the base of the second metacarpal; *innervation*—radial nerve, C6–C8.

extensor carpi ulnaris: *Function*—extends and adducts the wrist; *origin*—the lateral epicondyle; *insertion*—the tubercle on the medial side of the base of the fifth metacarpal; *innervation*—radial nerve, C6–C8.

extensor digiti minimi: *Function*—extends the fifth finger; *origin*—the common extensor tendon; *insertion*—the extensor hood (dorsal digital expansion) of the fifth digit; *innervation*—radial nerve, C6–C8.

extensor digitorum: *Function*—extends the fingers; *secondary function*—extends the wrist; *origin*—the lateral epicondyle of the humerus by a common extensor tendon; *insertion*—the middle and distal phalanges of the second through fifth digits; *innervation*—radial nerve, C6–C8.

extensor digitorum brevis: *Function*—extends the proximal phalanges of the great toe and the adjacent three toes; *origin*—the superolateral surface of the calcaneus; *insertion*—the first phalanx of the great toe and the tendons of the extensor digitorum longus; *innervation*—deep peroneal nerve, L5–S1.

extensor digitorum longus: *Function*—extends the proximal phalanges of the four toes; *secondary function*—dorsiflexes, abducts, and everts the foot; *origin*—the lateral condyle of the tibia, the proximal three-fourths of the anterior surface of the fibula, and the interosseous membrane; *insertion*—the middle and distal phalanges of the second through fifth digits; *innervation*—deep peroneal nerve, L4–S1.

extensor hallucis longus: *Function*—extends the proximal phalanx of the great toe; *secondary function*—dorsiflexes, adducts, and inverts the foot; *origin*—the middle two-fourths of the medial surface of the fibula; *insertion*—the dorsal aspect of the base of the distal phalanx of the great toe; *innervation*—deep peroneal nerve, L4–S1.

extensor indicis: *Function*—extends the index finger; *secondary function*—abducts the index finger; *origin*—the posterior surface of the ulna and the interosseous membrane; *insertion*—the extensor hood of the index finger; *innervation*—radial nerve, C6–C8.

extensor pollicis brevis: *Function*—extends the proximal phalanx of the thumb; *origin*—the posterior surface of the radius and interosseus membrane; *insertion*—the dorsal surface of the base of the proximal phalanx of the thumb; *innervation*—radial nerve, C6–C7.

extensor pollicis longus: *Function*—extends the second phalanx of the thumb; *origin*—the middle third of the posterior surface of the shaft of the ulna; *insertion*—the base of the distal phalanx of the thumb; *innervation*—radial nerve, C6–C8.

external intercostals: See *intercostales externi.*

external oblique: See *obliquus externus abdominis.*

extrinsic muscles of the eye: See *levator palpebrae superioris, obliquus inferior, obliquus superior, rectus inferior, rectus lateralis, rectus medialis,* and *rectus superior.*

fibularis brevis: *Function*—everts and abducts the foot; *secondary function*—plantar flexes the foot; *origin*—the distal two-thirds of the lateral surface of the fibula and the crural intermuscular septa; *insertion*—the tubercle on the base of the fifth metatarsal bone on its lateral side; *innervation*—superficial peroneal nerve, L4–S1.

fibularis longus: *Function*—everts and abducts the foot; *secondary function*—plantar flexes the foot; *origin*—the head and the proximal two-thirds of the lateral surface of the fibula and the crural intermuscular septa; *insertion*—lateral side of the base of the first metatarsal bone and the medial cuneiform; *innervation*—superficial peroneal nerve, L4–S1.

fibularis tertius: *Function*—abducts, dorsiflexes, and everts the foot; *origin*—the lower (distal) third of the anterior surface of the fibula and the crural intermuscular septum; *insertion*—the dorsal surface of the base of the fifth metatarsal bone; *innervation*—deep peroneal nerve, L5–S1.

flexor carpi radialis: *Function*—flexes and abducts the wrist; *origin*—the common flexor tendon from the medial epicondyle of the humerus; *insertion*—the palmar surface of the base of the second metacarpal; *innervation*—median nerve, C6–C7.

flexor carpi ulnaris: *Function*—flexes and adducts the wrist; *origin*—one head arises from the common flexor tendon of the medial epicondyle of the humerus, and the other head arises from the medial margins of the olecranon and the proximal two-thirds of the posterior border of the ulna; *insertion*—the pisiform bone and the fifth metacarpal; *innervation*—ulnar nerve, C8–T1.

flexor digiti minimi brevis of the foot: *Function*—flexes the proximal phalanx of small toe; *origin*—the plantar surface of the base of the fifth metatarsal; *insertion*—the lateral side of the base of the proximal phalanx of the fifth toe; *innervation*—lateral plantar nerve, S2–S3.

flexor digiti minimi brevis of the hand: *Function*—flexes the fifth finger; *origin*—the hamulus (hook) of the hamate and the flexor retinaculum; *insertion*—the ulnar side of the base of the proximal phalanx of the little finger; *innervation*—ulnar nerve, C8–T1.

flexor digitorum accessorius: See *quadratus plantae*.

flexor digitorum brevis: *Function*—flexes the second phalanges of the four toes; *origin*—the medial process of the tuberosity of the calcaneus, the plantar aponeurosis, and the intermuscular septa; *insertion*—the tendons divide and attach to both sides of the middle phalanges of the second through fifth toes; *innervation*—medial plantar nerve, L5–S1.

flexor digitorum longus: *Function*—flexes the four toes; *secondary function*—plantar flexes the ankle and flexes, adducts, and inverts the foot; *origin*—the posterior surface of the tibia; *insertion*—the distal phalanges of the second through fifth toes; *innervation*—tibial nerve, L5–S1.

flexor digitorum profundus: *Function*—flexes the distal phalanx of each finger; *secondary function*—flexes the more proximal phalanges of each finger and flexes the wrist; *origin*—the proximal three-fourths of the anterior and medial surfaces of the ulna, the interosseous membrane, and a depression on the medial side of the coronoid process; *insertion*—the palmar surface of the base of the distal phalanx of the second through fifth digits; *innervation*—median and ulnar nerves, C8–T1.

flexor digitorum superficialis: *Function*—flexes the second phalanx of each finger; *secondary function*—flexes the first phalanx of each finger and flexes the wrist; *origin*—the medial epicondyle of the humerus by the common flexor tendon, the intermuscular septa, the medial side of the coronoid process, and the anterior border of the radius from the radial tuberosity to the insertion of the pronator teres; *insertion*—tendons divide and insert into the sides of the shaft of the middle phalanx of the second through fifth digits; *innervation*—median nerve, C7–C8.

flexor hallucis brevis: *Function*—flexes the proximal phalanx of the great toe; *origin*—the medial part of the plantar surface of the cuboid, the lateral cuneiform, and the medial intermuscular septum; *insertion*—the tendon divides and attaches to the sides of the base of the proximal phalanx of the hallux (a sesamoid bone is usually in each of the attachments); *innervation*—medial plantar nerve, L5–S1.

flexor hallucis longus: *Function*—flexes the distal (second) phalanx of the great toe; *secondary function*—flexes, adducts, and inverts the foot; *origin*—the inferior two-thirds of the posterior surface of the fibula, the distal part of the interosseous membrane, the posterior crural intermuscular septum, and the fascia; *insertion*—the plantar aspect of the base of the distal phalanx of the great toe; *innervation*—tibial nerve, L5–S2.

flexor pollicis brevis: *Function*—flexes the proximal phalanx of the thumb and adducts the thumb; *origin*—the superficial head arises from the distal border of the flexor retinaculum and the tubercle of the trapezium, and the deep head arises from the trapezoid and capitate; *insertion*—the superficial head attaches by a tendon containing a sesamoid bone to the radial side of the base of the proximal phalanx of the thumb, and the deep head attaches by a tendon that unites with the superficial head on the sesamoid bone and base of the first phalanx; *innervation*—superficial head: median nerve, C8–T1; deep head: ulnar nerve, C8–T1.

flexor pollicis longus: *Function*—Flexes the second phalanx of the thumb; *origin*—the grooved anterior surface of the radius, the interosseous membrane; *insertion*—the palmar surface of the base of the distal phalanx of the thumb; *innervation*—median nerve, C8–T1.

gastrocnemius: *Function*—plantar flexes the foot and flexes the leg; *origin*—the medial head arises from the posterior part of the medial femoral condyle, and the lateral head arises from the lateral surface of the lateral femoral condyle; *insertion*—both heads form a tendon that joins the tendon of the soleus to form the tendocalcaneus, which inserts on the posterior surface of the calcaneus; *innervation*—tibial nerve, S1–S2.

gemelli (superior and inferior): *Function*—laterally rotates the extended thigh and abducts the flexed thigh; *origin*—the superior gemellus arises from the dorsal surface of the spine of the ischium, and the inferior gemellus arises from the upper part of the tuberosity of the ischium; *insertion*—both the superior and inferior gemelli attach to the medial surface of the greater trochanter; *innervation*—superior gemellus: nerve to obturator internus, L5–S2; inferior gemellus: nerve to quadratus femoris, L4–S1.

genioglossus: *Function*—protrudes or retracts the tongue and elevates the hyoid bone; *innervation*—hypoglossal nerve.

geniohyoid: *Function*—brings the hyoid bone anteriorly; *innervation*—branch of first cervical nerve via the hypoglossal nerve.

gluteus maximus: *Function*—extends and laterally rotates the thigh; *origin*—the posterior gluteal line of the ilium, the iliac crest, the aponeurosis of the erector spinae, the dorsal surface of the lower part of the sacrum, the side of the coccyx, the sacrotuberous ligament, and the intermuscular fascia; *insertion*—the iliotibial tract of the fascia lata and the gluteal tuberosity of the femur; *innervation*—inferior gluteal nerve, L5–S2.

gluteus medius: *Function*—abducts and medially rotates the thigh; *secondary function*—the anterior portion flexes the thigh, and the posterior portion extends the thigh; *origin*—the outer surface of the ilium between the iliac crest and the posterior gluteal line, the anterior gluteal line, and the fascia; *insertion*—the lateral surface of the greater trochanter; *innervation*—superior gluteal nerve, L4–S1.

gluteus minimus: *Function*—abducts and medially rotates the thigh; *origin*—the outer surface of the ilium between the anterior and inferior gluteal lines, and the margin of the greater sciatic notch; *insertion*—the ridge laterally situated on the anterior surface of the greater trochanter; *innervation*—superior gluteal nerve, L4–S1.

gracilis: *Function*—adducts the thigh; *secondary function*—flexes the leg and rotates the tibia medially; *origin*—the thin aponeurosis from the medial margins of the lower half of the body of the pubis and the whole of the inferior ramus; *insertion*—the proximal part of the medial surface of the tibia, below the tibial condyle and just proximal to the tendon of the semitendinosus; *innervation*—obturator nerve, L2–L3.

hamstrings muscles: See *biceps femoris, semitendinosus,* and *semimembranosus.*

hyoglossus (chondroglossus): *Function*—depresses the side of tongue and retracts the tongue; *innervation*—hypoglossal nerve.

iliacus: *Function*—flexes the thigh; *origin*—the superior two-thirds of the iliac fossa and the upper surface of the lateral part of the sacrum; *insertion*—fibers converge with tendon of the psoas major; *innervation*—femoral nerve, L2–L3.

iliocostalis (cervicis, thoracis, lumborum): See individual muscles.

iliocostalis cervicis: *Function*—extends the vertebral column and bends it to one side; *origin*—angles of the third through sixth ribs; *insertion*—posterior tubercles of the transverse processes of the fourth, fifth, and sixth cervical vertebrae; *innervation*—dorsal primary divisions of the spinal nerves.

iliocostalis lumborum: *Function*—extends the vertebral column and bends it to one side and draws the ribs down; *origin*—the broad erector spinae tendon from the median sacral crest; the spines of the lumbar and lower thoracic vertebrae, and the iliac crest; *insertion*—lumbar borders of the angles of the lower six or seven ribs; *innervation*—dorsal primary divisions of the spinal nerves.

iliocostalis thoracis: *Function*—extends the vertebral column, bends it to one side, and draws the ribs down; *origin*—upper borders of the angles of the lower six ribs; *insertion*—upper borders of the angles of the upper six ribs; *innervation*—dorsal primary divisions of the spinal nerves.

inferior constrictor: *Function*—narrows the pharynx for swallowing; *innervation*—pharyngeal plexus and external laryngeal and recurrent nerves.

inferior gemellus: See *gemelli.*

inferior oblique: See *obliquus inferior.*

inferior rectus: See *rectus inferior.*

infraspinatus: *Function*—laterally rotates the arm; *secondary function*—the upper fibers abduct and the lower fibers adduct the arm; *origin*—the medial two-thirds of the infraspinatus fossa; *insertion*—the middle impression (facet) on the greater tubercle of the humerus; *innervation*—suprascapular nerve, C5–C6.

intercostal muscles: See *intercostales externi* and *intercostales interni.*

intercostales externi: *Function*—elevates the ribs to increase the volume of the thoracic cavity; *origin*—the inferior border of the rib above; *insertion*—the superior border of the rib below; *innervation*—intercostal nerves.

intercostales interni: *Function*—elevates the ribs to decrease the volume of the thoracic cavity; *origin*—the floor of the costal grooves; *insertion*—the upper border of the rib below; *innervation*—intercostal nerves.

internal intercostals: See *intercostales interni.*

internal oblique: See *obliquus internus abdominis.*

interossei of the foot (dorsal): *Function*—abducts the toes; *secondary function*—flexes the proximal phalanges and extends the distal phalanges; *origin*—the dorsal interossei arise via two heads from the adjacent sides of two metatarsal bones; *insertion*—bases of the proximal phalanges and to the dorsal digital expansions, the first reaching the medial side of the second toe and the other three passing to the lateral sides of the second, third, and fourth toes; *innervation*—lateral plantar nerve, S2–S3.

interossei of the foot (plantar): *Function*—adduct the third through fifth digits; *secondary function*—flexes proximal phalanges and extends the distal phalanges; *origin*—bases and medial sides of the third, fourth, and fifth metatarsal bones; *insertion*—medial sides of the bases of the proximal phalanges of the same toes and into their dorsal digital expansions; *innervation*—lateral plantar nerve, S2–S3.

interossei of the hand (dorsal): *Function*—abducts the fingers; *secondary function*—flexes the metacarpophalangeal joints and extends the interphalangeal joints; *origin*—adjacent sides of two metacarpal bones; *insertion*—bases of the proximal phalanges and extensor hoods (dorsal digital expansions), the first interosseus is attached to the radial side of the proximal phalanx of the index finger; the second and third interossei are attached to the middle finger, the second to the radial side and the third to the ulnar side; and the fourth interosseus attaches to the dorsal digital expansion of the ring finger; *innervation*—ulnar nerve, C8–T1.

interossei of the hand (palmar): *Function*—adducts fingers; *secondary function*—flexes the metacarpophalangeal joints and extends the interphalangeal joints; *origin*—with the exception of the first, each of the four arises from the entire length of the metacarpal bone of one finger, and the first interosseus arises from the ulnar side of the palmar surface of the base of the first metacarpal bone; *insertion*—the first interosseus inserts into a sesamoid bone on the ulnar side of the proximal phalanx of the thumb and into the thumb's dorsal digital expansion, and the remaining three interossei pass to the dorsal digital expansion of the same digit; *innervation*—ulnar nerve, C8–T1.

MUSCULO

MUSCULO

intertransversarii: *Function*—bends the vertebral column laterally; *origin*—transverse processes of the vertebrae; *insertion*—adjacent transverse processes; *innervation*—anterior, lateral, and posterior branches of the ventral primary divisions of the spinal nerves.

ischiocavernosus: *Function*—in the male compresses the crus of the penis and in the female compresses the crus of the clitoris; *innervation*—perineal branch of the pudendal nerve, S2–S4.

lateral cricoarytenoid: *Function*—narrows the glottis; *innervation*—recurrent laryngeal nerve of the vagus nerve.

lateral pterygoid: *Function*—opens the jaw, protrudes the mandible, and moves the mandible from side to side; *origin*—the upper head arises from the infratemporal surface and infratemporal crest of the greater wing of the sphenoid bone, and the lower head arises from the lateral surface of the lateral pterygoid plate; *insertion*—a depression on the front of the neck of the mandible, the articular capsule, and the disk of the temporomandibular joint; *innervation*—lateral pterygoid nerve of the mandibular division of the trigeminal nerve.

lateral rectus: See *rectus lateralis*.

latissimus dorsi: *Function*—adducts, extends, and medially rotates the arm; *origin*—spines of the lower six thoracic vertebrae, the posterior layer of the thoracolumbar fascia, and the posterior part of the crest of the ilium; *insertion*—the bottom of the intertubercular sulcus of the humerus; *innervation*—thoracodorsal nerve, C6–C8.

levator anguli oris: *Function*—raises the angle of the upper lip; *innervation*—buccal branches of the facial nerve.

levator ani iliococcygeus: *Function*—supports and raises the pelvic floor and resists any increase in intra-abdominal pressure; *innervation*—pudendal plexus, including S3–S5.

levator ani pubococcygeus: *Function*—brings the anus toward the pubis and constricts it; *innervation*—pudendal plexus, including S3–S5.

levator labii superioris: *Function*—elevates the upper lip; *innervation*—buccal branches of the facial nerve.

levator labii superioris alaeque nasi: *Function*—elevates the upper lip and dilates the naris; *innervation*—buccal branches of the facial nerve.

levator palpebrae superioris: *Function*—raises the upper eyelid; *innervation*—oculomotor nerve.

levator scapulae: *Function*—elevates the scapula; *secondary function*—rotates the scapula downward; *origin*—transverse processes of the atlas and axis and posterior tubercles of the transverse processes of the third and fourth cervical vertebrae; *insertion*—medial border of the scapula between the superior angle and the spine; *innervation*—C3–C4 and frequently the dorsal scapular nerve, C5.

levator veli palatini: *Function*—elevates the soft palate; *innervation*—pharyngeal plexus.

levatores costarum: *Function*—raises the ribs to increase the thoracic cavity and extends the vertebral column, bending it laterally with slight rotation to opposite side; *origin*—ends of the transverse processes of the seventh cervical and first to eleventh thoracic vertebrae; *insertion*—the upper edge and external surfaces of the rib immediately below the vertebrae, from which it takes origin between the tubercle and the angle; *innervation*—intercostal nerves.

longissimus capitis: *Function*—extends the head and bends it to the same side, rotating the face to that side; *origin*—transverse processes of the upper four or five thoracic vertebrae; *insertion*—the posterior margin of the mastoid process; *innervation*—dorsal primary divisions of spinal nerves.

longissimus cervicis: *Function*—extends the vertebral column and bends it to one side while drawing the ribs down; *origin*—transverse process of the upper four or five thoracic vertebrae; *insertion*—posterior tubercles of the transverse processes of C2–C6; *innervation*—dorsal primary divisions of spinal nerves.

longissimus thoracis: *Function*—extends the vertebral column and bends it to one side while drawing the ribs down; *origin*—the whole length of the posterior surfaces of the transverse processes of the lumbar vertebrae; *insertion*—to the tips of the transverse processes of all the thoracic vertebrae and lower 9 or 10 ribs; *innervation*—dorsal primary divisions of spinal nerves.

longus capitis: *Function*—flexes head; *origin*—the anterior tubercles of the transverse processes of the third, fourth, fifth, and sixth cervical vertebrae; *insertion*—the inferior surface of the basilar part of the occipital bone; *innervation*—branches of spinal nerves C1–C3.

longus colli: *Function*—flexes the neck with slight cervical rotation; *origin*—the superior oblique portion arises from the anterior tubercles of the transverse processes of the third, fourth, and fifth cervical vertebrae; the inferior oblique portion arises from the anterior surfaces of the first two thoracic vertebrae; and the vertical portion arises from the anterolateral surface of the bodies of the first three thoracic and last three cervical vertebrae; *insertion*—the superior oblique portion inserts on the tubercle of the atlas, the inferior oblique portion inserts on the anterior tubercles of the transverse processes of the fifth and sixth cervical vertebrae, and the vertical portion inserts into the anterior surface of the bodies of the second through fourth cervical vertebrae; *innervation*—ventral branches of the C2–C6 spinal nerves.

lower trapezius: See *trapezius*.

lumbricals of the foot: *Function*—flexes the proximal phalanges and extends the distal phalanges of the four toes; *origin*—tendons of the flexor digitorum longus; *insertion*—the extensor hoods (dorsal digital expansions) on the proximal phalanges of the second through fifth digits; *innervation*—first lumbrical is by the medial plantar nerve, L5–S1, and second through fourth lumbricals by the lateral plantar nerve, S2–S3.

lumbricals of the hand: *Function*—flexes the metacarpophalangeal joints and extends the interphalangeal joints; *origin*—tendons of the flexor digitorum profundus; *insertion*—lateral margins of the extensor hoods (dorsal digital expansions) of the second through fifth digits; *innervation*—first and second lumbricals by the median nerve, C8–T1, and third and fourth lumbricals by the ulnar nerve, C8–T1.

masseter: *Function*—closes the jaw; *origin*—the zygomatic process of the maxilla and from the anterior two-thirds of the lower border of the zygomatic arch; *insertion*—the angle and ramus of the mandible; *innervation*—masseteric branch of the mandibular division of the trigeminal nerve.

MUSCULO

medial pterygoid: *Function*—closes the jaw; *origin*—the medial surface of the lateral pterygoid plate and the pyramidal process of the palatine bone; *insertion*—the posterior part of the medial surfaces of the ramus and angle of the mandible; *innervation*—medial pterygoid branch of the mandibular division of the trigeminal nerve.

medial rectus: See *rectus medialis*.

mentalis: *Function*—raises and protrudes the lower lip and wrinkles the chin; *origin*—the incisive fossa of the mandible; *insertion*—the skin of the chin; *innervation*—mandibular and buccal branches of the facial nerve.

middle constrictor: *Function*—narrows the pharynx for swallowing; *innervation*—pharyngeal plexus.

middle deltoid: See *deltoid*.

multifidus: *Function*—extends the vertebral column and rotates it toward opposite side; *origin*—the sacral portion arises from the posterior superior iliac spine and the dorsal sacroiliac ligaments, the lumbar portion arises from the mamillary processes, the thoracic portion arises from all thoracic transverse processes, and the cervical portion arises from the articular processes of the lower four vertebrae; *insertion*—the whole length of the spine of the vertebrae above; *innervation*—dorsal primary divisions of the spinal nerves.

musculus uvulae: *Function*—elevates the uvula; *innervation*—pharyngeal plexus of the accessory nerve.

mylohyoid: *Function*—raises the hyoid bone and tongue; *innervation*—mylohyoid nerve of the mandibular division of the trigeminal nerve.

nasalis: *Function*—enlarges the opening of nares; *innervation*—buccal branches of the facial nerve.

obliques: See *obliquus externus abdominis* and *obliquus internus abdominis*.

obliquus capitis inferior: *Function*—rotates the atlas and turns the head to the same side; *origin*—the spine of the axis; *insertion*—the transverse process of the atlas; *innervation*—dorsal primary ramus of the suboccipital nerve.

obliquus capitis superior: *Function*—extends and bends the head laterally; *origin*—the transverse process of the atlas; *insertion*—the occipital bone between the superior and inferior nuchal lines; *innervation*—dorsal primary ramus of the suboccipital nerve.

obliquus externus abdominis: *Function*—compresses the abdominal contents, flexes the vertebral column, and rotates the column to bring forward the shoulder on the same side as the active muscle; *origin*—inferior borders of the lower eight ribs; *insertion*—the iliac crest, the aponeurosis; *innervation*—intercostal nerves, T7–T12.

obliquus inferior: *Function*—elevates, abducts, and rotates the eye laterally; *innervation*—oculomotor nerve.

obliquus internus abdominis: *Function*—compresses abdominal contents, flexes the vertebral column, and rotates the column to bring the shoulder forward on the side opposite from the active muscle; *origin*—the lateral two-thirds of the upper surface of the inguinal ligament, the iliac crest, and the thoracolumbar fascia; *insertion*—posterior fibers pass upward and laterally to the inferior borders of the lower three or four ribs, the inguinal ligament fibers attach to the crest of the pubis, and the remainder of the fibers end in an aponeurosis that forms the linea alba; *innervation*—branches of the intercostal nerves from T8–T12 and the iliohypogastric and ilioinguinal branches of L1.

obliquus superior: *Function*—depresses, abducts, and rotates the eye laterally; *innervation*—trochlear nerve.

obturator externus: *Function*—laterally rotates the thigh; *origin*—rami of the pubis, the ramus of the ischium, and the medial two-thirds of the outer surface of the obturator membrane; *insertion*—the trochanteric fossa of the femur; *innervation*—obturator nerve, L3–L4.

obturator internus: *Function*—laterally rotates the thigh; *secondary function*—abducts when the thigh is flexed; *origin*—the internal surface of the anterolateral wall of the pelvis and the obturator membrane; *insertion*—the medial surface of the greater trochanter; *innervation*—nerve to obturator internus, L5–S2.

occipitofrontalis: *Function*—draws scalp back to raise the eyebrows and wrinkles forehead; *origin*—the superior nuchal line of the occipital bone and intermuscular attachments with the orbicularis oculi; *insertion*—the galea aponeurotica; *innervation*—temporal and posterior auricular branches of the facial nerve.

omohyoid: *Function*—draws the hyoid bone downward; *innervation*—ansa cervicalis containing fibers of C1–C3.

opponens digiti minimi: *Function*—abducts, flexes, and laterally rotates the fifth finger; *origin*—the hamulus (hook) of the hamate bone and the flexor retinaculum; *insertion*—the whole length of the ulnar margin and the fifth metacarpal bone; *innervation*—ulnar nerve, T1.

opponens pollicis: *Function*—abducts, flexes, and medially rotates the thumb; *origin*—the ridge of the trapezium and the flexor retinaculum; *insertion*—the whole length of the lateral border of the metacarpal bone of the thumb; *innervation*—median nerve (sometimes by branch of the ulnar nerve), C8–T1.

orbicularis oculi: *Function*—closes the eyelids; *innervation*—temporal and zygomatic branches of the facial nerve.

orbicularis oris: *Function*—closes the lips; *innervation*—buccal branches of the facial nerve.

palatoglossus: *Function*—elevates the posterior tongue and constricts the fauces; *innervation*—pharyngeal plexus of the accessory nerve.

palatopharyngeus: *Function*—constricts the fauces and closes off the nasopharynx; *innervation*—pharyngeal plexus.

palmar interossei of the foot: See *interossei.*

palmar interossei of the hand: See *interossei.*

palmaris brevis: *Function*—wrinkles the skin of the ulnar side of the palm; *origin*—the flexor retinaculum and the palmar aponeurosis; *insertion*—the dermis on the ulnar border of the hand; *innervation*—ulnar nerve, C8–T1.

palmaris longus: *Function*—flexes the hand; *origin*—the palmar longus arises from the common flexor tendon on the medial epicondyle of the humerus; *insertion*—the palmar aponeurosis; *innervation*—median nerve, C6–C7.

pectineus: *Function*—flexes and adducts the thigh; *secondary function*—rotates the thigh medially; *origin*—the pecten of the pubis; *insertion*—along a line leading from the lesser trochanter to the linea aspera; *innervation*— femoral, obturator, or accessory obturator nerves, L2–L4.

pectoralis major: *Function*—flexes and adducts the arm; *secondary function*— rotates the arm medially; *origin*—the anterior surface of the sternal half of the clavicle, the anterior surface of the sternum as low as the attachment of the cartilage of the sixth rib, from the cartilages of all true ribs, and from the aponeurosis of the obliquus externus abdominis; *insertion*—the lateral lip of the intertubercular sulcus of the humerus; *innervation*—medial and lateral pectoral nerves, C5–T1.

pectoralis minor: *Function*—rotates the scapula downward and forward; *secondary function*—raises third, fourth, and fifth ribs; *origin*—third, fourth, and fifth ribs; *insertion*—the medial border of the coracoid process; *innervation*—medial pectoral nerve, C8–T1.

piriformis: *Function*—laterally rotates and abducts thigh; *origin*—anterior sacrum, the gluteal surface of the ilium, the capsule of the sacroiliac joint, and the sacrotuberus ligament; *insertion*—the upper border of the greater trochanter of the femur; *innervation*—sacral plexus, S1.

plantar interossei: See *interossei*.

plantaris: *Function*—flexes the leg; plantar flexes the foot; *origin*—the distal linea aspera (lower part of the lateral supracondylar line) and from the oblique popliteal ligament; *insertion*—inserts with the tendocalcaneus into the calcaneus; *innervation*—tibial nerve, L4–S1.

platysma: *Function*—retracts and depresses the angle of the mouth; *innervation*—cervical branch of the facial nerve.

popliteus: *Function*—flexes the leg, rotates the leg (tibia) medially; *origin*— the lateral condyle of the femur and the arcuate popliteal ligament; *insertion*—the medial two-thirds of the triangular area above the soleal line on the posterior surface of the tibia; *innervation*—tibial nerve, L4–S1.

posterior cricoarytenoid: *Function*—opens the glottis; *innervation*—recurrent laryngeal nerve of the vagus nerve.

posterior deltoid: See *deltoid*.

procerus: *Function*—wrinkles the nose and draws the medial eyebrow downward; *origin*—the fascia covering the lower part of the nasal bone; *insertion*—the skin over the lower part of the forehead between the eyebrows; *innervation*—buccal branches of the facial nerve.

pronator quadratus: *Function*—pronates the forearm; *origin*—the oblique ridge on the distal part of the anterior surface of the shaft of the ulna; *insertion*—the distal fourth of the anterior border and the surface of the shaft of the radius; *innervation*—median nerve, C8–T1.

pronator teres: *Function*—pronates the forearm; *origin*—the humeral head arises from the common flexor tendon on the medial epicondyle of the humerus, and the ulnar head arises from the medial side of the coronoid process of the ulna; *insertion*—the rough area midway along the lateral surface of the radial shaft; *innervation*—median nerve, C6–C7.

psoas major: *Function*—flexes the thigh; *secondary function*—flexes the lumbar vertebrae and bends them laterally; *origin*—transverse processes of all the lumbar vertebrae, bodies and intervertebral disks of the lumbar vertebrae; *insertion*—lesser trochanter of the femur; *innervation*—lumbar plexus, L2–L3.

psoas minor: *Function*—flexes the pelvis and the lumbar vertebrae; *origin*—sides of the bodies of the 12th thoracic and 1st lumbar vertebrae and from the disk between them; *insertion*—the pecten pubis (pectineal line) and iliopectineal eminence; *innervation*—lumbar plexus, L1.

pyramidalis: *Function*—tightens the linea alba; *origin*—the pubic crest; *insertion*—linea alba; *innervation*—branch of 12th thoracic nerve.

quadratus femoris: *Function*—rotates the thigh laterally; *origin*—the ischial tuberosity; *insertion*—the quadrate tubercle of the femur; *innervation*—nerve to quadratus femoris, L4–S1.

quadratus lumborum: *Function*—laterally flexes the lumbar vertebral column; *origin*—the iliolumbar ligament and the iliac crest; *insertion*—the inferior border of the last rib and the transverse processes of the first four lumbar vertebrae; *innervation*—T12–L3 (or L4).

quadratus plantae (flexor digitorum accessorius): *Function*—flexes the distal phalanges of the third through fifth digits; *origin*—a medial head arises from the medial concave surface of the calcaneus, and a lateral head arises from the lateral border of the calcaneus and long plantar ligament; *insertion*—tendons of the flexor digitorum longus; *innervation*—lateral plantar nerve, S2–S3.

quadriceps femoris: See *rectus femoris, vastus intermedius, vastus lateralis,* and *vastus medialis.*

rectus abdominis: *Function*—flexes the vertebral column, tenses the anterior abdominal wall, and assists in compressing the abdominal contents; *origin*—the crest of the pubis; *insertion*—fifth, sixth, and seventh costal cartilages; *innervation*—T7–T12 and ilioinguinal (L1) and iliohypogastric nerves (T12–L1).

rectus capitis anterior: *Function*—flexes the head; *origin*—the anterior surface of the lateral mass of the atlas; *insertion*—the basilar part of the occipital bone in front of the occipital condyle; *innervation*—fibers from cervical nerve of C1 and C2.

rectus capitis lateralis: *Function*—bends the head laterally; *origin*—the upper surface of the transverse process of the atlas; *insertion*—the inferior surface of the jugular process of the occipital bone; *innervation*—fibers from cervical nerves, C1–C2.

rectus capitis posterior major: *Function*—extends and rotates the head to the same side; *origin*—the spine of the axis; *insertion*—the lateral part of the inferior nuchal line of the occipital bone; *innervation*—dorsal ramus of C1 (suboccipital nerve).

rectus capitis posterior minor: *Function*—extends the head; *origin*—the tubercle on the posterior arch of the atlas; *insertion*—the medial part of the inferior nuchal line of the occipital bone; *innervation*—dorsal ramus of C1 (suboccipital nerve).

rectus femoris: *Function*—flexes the thigh and extends the leg; *origin*—by two heads, from the anterior inferior iliac spine, and a reflected head from the groove above the acetabulum; *insertion*—the base of the patella; *innervation*—femoral nerve, L2–L4.

rectus inferior: *Function*—depresses, adducts, and rotates the eye medially; *innervation*—oculomotor nerve.

rectus lateralis: *Function*—abducts the eye; *innervation*—abducens nerve.

MUSCULO

rectus medialis: *Function*—adducts the eye; *innervation*—oculomotor nerve.

rectus superior: *Function*—elevates, adducts, and rotates the eye medially; *innervation*—oculomotor nerve.

rhomboid major: *Function*—adducts the scapula; *secondary function*—rotates the scapula down; *origin*—spines of the second through fifth thoracic vertebrae and supraspinous ligaments; *insertion*—medial border of the scapula between the root of the spine and the inferior angle; *innervation*—dorsal scapular nerve, C5.

rhomboid minor: *Function*—adducts the scapula; *secondary function*—rotates the scapula down; *origin*—the lower part of the ligamentum nuchae and from the spines of the seventh cervical and first thoracic vertebrae; *insertion*—the triangular smooth surface at the medial end of the spine of the scapula; *innervation*—dorsal scapular nerve, C5.

risorius: *Function*—retracts the angle of the mouth; *origin*—parotid fascia; *insertion*—the skin at the angle of the mouth; *innervation*—mandibular and buccal branches of the facial nerve.

rotatores: *Function*—extends vertebral column and rotates it toward the opposite side; *origin and insertion*—each of the rotatores connects the upper and posterior part of the transverse process of one vertebra to the lower border and lateral surface of the spine of the one or two vertebrae above; *innervation*—dorsal primary divisions of the spinal nerves.

salpingopharyngeus: *Function*—elevates the nasopharynx; *innervation*—pharyngeal plexus.

sartorius: *Function*—flexes, abducts, and laterally rotates the thigh, and also flexes and rotates the tibia medially; *origin*—the anterior superior iliac spine and the notch below the anterior superior iliac spine; *insertion*—the upper part of the medial surface of the tibia anterior to the gracilis; *innervation*—femoral nerve, L2–L3.

scalenus anterior: *Function*—raises the first rib; *origin*—anterior tubercles of the transverse processes of the third, fourth, fifth, and sixth cervical vertebrae; *insertion*—the scalene tubercle on the inner border of the first rib; *innervation*—branches from the anterior rami of C5–C6.

scalenus medius: *Function*—raises the first rib; *origin*—the transverse process of the atlas and the posterior tubercles of the transverse processes of the lower six cervical vertebrae; *insertion*—the upper surface of the first rib; *innervation*—branches from the anterior rami of C3–C8.

scalenus posterior: *Function*—raises the second rib; *origin*—posterior tubercles of the transverse processes of the fourth, fifth, and sixth cervical vertebrae; *insertion*—the second rib; *innervation*—ventral primary rami of C6–C8.

semimembranosus: *Function*—flexes the leg and extends the thigh; *secondary function*—medially rotates the flexed leg; *origin*—the ischial tuberosity; *insertion*—medial tibial condyle; *innervation*—tibial portion of the sciatic nerve, L5–S2.

semispinalis capitis: *Function*—extends the head and rotates it toward opposite side; *origin*—transverse processes of the upper six or seven thoracic and the seventh cervical vertebrae; *insertion*—the medial part of the area between the superior and inferior nuchal lines of the occipital; *innervation*—dorsal primary divisions of cervical nerves.

semispinalis cervicis: *Function*—extends the vertebral column and rotates it toward opposite side; *origin*—transverse processes of the upper five or six thoracic vertebrae; *insertion*—spines of the cervical vertebrae; *innervation*—dorsal primary divisions of spinal nerves.

semispinalis thoracis: *Function*—extends the vertebral column and rotates it toward opposite side; *origin*—transverse processes of the 6th to 10th thoracic vertebrae; *insertion*—spines of the upper four thoracic and lower two cervical vertebrae; *innervation*—dorsal primary divisions of spinal nerves.

semitendinosus: *Function*—flexes the leg and extends the thigh; *secondary function*—medially rotates the flexed leg; *origin*—the ischial tuberosity; *insertion*—the upper part of the medial surface of the tibia behind the attachment of the sartorius and below that of the gracilis; *innervation*—tibial portion of the sciatic nerve, L5–S2.

serratus anterior: *Function*—rotates the scapula upward and abducts the scapula; *origin*—outer surfaces of the upper eight or nine ribs; *insertion*—the costal aspect of the medial border of the scapula; *innervation*—long thoracic nerve, C5–C7.

serratus posterior inferior: *Function*—draws the ribs down and out; *origin*—spines of the lower two thoracic and upper two lumbar vertebrae; *insertion*—inferior borders of the lower four ribs; *innervation*—ventral primary divisions of T9–T12.

serratus posterior superior: *Function*—raises the ribs to increase the size of the thoracic cavity; *origin*—the lower part of the ligamentum nuchae and the spines of the seventh cervical and the upper two thoracic vertebrae; *insertion*—upper borders of the second, third, fourth, and fifth ribs; *innervation*—ventral primary divisions of T1–T4.

soleus: *Function*—plantar flexes the foot; *origin*—the head and proximal third of the posterior surface of the fibula, and from the soleal line and middle third of the medial border of the tibia; *insertion*—the soleus joins the tendon of gastrocnemius to form the tendocalcaneus inserting on the calcaneus; *innervation*—tibial nerve, S1–S2.

sphincter pupillae: *Function*—constricts the pupil; *innervation*—motor root of the ciliary ganglion from the oculomotor nerve.

sphincter urethrae: *Function*—compresses the urethra; *innervation*—perineal branch of the pudendal nerve, S2–S4.

spinalis (capitis, cervicis, thoracis): *Function*—extends the vertebral column; *origin*—arises from the spines of vertebrae in each region; *insertion*—on vertebral spines a few segments above; *innervation*—dorsal primary divisions of the spinal nerves.

splenius capitis: *Function*—brings the head and neck posteriorly and laterally with some rotation; *origin*—the lower half of the ligamentum nuchae, the spine of the seventh cervical vertebra, and the spines of the upper three or four thoracic vertebrae; *insertion*—the occipital bone inferior to the superior nuchal line and the mastoid process of the temporal bone; *innervation*—dorsal primary divisions of the middle cervical roots.

splenius cervicis: *Function*—brings the head and neck posteriorly and laterally with some rotation; *origin*—spines of the third to sixth thoracic vertebrae; *insertion*—posterior tubercles of the transverse processes of the upper two

MUSCULO

cervical vertebrae; *innervation*—dorsal primary divisions of the lower cervical roots.

stapedius: *Function*—pulls the head of the stapes posteriorly to increase tension of fluid in ear; *innervation*—the tympanic branch of the facial nerve.

sternocleidomastoid (sternomastoid): *Function*—rotates the head; *origin*—the upper part of the anterior surface of the manubrium sterni and the medial third of the clavicle; *insertion*—the mastoid process of the temporal bone; *innervation*—spinal part of the accessory nerve.

sternohyoid: *Function*—draws the hyoid bone inferiorly; *innervation*—branches of ansa cervicalis hypoglossi, including fibers from C1–C3.

sternomastoid: See *sternocleidomastoid.*

sternothyroid: *Function*—draws the larynx downward; *innervation*—branches of ansa cervicalis hypoglossi, including fibers from C1–C3.

styloglossus: *Function*—retracts and elevates the tongue; *innervation*—hypoglossal nerve.

stylohyoid: *Function*—elevates and retracts the hyoid bone; *innervation*—facial nerve.

stylopharyngeus: *Function*—elevates and dilates the pharynx; *innervation*—glossopharyngeal nerve.

subclavius: *Function*—depresses and pulls forward (anteriorly) the lateral end of the clavicle; *origin*—the junction of the first rib and its costal cartilage; *insertion*—the groove on the inferior surface of middle third of the clavicle; *innervation*—nerve to subclavius, C5–C6.

subscapularis: *Function*—medially rotates the arm; *secondary function*—flexes, extends, abducts, and adducts the arm, depending on the arm position; *origin*—the medial two-thirds of subscapular fossa; *insertion*—the lesser tubercle of the humerus; *innervation*—upper and lower subscapular nerves, C5–C6.

superior constrictor: *Function*—narrows the pharynx for swallowing; *innervation*—pharyngeal plexus.

superior gemellus: See *gemelli.*

superior oblique: See *obliquus superior.*

superior rectus: See *rectus superior.*

supinator: *Function*—supinates the forearm; *origin*—the lateral epicondyle of the humerus and the supinator crest of the ulna; *insertion*—the lateral surface of the proximal third of the radius; *innervation*—radial nerve, C6.

supraspinatus: *Function*—abducts the arm; *secondary function*—flexes and laterally rotates the arm; *origin*—the medial two-thirds of the supraspinatus fossa; *insertion*—the superior facet of the greater tubercle of the humerus; *innervation*—suprascapular nerve, C5.

temporalis: *Function*—closes the jaw, and the posterior portion retracts the mandible; *origin*—the temporalis fossa; *insertion*—medial surface, apex, anterior, and posterior borders of the coronoid process and the anterior border of the ramus of the mandible; *innervation*—anterior and posterior deep temporal nerves of the mandibular division of the trigeminal nerve.

temporoparietalis: *Function*—draws the skin backward over temples and wrinkles the forehead; *innervation*—temporal branches of the facial nerve.

tensor fasciae latae: *Function*—flexes and abducts the thigh; *secondary function*—medially rotates the thigh; *origin*—the outer lip of the iliac crest and the lateral surface of the anterior superior iliac spine; *insertion*—iliotibial tract; *innervation*—superior gluteal nerve, L4–S1.

tensor tympani: *Function*—draws the tympanic membrane medially to increase tension on the membrane; *innervation*—mandibular division of the trigeminal nerve through the otic ganglion.

tensor veli palatini: *Function*—stretches the soft palate; *innervation*—trigeminal nerve.

teres major: *Function*—adducts and extends the arm; *secondary function*—medially rotates the arm; *origin*—the dorsal surface of the inferior angle of the scapula; *insertion*—the medial lip of the intertubercular sulcus of the humerus; *innervation*—lower subscapular nerve, C5–C6.

teres minor: *Function*—laterally rotates the arm; *secondary function*—adducts the arm; *origin*—the proximal two-thirds of the lateral border of the scapula; *insertion*—inferior facet of the greater tubercle of the humerus; *innervation*—axillary nerve, C5.

thyroarytenoid (thyroarytenoideus): *Function*—relaxes the vocal cords; *innervation*—recurrent laryngeal nerve of the vagus nerve.

thyroepiglotticus: *Function*—depresses the epiglottis; *innervation*—recurrent laryngeal nerve of the vagus nerve.

thyrohyoid (thyroideus): *Function*—brings the hyoid bone inferiorly or raises the thyroid cartilage; *innervation*—fibers from C1.

tibialis anterior: *Function*—dorsiflexes, adducts, and inverts foot; *origin*—the lateral condyle and proximal half of the lateral surface of the tibial shaft; *insertion*—the medial cuneiform and the base of the first metatarsal bone; *innervation*—deep peroneal nerve, L4–S1.

tibialis posterior: *Function*—plantar flexes, adducts, and inverts the foot; *origin*—the posterior surface of the tibia and fibula; *insertion*—the tuberosity of the navicular, the three cuneiforms, the cuboid, and the bases of the second, third, and fourth metatarsals; *innervation*—tibial nerve, L5–S1.

transversus abdominis: *Function*—compresses the abdomen to assist in defecation, emesis, parturition, and forced expiration; *origin*—the lateral third of the inguinal ligament, the iliac crest, and the lower costal cartilages; *insertion*—primarily to the linear alba; *innervation*—branches of T7–T12, iliohypogastric and ilio-inguinal nerves.

transversus menti: *Function*—depresses the angle of the mouth; *innervation*—mandibular and buccal branches of the facial nerve.

transversus perinei profundus: *Function*—compresses the urethra; *innervation*—perineal branch of the pudendal nerve.

transversus perinei superficialis: *Function*—fixes the central tendinous part of the perineum; *innervation*—perineal branch of the pudendal nerve.

transversus thoracis: *Function*—brings the ventral ribs downward to decrease the size of the thoracic cavity; *origin*—the distal third of the posterior surfaces of the body of the sternum and the xiphoid process; *insertion*—lower borders of the costal cartilages of the second, third, fourth, fifth, and sixth ribs; *innervation*—intercostal nerves.

trapezius: *Function*—lower trapezius draws the scapula down, middle trapezius adducts the scapula, and upper trapezius draws the scapular upward; *origin*—the medial third of the superior nuchal line of the occipital bone, the external occipital protuberance, the ligamentum nuchae, the seventh

cervical and all the thoracic vertebral spinous processes, and the corresponding supraspinous ligaments; *insertion*—the lateral third of the clavicle, the
acromion process, and the spine of the scapula; *innervation*—spinal part of
accessory nerve.

triceps brachii: *Function*—extends the forearm; *origin*—the long head arises
from the infraglenoid tubercle of the scapula, the lateral head arises
from the posterior surface of the shaft of the humerus along an oblique line
above the radial groove, and the medial head arises from the posterior
surface of the shaft of the humerus below the radial groove; *insertion*—the
upper surface of the olecranon process of the ulna; *innervation*—radial
nerve, C7–C8.

upper trapezius: See *trapezius.*

vastus intermedius: *Function*—extends the leg; *origin*—anterior and lateral
surfaces of the proximal two-thirds of the femoral shaft; *insertion*—the
patella, with some fibers passing over to blend with the ligamentum patellae;
innervation—femoral nerve, L2–L4.

vastus lateralis: *Function*—extends the leg; *origin*—by a broad aponeurosis
to the proximal part of the intertrochanteric line, anterior and inferior
borders of the greater trochanter, the lateral lip of the gluteal tuberosity, and
the proximal half of the lateral lip of the linea aspera; *insertion*—the lateral
border of the patella; *innervation*—femoral nerve, L2–L4.

vastus medialis: *Function*—extends the leg; *origin*—the distal part of the intertrochanteric line, spiral line, the medial lip of the linea aspera, and the
medial intermuscular septum; *insertion*—the medial border of the patella;
innervation—femoral nerve, L2–L4.

vocalis: *Function*—closes the glottis; *innervation*—recurrent laryngeal branch
of the vagus nerve.

zygomaticus major: *Function*—draws angle of mouth upward and backward;
origin—the zygomatic bone in front of the zygomaticotemporal suture;
insertion—the angle of the mouth; *innervation*—buccal branches of the
facial nerve.

zygomaticus minor: *Function*—forms the nasolabial furrow; *origin*—the
lateral surface of the zygomatic bone immediately behind the zygomatico-
maxillary suture; *insertion*—the muscular substance of the upper lip;
innervation—buccal branches of the facial nerve.

MUSCULO

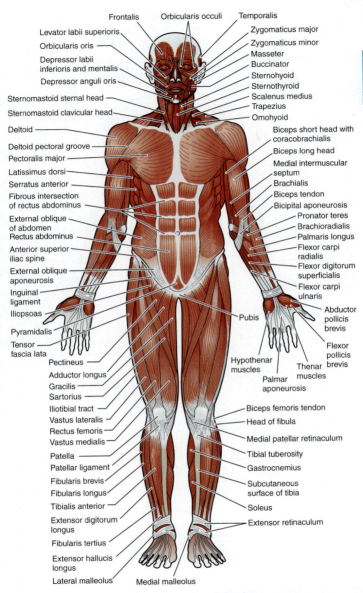

Frontalis
Orbicularis occuli
Temporalis
Levator labii superioris
Orbicularis oris
Depressor labii inferioris and mentalis
Depressor anguli oris
Sternomastoid sternal head
Sternomastoid clavicular head
Deltoid
Deltoid pectoral groove
Pectoralis major
Latissimus dorsi
Serratus anterior
Fibrous intersection of rectus abdominus
External oblique of abdomen
Rectus abdominus
Anterior superior iliac spine
External oblique aponeurosis
Inguinal ligament
Iliopsoas
Pyramidalis
Tensor fascia lata
Pectineus
Adductor longus
Gracilis
Sartorius
Iliotibial tract
Vastus lateralis
Rectus femoris
Vastus medialis
Patella
Patellar ligament
Fibularis brevis
Fibularis longus
Tibialis anterior
Extensor digitorum longus
Fibularis tertius
Extensor hallucis longus
Lateral malleolus

Zygomaticus major
Zygomaticus minor
Masseter
Buccinator
Sternohyoid
Sternothyroid
Scalenus medius
Trapezius
Omohyoid
Biceps short head with coracobrachialis
Biceps long head
Medial intermuscular septum
Brachialis
Biceps tendon
Bicipital aponeurosis
Pronator teres
Brachioradialis
Palmaris longus
Flexor carpi radialis
Flexor digitorum superficialis
Flexor carpi ulnaris
Abductor pollicis brevis
Flexor pollicis brevis
Thenar muscles
Hypothenar muscles
Palmar aponeurosis
Pubis
Biceps femoris tendon
Head of fibula
Medial patellar retinaculum
Tibial tuberosity
Gastrocnemius
Subcutaneous surface of tibia
Soleus
Extensor retinaculum
Medial malleolus

Muscles of the body, anterior view.

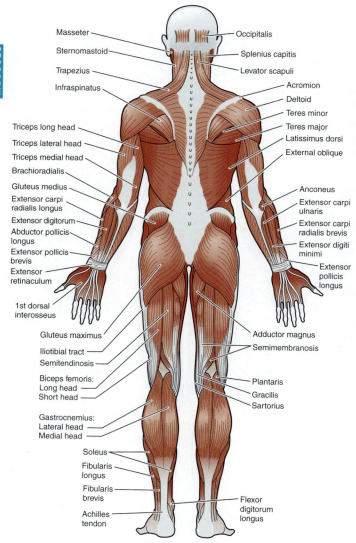

Masseter

Sternomastoid

Trapezius

Infraspinatus

Triceps long head

Triceps lateral head

Triceps medial head

Brachioradialis

Gluteus medius

Extensor carpi radialis longus

Extensor digitorum

Abductor pollicis longus

Extensor pollicis brevis

Extensor retinaculum

1st dorsal interosseus

Gluteus maximus

Iliotibial tract

Semitendinosis

Biceps femoris: Long head Short head

Gastrocnemius: Lateral head Medial head

Soleus

Fibularis longus

Fibularis brevis

Achilles tendon

Occipitalis

Splenius capitis

Levator scapuli

Acromion

Deltoid

Teres minor

Teres major

Latissimus dorsi

External oblique

Anconeus

Extensor carpi ulnaris

Extensor carpi radialis brevis

Extensor digiti minimi

Extensor pollicis longus

Adductor magnus

Semimembranosis

Plantaris

Gracilis

Sartorius

Flexor digitorum longus

Muscles of the body, posterior view.

Muscles Listed by Function

For a more detailed description of muscle action, look under the muscle's name in the reference (alphabetized) list of muscles (beginning on page 69). Here muscles are listed in the order of their relative importance in contributing to the movement listed. Nerves and innervating roots are in parentheses.

● TABLE 3.4 Muscles Used in Movement or Stabilization of the Scapula

Adduction	Trapezius (spinal part of accessory nerve, sensory branches, C3–C4)
Abduction	Serratus anterior (long thoracic nerve, C5–C7)
Upward rotation	Upper trapezius (spinal accessory nerve, sensory branches C3–C4) Serratus anterior (long thoracic nerve, C5–C7)
Downward rotation	Lower trapezius (spinal accessory nerve, sensory branches, C3–C4) Rhomboid major (dorsal scapular nerve, C5) Rhomboid minor (dorsal scapular nerve, C5) Levator scapulae (branches of C3 and C4, also frequently by the dorsal scapular nerve, C5) Pectoralis minor (medial pectoral nerve, C8–T1)

● TABLE 3.5 Muscles Primarily Active at the Glenohumeral Joint

Extension	Latissimus dorsi (thoracodorsal nerve, C6–C8) Triceps brachii long head (radial nerve, C7–C8) Posterior deltoid (axillary nerve, C5–C6) Teres major (lower subscapular nerve, C5–C6) Subscapularis (upper and lower subscapular nerves, C5–C6)
Flexion	Pectoralis major (medial and lateral pectoral nerves, C5–T1) Anterior deltoid (axillary nerve, C5–C6) Supraspinatus (suprascapular nerve, C5) Biceps brachii (musculocutaneous nerve, C5–C6) Coracobrachialis (musculocutaneous nerve, C6–C7) Subscapularis (upper and lower subscapular nerves, C5–C6)
Abduction	Middle deltoid (axillary nerve, C5–C6) Supraspinatus (suprascapular nerve, C5) Infraspinatus upper fibers C5 (suprascapular nerve, C5–C6)
Adduction	Latissimus dorsi (thoracodorsal nerve, C6–C8) Pectoralis major (medial and lateral pectoral nerves, C5–T1) Teres major (lower subscapular nerve, C5–C6) Triceps brachii long head (radial nerve, C7–C8) Teres minor (axillary nerve, C5) Infraspinatus lower fibers (suprascapular nerve, C5–C6)
Medial Rotation	Latissimus dorsi (thoracodorsal nerve, C6–C8) Pectoralis major (medial and lateral pectoral nerves, C5–T1) Subscapularis (upper and lower subscapular nerves, C5–C6) Teres major (lower subscapular nerve, C5–C6) Deltoid ventral fibers (axillary nerve, C5–C6)

(table continues on page 92)

TABLE 3.5 Muscles Primarily Active at the Glenohumeral Joint (continued)

Lateral Rotation	Deltoid dorsal fibers (axillary nerve, C5–C6) Infraspinatus (suprascapular nerve, C5–C6) Supraspinatus (suprascapular nerve, C5) Teres minor (axillary nerve, C5)

Muscles of the Right Shoulder and Arm, Anterior View

Anterior view

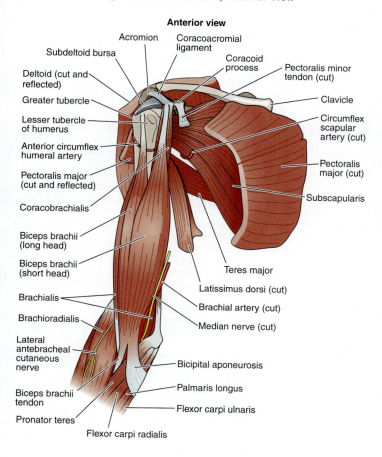

Acromion
Coracoacromial ligament
Coracoid process
Pectoralis minor tendon (cut)
Subdeltoid bursa
Pectoralis minor tendon (cut)
Deltoid (cut and reflected)
Clavicle
Greater tubercle
Circumflex scapular artery (cut)
Lesser tubercle of humerus
Anterior circumflex humeral artery
Pectoralis major (cut)
Pectoralis major (cut and reflected)
Subscapularis
Coracobrachialis
Biceps brachii (long head)
Biceps brachii (short head)
Teres major
Brachialis
Latissimus dorsi (cut)
Brachial artery (cut)
Brachioradialis
Median nerve (cut)
Lateral antebracheal cutaneous nerve
Bicipital aponeurosis
Biceps brachii tendon
Palmaris longus
Flexor carpi ulnaris
Pronator teres
Flexor carpi radialis

Muscles of the Right Shoulder and Arm, Posterior View

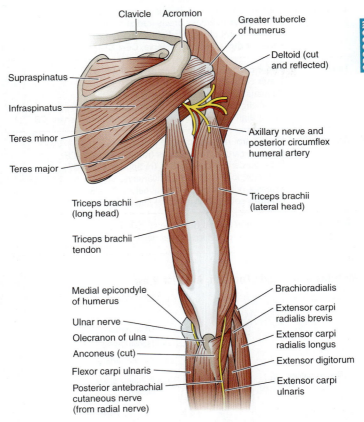

Posterior view

- Clavicle
- Acromion
- Greater tubercle of humerus
- Deltoid (cut and reflected)
- Supraspinatus
- Infraspinatus
- Teres minor
- Teres major
- Axillary nerve and posterior circumflex humeral artery
- Triceps brachii (long head)
- Triceps brachii (lateral head)
- Triceps brachii tendon
- Medial epicondyle of humerus
- Brachioradialis
- Extensor carpi radialis brevis
- Ulnar nerve
- Extensor carpi radialis longus
- Olecranon of ulna
- Anconeus (cut)
- Extensor digitorum
- Flexor carpi ulnaris
- Extensor carpi ulnaris
- Posterior antebrachial cutaneous nerve (from radial nerve)

🔴 TABLE 3.6 Muscles of the Elbow and Radioulnar Joints

Extension	Triceps brachii long head (radial nerve, C7–C8)
	Anconeus (radial nerve, C7–C8)
Flexion	Biceps brachii (musculocutaneous nerve, C5–C6)
	Brachialis (musculocutaneous nerve, C5–C6, and radial nerve for sensory)
	Brachioradialis (radial nerve, C5–C6)
Supination	Biceps brachii (musculocutaneous nerve, C6–C7)
	Supinator (radial nerve, C6)
Pronation	Pronator teres (median nerve, C5–C6)
	Pronator quadratus (median nerve, C8–T1)

MUSCULO

TABLE 3.7 **Muscles of the Wrist**

Extension	Extensor carpi radialis longus (radial nerve, C6–C8) Extensor carpi radialis brevis (radial nerve, C6–C7) Extensor carpi ulnaris (radial nerve, C6–C8) Extensor digitorum (radial nerve, C6–C8)
Flexion	Flexor carpi radialis (median nerve, C6–C7) Flexor carpi ulnaris (ulnar nerve, C8–T1) Palmaris longus (median nerve, C6–C7) Flexor digitorum superficialis (median nerve, C7–C8) Flexor digitorum profundus (median and ulnar nerves, C8–T1)
Abduction	Flexor carpi radialis (median nerve, C6–C7) Extensor carpi radialis longus (radial nerve, C6–C8) Extensor carpi radialis brevis (radial nerve, C6–C7) Abductor pollicis longus (radial nerve, C6–C7) Extensor pollicis longus (radial nerve, C6–C8) Extensor pollicis brevis (radial nerve, C6–C7)
Adduction	Flexor carpi ulnaris (ulnar nerve, C8–T1) Extensor carpi ulnaris (radial nerve, C6–C8)

Muscles of the Right Forearm, Anterior View

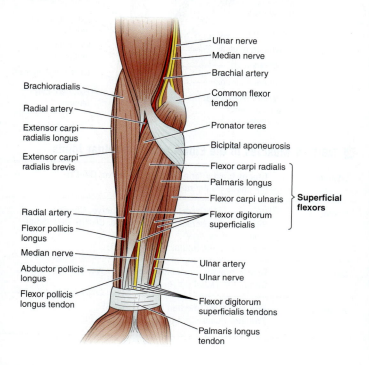

Ulnar nerve
Median nerve
Brachial artery
Brachioradialis
Common flexor tendon
Radial artery
Pronator teres
Extensor carpi radialis longus
Bicipital aponeurosis
Extensor carpi radialis brevis
Flexor carpi radialis
Palmaris longus
Flexor carpi ulnaris
Superficial flexors
Radial artery
Flexor digitorum superficialis
Flexor pollicis longus
Median nerve
Ulnar artery
Abductor pollicis longus
Ulnar nerve
Flexor pollicis longus tendon
Flexor digitorum superficialis tendons
Palmaris longus tendon

Muscles of the Right Forearm, Posterior View

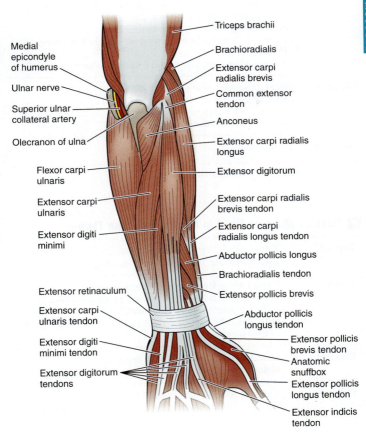

Triceps brachii

Brachioradialis

Extensor carpi radialis brevis

Common extensor tendon

Anconeus

Extensor carpi radialis longus

Extensor digitorum

Extensor carpi radialis brevis tendon

Extensor carpi radialis longus tendon

Abductor pollicis longus

Brachioradialis tendon

Extensor pollicis brevis

Abductor pollicis longus tendon

Extensor pollicis brevis tendon

Anatomic snuffbox

Extensor pollicis longus tendon

Extensor indicis tendon

Medial epicondyle of humerus

Ulnar nerve

Superior ulnar collateral artery

Olecranon of ulna

Flexor carpi ulnaris

Extensor carpi ulnaris

Extensor digiti minimi

Extensor retinaculum

Extensor carpi ulnaris tendon

Extensor digiti minimi tendon

Extensor digitorum tendons

🟠 **TABLE 3.8 Muscles Used in Movement of the Fingers**

Extension	Extensor digitorum (radial nerve, C6–C8)
	Extensor indicis (proprius) (radial nerve, C6–C8)
	Extensor digiti minimi (radial nerve, C6–C8)
	Lumbricals (1 and 2 by median nerve, C8–T1; 3 and 4 by ulnar nerve, C8–T1)
	Interossei (dorsal and palmar, IP extension) (ulnar nerve, C8–T1)

(table continues on page 96)

TABLE 3.8 Muscles Used in Movement of the Fingers (continued)

Flexion	Flexor digitorum superficialis (median nerve, C7–C8)
	Flexor digitorum profundus (median and ulnar nerves, C8–T1)
	Flexor digiti minimi (ulnar nerve, C8–T1)
	Opponens digiti minimi (ulnar nerve, T1)
	Lumbricals (1 and 2 by median nerve, C8–T1; 3 and 4 by ulnar nerve, C8–T1)
	Interossei (dorsal and palmar, MTP flexion) (ulnar nerve, C8–T1)
Abduction	Dorsal interossei (ulnar nerve, C8–T1)
	Abductor digiti minimi (ulnar nerve, C8–T1)
	Opponens digiti minimi (ulnar nerve, T1)
	Extensor indicis (radial nerve, C6–C8)
Adduction	Palmar interossei (ulnar nerve, C8–T1)

IP = interphalangeal, MTP = metatarsophalangeal.

TABLE 3.9 Muscles Used in Movement of the Thumb

Extension	Extensor pollicis longus (radial nerve, C6–C8)
	Extensor pollicis brevis (radial nerve, C6–C7)
Flexion	Flexor pollicis longus (median nerve, C8–T1)
	Flexor pollicis brevis (median nerve to superficial head, C8–T1; ulnar nerve to deep head, C8–T1)
	Opponens pollicis (median nerve and sometimes by a branch of the ulnar, C8–T1)
Abduction	Abductor pollicis longus (radial nerve, C6–C7)
	Abductor pollicis brevis (median nerve, C8–T1)
Adduction	Adductor pollicis (ulnar nerve, C8–T1)
	Opponens pollicis (median nerve and sometimes by a branch of the ulnar, C8–T1)
	Flexor pollicis longus (median nerve, C8–T1)
	Flexor pollicis brevis (median nerve to superficial head, C8–T1; ulnar nerve to deep head, C8–T1)

MUSCULO

Muscles of the Right Hand, Palmar View

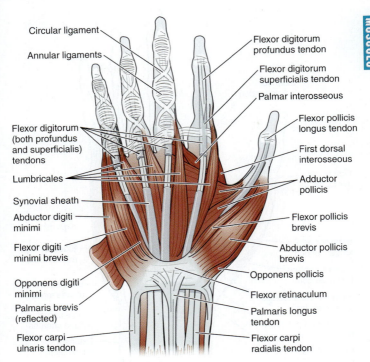

Circular ligament

Annular ligaments

Flexor digitorum (both profundus and superficialis) tendons

Lumbricales

Synovial sheath

Abductor digiti minimi

Flexor digiti minimi brevis

Opponens digiti minimi

Palmaris brevis (reflected)

Flexor carpi ulnaris tendon

Flexor digitorum profundus tendon

Flexor digitorum superficialis tendon

Palmar interosseous

Flexor pollicis longus tendon

First dorsal interosseous

Adductor pollicis

Flexor pollicis brevis

Abductor pollicis brevis

Opponens pollicis

Flexor retinaculum

Palmaris longus tendon

Flexor carpi radialis tendon

MUSCULO

Muscles of the Right Hand, Posterior View

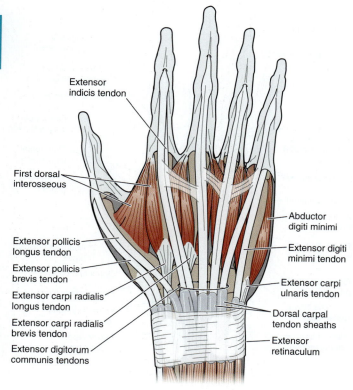

Extensor
indicis tendon

First dorsal
interosseous

Abductor
digiti minimi

Extensor digiti
minimi tendon

Extensor pollicis
longus tendon

Extensor pollicis
brevis tendon

Extensor carpi
ulnaris tendon

Extensor carpi radialis
longus tendon

Dorsal carpal
tendon sheaths

Extensor carpi radialis
brevis tendon

Extensor
retinaculum

Extensor digitorum
communis tendons

TABLE 3.10 Muscles Used in Movement of the Hip

Flexion	Psoas major (lumbar plexus, L2–L3)
	Psoas minor (lumbar plexus, L1)
	Iliacus (femoral nerve, L2–L3)
	Sartorius (femoral nerve, L2–L3)
	Rectus femoris (femoral nerve, L2–L4)
	Pectineus (femoral, obturator, or accessory obturator nerves, L2–L4)
	Gluteus medius (anterior portion) (superior gluteal nerve, L4–S1)
	Gluteus minimus (superior gluteal nerve, L4–S1)
	Adductor longus (obturator nerve, L2–L4)
	Adductor brevis (obturator nerve, L2–L4)
	Adductor magnus (upper portion) (obturator nerve, L2–L4; tibial portion of sciatic nerve, L2–L4)

MUSCULO

Extension	Gluteus maximus (inferior gluteal nerve, L5–S2)
	Gluteus medius (posterior portion) (superior gluteal nerve, L4–S1)
	Biceps femoris (long head) (tibial portion of sciatic nerve, S1–S3)
	Semimembranosus (tibial portion of sciatic nerve, L5–S2)
	Semitendinosus (tibial portion of sciatic nerve, L5–S2)
	Adductor magnus (lower portion) (obturator nerve, L2–L4; tibial portion of sciatic nerve, L2–L4)
	Piriformis (sacral plexus, S1)
	Obturator internus (nerve to obturator internus, L5–S2)
Abduction	Gluteus medius (superior gluteal nerve, L4–S1)
	Gluteus minimus (superior gluteal nerve, L4–S1)
	Piriformis (sacral plexus, S1)
	Obturator internus (nerve to obturator internus, L5–S2)
Adduction	Adductor magnus (upper portion) (obturator nerve, L2–L4; tibial portion of sciatic nerve, L2–L4)
	Gracilis (obturator nerve, L2–L3)
	Adductor longus (obturator nerve, L2–L4)
	Adductor brevis (obturator nerve, L2–L4)
	Pectineus (femoral, obturator, or accessory obturator nerves, L2–L4)
Medial Rotation	Gluteus medius (superior gluteal nerve, L4–S1)
	Gluteus minimus (superior gluteal nerve, L4–S1)
	Tensor fasciae latae (superior gluteal nerve, L4–S1)
	Adductor longus (obturator nerve, L2–L4)
	Pectineus (femoral, obturator, or accessory obturator nerves, L2–L4)
	Adductor brevis (obturator nerve, L2–L4)
	Adductor magnus (obturator nerve, L2–L4; tibial portion of sciatic nerve, L2–L4)
Lateral Rotation	Gluteus maximus (inferior gluteal nerve, L5–S2)
	Sartorius (femoral nerve, L2–L3)
	Piriformis (sacral plexus, S1)
	Obturator internus (nerve to obturator internus, L5–S2)
	Gemellus superior (nerve to obturator internus, L5–S2)
	Adductor magnus (lower portion) (obturator nerve, L2–L4; tibial portion of sciatic nerve, L2–L4)
	Gemellus inferior (nerve to quadratus femoris, L4–S1)
	Obturator externus (obturator nerve, L3–L4)

Muscles of the Right Thigh, Anterior View

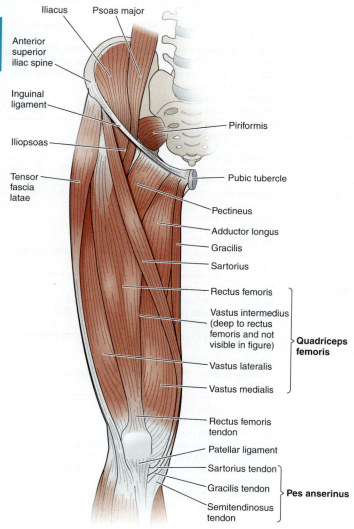

- Iliacus
- Psoas major
- Anterior superior iliac spine
- Inguinal ligament
- Iliopsoas
- Tensor fascia latae
- Piriformis
- Pubic tubercle
- Pectineus
- Adductor longus
- Gracilis
- Sartorius
- Rectus femoris
- Vastus intermedius (deep to rectus femoris and not visible in figure)
- Vastus lateralis
- Vastus medialis
- **Quadriceps femoris**
- Rectus femoris tendon
- Patellar ligament
- Sartorius tendon
- Gracilis tendon
- Semitendinosus tendon
- **Pes anserinus**

MUSCULO

Muscles of the Right Thigh, Posterior View

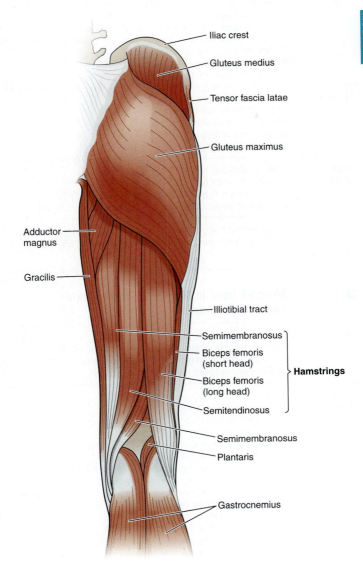

- Iliac crest
- Gluteus medius
- Tensor fascia latae
- Gluteus maximus
- Adductor magnus
- Gracilis
- Illiotibial tract
- Semimembranosus
- Biceps femoris (short head)
- Biceps femoris (long head)
- Semitendinosus

Hamstrings

- Semimembranosus
- Plantaris
- Gastrocnemius

🔶 TABLE 3.11 Muscles Used in Movement of the Knee

Flexion	Biceps femoris (long head: tibial portion of sciatic nerve, S1–S3; and short head: peroneal portion of sciatic nerve, L5–S2) Semitendinosus (tibial portion of sciatic nerve, L5–S2) Semimembranosus (tibial portion of sciatic nerve, L5–S2) Gastrocnemius (tibial nerve, S1–S2) Plantaris (tibial nerve, L4–S1) Sartorius (femoral nerve, L2–L3)
Extension	Rectus femoris (femoral nerve, L2–L4) Vastus medialis (femoral nerve, L2–L4) Vastus intermedius (femoral nerve, L2–L4) Vastus lateralis (femoral nerve, L2–L4) Articularis genus (femoral nerve, L3–L4)
Medial Rotation of the Tibia	Sartorius (femoral nerve, L2–L3) Gracilis (obturator nerve, L2–L3) Semitendinosus (tibial portion of sciatic nerve, L5–S2) Semimembranosus (tibial portion of sciatic nerve, L5–S2)
Lateral Rotation of the Tibia	Biceps femoris (long head: tibial portion of sciatic nerve, S1–S3; and short head: peroneal portion of sciatic nerve, L5–S2)

🔶 TABLE 3.12 Muscles Used in Movement of the Ankle and Subtalar Joints

Dorsiflexion	Tibialis anterior (deep peroneal nerve, L4–S1) Extensor hallucis longus (deep peroneal nerve, L4–S1) Extensor digitorum longus (deep peroneal nerve, L4–S1) Fibularis tertius (deep peroneal nerve, L5–S1)
Plantar Flexion	Gastrocnemius (tibial nerve, S1–S2) Soleus (tibial nerve, S1–S2) Flexor hallucis longus (tibial nerve, L5–S2) Flexor digitorum longus (tibial nerve, L5–S1) Tibialis posterior (tibial nerve, L5–S1) Plantaris (tibial nerve, L4–S1) Fibularis longus (superficial peroneal nerve, L4–S1) Fibularis brevis (superficial peroneal nerve, L4–S1)
Inversion	Tibialis posterior (tibial nerve, L5–S1) Flexor digitorum longus (tibial nerve, L5–S1) Flexor hallucis longus (tibial nerve, L5–S2) Tibialis anterior (deep peroneal nerve, L4–S1) Extensor hallucis longus (deep peroneal nerve, L4–S1)
Eversion	Fibularis longus (superficial peroneal nerve, L4–S1) Fibularis brevis (superficial peroneal nerve, L4–S1) Fibularis tertius (deep peroneal nerve, L5–S1) Extensor digitorum longus (deep peroneal nerve, L4–S1) Extensor digitorum brevis (deep peroneal nerve, L5–S1)

Adduction	Tibialis anterior (deep peroneal nerve, L4–S1)
	Tibialis posterior (tibial nerve, L5–S1)
	Flexor hallucis longus (tibial nerve, L5–S2)
	Flexor digitorum longus (tibial nerve, L5–S2)
	Extensor hallucis longus (deep peroneal nerve, L5–S1)
Abduction	Extensor digitorum longus (deep peroneal nerve, L4–S1)
	Fibularis longus (superficial peroneal nerve, L4–S1)
	Fibularis brevis (superficial peroneal nerve, L4–S1)
	Fibularis tertius (deep peroneal nerve, L5–S1)

MUSCULO

Muscles of the Right Leg, Anterior View

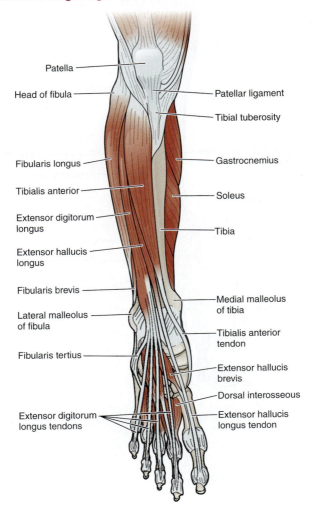

Muscles of the Right Leg, Posterior View

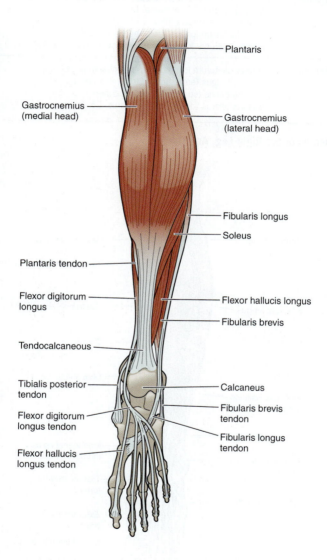

Plantaris

Gastrocnemius (medial head)

Gastrocnemius (lateral head)

Fibularis longus

Soleus

Plantaris tendon

Flexor digitorum longus

Flexor hallucis longus

Fibularis brevis

Tendocalcaneous

Tibialis posterior tendon

Calcaneus

Fibularis brevis tendon

Flexor digitorum longus tendon

Fibularis longus tendon

Flexor hallucis longus tendon

Muscles of the Right Foot, Anterior View

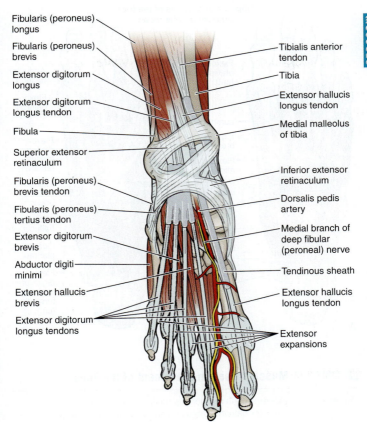

Fibularis (peroneus) longus

Fibularis (peroneus) brevis

Extensor digitorum longus

Extensor digitorum longus tendon

Fibula

Superior extensor retinaculum

Fibularis (peroneus) brevis tendon

Fibularis (peroneus) tertius tendon

Extensor digitorum brevis

Abductor digiti minimi

Extensor hallucis brevis

Extensor digitorum longus tendons

Tibialis anterior tendon

Tibia

Extensor hallucis longus tendon

Medial malleolus of tibia

Inferior extensor retinaculum

Dorsalis pedis artery

Medial branch of deep fibular (peroneal) nerve

Tendinous sheath

Extensor hallucis longus tendon

Extensor expansions

Muscles of the Right Foot, Plantar View

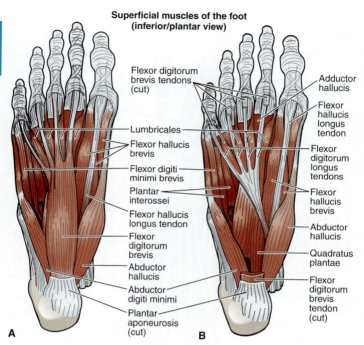

Superficial muscles of the foot
(inferior/plantar view)

Flexor digitorum brevis tendons (cut)

Lumbricales

Flexor hallucis brevis

Flexor digiti minimi brevis

Plantar interossei

Flexor hallucis longus tendon

Flexor digitorum brevis

Abductor hallucis

Abductor digiti minimi

Plantar aponeurosis (cut)

A

Adductor hallucis

Flexor hallucis longus tendon

Flexor digitorum longus tendons

Flexor hallucis brevis

Abductor hallucis

Quadratus plantae

Flexor digitorum brevis tendon (cut)

B

MUSCULO

🟠 TABLE 3.13 Muscles Used in Movement of the Toes

Extension	Extensor digitorum longus (deep peroneal nerve, L4–S1) Extensor hallucis longus (deep peroneal nerve, L4–S1) Extensor digitorum brevis (deep peroneal nerve, L5–S1) Lumbricals (distal IP extension) (first lumbrical by medial plantar nerve, L5–S1; and second through fourth lumbricals by the lateral plantar nerve S2–S3) Interossei, dorsal and plantar (IP extension) (lateral plantar nerve, S2–S3)
Flexion	Flexor digitorum longus (tibial nerve, L5–S1) Flexor hallucis longus (tibial nerve, L5–S2) Flexor digitorum brevis (medial plantar nerve, L5–S1) Flexor hallucis brevis (medial plantar nerve, L5–S1) Lumbricals (MTP flexion) (first lumbrical by medial plantar nerve, L5–S1; and second through fourth lumbricals by the lateral plantar nerve, S2–S3) Interossei (MTP flexion) (lateral plantar nerve, S2–S3) Flexor digiti minimi (lateral plantar nerve, S2–S3) Quadratus plantae (lateral plantar nerve, S2–S3)

Abduction	Abductor hallucis (medial plantar nerve, L5–S1) Abductor digiti minimi (lateral plantar nerve, S2–S3) Dorsal interossei (lateral plantar nerve, S2–S3)
Adduction	Adductor hallucis (lateral plantar nerve, S2–S3) Plantar interossei (lateral plantar nerve, S2–S3)

MUSCULO

IP = interphalangeal, MTP = metatarsophalangeal.

Muscles Listed by Region

Muscles are listed by body region. See the alphabetized reference list of muscles (starting on page 69) for descriptions that include function, innervation, origin, and insertion.

Muscles of the External Ear
Auricularis anterior
Auricularis posterior

Auricularis superior

Muscles of Facial Expression
Buccinator
Corrugator supercilii
Depressor anguli oris
Depressor labii inferioris
Depressor septi
Levator anguli oris
Levator labii superioris
Levator labii superioris alaeque nasi
Levator palpebrae superioris
Mentalis
Nasalis

Occipitofrontalis
Orbicularis oculi
Orbicularis oris
Platysma
Procerus
Risorius
Temporoparietalis
Transversus menti
Zygomaticus major
Zygomaticus minor

Muscles of Mastication
Buccinator
Lateral pterygoid
Masseter

Medial pterygoid
Temporalis

Muscles of the Eye
Ciliaris
Dilator pupillae
Levator palpebrae superioris
Obliquus inferior (inferior oblique)
Obliquus superior (superior oblique)

Rectus inferior (inferior rectus)
Rectus lateralis (lateral rectus)
Rectus medialis (medial rectus)
Rectus superior (superior rectus)
Sphincter pupillae

Muscles of the Internal Ear
Stapedius

Tensor tympani

Muscles of the Tongue
Chondroglossus
Genioglossus
Hyoglossus

Palatoglossus
Styloglossus

MUSCULO

Muscles of the Palate
Levator veli palatini
Musculus uvulae
Palatoglossus
Palatopharyngeus
Tensor veli palatini

Muscles of the Pharynx
Inferior constrictor (constrictor inferior)
Middle constrictor (constrictor medius)
Palatopharyngeus
Salpingopharyngeus
Stylopharyngeus
Superior constrictor (constrictor superior)

Muscles of the Larynx
Aryepiglotticus
Arytenoid (arytenoideus)
Cricothyroid (cricothyroideus)
Lateral cricoarytenoid
Posterior cricoarytenoid (cricoarytenoideus posterior)
Thyroarytenoid (thyroartenoideus)
Thyroepiglotticus
Vocalis

Muscles of the Neck
Digastricus (anterior and posterior bellies)
Geniohyoid
Longus capitis
Longus colli
Mylohyoid
Omohyoid
Rectus capitis anterior
Rectus capitis lateralis
Scalenus anterior
Scalenus medius
Scalenus posterior
Sternohyoid
Sternothyroid
Stylohyoid
Thyrohyoid

Muscles Behind the Cranium
Obliquus capitis inferior
Obliquus capitis superior
Rectus capitis posterior major
Rectus capitis posterior minor

Muscles of the Back
Iliocostalis cervicis
Iliocostalis lumborum
Iliocostalis thoracis
Intertransversarii
Longissimus capitis
Longissimus cervicis
Longissimus thoracis
Multifidus
Rotatores
Semispinalis capitis
Semispinalis cervicis
Semispinalis thoracis
Spinalis capitis
Spinalis cervicis
Spinalis thoracis
Splenius capitis
Splenius cervicis

Muscles of the Thorax
Diaphragm
Innermost intercostals
Intercostales externi (external intercostals) (cricoarytenoideus lateralis)
Intercostales interni (internal intercostals)
Levatores costarum
Serratus anterior
Serratus posterior inferior
Serratus posterior superior
Transversus thoracis

Muscles of the Abdominal Region

Cremaster
Obliquus externus abdominis
  (external oblique)
Obliquus internus abdominis
  (internal oblique)

Rectus abdominis
Transversus abdominis

Muscles of the Pelvis

Coccygeus
Levator ani iliococcygeus

Levator ani pubococcygeus

Muscles of the Perineum

Anal sphincter (external)
Anal sphincter (internal)
Bulbospongiosus (bulbocavernosus)
Ischiocavernosus

Sphincter urethrae
Transversus perinei profundus
Transversus perinei superficialis

Muscles Connecting the Trunk or the Head to the Scapula

Levator scapulae
Lower trapezius
Pectoralis minor
Rhomboid major

Rhomboid minor
Serratus anterior
Sternocleidomastoid (sternomastoid)
Upper trapezius

Muscles of the Shoulder

Deltoid (anterior, middle, posterior)
Infraspinatus
Latissimus dorsi
Pectoralis major

Subscapularis
Supraspinatus
Teres major
Teres minor

Muscles of the Arm

Anconeus
Biceps brachii
Brachialis

Coracobrachialis
Triceps brachii

Muscles of the Forearm

Abductor pollicis longus
Brachioradialis
Extensor carpi radialis brevis
Extensor carpi radialis longus
Extensor carpi ulnaris
Extensor digiti minimi
Extensor digitorum
Extensor indicis
Extensor pollicis brevis
Extensor pollicis longus

Flexor carpi radialis
Flexor carpi ulnaris
Flexor digitorum profundus
Flexor digitorum superficialis
Flexor pollicis longus
Palmaris longus
Pronator quadratus
Pronator teres
Supinator

Muscles of the Hand

Abductor digiti minimi
Abductor pollicis brevis
Adductor pollicis
Flexor digiti minimi
Flexor pollicis brevis

Interossei (dorsal and palmar)
Lumbricales
Opponens digiti minimi
Opponens pollicis
Palmaris brevis

MUSCULO

Muscles of the Iliac Region

Iliacus
Psoas major

Psoas minor
Quadratus lumborum

Muscles of the Thigh

Adductor brevis
Adductor longus
Adductor magnus
Articularis genus
Biceps femoris
Gemelli (superior and inferior)
Gluteus maximus
Gluteus medius
Gluteus minimus
Gracilis
Obturator externus

Obturator internus
Pectineus
Piriformis
Rectus femoris
Sartorius
Semimembranosus
Semitendinosus
Tensor fasciae latae
Vastus intermedius
Vastus lateralis
Vastus medialis

Muscles of the Leg

Extensor digitorum longus
Extensor hallucis longus
Fibularis brevis
Fibularis longus
Fibularis tertius
Flexor digitorum longus
Flexor hallucis longus

Gastrocnemius
Plantaris
Popliteus
Soleus
Tibialis anterior
Tibialis posterior

Muscles of the Foot

Abductor digiti minimi
Abductor hallucis
Adductor hallucis
Extensor digitorum brevis
Flexor digiti minimi brevis
Flexor digitorum brevis

Flexor hallucis brevis
Interossei (dorsal and plantar)
Lumbricales
Quadratus plantae (flexor digitorum
    accessorius)

Joints and Ligaments

Classification System Used for Joints

Fibrous

syndesmosis: A union via cordlike ligamentous fibers.
suture: Alignment of the growing edges of two bones with thin, fibrous tissue.
gomphosis: Tooth and periodontal membrane (membranous union).

Cartilaginous

synchondrosis: Residual cartilage plate between two bones.
symphysis: Two bones united by a coating of fibrocartilage and reinforced.

Synovial

Plane
arthrodial: Gliding articulations with flat surfaces.
amphiarthrodial: Bony articulating surfaces connected by cartilage.

synarthrodial: Skeletal articulations are maintained by a continuous intervening cartilage, fibrous tissue, or bone.

Uniaxial
ginglymus: Hinge.
trochoid: Pivot.

Biaxial
Allows circumduction.
condyloid: Ball and socket without rotation.
ellipsoid: Oval and socket.

Multiaxial
True ball and socket.

TABLE 3.14 Classifications of the Joints of the Body (in alphabetical order)

Joint	Classification
Acromioclavicular	Arthrodial
Ankle	Ginglymus
Atlantoaxial	Trochoid and arthrodial
Calcaneocuboid	Arthrodial
Capitate and hamate with scaphoid	Condyloid and lunate
Carpometacarpal	Condyloid
Cranial bones	Sutures
Distal carpal bones	Arthrodial
Elbow	Ginglymus
Hip	Multiaxial
Intercarpal joints	Arthrodial
Intermetatarsal	Arthrodial
Interphalangeal	Ginglymus
Knee	Ginglymus
Manubrium and sternum	Symphysis
Metacarpophalangeal	Condyloid

(table continues on page 112)

■ TABLE 3.14 Classifications of the Joints of the Body (in alphabetical order) (continued)

Joint	Classification
Metatarsophalangeal	Condyloid
Proximal carpal bones	Arthrodial
Pubic rami	Symphysis
Radioulnar (middle)	Syndesmosis
Radioulnar (proximal and distal)	Trochoid
Sacrococcygeal	Amphiarthrodial
Sacroiliac	Synchondrosis
Shoulder	Multiaxial
Sphenoid-ethmoid	Synchondrosis
Sternoclavicular	Double arthrodial
Sternocostal	Arthrodial
Subtalar	Arthrodial
Talocalcaneonavicular	Arthrodial
Tarsometatarsal	Arthrodial
Teeth and surrounding membrane	Gomphosis
Temporomandibular	Ginglymus and arthrodial
Tibiofibular	Arthrodial
Tibiofibular with interosseous membrane	Syndesmosis
Tubercles and necks of ribs	Arthrodial
Vertebral arches	Arthrodial and syndesmosis
Vertebral bodies	Amphiarthrodial
Vertebral column with cranium	Condyloid
Wrist (radiocarpal)	Condyloid

MUSCULO

Close-Packed and Loose-Packed Positions for the Joints
Definitions of Terms

close-packed position: The position in which opposing joint surfaces are fully congruent, the area of contact between joint surfaces is maximal, and the surfaces are tightly compressed.

loose-packed position: The position in which opposing joint surfaces are not congruent and some parts of the articular capsule are lax. The maximum loose-packed position is the position in which the capsule and ligaments are most lax and separation of joint surfaces is greatest.

TABLE 3.15 Close-Packed Position of Joints (in alphabetical order)

Joint	Close-Packed Position
Acromioclavicular	Shoulder abducted to 30°
Ankle	Maximal dorsiflexion
Elbow (radiohumeral)	Elbow flexed 90°, 5° of supination
Elbow (ulnohumeral)	Maximal elbow extension
Facet (spine)	Maximal extension
Glenohumeral	Maximal shoulder abduction and lateral rotation
Hip	Maximal extension of the hip and maximal medial rotation of the hip
Interphalangeal (fingers)	Maximal extension of IP joints
Interphalangeal (toes)	Maximal extension of IP joints
Metacarpophalangeal (fingers)	Maximal flexion
Metacarpophalangeal (thumb)	Maximal opposition
Metatarsophalangeal (toes)	Maximal extension of MTP joints
Midtarsal	Maximal supination
Radiocarpal	Maximal extension and maximal ulnar deviation
Radioulnar (distal)	5° of supination
Radioulnar (proximal)	5° of supination
Sternoclavicular	Maximal shoulder elevation

(table continues on page 114)

MUSCULO

MUSCULO

■ TABLE 3.15 Close-Packed Position of Joints (in alphabetical order) (continued)

Joint	Close-Packed Position
Subtalar	Maximal supination
Tarsometatarsal	Maximal supination
Temporomandibular	Teeth clenched
Tibiofemoral	Maximal extension and maximal lateral rotation

■ TABLE 3.16 Maximum Loose-Packed Positions of Joints (in alphabetical order)

Joint	Loose-Packed Position
Acromioclavicular	Shoulder in anatomic position
Ankle	10° of plantar flexion
Carpometacarpal	Anatomic position of the wrist
Elbow (radiohumeral)	Anatomic position
Elbow (ulnohumeral)	70° of elbow flexion, 10° of supination
Facet (spine)	Midway between flexion and extension
Glenohumeral	55° of shoulder abduction, 30° of horizontal adduction
Hip	30° of hip flexion, 30° of hip abduction, and slight lateral rotation of the hip
Interphalangeal (fingers)	Slight flexion of IP joints
Interphalangeal (toes)	Slight flexion of IP joints
Metacarpophalangeal	Slight flexion of MCP joints
Metatarsophalangeal	Midrange position
Midtarsal	Midrange position
Radiocarpal	Anatomic position relative to flexion and extension with slight ulnar deviation
Radioulnar (distal)	10° of supination

Joint	Loose-Packed Position
Radioulnar (proximal)	70° of elbow flexion, 35° of supination
Sternoclavicular	Shoulder in anatomic position
Subtalar	Midrange position
Tarsometatarsal	Midrange position
Temporomandibular	Mouth slightly open
Tibiofemoral	25° of knee flexion

■ TABLE 3.17 Major Ligaments and Their Functions

Joint	Ligament	Function
Upper Extremity (Proximal to Distal)		
Shoulder girdle	Coracoclavicular	Binds the clavicle to the coracoid process
	Costoclavicular	Binds the clavicle to the costal cartilage of the first rib
Shoulder	Coracohumeral	Strengthens the upper portion of the joint capsule
	Glenohumeral	Reinforces the anterior aspect of the joint capsule
	Coracoacromial	Protects the superior aspect of the joint
Elbow	Annular	Holds the head of radius in position
	Ulnar collateral	Restricts medial displacement of the elbow joint
	Radial collateral	Restricts lateral displacement of the elbow joint
Wrist	Volar and dorsal radioulnar	Holds the distal ends of the radius and ulna in place
	Flexor and extensor retinacula	Holds tendons against fingers
	Interosseous	Binds the carpal bones together
	Dorsal and volar collateral	Connects articulations between the rows of carpal bones
Fingers	Volar and collateral interphalangeal	Prevents displacements of the interphalangeal joints

(table continues on page 116)

TABLE 3.17 Major Ligaments and Their Functions (continued)

Joint	Ligament	Function
Lower Extremity (Proximal to Distal)		
Ischium	Sacrospinous	Runs from sacrum to ischial spine to create the greater sciatic foramen
	Sacrotuberous	Runs from the sacrum to the ischial tuberosity and prevents the sacrum from tilting excessively; creates lesser sciatic foramen
Pubis	Transverse	Converts the acetabular notch into a foramen
	Superior pubic	Holds the pubic bones together
	Arcuate pubic	Holds the pubic bones together
Hip	Ligamentum teres	Carries nutrient vessels into the head of the femur
	Transverse	Holds the femoral head in place
	Iliofemoral	Limits extension of the hip joint
	Ischiofemoral	Limits anterior displacement of the hip joint
	Pubofemoral	Limits extension of the hip joint
Tibiofemoral	Medial collateral	Stabilizes the medial aspect of the knee joint (tibial-femoral articulation)
	Lateral collateral	Stabilizes the lateral aspect of the knee joint (tibial-femoral articulation)
	Medial and lateral menisci	Cartilages that provide stability and cushioning to the tibial-femoral articulation
	Anterior cruciate	Prevents backward sliding of the femur and hyperextension of the knee
	Posterior cruciate	Prevents forward sliding of the femur
	Oblique and arcuate popliteal	Provides lateral and posterior support to the knee joint
Ankle	Deltoid	Provides stability between the medial malleolus, navicular, talus, and calcaneus
	Anterior and posterior talofibular	Secures the fibula to the talus
	Calcaneofibular	Secures the fibula to the calcaneus

Joint	Ligament	Function
Lower Extremity (Proximal to Distal)		
Intertarsal	Long plantar	Provides a groove for the peroneus longus tendon and runs from the calcaneus to the metatarsals
	Calcaneonavicular	Supports the head of the talus between the navicular and the calcaneus
Tarsometatarsal	Dorsal and plantar interosseus	Limits movement of the tarsal bones
Intermetatarsal	Dorsal and plantar metatarsal	Limits movement of the metatarsal bones
Metatarsophalangeal	Plantar and transverse metatarsal	Holds the metatarsophalangeal joints in place
Vertebral (caudal to cephalad)		
Vertebral column	Iliolumbar	Provides stability between L4–L5 and the iliac crest
	Interspinous	Limits movement between the spinous processes
	Lateral odontoid	Stabilizes the odontoid process of the axis with respect to the occipital condyles
	Lateral occipitoatlantal	Stabilizes the transverse process of the atlas and the jugular processes of the occipital bone
	Sacroiliac	Consists of two ligaments that hold the sacrum to the ilium
	Flava	Holds adjacent lamina together
	Nuchae	Runs from C7 to the occipital bone for reinforced neck stability; limits movement between cervical spinous processes
	Anterior and posterior longitudinal	Reinforces and strengthens the vertebral bodies and disks

Terminology Related to Joint Injuries

dislocation: A complete displacement of a bone from its normal position at a joint.

sprain: A stretching or tearing of a ligament or joint capsule.

strain: A stretching or tearing of a muscle or tendon.

subluxation: An incomplete or partial displacement of a bone from its normal position at a joint.

Grading of Sprains/Strains

Grade I: Stretching or a microscopic tearing with no loss of function.

Grade II: Partial disruption or stretching with some loss of function.

Grade III: Complete tear with complete loss of function.

Beighton Hypermobility Score

Scored from 0 to 9. Each of the following is scored one point if present:

- Passively appose right thumb to forearm
- Passively appose left thumb to forearm
- Passively extend right fifth metacarpal phalangeal joint more than 90°
- Passively extend left fifth metacarpal phalangeal joint more than 90°
- Hyperextend right elbow more than 10°
- Hyperextend left elbow more than 10°
- Hyperextend right knee more than 10°
- Hyperextend left knee more than 10°
- Place palms on floor by flexing the trunk and keeping knees straight

Examination

Posture

Ideal Plumb Line Alignment

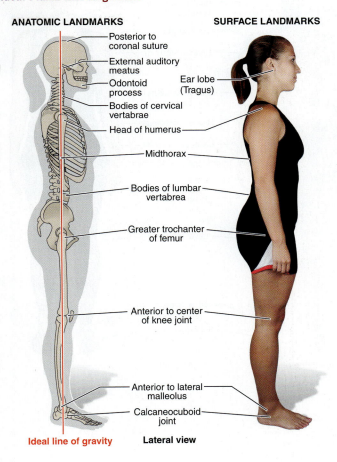

ANATOMIC LANDMARKS

SURFACE LANDMARKS

- Posterior to coronal suture
- External auditory meatus
- Odontoid process
- Ear lobe (Tragus)
- Bodies of cervical vertabrae
- Head of humerus
- Midthorax
- Bodies of lumbar vertabrea
- Greater trochanter of femur
- Anterior to center of knee joint
- Anterior to lateral malleolus
- Calcaneocuboid joint

Ideal line of gravity

Lateral view

MUSCULO

ANATOMIC LANDMARKS   SURFACE LANDMARKS

- Bilateral symmetry of head and facial bones
- Bisects cervical vertebral bodies
- Level shoulders
- Bisects sternum
- Bisects vertebral bodies
- Bisects umbilicus
- Level pelvic crest
- Level ASIS
- Bisects pubic symphysis
- Level midpole patellae
- Bisects base of support
- 8-10 degrees of forefoot abduction

Ideal line of gravity   Anterior view

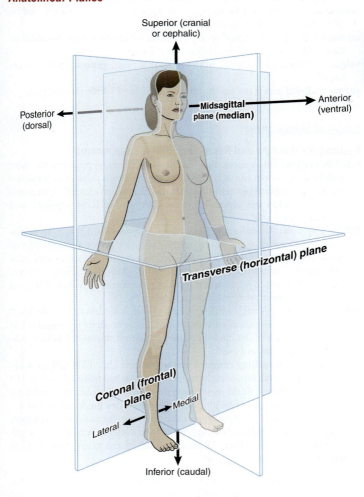

Anatomical Planes

MUSCULO

Superior (cranial or cephalic)

Posterior (dorsal)

Midsagittal plane (median)

Anterior (ventral)

Transverse (horizontal) plane

Coronal (frontal) plane

Medial

Lateral

Inferior (caudal)

Terms Used to Describe Positional Deformities of Joints

anteversion: an anterior rotation, e.g., femoral anteversion (a forward rotation of the femoral neck in relation to the femur)

retroversion: a posterior rotation, e.g., femoral retroversion (a backward rotation of the femoral neck in relation to the femur)

valgus: the distal part is away from the midline, e.g., genu valgum (knock-kneed)

varus: the distal part is toward the midline, e.g., genu varum (bowlegged)

Range of Motion (ROM)

Systems for Notating and Recording ROM Measurements

0 to 180 system: This system, first described by Silver, is probably the most widely used system of notating and recording range of motion measurements. The starting position (the anatomical position) for all movements except pronation and supination is considered to be 0. Movements then proceed toward 180°.

180 to 0 system: According to Clark, who first described this system, the anatomical position is designated as the 180° position for all joints. Movements toward flexion approach 180°, and movements toward extension or past the 180° or neutral position approach 0°. Movements in the frontal plane also approach 0°. External rotation movements approach 180°, and internal rotation movements approach zero.

360° system: This system, first described by West, is similar to the 180° to 0° system in that the neutral starting position for most joints is designated as 180°. Movements of flexion are toward 0°, and movements beyond the neutral position are toward 360°.

SFTR system of recording range of motion values: The SFTR (abbreviation for sagittal, frontal, transverse, and rotation) system combines the 0 to 180 method for notating ROM measurements with a systematic set of rules for recording these measurements. The following rules guide the use of the SFTR system. All joint motions are measured from the anatomical position. All joint motions and positions are recorded in the three basic planes (sagittal, frontal, and transverse). Motions of internal and external rotation are recorded as rotations.

All motions are recorded with three numbers. Motions leading away from the body are recorded first, and motions leading toward the body are recorded last. The starting position is recorded in the middle and is usually 0. For example, an elbow that can be hyperextended 10° and flexed 140° would be recorded as S 10–0–140. The S indicates motion in the sagittal plane. All fixed positions, such as ankyloses, are recorded with two numbers. For example, an elbow that is ankylosed at a position of 30° of flexion would be recorded as S 0–30. Lateral bending and rotation of the spine to the left is recorded first and motions to the right are recorded last.

Based on:

Clark, WA: A system of joint measurements. J Orthop Surg 2:687, 1920.
Gerhardt, JJ: Clinical measurements of joint motion and position in the neutral-zero method and SFTR recording: Basic principles. Int Rehab Med 5:161, 1983.
Gerhardt, JJ, and Russe, OA: International SFTR Method of Measuring and Recording Joint Motion. Huber, Bern, Switzerland, 1975.
Silver, D: Measurement of the range of motion in joints. J Bone Joint Surg 21:569, 1923.
West, CC: Measurement of joint motion. Arch Phys Med 26:414, 1945.

MUSCULO

◗ TABLE 3.18 Cervical Spine Range of Motion for Adults (in degrees)

Motion	AAOS	AMA
Flexion	45	50
Extension	45	60
Lateral flexion	45	45
Rotation	60	80

Data from American Academy of Orthopedic Surgeons: *Joint Motion: Method of Measuring and Recording.* AAOS, Chicago, 1965; American Medical Association: *Guides to the Evaluation of Permanent Impairment*, ed. 5. AMA, Chicago, 2001.
AAOS = American Academy of Orthopaedic Surgeons, AMA = American Medical Association.

◗ TABLE 3.19 Thoracolumbar and Lumbosacral Range of Motion for Adults (in degrees)

Motion	AAOS (thoracolumbar)	AMA (lumbosacral)	AMA (thoracic)
Flexion	80	60	45
Extension	20–30	25	0
Lateral flexion	35	25	45
Rotation	45		30

Data from Greene, WB, and Heckman, JD: *The Clinical Measurement of Joint Motion.* American Academy of Orthopaedic Surgeons, Rosemont, IL 1994; and American Medical Association: *Guides to the Evaluation of Permanent Impairment*, ed. 5. AMA, Chicago, 2001.
AAOS = American Academy of Orthopaedic Surgeons, AMA = American Medical Association.

TABLE 3.20 Temporomandibular Motions for Adults (mean values in mm)

Motion	Walker et al 3 Men and 12 Women	Hirsch et al 486 Men	Hirsch et al 525 Women
Opening	43	51	51
Left lateral deviation	9	11	10
Right lateral deviation	9	10	10
Protrusion	7	8	8

Data from Walker, N, Bohannon, RW, and Cameron, D: Validity of temporomandibular joint range of motion measurements obtained with a ruler. *J Orthop Sports Phys Ther* 30:484, 2000; Hirsch, C, et al: Mandibular jaw movement capacity in 10–17-yr-old children and adolescents: Normative values and the influence of gender, age, and temporomandibular disorders. *Eur J Oral Sci* 114:465, 2006.

TABLE 3.21 Range of Motion for the Extremities of Adults According to Various Authors (in degrees)

Joint	AAOS	AMA	Boone and Azen
Shoulder			
Flexion	180	180	167
Extension	60	50	62
Abduction	180	170	184
Internal rotation	70	80	69
External rotation	90	60	104
Elbow			
Flexion	150	140	143
Radioulnar			
Pronation	80	80	76
Supination	80	80	82
Wrist			
Flexion	80	60	76
Extension	70	60	75
Radial deviation	20	20	22
Ulnar deviation	30	30	36

MUSCULO

Joint	AAOS	AMA	Boone and Azen
Finger MCP			
Flexion	90	90	
Extension	20	20	
Finger PIP			
Flexion	100	100	
Extension	0	0	
Finger DIP			
Flexion	70	70	
Extension	0	0	
Thumb CMC			
Abduction	70	50	
Flexion			
Extension			
Thumb MCP			
Flexion	50	60	
Extension	0	0	
Thumb IP			
Flexion	80	80	
Extension	20	10	
Hip			
Flexion	120	>100	122
Extension	20	<10 flexion contracture	10
Abduction	40	>25	46
Adduction	30	>15	27
Internal rotation	45	>20	47
External rotation	45	>30	47

(table continues on page 126)

MUSCULO

🔵 **TABLE 3.21 Range of Motion for the Extremities of Adults According to Various Authors (in degrees)** (continued)

Joint	AAOS	AMA	Boone and Azen
Knee			
Flexion	135	>110	143
Ankle			
Plantar flexion	50	>20	56
Dorsiflexion	20	>10	13
Subtalar Joint			
Inversion	35	>20	37
Eversion	15	>10	21
First MTP			
Flexion	45		
Extension	70	>30	

Data from: Greene, WB, and Heckman JD: *The Clinical Measurement of Joint Motion.* American Academy of Orthopaedic Surgeons, Rosemont, IL 1994; Rondinelli, RD: *Guides to the Evaluation of Permanent Impairment*, ed. 6. American Medical Association, Chicago 2008; Boone, DC, and Azen, SP: Normal range of motion of joints in male subjects. *J Bone Joint Surg Am* 61(5):756–759, 1979.
AAOS = American Academy of Orthopaedic Surgeons, AMA = American Medical Association.

Manual Muscle Testing

Manual Muscle Testing Positions

There are two major texts on muscle testing: Kendall, FP, et al: *Muscles: Testing and Function,* ed. 5, Williams & Wilkins, Baltimore, 2005; and Hislop, HJ, and Montgomery, J: *Daniels and Worthingham's Muscle Testing: Techniques of Manual Examination,* ed. 8, Saunders, St. Louis, MO, 2007. Each suggests different positions for testing. See manual muscle testing grading scales (on page 130) for differences in how they grade muscles. To facilitate testing patients once they have been positioned, the following tables list the positions suggested by the two texts.

TABLE 3.22 Supine Position

Hislop and Montgomery	Kendall et al
Cervical flexion—all tests	Toe extensors
Cervical rotation—normal, good, and fair	Toe flexors Tibialis anterior
Trunk flexion—all tests	Tibialis posterior
Trunk rotation—all tests	Peroneals
Elevation of pelvis—all tests	Tensor fasciae latae
Hip flexion—trace and zero	Sartorius
Hip flexion, abduction and external rotation with knee flexion—poor, trace, and zero	Iliopsoas Abdominals Neck flexors
Hip abduction—poor, trace, and zero	Finger flexors
Hip adduction—poor, trace, and zero	Finger extensors
Hip external rotation—poor, trace, and zero	Thumb muscles Wrist extensors
Hip internal rotation—poor, trace, and zero	Wrist flexors Supinators
Knee extension—trace and zero	Pronators
Shoulder horizontal adduction—normal, good, and fair	Biceps brachii Brachioradialis
Elbow flexion—trace and zero	Triceps brachii—supine test Pectoralis major—upper part Pectoralis major—lower part Pectoralis minor Shoulder medial rotators—supine test Shoulder lateral rotators—supine test Serratus anterior Anterior deltoid—supine test

MUSCULO

MUSCULO

🔴 TABLE 3.23 Prone Position

Hislop and Montgomery	Kendall et al
Cervical extension—all tests	Gastrocnemius and plantaris soleus
Trunk extension—all tests	Hamstrings—medial and lateral
Hip extension—all tests except poor	Gluteus maximus
Knee flexion—all tests except poor	Neck extensors
Ankle plantar flexion—poor, trace, and zero	Back extensors
Scapular adduction—all tests	Quadratus lumborum
Scapular adduction and downward rotation—normal, good, and fair	Latissimus dorsi Lower trapezius
Scapular elevation—poor, trace, and zero	Middle trapezius Rhomboids
Scapular depression and adduction—all tests	Posterior deltoid—prone test Triceps brachii—prone test
Shoulder extension—all tests	Teres major
Shoulder horizontal abduction—normal, good, and fair Shoulder external rotation—all tests Shoulder internal rotation—all tests Elbow extension—normal, good, and fair	Shoulder medial rotators—prone test Shoulder lateral rotators—prone test

🔴 TABLE 3.24 Side-Lying Position

Hislop and Montgomery	Kendall et al
Hip flexion—poor	Gluteus medius
Hip extension—poor	Gluteus minimus
Hip abduction—normal, good, and fair	Hip adductors
Hip abduction from the flexed position—normal, good, and fair Hip adduction—normal, good, and fair Knee flexion—poor Knee extension—poor	Lateral abdominals

🟥 TABLE 3.25 Sitting Position

Hislop and Montgomery	Kendall et al
Cervical rotation—poor, trace, and zero	Quadriceps
Hip flexion—normal, good, and fair	Hip medial rotators
Hip flexion, abduction, and external rotation with knee flexion—normal, good, and fair	Hip lateral rotators Hip flexors—group test
Hip abduction from the flexed position—poor, trace, and zero	Deltoid, anterior, middle, and posterior
Hip external rotation—normal, good, and fair	Coracobrachialis Upper trapezius
Hip internal rotation—normal, good, and fair Knee extension—normal, good, and fair Foot dorsiflexion and inversion—all tests Foot inversion—all tests Foot eversion with plantar flexion—all tests Toe motions—all tests Hallux motions—all tests Scapular abduction and upward rotation—all tests Scapular adduction and downward rotation—poor, trace, and zero Scapular elevation—normal, good, and fair Shoulder flexion—all tests Shoulder abduction—all tests Shoulder horizontal abduction—poor, trace, and zero Shoulder horizontal adduction—poor, trace, and zero Elbow flexion—normal, good, fair, and poor Elbow extension—poor, trace, and zero Forearm motions—all tests Wrist motions—all tests Finger motions—all tests Thumb motions—all tests Muscles innervated by cranial nerves	Serratus anterior—preferred test

🟥 TABLE 3.26 Standing Position

Hislop and Montgomery	Kendall et al
Ankle plantar flexion—normal, good, and fair	Serratus anterior Ankle plantar flexors

Grading Systems for Manual Muscle Testing

Manual muscle testing has been used to describe the performance of muscles and muscle groups. Three systems are in common use for testing and grading, and their grading scales are presented here.

Kendall and coauthors initially utilized a percentage-based system for "muscle grading." In the 1993 edition of their text, the percentage-based system was dropped. A 0–10 numeric grading scale was introduced and attempts were made to standardize this system with other muscle grading systems.

◖ TABLE 3.27 Grading System of Kendall et al

Numeric Grade	Grade	Definition
10	Normal	In antigravity position holds test position against strong pressure.
9	Good+	In antigravity position holds test position against moderate to strong pressure.
8	Good	In antigravity position holds test position against moderate pressure.
7	Good-	In antigravity position holds test position against slight to moderate pressure.
6	Fair+	In antigravity position holds test position against slight pressure.
5	Fair	In antigravity position holds position (no added pressure).
4	Fair–	In antigravity position a gradual release from test position.
3	Poor+	In horizontal plane: Moves to completion of range against resistance or moves to completion of range and hold against pressure.
		In antigravity position: Moves through partial range of motion.
2	Poor	Moves through complete range of motion in horizontal plane.
1	Poor–	Moves through partial range of motion in horizontal plane.
T	Trace	Tendon becomes prominent or feeble contraction felt in the muscle, but no visible movement of the part.
0	Zero	No contraction felt in the muscle.

Based on Kendall, FP, et al: *Muscles: Testing and Function*, ed. 5. Williams & Wilkins, Baltimore, 2005, p 23.

🔴 TABLE 3.28 Grading System of Hislop and Montgomery

Grade	Definition
5 (Normal)	Completes full range of motion against gravity; maintains end-range position against maximal resistance
4 (Good)	Completes full range of motion against gravity; maintains end-range position against strong resistance
3+ (Fair+)	Completes full range of motion against gravity; maintains end-range position against mild resistance
3 (Fair)	Completes full range of motion against gravity; unable to maintain end-range position against any resistance
2 (Poor)	Completes full range of motion in a gravity-eliminated position
2– (Poor–)	Completes partial range of motion in a gravity-eliminated position
1 (Trace)	The examiner observes or palpates contractile activity in the muscle; no movement
0 (Zero)	No activity detected in the muscle

Based on Hislop, HJ, and Montgomery, J: *Daniels and Worthingham's Muscle Testing: Techniques of Manual Examination*, ed. 8. WB Saunders, Philadelphia, 2007, pp 2–8.

🔴 TABLE 3.29 Medical Research Council's Grading System

Grade	Definition
5	Normal power
4+	Active movement against gravity and strong resistance
4	Active movement against gravity and moderate resistance
4–	Active movement against gravity and slight resistance
3	Active movement against gravity
2	Active movement, with gravity eliminated
1	Flicker or trace of contraction
0	No contraction

From Medical Research Council: *Aids to the Examination of the Peripheral Nervous System: Memorandum No. 45*. Her Majesty's Stationary Office, London, England, 1976, p 1, with permission.

Orthopedic Tests by Body Region

The following table lists a selection of orthopedic tests by body region. Regions are listed from cephalad to caudal.

⬤ TABLE 3.30 Orthopedic Tests by Body Region

Body Region and Pathology	Test
Cervical Region	
Cranial nerve tests	See neuromuscular section, pages 225–231.
Dural irritation	Lhermitte's sign
Nerve root lesions	Distraction test Foraminal compression test Upper limb tension tests Valsalva test
Subluxation of the axis	Sharp-Purser test
Vascular compression	Vertebral artery test
Thoracic Outlet	
Neurovascular compression syndromes	Adson's maneuver (for thoracic outlet syndrome) Allen maneuver (for thoracic outlet syndrome) Halstead maneuver (for thoracic outlet syndrome) Costoclavicular syndrome test (for thoracic outlet syndrome)
Shoulder	
Anterior shoulder dislocation	Apprehension test
Glenoid labrum tear	Active compression test Clunk test
Nerve entrapment	Suprascapular nerve entrapment test
Rotator cuff tendinitis	Hawkins-Kennedy impingement test Neer impingement sign
Elbow	
Ligamentous instability	Ligamentous instability tests (for medial and lateral collateral ligaments)
Neurovascular compression	Elbow flexion test (for cubital tunnel syndrome)
Tendinitis	Golfer's elbow test Tennis elbow tests

MUSCULO

Body Region and Pathology	Test
Wrist and Hand	
Contractures	Bunnel-Littler test (for limitations at the PIP joints)
	Tight retinacular ligament test (PIP, DIP joint, or collateral ligaments)
Neurovascular compression	Allen test (for vascular insufficiency to the hand)
	Froment's sign (for ulnar nerve damage)
	Phalen's test (wrist flexion test) (for carpal tunnel syndrome)
	Tinel's sign (for carpal tunnel syndrome)
Rheumatoid arthritis	Intrinsic-plus test (for limitations of the intrinsic hand muscles)
Tendinitis	Finkelstein's test (for de Quervain's disease)
Low Back	
Instability	Prone instability test
Malingering	Hoover's test (for differentiating lower limb weakness from malingering)
Nerve compression	Femoral nerve traction test (for roots L2 to L4)
	Prone knee flexion test (reverse Lasègue test) (for roots L2, L3)
	Sitting root test (slump test) (for the sciatic nerve)
	Straight leg raising test (Lasègue's test) (for the sciatic nerve)
Sacroiliac Joint	
	Side-lying iliac approximation (transverse posterior stress) test
	Sitting flexion test
	Standing flexion test
	Standing Gillet test
	Supine iliac gapping (transverse anterior stress) test
	Supine to long sitting test
Hip	
Arthritis	Patrick's test (Fabere test, Faber test, or figure-of-four test)
Contractures	Ober's test (for a tight iliotibial band)
	Thomas test (for tight hip flexor muscles)

(table continues on page 134)

⬤ TABLE 3.30 Orthopedic Tests by Body Region (continued)

Body Region and Pathology	Test
Hip	
Dislocation	Ortolani's test Galeazzi's test Barlow's provocative test Trendelenburg's test (for detecting disloca-tion, weakness of the gluteus medius muscle, or extreme coxa vara)
Knee	
Anterior instability	Anterior drawer test (for anterior instability) Lachman's test (for anterior instability)
Lateral instability	Adduction (varus) stress test
Medial instability	Abduction (valgus) stress test
Meniscus and tibiofemoral joint lesions	Apley grinding test (for meniscal or ligamentous lesions) McMurray test (for meniscal lesions) Wilson test (for osteochondritis dissecans)
Patellar lesions	Apprehension test (for a dislocating patella) Clarke's sign (for hondromalacia of the patella)
Posterior instability	Posterior drawer test (for posterior instability) Posterior sag sign (gravity drawer test) (for posterior instability)
Ankle and Foot	
Achilles tendon	Thompson's test (for Achilles tendon rupture)
Deep vein thrombosis	Homans' sign (for deep vein thrombosis of the leg)
Ligamentous instability	Anterior drawer test (for anterior ankle instability) Kleiger test (for medial instability) Talar tilt (for the calcaneofibular ligament)
Plantar fasciitis	Windlass test

MUSCULO

Orthopedic Tests by Body Region

A selection of common orthopedic tests are described and listed by body region. The more proximal regions are listed first. Within body regions, the tests are listed in alphabetical order.

Cervical Spine

cranial nerve tests: See neuromuscular section, pages 225–231.

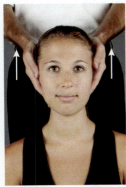

distraction test: A test designed to identify nerve root compression. The examiner places one hand under the patient's chin and the other under the occiput. The head is slowly lifted (distraction), and the test is considered positive if the radiating pain is decreased.

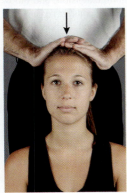

foraminal compression test (Spurling's test): A test designed to identify nerve root compression. The patient laterally flexes the head. The examiner carefully presses down (compression) on the head. The test result is positive if pain radiates into the arm toward the flexed side.

Lhermitte's sign: A test designed to identify dural irritation. The patient is in the long leg sitting position. While keeping the patient's knees extended, the examiner flexes the patient's head and hips simultaneously. The test result is positive if there is a sharp pain down the spine and into the upper or lower extremities.

Sharp-Purser test: A test designed to determine subluxation of the atlas on the axis. The examiner places one hand on the patient's forehead while 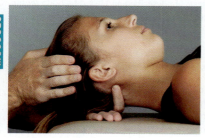 the thumb of the other hand is placed over the spinous process of the axis to stabilize it. The patient is asked to slowly flex the head; at the same time the examiner presses backward with the palm. A positive test is indicated if the examiner feels the head slide backward during the movement.

Spurling's test: See *foraminal compression test.*

upper limb tension test: A test designed to stress all the tissues of the upper limb, especially the neurological structures. The patient lies supine, with the cervical spine laterally flexed to the contralateral side. Each joint of the upper limb is positioned in sequence of shoulder, forearm, wrist, fingers, and elbow until symptoms are reproduced. Modification of the joint positions is believed to place great stress on specific nerves. Position to bias median nerve and anterior interosseus nerve: shoulder depression and abduction to 110°; forearm supination, wrist, finger, and thumb extension; and elbow extension. Position to bias median nerve, musculocutaneous nerve, and axillary nerve: shoulder depression; abduction to 10° and lateral rotation; forearm supination; wrist, fingers, and thumb extension; and elbow extension. Position to bias radial nerve: shoulder depression; abduction to 10° and medial rotation; forearm pronation; wrist flexion and ulnar deviation; fingers and thumb flexion; and elbow extension. Position to bias ulnar nerve: shoulder depression; abduction between 10 and 90°, and lateral rotation, forearm supination, wrist extension and ulnar deviation; fingers and thumb extension; and elbow flexion.

Valsalva test: A test designed to detect a space-occupying lesion in the cervical spine, such as a herniated disk or an osteophyte. The examiner instructs the patient to take a deep breath and hold the breath, as if the patient is having a bowel movement. The test result is positive if symptoms are reproduced or increased.

vertebral artery test: A test designed to detect compression of the vertebral artery. The patient is in a supine position. The examiner places the patient's 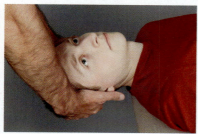 head into a position of extension, lateral flexion, and rotation and holds that position for 30 seconds. Each side is tested separately. The test is positive if the patient reports having a feeling of dizziness or nausea, or if nystagmus is observed.

Thoracic Outlet

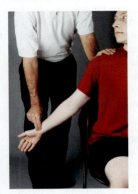

Adson's maneuver: A test designed to determine the presence of thoracic outlet syndrome. The patient turns the head toward the shoulder on the side being tested. The examiner externally rotates and extends the shoulder while the patient extends the head. The test result is positive if the radial pulse disappears while the patient holds a deep breath.

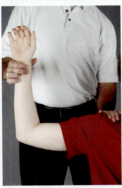

Allen maneuver: A test designed to identify the presence of thoracic outlet syndrome. With the patient seated, the examiner flexes the patient's elbow to 90° while the patient's shoulder is abducted 90° and externally rotated. The examiner then palpates the radial pulse while the patient rotates the head away from the test side. The test result is positive if the pulse disappears.

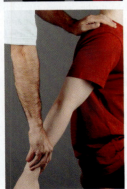

costoclavicular syndrome test: A test designed to determine the presence of thoracic outlet syndrome. The patient is asked to adduct the scapula while the examiner extends the patient's shoulder. For a positive test, symptoms should be reproduced with a decreased radial pulse to confirm the diagnosis.

Halstead maneuver: A test designed to determine the presence of thoracic outlet syndrome. With the patient seated, the examiner palpates the radial pulse and applies a downward force on the arm. The patient extends the neck and rotates the head toward the opposite side of the limb being tested. The test result is positive if the pulse disappears following this maneuver.

Shoulder

active compression test: A test designed to determine the presence of a tear of the glenoid labrum. The patient stands and the arm is flexed to 90° with the elbow in full extension. The arm is then adducted 10° to 15° medial to the sagittal plane of the body and internally rotated so that the thumb faces downward. The examiner stands behind the patient and applies a uniform downward force to the arm. With the arm in the same position, the palm is then fully supinated and the downward force is repeated. The test is considered positive if pain was elicited during the first part of the test and is eliminated or reduced during the second part.

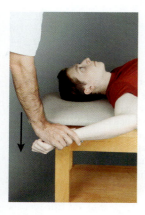

apprehension test for anterior shoulder dislocation: A test designed to determine whether a patient has a history of anterior dislocations. With the patient supine, the examiner slowly abducts and externally rotates the patient's arm. The test is positive if the patient becomes apprehensive and resists further motion.

clunk test: A test designed to determine the presence of a tear of the glenoid labrum. With the patient supine, the examiner places one hand on the posterior aspect of the shoulder over the humeral head. The examiner fully abducts the arm over the patient's head and then pushes anteriorly with the hand over the humeral head. The test is positive if a "clunk" or grinding is palpated. The test may also cause apprehension if anterior instability is present.

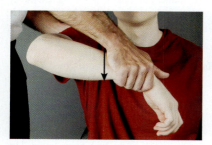

Hawkins-Kennedy impingement test: A test designed to identify supraspinatus tendinitis and/or impingement within the subacromial space. The patient stands while the examiner flexes the arm to 90° and then forcibly internally rotates the shoulder. The test result is positive if pain is present during the maneuver.

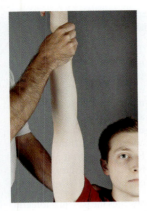

Neer impingement sign: A test designed to identify inflammation of tissues within the subacromial space. The patient's upper extremity is forcibly flexed forward by the examiner. The maneuver is thought to decrease the space between the head of the humerus and acromion process. The test result is positive if the patient reports pain.

MUSCULO

suprascapular nerve entrapment test: A test designed to identify entrapment of the suprascapular nerve in the suprascapular notch. Patients report pain when horizontally adducting their arm across their chest. The pain is poorly localized to the posterior aspect of the shoulder.

Elbow

elbow flexion test: A test designed to identify cubital tunnel syndrome. The patient is asked to hold his or her elbow fully flexed for up to 5 minutes. The test result is positive if tingling or paresthesias is felt in the ulnar nerve distribution of the forearm and hand.

golfer's elbow test: A test designed to identify the presence of inflammation in the area of the medial epicondyle of the humerus. The patient flexes the elbow and wrist. The examiner then passively supinates the forearm and extends the elbow and wrist. The test result is positive if the patient complains of pain over the medial epicondyle.

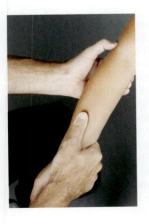

ligamentous instability tests: Tests designed to assess the integrity of the lateral and medial collateral ligaments of the elbow. The patient's arm is held by the examiner so that the examiner is supporting the elbow and wrist. The examiner tests the lateral collateral ligament by applying an adduction or varus force to the distal forearm with the patient's elbow held in 20° to 30° of flexion. The medial collateral ligament is similarly tested by the application of an abduction or valgus force at the distal forearm (see below). The test result is positive if pain or altered mobility is present.

tennis elbow tests: The following three tests are designed to determine the presence of inflammation in the area of the lateral epicondyle:

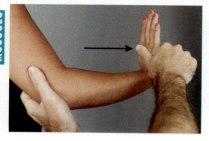

- The patient flexes the elbow to approximately 45° and fully supinates the forearm while making a fist. The patient is then asked to pronate the forearm and radially deviate and extend the wrist while the examiner resists these motions. For a positive test result, pain is elicited in the area of the lateral epicondyle. (Cozen's test)

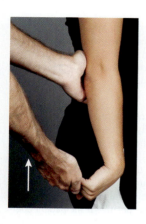

- The examiner pronates the patient's forearm, fully extends the elbow, and fully flexes the wrist. For a positive test result, pain is elicited in the area of the lateral epicondyle. (Mill's test)
- The examiner resists extension of the third digit of the hand distal to the proximal interphalangeal (PIP) joint. A positive test is indicated by pain in the area of the lateral epicondyle of the humerus.

Wrist and Hand

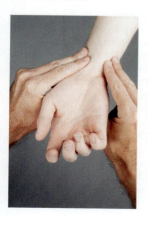

Allen test: A test designed to determine the patency of the vascular communication in the hand. The examiner first palpates and occludes the radial and ulnar arteries. The patient is then asked to open and close the fingers rapidly from three to five times to cause the palmar skin to blanch. Pressure is then released from either the radial or ulnar artery, and the rapidity with which the hand regains color is noted. The test is repeated with release of the other artery. A positive Allen test result indicates that there is a diminished or absent communication between the superficial ulnar arch and the deep radial arch.

MUSCULO

Bunnel-Littler test: A test designed to identify intrinsic muscle or joint contractures at the PIP joints. The examiner flexes the PIP joint maximally while maintaining the metacarpophalangeal (MCP) joint in slight extension. The test result is positive for a joint capsule contracture if the PIP joint cannot be flexed. The test is positive for intrinsic muscle contracture if the MCP is slightly flexed and the PIP flexes fully.

Finkelstein's test: A test designed to determine the presence of tenosynovitis of the abductor pollicis longus and extensor pollicis brevis tendons. The test is commonly used to determine the presence of de Quervain's disease.

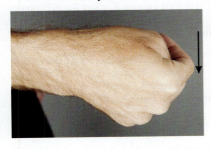

The patient makes a fist while holding the thumb inside the fingers. The patient then attempts to deviate ulnarly the first metacarpal and extend the proximal joint of the thumb. If the patient experiences pain, this is recorded as a positive test result.

Froment's sign: A test designed for determining the presence of adductor pollicis weakness from ulnar nerve paralysis. The patient attempts to grasp a piece of paper between the tips of the thumb and the radial side of the index finger. The test result is positive if the terminal phalanx of the patient's thumb flexes or if the MCP joint of the thumb hyperextends (Jeanne's sign) as the examiner attempts to pull the paper from the patient's grasp.

intrinsic-plus test: A test designed to identify shortening of the intrinsic muscles of the hand. This test is useful and specific when examining the hand of the patient with rheumatoid arthritis, particularly in the early stages prior to any destruction or deformity of the hand. In this test, the MCP joint of the finger being tested is hyperextended. The middle and distal joints flex slightly owing to passive action of tissues. The examiner then further attempts to flex passively the PIP joint of the finger. Any severe restriction to this movement is considered a positive sign.

Jeanne's sign: See *Froment's sign*.

Phalen's (wrist flexion) test: A test designed to determine the presence of carpal tunnel syndrome. The patient's wrists are maximally flexed by the examiner, who maintains this position by holding the patient's wrists together for 1 minute. The test result is positive if paresthesias are present in the thumb, index finger, and the middle and lateral half of the ring finger.

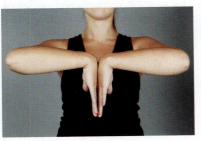

MUSCULO

tight retinacular ligament test: A test designed to determine the presence of shortened retinacular ligaments or a tight distal interphalangeal (DIP) joint

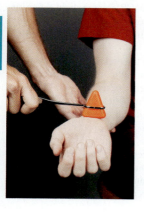

capsule. The examiner holds the patient's PIP joint in a fully extended position while attempting to flex the DIP joint. If the DIP joint does not flex, the test is positive for either a contracted collateral ligament or joint capsule. The test is positive for tight retinacular (collateral) ligaments and a normal joint capsule if, when the PIP joint is flexed, the DIP joint flexes easily.

Tinel's sign: A test designed to detect carpal tunnel syndrome. The examiner taps over the median nerve in the carpal tunnel region of the wrist. The test result is positive if the patient reports paresthesia distal to the wrist.

wrist flexion test: See *Phalen's test.*

Low Back

femoral nerve traction test: A test designed to identify nerve root compression of the midlumbar area (L2, L3, and L4). The patient lies on the unaffected side with the unaffected limb flexed slightly for support. The examiner grasps the affected limb and extends the knee while gently extending the hip approximately 15°, being sure not to extend the back. The patient's knee is then flexed, further stretching the femoral nerve. The test result is positive if pain radiates down the anterior thigh.

Hoover's test: A test designed to discriminate lower limb weakness from possible malingering. The patient relaxes in a supine position while the examiner places one hand under each heel. The patient is then asked to do a straight leg raise (knee extended). The test result is positive if the patient is unable to lift the leg and there is no downward pressure from the opposite leg.

Lasègue's test: See *straight leg raising test.*

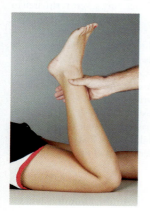

prone knee flexion test (reverse Lasègue test): A test designed to identify L2 or L3 nerve root lesions. The patient lies prone while the examiner passively flexes the knee so that the patient's heel touches the patient's buttocks. The test result is positive if unilateral symptoms are elicited or increased in the lumbar area or anterior thigh. Pain in the anterior thigh may indicate a tight quadriceps muscle.

prone instability test: A test designed to identify persons likely to respond to a stabilization exercise program. The patient lies prone with their legs over the edge of the examining table and feet on the floor. The examiner applies a posterior to anterior mobilization over the spinous process of the symptomatic lumbar vertebrae and notes the response of pain. The patient then lifts and holds their legs off the floor and the posterior to anterior mobilization is repeated. The test is considered positive if pain is present to the first mobilization but subsides in the second position (see figures below).

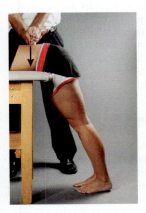 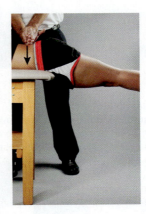

reverse Lasègue test: See *prone knee flexion test*.

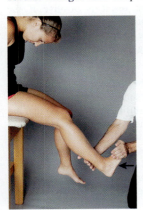

sitting root test (slump test): A test designed to identify compression of the sciatic nerve. The patient is seated with neck flexed. The knee is actively extended while the hip remains flexed. The test result is positive if pain increases.

slump test: See *sitting root test.*

straight leg raising test (Lasègue test): A test designed to identify sciatic nerve root compression. With the patient supine, the examiner raises the patient's extended leg while watching the patient's reaction. The examiner stops when

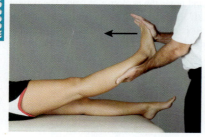

the patient complains of back or leg pain (and not hamstring tightness). The examiner may also dorsiflex the ankle to further increase the traction on the sciatic nerve. Back pain suggests a central herniation, and leg pain suggests a lateral disk protrusion. The test is repeated for both sides.

Sacroiliac Joint

side-lying iliac approximation (transverse posterior stress) test: A test designed to identify the presence of sacroiliac joint dysfunction. The patient lies on the side. The examiner stands above the patient and, with

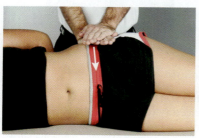

elbows fully extended, interlocks palms and places them over the most cephalad margin of the iliac crest. The examiner then exerts a downward and cephalad-directed force on the crest. The test result is positive if the patient's painful symptoms in the sacroiliac, gluteal, or crural regions are reproduced.

sitting flexion test: A test designed to identify the presence of sacroiliac joint dysfunction. The patient sits erect on a flat surface, with feet flat on the floor and knees flexed to 90°. The hips are sufficiently abducted that the patient can bend forward between them. The examiner, who is kneeling or squatting behind the patient, places his or her thumbs on the inferior margin of the posterior superior iliac spines (PSISs). The patient bends forward as far as possible, reaching the hands toward the floor. A positive test result occurs when one PSIS moves more in a cranial direction than does the other. The side with the greater movement is said to have articular restriction.

standing flexion test: A test designed to identify the presence of sacroiliac joint dysfunction. The patient stands with feet 12 in. apart. The examiner, who is standing or squatting behind the patient, places his or her thumbs on the inferior margin of the PSISs. The patient then bends forward while keeping the knees straight. A positive test result occurs when one PSIS moves more in a cranial direction than does the other. The side with the greater movement is said to have articular restriction. Because hamstring tightness may also cause these findings, the test is not considered positive until hamstring tightness has been ruled out.

standing Gillet test: A test designed to identify the presence of sacroiliac joint dysfunction. The patient stands with feet 12 in. apart. The examiner, who is standing behind the patient, places one thumb directly under one PSIS and the other thumb on the ipsilateral tubercle of S2 (which is on the sacrum at the level of the PSIS). The patient flexes the hip and knee on the side being palpated so that she or he is standing on one leg. A positive test result is one in which the PSIS does not dip downward as the extreme of hip flexion is reached. The test is repeated on the contralateral side (see figure at left).

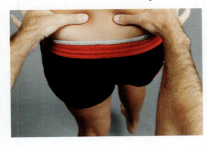

supine iliac gapping (transverse anterior stress) test: A test designed to identify sacroiliac joint dysfunction. The patient lies supine. The examiner crosses his or her arms, placing the palms of her or his hands on the patient's anterior superior iliac spines (ASISs). The examiner then presses down and laterally to strain the sacroiliac ligaments. A positive test result occurs when the patient reports pain in the gluteal or posterior crural areas. If pain is felt in the lumbar region, the test is repeated after using more support for the lumbar spine.

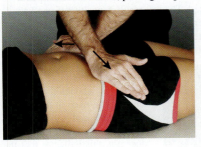

supine to long sitting test: A test designed to identify the presence of rotation of the innominate bones relative to the sacroiliac joint. The patient lies supine while the examiner places her or his thumbs on the inferior borders of the medial malleoli. The patient then sits up, being careful to do so in a symmetrical, nontwisting fashion. Changes in the relative positions of the medial malleoli are noted. If one leg appears to lengthen when the patient sits up, that is interpreted as indicating a posterior innominate rotation on that side. If one leg appears to shorten when the patient sits up, that is interpreted as indicating an anterior innominate rotation on that side.

Hip

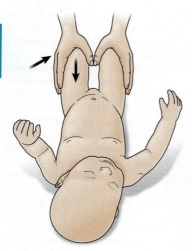

Barlow's provocative test: See also *Ortolani's test.* A test designed to identify hip instability in infants. The test is performed after the Ortolani test has been conducted. With the infant in the same position used for Ortolani's test, the examiner stabilizes the pelvis between the symphysis and sacrum with one hand. With the thumb of the other hand, the examiner attempts to dislocate the hip by gentle but firm posterior pressure.

faber test or Figure-of-four test: See *Patrick's test.*

Galeazzi's test: A test designed to detect unilateral congenital dislocations of the hip in children. The child is positioned supine with the hips flexed to 90° and the knees fully flexed. The test result is positive if one knee is positioned higher than the other.

Ober test: A test designed to determine the presence of a shortened (tight) iliotibial band. With the patient lying on one side, the lower limb closest to the table is flexed. The other

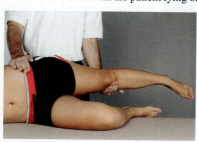

lower limb, which is being tested, is abducted and extended. The knee of the limb is flexed to 90° and is then allowed to drop to the table. If the limb does not, this indicates that the iliotibial band is shortened (tight).

MUSCULO

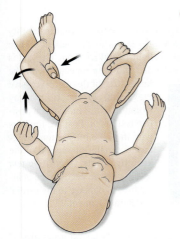

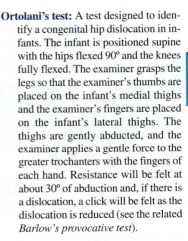

Ortolani's test: A test designed to identify a congenital hip dislocation in infants. The infant is positioned supine with the hips flexed 90° and the knees fully flexed. The examiner grasps the legs so that the examiner's thumbs are placed on the infant's medial thighs and the examiner's fingers are placed on the infant's lateral thighs. The thighs are gently abducted, and the examiner applies a gentle force to the greater trochanters with the fingers of each hand. Resistance will be felt at about 30° of abduction and, if there is a dislocation, a click will be felt as the dislocation is reduced (see the related *Barlow's provocative test*).

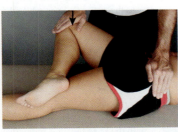

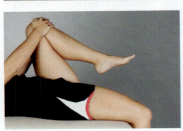

Patrick's test (Fabere test, Faber test, or figure-of-four test): A test designed to identify arthritis of the hip. With the patient lying supine, the knee is flexed and the hip is flexed, abducted, and externally rotated until the lateral malleolus rests on the opposite knee just above the patella. In this position the knee on the side being tested is gently forced downward; if pain is produced, the test result is positive for the presence of osteoarthritis of the hip.

Thomas test: A test designed to test for contracture of the hip flexor muscles. In supine position, the patient holds one flexed hip against the chest. The test is positive if the other thigh does not remain against the surface.

Trendelenburg's test: A test designed to identify the presence of an unstable hip. The patient stands on the leg to be tested. The test is positive if the non-weight-bearing side does not rise as the patient stands on one lower extremity. A positive test result may be caused by a hip dislocation, weakness of the hip abductors, or coxa vara.

Knee

abduction (valgus stress) test: A test designed to identify medial instability of the knee. The examiner applies a valgus stress to the patient's knee while the patient's ankle is stabilized in slight lateral rotation. The test is first conducted with the knee fully extended and then repeated with the

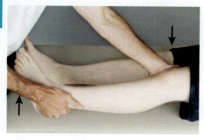

knee at 20° of flexion. Excessive movement of the tibia away from the femur indicates a positive test result. Positive findings with the knee fully extended indicate a major disruption of the knee ligaments. A positive test result with the knee flexed is indicative of damage to the medial collateral ligament.

adduction (varus stress) test: A test designed to identify lateral instability of the knee. The examiner applies a varus stress to the patient's knee while the

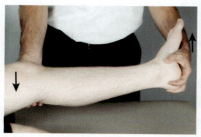

ankle is stabilized. The test is done with the patient's knee in full extension and then with the knee in 20°–30° of flexion. A positive test result with the knee extended suggests a major disruption of the knee ligaments, whereas a positive test result with the knee flexed is indicative of damage to the lateral collateral ligament.

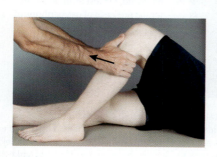

anterior drawer (sign) test: A test designed to detect anterior instability of the knee. The patient lies supine with the knee flexed 90°. The examiner sits across the forefoot of the patient's flexed lower limb. With the patient's foot in neutral rotation, the examiner pulls forward on the proximal part of the calf. Both lower limbs are tested. The test result is positive if there is excessive anterior movement of the tibia with respect to the femur.

MUSCULO

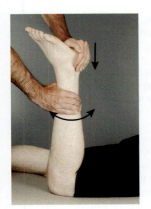

Apley grinding test: A test designed to detect meniscal lesions. The patient lies prone with the knees flexed 90°. The examiner applies a compressive force through the foot and rotates the tibia back and forth while palpating the joint line with the other hand feeling for crepitation. The test result is positive if the patient reports pain or the examiner feels crepitation. This test is then repeated by applying a distractive force to the leg, and if pain is elicited it is indicative of a ligamentous injury rather than a meniscal injury.

apprehension test: A test designed to identify dislocation of the patella. The patient lies supine with the knee resting at 30° flexion. The examiner carefully and slowly displaces the patella laterally. If the patient looks apprehensive and tries to contract the quadriceps muscle to bring the patella back to neutral, the test result is positive.

Clarke's sign: A test designed to identify the presence of chondromalacia of the patella. The patient lies relaxed with knees extended as the examiner presses down slightly proximal to the base of the patella with the web of the hand. The patient is then asked to contract the quadriceps muscle as the examiner applies more force. The test result is positive if the patient cannot complete the contraction without pain.

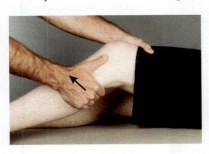

Lachman's test: A test designed to identify injury to the anterior cruciate ligament. The patient lies supine with the examiner stabilizing the distal femur with one hand and grasping the proximal tibia with the other hand. With the knee held in slight flexion, the tibia is moved forward on the femur. A positive test result is indicated by a soft end-feel and excessive observable movement of the tibia.

McMurray test: A test designed to identify meniscal lesions. The patient lies supine while the examiner grasps the foot with one hand and palpates the joint line with the other. The knee is fully flexed and the tibia rotated back and forth and then held alternately in internal and external rotation as the knee is extended. A click or crepitation may be felt over the joint line with a posterior meniscal lesion, as the knee is extended.

posterior drawer test: A test designed to identify posterior instability of the knee. The patient lies supine with the knee flexed to 90° as the foot is held in a neutral position by the examiner sitting on it. The examiner's hands grasp the leg around the proximal tibia and attempt to move the tibia backward on the femur. The test result is positive if there is excessive posterior movement of the tibia on the femur.

posterior sag sign (gravity drawer test): A test designed to identify posterior instability of the knee. The patient lies supine with the knees flexed to 90° and the feet supported. The test result is positive if the tibia sags back on the femur.

valgus stress test: See *abduction test.*

varus stress test: See *adduction test.*

Wilson test: A test designed to identify osteochondritis dissecans. The patient is seated with the leg in the dependent position. The patient extends the knee with the tibia medially rotated until the pain increases. The test is repeated with the tibia laterally rotated during extension. The test result is positive if the pain does not occur when the tibia is laterally rotated.

Ankle and Foot

Achilles tendon test: See *Thompson's test.*

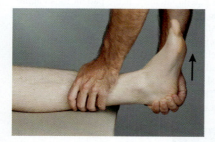

anterior drawer sign: A test designed to identify anterior ankle instability. The patient lies supine, and the examiner stabilizes the distal tibia and fibula with one hand while the examiner's other hand holds the foot in 20° of plantar flexion. The test result is positive if, while drawing the talus forward in the ankle mortise, there is straight anterior translation that exceeds that of the uninvolved side.

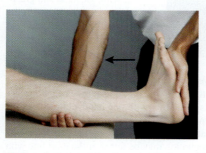

Homans' sign: A test designed to detect deep vein thrombosis in the lower part of the leg. The ankle is passively dorsiflexed, and any sudden increase of pain in the calf or popliteal space is noted.

Kleiger test: A test for detecting lesions of the deltoid ligament. The patient is seated with the knees flexed to 90°. The examiner holds the foot and attempts to abduct the forefoot. The test result is positive if the patient complains of pain medially and laterally. The talus may be felt to displace slightly from the medial malleolus.

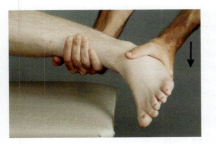

talar tilt: A test designed to identify lesions of the calcaneofibular ligament. The patient is supine or lying on one side with the knee flexed to 90°. With the foot in a neutral position, the talus is tilted medially. The test result is positive if the amount of adduction on the involved side is excessive. (See photo at left.)

MUSCULO

Thompson's test: A test designed to detect ruptures of the Achilles tendon. The patient is placed in a prone position or on the knees with the feet extended over the edge of the bed. The middle third of the calf muscle is squeezed by the examiner. If a normal plantar flexion response is not elicited, an Achilles tendon rupture is suspected.

Windlass test: A test to identify plantar fasciitis. The patient is standing with equal weight on both feet. The examiner passively dorsiflexes the big toe. The test is positive if pain is reproduced along the medial longitudinal arch of the foot.

Manual Therapy

According to the *Guide to Physical Therapist Practice,* the term *manual therapy* refers to "skilled hand movements intended to improve tissue extensibility; increase range of motion; induce relaxation; mobilize or manipulate soft tissues and joints; modulate pain; and reduce soft tissue swelling, inflammation, or restriction." Mobilization/manipulation is further defined as a "manual therapy technique comprising a continuum of skilled passive movements to the joints and/or related soft tissues that are applied at varying speeds and amplitudes, including a small-amplitude/high-velocity therapeutic movement." The following pages describe manual therapy terms according to different authors.

Cyriax Terms
End-Feels According to Cyriax
end-feel: The type of resistance felt by an examiner at the end-range of a passive range-of-motion test.

bone to bone: The abrupt halt to the movement that is felt when two hard surfaces meet, for example, at the extreme of passive extension of the normal elbow.

capsular: The feeling of immediate stoppage of movement with some give. It is the type of end-feel felt at the end of the range of normal shoulder extension or hip extension.

empty: The end-feel felt when the patient complains of considerable pain during passive movement but the examiner perceives no increase in resistance to joint movement.

spasm: The feeling of muscle "spasm" coming actively into play. It is said to indicate the presence of acute or subacute arthritis.

springy block: A rebound is seen and felt at the end of the range. It is said to occur with displacement of an intra-articular structure, for example, when a torn meniscus in the knee engages between the tibia and femur and prevents the last few degrees of extension.

tissue approximation: The end-feel felt when a limb segment cannot be moved further because the soft tissues surrounding the joint cannot be compressed any further. It is the sensation felt at the end-range of elbow or knee flexion.

Cyriax's Selective Tissue Tension Tests

The following terms, developed by Cyriax, relate to a method that can be used to identify the source of the patient's pain complaints. In his system the diagnosis depends on asking the patient to move or on applying forces. In either case, patients report what they feel. Equal importance is placed on determining which movements are painful and/or limited and which movements are full range and/or pain free.

active range of movements: These assess the patient's ability and willingness to perform the movements requested, the range of active movements available, and the patient's ability to produce the muscle forces required for active movement. These movements are also used to determine the region of the body from which the symptoms are originating and to determine which movements and muscles to examine in detail.

painful arc: The excursion (arc) near the midrange in which pain is felt during an active movement test. The pain disappears as this position is passed in either direction. The pain may reappear at the end-range. According to Cyriax, a painful arc implies that a structure is pinched between two bony surfaces.

passive range of movements: These assess the ability of the "inert" (noncontractile, according to Cyriax) tissues to allow motion at a joint. The patient states whether pain is provoked. Each motion possible for the joint being tested must be examined to distinguish between capsular and noncapsular patterns of movement restrictions. Any discrepancy between the range of movement obtained actively and passively is noted.

resisted movements: These are resisted isometric contractions with the limb segment near the midrange. These movements assess the tension-producing capabilities of specific muscle groups and whether the patient's pain is originating from these muscle groups.

Based on:

Cyriax, J: Textbook of Orthopaedic Medicine, ed. 11. Bailliere Tindall, London, England, 1984. Guide to Physical Practice, second edition. Phys Ther 2001; 81:9–744.

TABLE 3.31 Significance of Diagnostic Movements in Selective Tissue Tension Tests of Cyriax

Tests	Results of Tests	Conclusion According to Cyriax
Active and passive movements	Pain is felt in one direction during the passive movement and in the opposite direction during the active movement.	A contractile structure is at fault.
Passive movements	Excessive range of motion is found.	Capsular or ligamentous laxity is evident.
Active and passive movements, resisted movements	Pain is felt at the end-range of active and passive movements; resisted movements are pain free.	An "inert" noncontractile structure is at fault.
Resisted movements	Pain is not felt; strength is normal.	No lesion is present.
Resisted movements	Pain is felt; strength is normal.	A minor lesion of muscle or tendon may be present.
Resisted movements	Pain is felt; strength is decreased.	A serious lesion of the muscle or tendon may be present.
Resisted movements	Pain is not felt; strength is decreased.	A complete rupture of the muscle or tendon may be present.
Resisted movements	Pain is felt after a number of repetitions.	Intermittent claudication may be present.
Resisted movements	Pain is felt with all resisted movements.	There is evidence of emotional hypersensitivity or an organic cause of pain.

Based on Cyriax, J: *Textbook of Orthopaedic Medicine*, ed. 11. Bailliere Tindall, London, England, 1984.

MUSCULO

Capsular Patterns of the Joints According to Cyriax

capsular pattern: A limitation of movement or a pattern of pain at a joint that occurs in a predictable pattern. According to Cyriax, these patterns are due to lesions in either the joint capsule or the synovial membrane. Limitations of motion at a joint that do not fall into these predictable patterns are said to exhibit noncapsular patterns. Causes of noncapsular patterns are said to be ligamentous adhesions, internal derangements, and extra-articular lesions.

acromioclavicular joint: Pain only at the extremes of range.

ankle joint: If the calf muscles are of adequate length, there will be a greater limitation of plantar flexion than of dorsiflexion.

cervical spine (facet joints): Lateral flexion and rotation are equally limited, flexion is full range and painful, and extension is limited.

elbow: Greater limitation in flexion than in extension.

facet joints: See specific body region—*cervical spine, lumbar spine,* or *thoracic spine.*

finger joints: Greater limitation in flexion than in extension.

glenohumeral joint: Greatest limitation in external rotation, followed by abduction, with less limitation in internal rotation.

hip joint: Equal limitations in flexion, abduction, and medial rotation, with a slight loss in extension. There is little or no loss in lateral rotation.

knee joint: Greater limitation in flexion than in extension.

lumbar spine (facet joints): The capsular pattern for the joints of the lumbar spine cannot be determined because of the difficulty of assessing the amount of motion in these joints.

metatarsophalangeal joint (first): Greater limitation in extension than in flexion.

metatarsophalangeal joints (second through fifth): Variable.

midtarsal joint: Equal limitations in dorsiflexion, plantar flexion, adduction, and medial rotation.

radioulnar joint (distal): Full range of motion with pain at both extremes of rotation.

sacrococcygeal joints: Pain produced when forces are applied to these joints.

sacroiliac joint: Pain produced when forces are applied to these joints.

sternoclavicular joint: Pain only at the extremes of range.

symphysis pubis: Pain produced when forces are applied to this joint.

talocalcaneal joint: Limitation in varus.

thoracic spine (facet joints): The capsular pattern for the joints of the thoracic spine cannot be determined because of the difficulty of assessing the amount of motion in these joints.

thumb joints: Greater limitation in flexion than in extension.

trapeziometacarpal joint: Limitations in abduction and in extension with full flexion.

wrist: Equal limitation in flexion and extension.

Based on:

Cyriax, J: *Textbook of Orthopaedic Medicine,* ed. 11. London, England, Bailliere Tindall, 1984.

Kaltenborn Terms

Grading System for Classifying Joint Motion

Hypomobility	0 = No movement (ankylosis)
	1 = Considerable decrease in movement
	2 = Slight decrease in movement
Normal	3 = Normal
	4 = Slight increase in movement
Hypermobility	5 = Considerable increase in movement
	6 = Complete instability

convex-concave rule: The rule is used to guide therapists as to which direction they should move limb segments when examining joints with limitations in range of motion. When a therapist moves a convex joint surface on a concave joint surface, the convex joint surface is moved in a direction opposite the range-of-motion limitation. Conversely, when a therapist moves a concave joint surface on a convex joint surface, the concave joint surface is moved in the same direction as the range-of-motion limitation.

End-Feels According to Kaltenborn

end-feel: The type of resistance felt by an examiner at the end-range of a passive range-of-motion test.

firm end-feel: Results from capsular or ligamentous stretching. An example is the resistance felt by the examiner at the end-range of external rotation of the glenohumeral joint.

hard end-feel: Occurs when bone meets bone. An example is the resistance felt by the examiner at the end-range of extension of the elbow.

soft end-feel: Is due to soft tissue approximation or soft tissue stretching. An example is the resistance felt by the examiner at the end-range of knee flexion.

Grades of Movement According to Kaltenborn

Grade I traction: Movements are of small amplitude, and there is no appreciable joint separation. Traction force to nullify the compressive forces acting on the joint is applied.

Grade II traction and gliding: The slack of tissues surrounding the joint is taken up, and the tissues surrounding the joint are tightened.

Grade III traction and gliding: After the slack has been taken up, more force is applied, and the tissues crossing the joint are stretched.

Based on:

Kaltenborn, FM: Manual Mobilization of the Extremity Joints: Basic Examination and Treatment Techniques, ed. 4. Oslo, Norway, Olaf Norlis Bokhandel, 1989.

MacConnaill Terms

arthrokinematics: The study of movements within joints.

osteokinematics: The study of the movement of bony segments around a joint axis.

MUSCULO

roll: The movement that occurs when equidistant points on a convex surface come into contact with equidistant points on the concave surface. Roll also occurs when equidistant points on a concave surface come into contact with equidistant points on the convex surface.

slide: The movement that occurs when the same point on the convex surface comes into contact with new points on the concave surface. Slide also occurs when the same point on the concave surface comes into contact with new points on the convex surface.

spin: Rotation of a convex joint surface about a longitudinal axis on a concave joint surface. Spin also occurs when a concave surface rotates about a longitudinal axis on the convex surface.

Maitland Terms

comparable sign: Any form of joint movement testing that causes the patient to report symptoms comparable to those associated with the patient's chief complaint.

manipulation: Manipulation is a sudden movement or thrust, of small amplitude, performed at a speed that makes the patient unable to prevent the motion.

mobilization: Passive movement test performed by an examiner in such a way that the patient can prevent the movement if he or she so chooses. Two main types of movement include the following:
- Passive oscillatory movements that are done at a rate of two or three per second. They are of small or large amplitude and are applied anywhere in a range of movement.
- Sustained stretching that is performed with small-amplitude oscillations at the end of the range of motion.

Grades of Movement According to Maitland

Grade I: Small-amplitude movements performed at the beginning of the range.

Grade II: Large-amplitude movements that do not reach the limit of the range. If the movement is performed near the beginning of the range, it is a II–; if taken deeply into the range, yet still not reaching the limit, it is a II+.

Grade III: Large-amplitude movements performed up to the limit of the range. If the movement is applied forcefully at the limit of the range, it is a III+; if applied gently at the limit of the range, it is a III–.

Grade IV: Small-amplitude movements performed at the limit of the range. Depending on the vigor of the motion, the grades can be a IV– or IV+.

Grade V: Small-amplitude, high-velocity thrust performed at the end of range.

Based on:

Hengeveld, E, and Banks, K (eds): Maitland's Peripheral Manipulation, ed. 4. Edinburgh, Scotland, Elsevier, 2005.
Maitland, G, et al (eds): Maitland's Vertebral Manipulation, ed. 7. Edinburgh, Scotland, Elsevier, 2005.

Contraindications to Mobilization/Manipulation

Protective spasm
Medically unstable

Suspected joint hypermobility or instability
Malignancy in treatment region
Cauda equina syndrome
Bowel and bladder dysfunction
Fracture in treatment region
Vertebral basilar insufficiency
Joint ankylosis
Bone disease detectable on radiograph such as osteomyelitis and Paget's
   disease
Osteoporosis
Rheumatoid arthritis
Neurological changes
Radiological changes
Condition made worse by treatment

Massage Terminology

Massage

The definitions and categories given below are by no means universal. *Note:*
Massage strokes are listed in order of increasing vigor.

stroking (effleurage): Passing of the hands over a large body area with constant
   pressure.

superficial effleurage: Extremely light form, using palms of hands, described
   as little more than a caress.

deep effleurage: Strong enough stroking to evoke a mechanical as well as
   reflex effect on muscles.

compression: Use of intermittent pressure to lift, roll, press, squeeze, and
   stretch tissue and to hasten venous and lymphatic flow.

kneading (petrissage): Hands take a large fold of skin and underlying tissue
   and forcefully roll, raise, and squeeze it.

pinching (placement): Pinching using thumb and index finger.

rolling (roulement): Rolling of muscle belly.

wringing: Like twisting dry a wet towel.

fulling: Rippling of deeper muscle caused by asynchronous movement of hands.

fist kneading: Compression via knuckles of a partially closed fist.

digital kneading: Use of a single finger or three fingers positioned triangu-
   larly.

friction: Firm contact over a limited area to loosen adherent tissue.

crushing (ecrasement): Localized and vigorous.

tearing (dilaceration): Intense deep pressure, like connective tissue massage.

pleating (pleissate): Ends of finger perpendicular to veins.

sawing (sciage): Rapid and deep transverse movement of the ulnar border.

come-and-go: Reciprocal movement of the two index fingers or the thumbs.

vibration and shaking: Hands are kept in contact with the patient, and movement originates with the therapist's body and is transmitted to the patient
   via the therapist's outstretched arms. Shaking (secousses) is characterized
   by the alternate flexion and extension of the therapist's elbows, whereas in
   vibration the elbows remain fully extended.

point vibration: Use of a single digit.

percussion: Brief, brisk, rapid contacts reciprocally applied with relaxed wrists.

tapping (tapotement): Rapid series of blows, hands parallel and partially flexed, with the ulnar borders of the hand striking the patient. Sometimes *tapping* is used to describe percussion with the fingertips.

hammering (martelage): Soft percussion with the ulnar edges of the hand of the slightly flexed last four fingers, so that the little finger strikes first.

clapping (claquement): Use of fingers, palm, and thumb to form a concave surface.

hacking (hachure): Chopping strokes made by the ulnar surface hitting the patient; more vigorous than tapping.

beating (frappement): Striking with half-closed fists so that the ulnar side of the hand makes contact.

Soft Tissue Mobilization Techniques

bending: The muscle belly is held by approximating both thumb and index fingers in a triangular shape. Alternating compressive and distractive forces are applied to the muscle belly working toward the tendinous insertion.

C-stroke: While stabilizing with one hand, the index, middle, and ring fingers (interphalangeals flexed) of the other hand draw the skin away in a C fashion.

clearing: A rhythmical, rolling stroke, with successively increasing pressure. This technique is typically applied using the fingertips, movements of which are coordinated with the patient's expirations.

cross-fiber (a.k.a. deep friction or transverse friction): Deep pressure applied perpendicularly to muscle tendon, ligament, or fascia using fingertips.

deep perpendicular: With two middle fingers held together overlapping the index fingers, the therapist starts at the lateral border of the muscle and pushes toward the muscle belly while maintaining pressure.

distraction: Stretching of soft tissue using both hands to mobilize a joint or bony segment of the body.

forearm inhibition (a.k.a. cross hands technique): Proximal one-third of forearm is slowly swept longitudinally or laterally across the muscle in a repetitive motion. Strokes are typically synchronized with the patient's expirations when applied to the paraspinal musculature. Neuromuscular technique that incorporates stress relaxation to promote connective tissue changes.

inhibitive kneading: Using both hands with fingertips slightly flexed on either side of the muscle belly, the therapist alternately applies upward and downward rolling pressure.

release: Application of slow, firm, and deep pressure across a muscle belly using fingertips of one hand (or one hand placed over the other). Pressure is often held for an extended period.

skin rolling: Fingertips of both hands are placed in a V pattern with both thumbs and index fingers touching. The thumbs are gently but firmly pushed toward the index fingers, rolling the superficial skin layers toward the index fingers. This technique is typically applied to lumbar paraspinal muscles.

sweep: Sweeping motion with applied pressure along the length of a muscle held in either a stretched or shortened position. Contact is made by either the thumb, fingers (either singularly or in combination), knuckles, or forearm.

Orthopedic Conditions

Fractures

Salter's Fracture Classification

According to Salter, to describe a fracture completely, you must identify the site, extent, configuration, relationship of the fracture fragments to each other, the relationship of the fracture fragments to the external environment, and the presence or absence of complications.

Site

Classification. Diaphyseal, metaphyseal, epiphyseal, or intraarticular. A dislocation occurring in conjunction with a fracture is a fracture dislocation.

Extent

Classification. Complete or incomplete. Types of incomplete fractures are crack, hairline, buckle, and greenstick.

Configuration

Classification. Complete fractures can have a transverse, oblique, or spiral arrangement. If there are more than two fragments, the fracture is a comminuted fracture.

Relationship of the Fracture Fragments to Each Other

Classification. Fragments can be either displaced or nondisplaced. When the fragments are displaced, they can be shifted sideways, angulated, rotated, distracted, overriding, or impacted.

Relationship of the Fracture Fragments to the External Environment

Classification. Closed or open. A closed fracture is one in which the skin in the area of the fracture is intact. An open fracture is one in which the skin in the area of the fracture is not intact. The fracture fragment may have penetrated the skin, or an object may have penetrated the skin to cause the fracture. Closed fractures are also called *simple fractures* and open fractures are also called *compound fractures*.

Complications

Classification. Complicated or uncomplicated. A complicated fracture is one that results in either a local or systemic complication due to the fracture or the treatment of the fracture. An uncomplicated fracture is one that does not immediately result in a local or systemic complication and heals uneventfully.

Based on:

Salter, RB: *Textbook of Disorders and Injuries of the Musculoskeletal System*, ed. 3. Baltimore, Williams & Wilkins, 1999, pp 419–422.

Types of Fractures

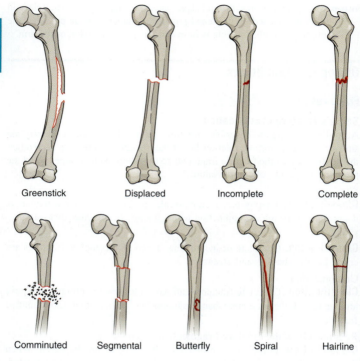

Greenstick Displaced Incomplete Complete

Comminuted Segmental Butterfly Spiral Hairline

Clinical Prediction Rules for Identification of Fractures

Ottawa Ankle Rules

- An ankle x-ray is required if there is pain in the malleolar zone AND any of the following:
  - Bone tenderness along the distal 6 cm of the posterior edge of the tibia or tip of the medial malleolus
  - Bone tenderness along the distal 6 cm of the posterior edge of the fibula or tip of the lateral malleolus
  - An inability to bear weight both immediately and in the emergency department for four steps

Ottawa Foot Rules

- A foot x-ray series is indicated if there is bony pain in the midfoot AND either:
  - Bone tenderness at the base of the fifth metatarsal or at the navicular bone
  - An inability to bear weight both immediately and in the emergency department for four steps.

Classification of Epiphyseal Plate Injuries

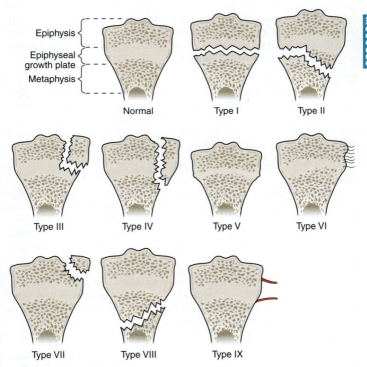

Epiphyseal Plate Injuries.

Types I through V were originally described by Salter and Harris and are referred to as the Salter-Harris Classification of Epiphyseal Plate Injuries.

Type I
Complete separation of the epiphysis from the metaphysis without fracture of the bone. Type I injuries are usually caused by shear forces and are most common in newborns (birth injuries) and young children. Closed reduction is not difficult, and the prognosis is excellent, provided that the blood supply to the epiphysis is intact.

Type II
The line of separation extends a variable distance along the epiphyseal plate and then out through the metaphysis to produce a triangular fragment. Type II injuries are the most common type of epiphyseal fracture and occur as a result of shearing and bending forces. These injuries tend to occur in the older child. Closed reduction is relatively easy to maintain. The prognosis for growth is excellent, provided that blood supply to the plate is intact.

Type III

Intra-articular fracture extending from the joint surface to the deep zone of the epiphyseal plate and then along the plate to the periphery. Type III injuries are uncommon. They are caused by an intra-articular shearing force and are usually limited to the distal epiphysis. Open reduction is usually necessary. The prognosis for growth is good, provided that the blood supply to the separated portion of the epiphysis has not been disrupted.

Type IV

An intra-articular fracture extending from the joint surface through the epiphysis, across the entire thickness of the plate, and through a portion of the metaphysis. Type IV injuries are commonly seen as fractures of the lateral condyle of the humerus. Except for undisplaced fractures, open reduction and internal skeletal fixation are necessary. Perfect reduction is necessary for a favorable prognosis of restored bone growth.

Type V

An uncommon injury that results from a severe crushing force applied through the epiphysis to one area of the plate. Type V injuries are most common in the ankle or the knee, resulting from a severe abduction or adduction injury to the joint. Weight-bearing must be avoided for 3 weeks in the hopes of preventing the almost inevitable premature cessation of growth. Prognosis for bone growth is usually poor.

Rang's Type VI

A rare injury resulting from damage to the periosteum or perichondral ring. Type VI injuries can be caused by direct blows or deep lacerations from sharp objects. Because a local bony bridge tends to form across the growth plate, the prognosis for subsequent growth is poor.

Ogden's Types VII, VIII, and IX

Three perichondral fractures do not directly damage the physis. They may subsequently disrupt the physeal blood supply and result in growth disturbances. Type VII is an osteochondral fracture of the articular portion of the epiphysis. Type VIII is a fracture of the metaphysis. Type IX is an avulsion fracture of the periosteum.

TABLE 3.32 Contribution of the Epiphyses to Bone Growth

Bone	Proximal End (%)	Distal End (%)
Femur	30	70
Fibula	60	40
Humerus	80	20
Radius	25	75
Tibia	55	45
Ulna	20	80

From Rang, M: *The Growth Plate and Its Disorders*. Williams & Wilkins, Baltimore, 1969.

Scoliosis

Systems Used to Measure Curves
Cobb Method

Upper end-vertebra for thoracic curve (highest vertebra with superior border inclined toward thoracic concavity)

Transitional vertebra (lowest vertebra with inferior border inclined toward thoracic concavity and highest vertebra with superior border inclined toward lumbar concavity

Lower end-vertebra for lumbar curve (lowest vertebra with inferior border inclined toward lumbar concavity)

A line is drawn perpendicular to the upper margin of the vertebra that inclines most toward the concavity. A line is also drawn on the inferior border of the lower vertebra with greatest angulation toward the concavity. The angle formed by these intersecting lines is the measure of curvature. The apical vertebra is also usually noted.

Risser-Ferguson Method

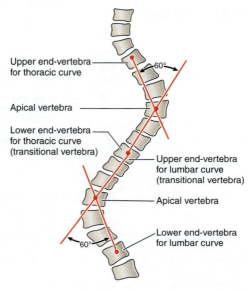

The midpoints of the proximal, distal, and apical vertebrae of the curvature are identified. The proximal vertebra is the highest vertebra whose superior surface tilts to the concavity of the curve. The distal vertebra is the lowest vertebra whose inferior surface tilts to the concavity of the curve. The apical vertebra is between the proximal and distal vertebrae and is parallel to the horizontal or transverse plane of the body. The angle formed by the two lines that intersect the apex from the proximal and distal midpoints is the measure of the curvature. The method is still used but is no longer accepted internationally.

Classification of Scoliotic Curves

Classifications of curves has been standardized by the Scoliosis Research Society. Their system bases the classification into seven groups, depending on the angle obtained by the Cobb method.

Group I:	0°–20°
Group II:	21°–30°
Group III:	31°–50°
Group IV:	51°–75°
Group V:	76°–100°
Group VI:	101°–125°
Group VII:	126° or greater

Nash-Moe Method of Measuring the Rotation of the Vertebrae

Vertebral rotation is measured by estimating the amount the pedicles of the vertebrae have rotated as seen on an anteroposterior radiograph.

Measurement of rotation

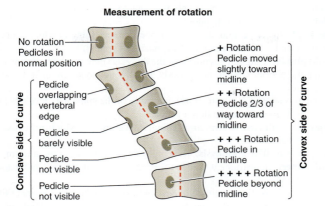

No rotation
Pedicles in
normal position

\+ Rotation
Pedicle moved
slightly toward
midline

Concave side of curve

Pedicle
overlapping
vertebral
edge

\+ + Rotation
Pedicle 2/3 of
way toward
midline

Pedicle
barely visible

\+ + + Rotation
Pedicle in
midline

Pedicle
not visible

\+ + + + Rotation
Pedicle beyond
midline

Pedicle
not visible

Convex side of curve

Glossary of Scoliosis Terms

adolescent scoliosis: Spinal curvature presenting at or about the onset of puberty and before maturity.

adult scoliosis: Spinal curvature existing after skeletal maturity.

angle of thoracic inclination: With the trunk flexed 90° at the hips, this is the angle between the horizontal plane and a plane across the posterior rib cage at the greatest prominence of a rib hump.

apical vertebra: The most rotated vertebra in a curve; the most deviated vertebra from the vertical axis of the patient.

body alignment, balance, compensation: (1) The alignment of the midpoint of the occiput over the sacrum in the same vertical plane as the shoulders over the hips. (2) In roentgenology, when the sum of the angular deviations of the spine in one direction is equal to that in the opposite direction.

café au lait spots: Light brown, irregular areas of skin pigmentation. If they are sufficient in number and have smooth margins, they suggest neurofibromatosis.

compensatory curve: A curve, which can be structural, above or below a major curve that tends to maintain normal body alignment.

congenital scoliosis: Scoliosis due to congenitally anomalous vertebral development.

curve measurement: Cobb method: Select the upper- and lower-end vertebrae. Erect lines perpendicular to their transverse axes. They intersect to form the angle of the curve. If the vertebral end plates are poorly visualized, a line through the bottom or top of the pedicles may be used.

double major scoliosis: Scoliosis with two structural curves.

double thoracic curves (scoliosis): Two structural curves within the thoracic spine.

end vertebra: (1) The most cephalad vertebra of a curve, whose superior surface tilts maximally toward the concavity of the curve. (2) The most

MUSCULO

caudad vertebra, whose inferior surface tilts maximally toward the concavity of the curve.

fractional curve: A compensatory curve that is incomplete because it returns to the erect position. Its only horizontal vertebra is its caudad or cephalad one.

full curve: A curve in which the only horizontal vertebra is at the apex.

gibbus: A sharply angular kyphos.

hyperkyphosis: A sagittal alignment of the thoracic spine in which there is more than the normal amount of kyphosis (a kyphos).

hypokyphosis: A sagittal alignment of the thoracic spine in which there is less than the normal amount of kyphosis, but it is not so severe as to be truly lordotic.

hysterical scoliosis: A nonstructural deformity of the spine that develops as a manifestation of a conversion reaction.

idiopathic scoliosis: A structural spinal curvature for which no cause is established.

iliac epiphysis, iliac apophysis: The epiphysis along the wing of an ilium.

inclinometer: An instrument used to measure the angle of thoracic inclination or rib hump.

infantile scoliosis: Spinal curvature developing during the first 3 years of life.

juvenile scoliosis: Spinal curvature developing between the skeletal age of 3 years and the onset of puberty.

kyphos: A change in alignment of a segment of the spine in the sagittal plane that increases the posterior convex angulation; an abnormally increased kyphosis.

kyphoscoliosis: A spine with scoliosis and a true hyperkyphosis. A rotatory deformity with only apparent kyphosis should not be described by this term.

kyphosing scoliosis: A scoliosis with marked rotation such that lateral bending of the rotated spine mimics kyphosis.

lordoscoliosis: A scoliosis associated with an abnormal anterior angulation in the sagittal plane.

major curve: Term used to designate the largest structural curve.

minor curve: Term used to refer to the smallest curve, which is always more flexible than the major curve.

nonstructural curve: A curve that has no structural component and that corrects or overcorrects on recumbent side-bending roentgenograms.

pelvic obliquity: Deviation of the pelvis from the horizontal in the frontal plane. Fixed pelvic obliquities can be attributable to contractures either above or below the pelvis.

primary curve: The first or earliest of several curves to appear, if identifiable.

rotational prominence: In the forward-bending position, the thoracic prominence on one side is usually due to vertebral rotation, causing rib prominence. In the lumbar spine, the prominence is usually due to rotation of the lumbar vertebrae.

skeletal age, bone age: The age obtained by comparing an anteroposterior roentgenogram of the left hand and wrist with the standards of the Greulich and Pyle Atlas.

structural curve: A segment of the spine with a lateral curvature that lacks normal flexibility. Radiographically, it is identified by the complete lack of a curve on a supine film or by the failure to demonstrate complete segmental mobility on supine side-bending films.

vertebral end plates: The superior and inferior plates of cortical bone of the vertebral body adjacent to the intervertebral disc.

vertebral growth plate: The cartilaginous surface covering the top and bottom of a vertebral body, which is responsible for the linear growth of the vertebra.

vertebral ring apophyses: The most reliable index of vertebral immaturity, seen best in lateral roentgenograms or in the lumbar region in side-bending anteroposterior views.

From:

Greulich, WW, and Pyle SI: *Atlas of the Development of the Hand and Wrist, ed 2. Stanford University Press, Stanford, CA, 1959.*

Winter, RB: *Classification and terminology. In Lonstein, JE, et al: Moe's Textbook of Scoliosis and Other Spinal Deformities, ed. 3. WB Saunders, Philadelphia, 1995, pp 41–42.*

Metabolic Bone Diseases

TABLE 3.33 Examples of Metabolic Bone Diseases

Disease	Pathophysiology	Drug Treatment
Hypoparathyroidism	Decreased parathyroid hormone secretion; leads to impaired bone resorption and hypocalcemia	Calcium supplements, vitamin D
Hyperparathyroidism	Increased parathyroid hormone secretion; usually caused by parathyroid tumors; leads to excessive bone resorption and hypercalcemia	Usually treated surgically by partial or complete resection of parathyroid gland
Osteoporosis	Generalized bone demineralization; often associated with effects of aging and hormonal changes in postmenopausal women	Calcium supplements, vitamin D, calcitonin, bisphosphonates, intermittent parathyroid hormone, estrogen, or selective estrogen receptor modulators (raloxifene)
Rickets	Impaired bone mineralization in children caused by a deficiency of vitamin D	Calcium supplements, vitamin D
Osteomalacia	Adult form of rickets	Calcium supplements, vitamin D

(table continues on page 168)

TABLE 3.33 Examples of Metabolic Bone Diseases (continued)

Disease	Pathophysiology	Drug Treatment
Paget disease	Excessive bone formation and resorption (turnover); leads to ineffective remodeling and structural abnormalities within the bone	Calcitonin, bisphosphonates
Renal osteodystrophy	Chronic renal failure; induces complex metabolic changes resulting in excessive bone resorption	Vitamin D, calcium supplements
Gaucher disease	Excessive lipid storage in bone leads to impaired remodeling and excessive bone loss	No drugs are effective
Hypercalcemia of malignancy	Many forms of cancer accelerate bone resorption, leading to hypercalcemia.	Calcitonin, bisphosphonates

From Ciccone, CD: *Pharmacology in Rehabilitation, ed.* 4. FA Davis, Philadelphia, 2007, p 467, with permission.

Rheumatoid Arthritis

TABLE 3.34 Criteria for the Classification of Rheumatoid Arthritis

The 1987 Revised Criteria for Classification of Rheumatoid Arthritis Traditional Format

Criterion	Definition
1. Morning stiffness	Morning stiffness in and around the joints lasting at least 1 hr before maximal improvement.
2. Arthritis of three or more joints	At least three joint areas have simultaneously had soft tissue areas' swelling or fluid (not bony overgrowth alone) observed by a physician. The 14 possible joint areas are right or left PIP, MCP, wrist, elbow, knee, ankle, and MTP joints.
3. Arthritis of hand joints	At least one joint area swollen as joints above in a wrist, MCP, or PIP.
4. Symmetric arthritis	Simultaneous involvement of the same joint areas (as in no. 2) on both sides of the body (bilateral involvement of PIPs, MCPs, or MTPs is acceptable without absolute symmetry).

Criterion	Definition
5. Rheumatoid nodules	Subcutaneous nodules, over bony prominences, or extensor surfaces, or in juxta-articular regions, observed by a physician.
6. Serum rheumatoid factor	Demonstration of abnormal amounts of serum "rheumatoid factor" by any method that has been positive in 5% of normal control subjects.
7. Radiological changes	Radiological changes typical of rheumatoid arthritis on PA hand and wrist roentgenograms, which must include erosions or unequivocal bony decalcification localized to or most marked adjacent to the involved joints (osteoarthritis changes alone do not qualify).

From Arnett, FC, et al: The American Rheumatological Association 1987 revised criteria for the classification of rheumatoid arthritis. *Arthritis & Rheum* 31:315, 1988.

For classification purposes, a patient shall be said to have rheumatoid arthritis if he/she has satisfied at least four of the above seven criteria. Criteria 1–4 must have been present for at least 6 weeks. Patients with two clinical diagnoses are not excluded. Designation as "classic," "definite," or "probable" rheumatoid arthritis is not to be made.

MCPs = metacarpophalangeal joints, MTP = metatarsophalangeal joints, PA = posteroanterior, PIPs = proximal interphalangeal joints.

TABLE 3.35 Classification of Rheumatoid Arthritis by Functional Capacity

Class	Functional Capacity
Class I	Completely able to perform usual activities of daily living (self-care, vocational, and avocational)
Class II	Able to perform usual self-care and vocational activities, but limited in avocational activities
Class III	Able to perform usual self-care activities, but limited in vocational and avocational activities
Class IV	Limited in ability to perform usual self-care, vocational, and avocational activities

From Hochberg, MC, et al: The American College of Rheumatology 1991 revised criteria for the classification of global functional status in rheumatoid arthritis. *Arthritis & Rheum* 35:498, 1992.

MUSCULO

● TABLE 3.36 Classification of Rheumatoid Arthritis by Stages of Progression

Stage I, Early
†1. No destructive changes on roentgenographic examination.
2. Roentgenologic evidence of osteoporosis may be present.

Stage II, Moderate
†1. Roentgenologic evidence of osteoporosis, with or without slight subchondral bone destruction; slight cartilage destruction may be present.
†2. No joint deformities, although limitation of joint mobility may be present.
3. Adjacent muscle atrophy.
4. Extra-articular soft-tissue lesions, such as nodules and tenosynovitis, may be present.

Stage III, Severe
†1. Roentgenologic evidence of cartilage and bone destruction, in addition to osteoporosis.
†2. Joint deformity, such as subluxation, ulnar deviation, or hyperextension, without fibrous or bony ankylosis.
3. Extensive muscle atrophy.
4. Extra-articular soft-tissue lesions, such as nodules and tenosynovitis, may be present.

Stage IV, Terminal
†1. Fibrous or bony ankylosis.
2. Criteria of stage III.

From *Primer on the Rheumatic Diseases*, ed. 10. Arthritis Foundation, Atlanta, 1993.
†The criteria prefaced by daggers are those that must be present to permit classification of a patient in any particular stage or grade.

Drugs Commonly Used in Treatment of Rheumatoid Arthritis

● TABLE 3.37 Drug Categories Used in Rheumatoid Arthritis

I. Nonsteroidal Anti-Inflammatory Drugs	
Aspirin (many trade names)	Ketoprofen (Orudis, others)
Celecoxib (Celebrex)*	Meclofenamate (Meclomen)
Diclofenac (Cataflam, Voltaren)	Nabumetone (Relafen)
Diflunisal (Dolobid)	Naproxen (Anaprox, Naprosyn)
Fenoprofen (Nalfon)	Oxaprozin (Daypro)

Flurbiprofen (Ansaid)	Piroxicam (Feldene)
Ibuprofen (many trade names)	Sulindac (Clinoril)
Indomethacin (Indocin)	Tolmetin (Tolectin)

II. Corticosteroids

Betamethasone (Celestone)	Methylprednisolone (Medrol, others)
Cortisone (Cortone acetate)	Prednisolone (Prelone, others)
Dexamethasone (Decadron, others)	Prednisone (Deltasone, others)
Hydrocortisone (Cortef, others)	Triamcinolone (Aristocort, others)

III. Disease-Modifying Antirheumatic Drugs

Adalimumab (Humira)	Etanercept (Enbrel)
Anakinra (Kineret)	Gold sodium thiomalate (Myochrysine)
Auranofin (Ridaura)	Hydroxychloroquine (Plaquenil)
Aurothioglucose (Solganal)	Infkiximab (Remicade)
Azathioprine (Imuran)	Leflunomide (Arava)
Chloroquine (Aralen)	Methotrexate (Rheumatrex, others)
Cyclophosphamide (Cytoxan)	Penicillamine (Cuprimine Depen)
Cyclosporine (Neoral, Sandimmune)	Sulfasalazine (Azulfidine)

From Ciccone, CD: *Pharmacology in Rehabilitation*, ed. 4. FA Davis, Philadelphia, 2007, p 219, with permission.
*Subclassified as cyclooxygenase type 2 (COX-2) inhibitors

TABLE 3.38 Disease-Modifying Antirheumatic Drugs

Drug	Trade Name	Usual Dosage	Special Considerations
Anakinra	Kineret	Subcutaneous injection: 100 mg/day.	Can be used alone or with other antiarthritic agents, but should not be used with tumor necrosis factor.

(table continues on page 172)

● **TABLE 3.38 Disease-Modifying Antirheumatic Drugs** (continued)

Drug	Trade Name	Usual Dosage	Special Considerations
Antimalarials			
Chloroquine	Aralen	Oral: Up to 4 mg/kg of lean body weight per day.	Periodic ophthalmic exams recommended to check for retinal toxicity.
Hydroxychloroquine	Plaquenil	Oral: Up to 6.5 mg/kg of lean body weight per day.	Similar to chloroquine.
Azathioprine	Imuran	Oral: 1 mg/kg body weight per day; can be increased after 6–8 wk up to maximum dose of 2.5 mg/kg body weight.	Relatively high toxicity; should be used cautiously in debilitated patients or patients with renal disease.
Cyclophosphamide	Cytoxan	Oral: 1.5–2mg/kg body weight per day; can be increased to a maximum dose of 3 mg/kg body weight.	Long-term use is limited because of potential for carcinogenicity
Cyclosporine	Neoral, Sandim-mune	Oral: 2.5 mg/kg body weight per day; can be increased after 8 wk by 0.5–0.75 mg/kg body weight per day. Dose can be increased after another 4 wk to a maximum daily dose of 4 mg/kg body weight per day.	May cause nephro-toxicity and gastrointestinal problems.

MUSCULO

Drug	Trade Name	Usual Dosage	Special Considerations
Gold Compounds			
Auranofin	Ridaura	Oral: 6 mg one each day or 3 mg bid.	May have a long latency (6–9 mo) before onset of benefits.
Aurothioglucose	Solganal	Intramuscular: 10 mg the 1st wk, 25 mg the 2nd and 3rd wk, then 25–50 mg each wk until total dose of 1 g. Mainte-nance doses of 25–50 mg every 2–4 wk can follow.	Effects occur somewhat sooner than oral gold, but still has long delay (4 mo).
Gold sodium thiomalate	Myochrysine	Similar to aurothioglucose.	Similar to auro-thioglucose.
Leflunomide	Arava	Oral: 100 mg/day for the first 3 days; continue with a maintenance dose of 20 mg/day thereafter.	May decrease joint erosion and destruction with relatively few side effects during long-term use; effects of long-term use remain to be determined.
Methotrexate	Rheumatrex, others	Oral: 2.5–5 mg every 12 h for total of 3 doses/wk or 10 mg once each week. Can be increased up to a maximum of 20–25 mg/wk.	Often effective in halting joint destruction, but long-term use limited by toxicity.
Penicillamine	Cuprimine, Depen	Oral: 125 or 250 mg/day; can be increased to a maximum of 1.5 g/day.	Relatively high incidence of toxicity with long-term use.

(table continues on page 174)

MUSCULO

● **TABLE 3.38** **Disease-Modifying Antirheumatic Drugs** (continued)

Drug	Trade Name	Usual Dosage	Special Considerations
Sulfasalazine	Azulfidine	Oral: 0.5–1.0 g/day for the first week; dose can be increased by 500 mg each week up to a maximum daily dose of 2–3 g/day.	Relatively high toxicity; may produce serious hypersensitivity reactions and blood dyscrasias.
Tumor Necrosis Factor Inhibitors			
Adalimumab	Humira	Subcutaneous injection: 40 mg every week if used alone; 40 mg every other week if used in combination with other antiarthritic agents such as methotrexate.	Relatively low incidence of serious side effects compared to other immunosuppressants.
Etanercept	Enbrel	Subcutaneous injection: 25 mg twice each day.	Relatively low incidence of side effects compared with other immunosuppressants.
Infliximab	Remicade	Slow intravenous infusion: 3 mg/kg body weight. Additional doses at 2 and 6 wk after first infusion, then every 8 wk thereafter.	Should be administered in combination with methotrexate.

From Ciccone, CD: *Pharmacology in Rehabilitation*, ed. 4. FA Davis, Philadelphia, 2007, pp 223–224, with permission.

MUSCULO

Osteoarthritis

Clinical Classification Criteria for Hip Osteoarthritis

Hip internal rotation greater than or equal to 15° with pain; morning stiffness less than or equal to 60 minutes; and age greater than 50 years, and pain on internal rotation, or

Hip pain and hip internal rotation less than 15°, and hip flexion less than 115°

From:

Altman, R et al: The American College of Rheumatology criteria for the classification and reporting of osteoarthritis of the hip. Arthritis Rheum 34:505–514, 1991.

Clinical Classification Criteria for Knee Osteoarthritis

Knee pain
Joint stiffness less than or equal to 30 minutes
Crepitus
Bony enlargement
Bony tenderness
No palpable warmth

From:

Altman, R et al: Development of criteria for the classification and reporting of osteoarthritis. Classification of osteoarthritis of the knee. Diagnostic and Therapeutic Criteria Committee of the American Rheumatism Association. Arthritis Rheum 29:1039–1049, 1986.

Kellgren-Lawrence Criteria for Osteoarthritis

Grade 0: normal radiograph
Grade 1: doubtful narrowing of the joint space and possible osteophytic lipping
Grade 2: definite osteophytes, definite narrowing of the joint space
Grade 3: moderate multiple osteophytes, definite narrowing of the joint space, some sclerosis, and possible deformity of bone contour
Grade 4: large osteophytes, marked narrowing of joint space, severe sclerosis, and definite bony deformity

From:

Kellgren, JH, and Lawrence, JS: Atlas of Standard Radiographs: The Epidemiology of Chronic Rheumatism, vol 2. Blackwell Scientific, Oxford, England, 1963.

TABLE 3.39 Common Nonsteroidal Anti-Inflammatory Drugs (NSAIDs)

Generic Name	Trade Name(s)	Specific Comments— Comparisons to Other NSAIDs
Aspirin	Many trade names	Most widely used NSAID for analgesic and anti-inflammatory effects; also used frequently for antipyretic and anticoagulant effects.
Diclofenac	Voltaren Dolobid	Substantially more potent than naproxen and several other NSAIDs; adverse side effects occur in 20% of patients.

(table continues on page 176)

TABLE 3.39 Common Nonsteroidal Anti-Inflammatory Drugs (NSAIDs) (continued)

Generic Name	Trade Name(s)	Specific Comments—Comparisons to Other NSAIDs
Diflunisal		Has potency 3–4 times greater than aspirin in terms of analgesic and anti-inflammatory effects but lacks antipyretic activity.
Etodolac	Lodine	Effective as analgesic/anti-inflammatory agent with fewer side effects than most NSAIDs; may have gastric-sparing properties.
Fenoprofen	Nalfon	GI side effects fairly common but usually less intense than those occurring with similar doses of aspirin.
Flurbiprofen	Ansaid	Similar to aspirin's benefits and side effects; also available as topical ophthalmic preparation (Ocufen).
Ibuprofen	Motrin, many others	First nonaspirin NSAID also available in nonprescription form; fewer GI side effects than aspirin but GI effects still occur in 5%–15% of patients.
Indomethacin	Indocin	Relative high incidence of dose-related side effects; problems occur in 25%–50% of patients.
Ketoprofen	Orudis, Oruvail, others	Similar to aspirin's benefits and side effects but has relatively short half-life (1–2 hr).
Ketorolac	Toradol	Can be administered orally or by intramuscular injection; parenteral doses provide postoperative analgesia equivalent to opioids.
Meclofenamate	Meclomen	No apparent advantages or disadvantages compared to aspirin and other NSAIDs.
Mefenamic acid	Ponstel	No advantages; often less effective and more toxic than aspirin and other NSAIDs.

MUSCULO

Generic Name	Trade Name(s)	Specific Comments—Comparisons to Other NSAIDs
Nabumetone	Relafen	Effective as analgesic/anti-inflammatory agent with fewer side effects than most NSAIDs.
Naproxen	Anaprox, Naprosyn, others	Similar to ibuprofen in terms of benefits and adverse effects.
Oxaprozin	Daypro	Analgesic and anti-inflammatory effects similar to aspirin; may produce fewer side effects than other NSAIDs.
Phenylbutazone	Cotylbutazone	Potent anti-inflammatory effects but long-term use limited by high incidence of side effects (10%–45% of patients).
Piroxicam	Feldene	Long half-life (45 hr) allows once-daily dosing; may be somewhat better tolerated than aspirin.
Sulindac	Clinoril	Relatively little effect on kidneys (renal-sparing), but may produce more GI side effects than aspirin.
Tolmetin	Tolectin	Similar to aspirin's benefits and side effects but must be given frequently (qid) because of short half-life (1 hr).

From Ciccone, CD: *Pharmacology in Rehabilitation*, ed. 4. FA Davis, Philadelphia, 2007, pp 207–208, with permission.

TABLE 3.40 Dosages of Common Nonsteroidal Anti-Inflammatory Drugs (NSAIDs)

Classes	Analgesia	Anti-inflammation
Aspirin (many trade names)	325–650 mg every 4 hr	3.6–5.4 g/day in divided doses
Diclofenac (Voltaren)	Up to 100 mg for the first dose; then up to 50 mg tid thereafter	Initially: 150–200 mg/day in 3–4 divided doses; try to reduce to 75–100 mg/day in 3 divided doses

(table continues on page 178)

TABLE 3.40   Dosages of Common Nonsteroidal Anti-Inflammatory Drugs (NSAIDs) (continued)

Classes	Analgesia	Anti-inflammation
Diflunisal (Dolobid)	1 g initially; 500 mg every 8–12 hr as needed	250–500 mg bid
Etodolac (Lodine)	400 mg initially; 200–400 mg every 6–8 hr as needed	400 mg bid or tid or 300 mg tid or qid; total daily dose is typically 600–1,200 mg/day
Fenoprofen (Nalfon)	200 mg every 4–6 hr	300–600 mg tid or qid
Flurbiprofen (Ansaid)	—	200–300 mg/day in 2–4 divided doses
Ibuprofen (Advil, Motrin, Nuprin, others)	200–400 mg every 4–6 hr as needed	1.2–3.2 g/day in 3–4 divided doses
Indomethacin (Indocin)	—	25–50 mg 2–4 times each day initially; can be increased up to 200 mg/day as tolerated
Ketoprofen (Orudis)	25–50 mg every 6–8 hr	150–300 mg/day in 3–4 divided doses
Meclofenamate (Meclomen)	50 mg every 4–6 hr	200–400 mg/day in 3–4 divided doses
Mefenamic acid (Ponstel)	500 mg initially; 250 mg every 6 hr as needed	—
Nambutone (Relafen)	—	Initially: 1,000 mg/day in a single dose or 2 divided doses; can be increased to 1,500–2,000 mg/day in 2 divided doses if needed
Naproxen (Naprosyn)	500 mg initially; 250 mg every 6–8 hr	250, 375, or 500 mg bid
Naproxen sodium (Aleve, Anaprox, others)	500–650 mg initially; 275 mg every 6–8 hr	275 or 550 mg bid

MUSCULO

Classes	Analgesia	Anti-inflammation
Oxaprozin (Daypro)	—	Initially: 1,200 mg/day, then adjust to patient tolerance
Phenylbutazone (Butazolidin, Cotylbutazone)	—	300–600 mg/day in 3–4 divided doses initially; reduce as tolerated to lowest effective dose
Piroxicam (Feldene)	—	20 mg/day single dose; or 10 mg bid
Sulindac (Clinoril)	—	150 or 200 mg bid
Tolmetin (Tolectin)	—	400 mg tid initially; 600 mg–1.8 g/day in 3–4 divided doses

From Ciccone, CD: *Pharmacology in Rehabilitation*, ed. 4. FA Davis, Philadelphia, 2007, pp 208–209, with permission.

Cervical Spine

Criteria for Classification Into the Cervical Syndromes According to McKenzie

The following describes the common findings associated with each syndrome. Information usually obtained during the history is listed first, followed by the information obtained during the physical examination (which consists of assessing posture in sitting and standing, movement loss, and the use of repeated movements).

Postural Syndrome

History
- Patients are usually 30 years of age or younger.
- Patients frequently have sedentary occupations.
- Local pain that is always intermittent (can be in cervical, thoracic, and lumbar regions simultaneously).
- Pain ceases with movement and activity.
- Pain produced with static loading only (sitting, standing, or lying).
- No pain with movement or activity.
- Posture correction abolishes pain.

Physical Examination
- Poor sitting or standing posture.
- No loss of motion is noted.
- All repeated movements are pain free.
- Pain cannot be reproduced with repeated movements. The patient must assume and maintain a static position to expose the pain.

Dysfunction Syndrome

History

- Patients tend to be older than 30 years of age.
- Dysfunctions are named by the direction(s) of movement that are painfully limited.
- Time is a factor; must be at least 6 to 8 weeks since onset of low back pain.
- Causes of dysfunctions can include, but not limited to, previous surgery, mechanical low back pain, trauma, years of poor posture, or degenerative changes.
- Intermittent local pain that is felt at the end-range of a certain movement, either protrusion, flexion, retraction, extension, rotation, or side bending.
- Pain will be produced in the upper extremity in the presence of an adherent nerve root.
- Pain does not last once patient is off end-range.
- Rapid changes in symptoms or range of motion does not occur.
- Consistent reproduction of pain with certain movements (flexion, extension, and rarely rotation or side bending).
- Patients often feel better when active and moving as long as movement does not achieve end-range or with movement that keeps the spine in midrange.

Physical Examination

- The sitting posture is fair to poor.
- A loss of movement is present in the direction of the dysfunction.
- Pain is reproduced with repeated movements in the direction of the dysfunction.
- Pain is elicited as soon as the end-range of limited movement is reached, but the pain ceases when the patient returns to the neutral position.
- Patients who have an adherent nerve root will have pain reproduced in the upper extremity only when the upper extremity is in a position of dural tension and symptoms increase with flexion or contralateral bending of the cervical spine.

Derangement Syndromes

History for All Derangement Syndromes

- Patients are likely to be between 20 and 55 years of age. However, the age can fall outside of this range.
- Derangements may arise from a single incident, sustained postures, or for no identifiable reason.
- Pain may be felt adjacent to the midline of the spine and may refer distally into the upper extremity in the form of pain or paresthesia.
- Patients with derangement syndromes can have constant/intermittent pain that varies in intensity, frequency, or duration, whereas patients with postural and dysfunction syndromes always have intermittent pain.
- Varied clinical presentation typically responds to dynamic or static loading strategies.
- Pain is usually worse when the patient assumes certain postures/positions.
- Pain is often increased when patients are in the sitting position.
- Patients can have difficulty finding a comfortable sleeping position.
- Patients have a loss of movement that can occur in more than one plane of movement.

- Deformity may be present (wry neck or kyphotic).
- Patients often have a history of recurring episodes of cervical pain.
- Centralization of symptoms occurs *only* in derangement syndromes.
- Repeated movements can have a rapid effect on the condition. If a patient with derangement describes changes in the pain pattern after repeated movements, there should also be observable changes in range of motion and deformity (if present) which corresponds to the symptomatic changes.
- Symptoms are changed as a result of the repeated movements.

MUSCULO

History and Physical Examination for Central/Symmetrical (Previously Derangement One)
- Central or symmetrical symptoms occur around the lower cervical spine.
- Sometimes symptoms radiate to the shoulders or scapula.
- Gross loss of movement may occur and extension is limited.

History and Physical Examination for Central/Symmetrical With Kyphotic Deformity (Previously Derangement Two)
- Central or symmetrical symptoms occur around the lower cervical spine.
- Symptoms may radiate bilaterally into the arms.
- Extension is majorly limited.
- Deformity of kyphosis (protruded head) occurs.

History and Physical Examination for Unilateral/Asymmetrical Above the Elbow Without Deformity (Previously Derangement Three)
- Unilateral or asymmetrical symptoms occur in the neck.
- Symptoms occur with or without radiating pain into the scapula, shoulder, or upper arm.
- No deformity (wry neck) is present.
- Loss of range of motion in extension may have minor loss of flexion and possible asymmetric loss of side bending and/or rotation.

History and Physical Examination for Unilateral/Asymmetrical Above the Elbow With Deformity (Previously Derangement Four)
- Unilateral or asymmetrical symptoms occur in the neck.
- Symptoms occur with or without radiating pain into the scapula, shoulder, or upper arm.
- Wry neck deformity is present. Deformity of flexion, lateral flexion, rotation, or a combination is present can be toward or away from the side of pain.
- Loss of range of motion in extension, loss of flexion and asymmetric loss of side bending and/or rotation.
- This is relatively rare.

History and Physical Examination for Unilateral/Asymmetrical Below the Elbow Without Deformity (Previously Derangement Five)
- Unilateral or asymmetrical symptoms occur in the neck.
- Symptoms (pain and/or paresthesia) occur in the forearm that may be accompanied by pain in the shoulder, scapula arm, and neck regions.
- No deformity (wry neck) is present.
- Loss of range of motion in extension, may have minor loss of flexion and possible asymmetric loss of side bending and/or rotation.

History and Physical Examination for Unilateral/Asymmetrical Below the Elbow With Deformity (Previously Derangement Six)

- Unilateral or asymmetrical symptoms occur in the neck.
- Symptoms (pain, and/or paresthesia) occur the forearm that may be accompanied by pain in the shoulder, scapula arm, and neck regions.
- Wry neck deformity is present in one plane or a combination of lateral and sagittal. This can be fixed in protrusion or a combination of lateral bending and rotation.
- Constant radicular symptoms with neurological deficit are often present.
- Loss of range of motion in extension, may have minor loss of flexion and possible asymmetric loss of side bending and/or rotation.

History and Physical Examination for Symmetrical or Assymmetrical Above the Elbow (Previously Derangement Seven)

- Symmetrical or asymmetrical cervical pain occurs with or without symptoms above the elbow.
- The patient may have symptoms in the anterior neck region and difficulty swallowing.
- There will be a gross loss of flexion, but the patient may have full extension.
- The condition is rapidly reversible.
- Presentation is rare.

Quebec Classification of Whiplash-Associated Disorders

TABLE 3.41 Quebec Classification of Whiplash-Associated Disorders

Grade	Clinical Presentation
0	No complaints about the neck No physical signs
I	Neck complaint of pain, stiffness, or tenderness only No physical signs
II	Neck compaint AND Musculoskeltetal signs, such as decreased range of motion and point tenderness
III	Neck complaint AND Neurological signs, such as decreased or absent deep tendon reflexes, weakness, and sensory deficits
IV	Neck complaint AND Fracture or dislocation

Based on:

Scientific monograph of the Quebec task force on whiplash-associated disorders: Redefining "whiplash" and its management. Spine 20(8), 1995.

Low Back

Criteria for Classification Into the Lumbar Syndromes According to McKenzie

The following describes the common findings associated with each syndrome. Information usually obtained during the history is listed first, followed by the information obtained during the physical examination (which consists of assessing posture in sitting and standing, movement loss, and the use of repeated movements).

Postural Syndrome

History

- Patients are usually 30 years of age or younger.
- Patients frequently have sedentary occupations.
- Local pain is present that is always intermittent (can be in cervical, thoracic, and lumbar regions simultaneously).
- Pain ceases with movement and activity.
- Pain is produced with static loading only (sitting, standing, or lying).
- No pain is experienced with movement or activity.
- Posture correction abolishes pain.

Physical Examination

- Poor sitting or standing posture.
- No loss of motion is noted.
- All repeated movements are pain free.
- Pain cannot be reproduced with repeated movements. The patient must assume and maintain a static position to expose the pain.

Dysfunction Syndrome

History

- Patients tend to be older than 30 years of age.
- Dysfunctions are named by the direction(s) of movement that are painfully limited.
- Time is a factor; there must be at least 6 to 8 weeks since onset of low back pain.
- Causes of dysfunctions can include, but are not limited to, previous surgery, mechanical low back pain, trauma, years of poor posture, or degenerative changes.
- Intermittent local pain is present that is felt at the end-range of a certain movement, either flexion, extension, or side gliding.
- Pain will be produced in the lower extremity in the presence of an adherent nerve root.
- Pain does not last once patient is off end-range.
- Rapid changes in symptoms or range of motion does not occur.
- Consistent reproduction of pain occurs with certain movements (flexion, extension, and rarely, side gliding).
- Patients often feel better when active and moving as long as the movements do not achieve end-range or with movements that keep the spine in midrange.

MUSCULO

Physical Examination
- The sitting posture is fair to poor.
- A loss of movement is present in the direction of the dysfunction.
- Patients who have an adherent nerve root may laterally deviate during flexion toward the painful side.
- Pain is reproduced with repeated movements in the direction of the dysfunction.
- Pain is elicited as soon as the end-range of limited movement is reached, but the pain ceases when the patient returns to the neutral position.
- Patients who have an adherent nerve root will have pain reproduced in the lower extremity with flexion in standing but not with flexion in lying.

Derangement Syndromes

History for All Derangement Syndromes
- Patients are likely to be between 20 and 55 years of age. The age range can fall outside of this range.
- Derangements may arise from a single incident, sustained postures, or for no identifiable reason.
- Pain may be felt adjacent to the midline of the spine and may refer distally into the lower extremity in the form of pain or paresthesia.
- Patients with derangement syndromes can have constant/intermittent pain that varies in intensity, frequency, or duration, whereas patients with postural and dysfunction syndromes always have intermittent pain.
- Varied clinical presentations typically respond to dynamic or static loading strategies.
- Pain is usually worse when the patient assumes certain postures/positions.
- Pain is often increased when patients are in the sitting position.
- Patients can have difficulty finding a comfortable sleeping position.
- Patients have a loss of movement that can be in more than one plane of movement.
- Deformity may be present (lateral shift, kyphotic, or lordotic).
- During the assessment of sagittal pain movements (flexion and extension), the patient's trunk may deviate to one side.
- Patients often have a history of recurring episodes of low back pain.
- Centralization of symptoms occurs *only* in derangement syndromes.
- Repeated movements can have a rapid effect on the condition. If a patient with derangement describes changes in the pain pattern after repeated movements, there should also be observable changes in range of motion and deformity (if present) that corresponds to the symptomatic changes.
- Symptoms are changed as a result of the repeated movements.

History and Physical Examination for Central or Symmetrical (Previously Derangement One)
- Central or symmetrical low back pain is present.
- Patients may have radiating symptoms bilaterally into both buttocks equally.
- Patients rarely have radiating symptoms bilaterally down both thighs and legs (considered symmetrical symptoms as long as symptoms are relatively equal in both extremities).
- Gross loss of movement may occur and extension is limited.
- The lumbar lordosis is reduced without any deformity.

History and Physical Examination for Central or Symmetrical With Kyphotic Deformity (Previously Derangement Two)
- Central or symmetrical low back pain is present.
- Patients may have radiating symptoms bilaterally into both buttocks equally.
- Patients rarely have radiating symptoms bilaterally down both thighs and legs (considered symmetrical symptoms as long as symptoms are relatively equal in both extremities).
- Extension is majorly limited and the patient is unable to stand fully erect.
- Deformity of kyphosis is present.

History and Physical Examination for Unilateral or Asymmetrical Above the Knee Without Deformity (Previously Derangement Three)
- Unilateral or asymmetrical low back pain is present.
- Unilateral or asymmetrical buttock and/or thigh pain may be present.
- No deformity (i.e., a lateral shift, reduced, or accentuated lumbar lordosis) is present.

History and Physical Examination for Unilateral or Asymmetrical Above the Knee With Deformity (Previously Derangement Four)
- Unilateral or asymmetrical low back pain is present.
- Unilateral or asymmetrical buttock and/or thigh pain may be present.
- A lateral shift deformity is present while the patient is standing (either toward or away from the side of pain).
- Often a loss of the lumbar lordosis is present. There is a loss of extension and sidegliding.

History and Physical Examination for Unilateral or Asymmetrical Below the Knee Without Deformity (Previously Derangement Five)
- Unilateral or asymmetrical low back pain is present.
- Intermittent or constant pain extends into the calf with or without neurological signs.
- No deformity (i.e., a lateral shift,) is present.
- Extension is limited and may have an asymmetrical loss of sidegliding.

History and Physical Examination for Unilateral or Asymmetrical Below the Knee With Deformity (Previously Derangement Six)
- Unilateral or asymmetrical low back pain is present.
- Usually constant pain or paresthesia extending into the calf is present.
- A lateral shift deformity (toward or away from pain) is present with a reduced lumbar lordosis.
- Neurological deficit is often present.
- May have gross loss of range of motion in flexion, extension, and sidegliding.

History and Physical Examination for Symmetrical or Assymmetrical Above the Knee (Previously Derangement Seven)
- Symmetrical or asymmetrical low back pain is present.
- Asymmetrical buttock and/or anterior thigh pain may be present.
- Lordotic deformity is present.
- Gross loss of flexion, extension may be full.
- The condition is rapidly reversible.

MUSCULO

Treatment-Based Classification of Delitto and Colleagues

A proposed classification system for persons with acute low back pain and acute exacerbations of low back pain was proposed by Delitto, Erhard, and Bowling in 1995 and has undergone further testing and revision. After screening for red flags, information from the history and examination is used to classify patients into one of four treatment-based categories. The following criteria for the proposed categories are based on Fritz, Cleland, and Childs, 2007.

Lumbosacral Manipulation

- Duration of symptoms less than 16 days
- At least one hip with internal rotation of greater than 35°
- Lumbar hypomobility
- No symptoms distal to the knee
- Fear Avoidance Beliefs Questionnaire, Work Subscale Score Less Than 19

Stabilization Exercises

- Positive prone instability test
- Aberrant motion present during lumbar flexion/extension
- Average straight leg raise (>91°)
- Age younger than 40 years
- Postpartum with positive posterior pelvic pain provocation, active straight leg raise and modified Trendelenburg tests, pain provocation with palpation of the long dorsal sacroiliac ligament or pubic symphysis

Specific Exercises

Extension

- Symptoms distal to the buttocks
- Symptoms centralize with lumbar extension
- Symptoms peripheralize with lumbar flexion
- Directional preference for extension

Flexion

- Age older than 50 years
- Directional preference for flexion
- Imaging evidence of lumbar spinal stenosis

Lateral Shift

- Visible frontal plane deviation of the shoulders relative to the pelvis
- Directional preference for lateral translation movements of the pelvis

Traction

- Signs and symptoms of nerve root compression
- No movements centralize symptoms

Clinical Prediction Rules for Persons With Low Back Pain Related to the Classification Scheme of Delitto and Colleagues

Clinical prediction rule for success with spinal manipulation

- Criterion 50% improvement in Oswestry score in 1 week
  - Duration of symptoms less than 16 days
  - At least one hip with internal rotation of greater than 35°
  - Lumbar hypomobility
  - No symptoms distal to the knee
  - Fear Avoidance Beliefs Questionnaire, Work Subscale score less than 19

- Four of five factors present positive likelihood ratio = 24.4
- Three factors present positive likelihood ratio = 2.6

Clinical prediction rule for success with lumbar stabilization exercises

- Criterion 50% improvement in Oswestry score after 8 weeks of exercise
  - Positive prone instability test
  - Aberrant motion present
  - Average straight leg raise (greater than 91°)
  - Age younger than 40 years
- Three of four factors present positive likelihood ratio = 4.0

Waddell's Nonorganic Physical Signs in Low Back Pain

tenderness: Tenderness not related to a particular skeletal or neuromuscular structure, may be either superficial or nonanatomic.

   superficial: The skin is tender to light pinch over a wide area of lumbar skin not in a distribution associated with a posterior primary ramus.

   nonanatomic: Deep tenderness, which is not localized to one structure, is felt over a wide area and often extends to the thoracic spine, sacrum, or pelvis.

simulation tests: These tests give the patient the impression that a particular examination is being carried out when in fact it is not.

   axial loading: Low back pain is reported when the examiner presses down on the top of the patient's head. Neck pain is common and should not be considered indicative of a nonorganic sign.

   rotation: Back pain is reported when the shoulders and pelvis are passively rotated in the same plane as the patient stands relaxed with the feet together. In the presence of root irritation, leg pain may be produced and should not be considered indicative of a nonorganic sign.

distraction tests: A positive physical finding is demonstrated in the routine manner; this finding is then checked while the patient's attention is distracted. A nonorganic component may be present if the finding disappears when the patient is distracted.

   straight leg raising: The examiner lifts the patient's foot as when testing the plantar reflex in the sitting position. A nonorganic component may be present if the leg is lifted higher than when tested in the supine position.

regional disturbances: Dysfunction (e.g., sensory or motor) involving a widespread region of body parts in a manner that cannot be explained based on anatomy. Care must be taken to distinguish from multiple nerve root involvement.

   weakness: Demonstrated on testing by a partial cogwheel "giving way" of many muscle groups that cannot be explained on a localized neurologic basis.

   sensory: Include diminished sensation to light touch, pinprick, or other neurological tests fitting a "stocking" rather than a dermatomal pattern.

overreaction: May take the form of disproportionate verbalization, facial expression, muscle tension and tremor, collapsing, or sweating. Judgments should be made with caution, minimizing the examiner's own emotional reaction.

Scoring. Any individual sign counts as a positive sign for that type; a finding of three or more of the five types is clinically significant.

Based on:
Waddell, G, et al: Nonorganic physical signs in low-back pain. Spine 5:117, 1980.

MUSCULO

TABLE 3.42 Quebec Task Force Classification of Activity-Related Spinal Disorders

Classification	Symptoms	Duration of Symptoms From Onset	Working Status at Time of Evaluation
1	Pain without radiation	a (<7 day)	
2	Pain + radiation to extremity, proximally	b (7 d–7 wk)	W (working)
3	Pain + radiation to extremity, distally*	c (>7 wk)}	I (idle)
4	Pain + radiation to upper/lower limb neurological signs		
5	Presumptive compression of a spinal nerve root on a simple roentgenogram (i.e., spinal instability or fracture)		
6	Compression of a spinal nerve root confirmed by Specific imaging techniques (i.e., computerized axial tomography, myelography, or magnetic resonance imaging) Other diagnostic techniques (e.g., electromyography, venography)		
7	Spinal stenosis		
8	Postsurgical status, 1–6 mo after intervention		
9	Postsurgical status, >6 mo after intervention		
	9.1 Asymptomatic		
	9.2 Symptomatic		

Classification	Symptoms	Duration of Symptoms From Onset	Working Status at Time of Evaluation
10	Chronic pain syndrome		W (working)
11	Other diagnoses		I (idle)

Based on Quebec Task Force on Spinal Disorders: Scientific approach to the assessment and management of activity-related spinal disorders; a monograph for clinicians. Report of the Quebec Task Force on Spinal Disorders. *Spine* 12:S17, 1987.
*Not applicable to the thoracic segment.

Warning Signs ("Red Flags") to Guide in Assessment of Acute Low Back Problems in Adults

According to Clinical Practice Guideline No. 14 of the Agency for Health Care Policy and Research

Red flags are indicators of potentially serious pathology. The identification of red flags indicates the need for additional inquiry or investigations.

TABLE 3.43 Assessment of Acute Low Back Pain

Red Flag	Reason Information Is Important
Past history of: Cancer Unexplained weight loss Immunosuppression IV drug use Urinary infection Pain increasing with rest	Indications of possible cancer or infections
Presence of fever	Indications of possible cancer or infections
Presence of bladder dysfunction	Indication of cauda equina syndrome
Presence of saddle anaesthesia	Indication of cauda equina syndrome
Presence of major weakness in the limb of the lower extremity	Indication of cauda equina syndrome
Trauma that could have caused a fracture, taking into account consideration of the patient's age and likelihood of having osteoporosis	Avoidance of delays in diagnosing possible fracture

MUSCULO

Spondylolisthesis

A forward displacement of one vertebral body over another usually occurs as a result of a defect of the pars interarticularis. It is evaluated on a lateral radiograph and the amount of forward slippage is graded from the posterior edge of the superior vertebral body to the posterior edge of the adjacent inferior vertebral body. This distance is then reported as a percentage of the total superior vertebral body length:

Grade 1 is 0%–25%
Grade 2 is 25%–50%
Grade 3 is 50%–75%
Grade 4 is 75%–100%

Pain

Pain From Viscera

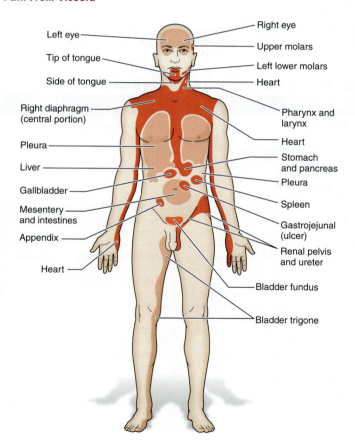

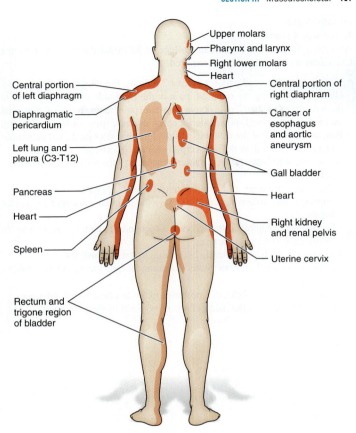

Upper molars

Pharynx and larynx

Right lower molars

Heart

Central portion of left diaphragm

Central portion of right diaphram

Diaphragmatic pericardium

Cancer of esophagus and aortic aneurysm

Left lung and pleura (C3-T12)

Gall bladder

Pancreas

Heart

Heart

Right kidney and renal pelvis

Spleen

Uterine cervix

Rectum and trigone region of bladder

Fibromyalgia

Diagnostic Criteria

According to the 1990 American College of Rheumatology Criteria for the Classification the following are required:

- History of widespread pain for at least 3 months. For pain to be widespread, all of the following are required: pain in the right side of the body, pain in the left side of the body, pain above the waist, pain below the waist, and axial skeletal pain (cervical spine, anterior chest, thoracic spine, or low back pain).
- Pain in at least 11 of the following 18 tender-point sites on digital palpation:
  - Occiput: Bilateral, at the suboccipital muscle insertions
  - Low cervical: Bilateral, at the anterior aspects of the intertransverse spaces at C5–C7
  - Trapezius: Bilateral, at the midpoint of the upper border
  - Supraspinatus: Bilateral, at origins above the scapular spine near the medial border
  - Second rib: Bilateral, at the second costochondral junctions, just lateral to the junctions on upper surfaces
  - Lateral epicondyle: Bilateral, 2 cm distal to the epicondyles
  - Gluteal: Bilateral, in upper outer quadrants of buttocks in anterior fold of muscle
  - Greater trochanter: Bilateral, posterior to the trochanteric prominence
  - Knees: Bilateral, at the medial fat pad proximal to the joint line

NEUROMUSCULAR

NEURO

NEURO

Neuroanatomy

The Brain

Lateral View—Major Areas by Function

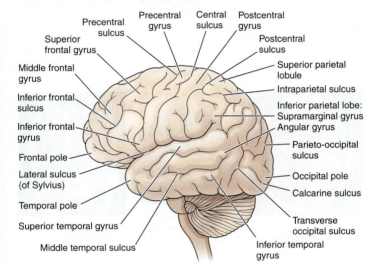

Lateral View—Major Gyri and Sulci

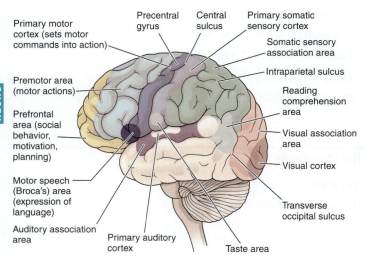

- Primary motor cortex (sets motor commands into action)
- Precentral gyrus
- Central sulcus
- Primary somatic sensory cortex
- Somatic sensory association area
- Intraparietal sulcus
- Premotor area (motor actions)
- Reading comprehension area
- Prefrontal area (social behavior, motivation, planning)
- Visual association area
- Visual cortex
- Motor speech (Broca's) area (expression of language)
- Transverse occipital sulcus
- Auditory association area
- Primary auditory cortex
- Taste area

Cortical Areas by Function

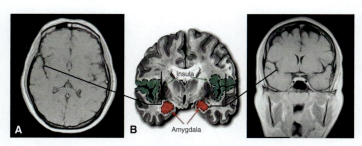

Two views: **(A)** horizontal section and **(B)** tranverse section with amygdala and insula identified, of deep brain structures oriented to identifications of amygdala.

Cortical Gyri and Sulci

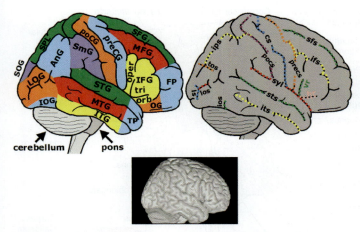

NEURO

Right lateral views of brain (upper) with gyrus and key structures labeled.

SFG: superior frontal gyrus
FP: frontal pole
MFG: middle frontal gyrus
preCG: precentral gyrus
poCG: postcentral gyrus
IFG: inferior frontal gyrus
SMG: supplemental motor gyrus
SPL: splenius
ANG: angularis
SOG: superior occipital gyrus
LOG: lateral occipital gyrus
IOG: inferior occipital gyrus
STG, MTG, ITG: superior, middle, inferior temporal gyrus
OG: orbital gyrus
ORB: orbitofrontal cortex
Oper: pars opercularis

Left Sagittal View—Brain

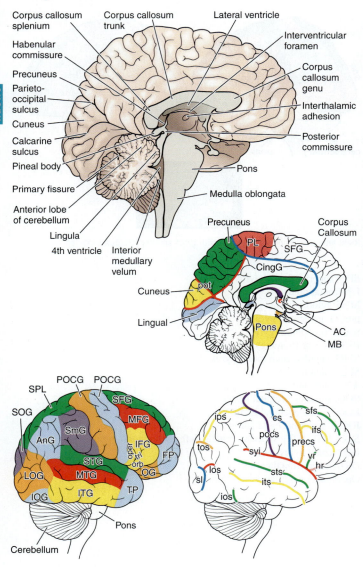

Corpus callosum splenium
Corpus callosum trunk
Lateral ventricle
Interventricular foramen
Habenular commissure
Corpus callosum genu
Precuneus
Parieto-occipital sulcus
Interthalamic adhesion
Cuneus
Posterior commissure
Calcarine sulcus
Pineal body
Pons
Primary fissure
Medulla oblongata
Anterior lobe of cerebellum
Lingula
4th ventricle
Interior medullary velum

Precuneus
Corpus Callosum
PL
SFG
CingG
Cuneus
pot
Lingual
Pons
AC
MB

SPL
POCG
POCG
SOG
SFG
MFG
SmG
AnG
IFG
oper
tri
FP
STG
orb
OG
LOG
MTG
IOG
ITG
T-P
Pons
Cerebellum

ips
cs
sfs
tos
pocs
precs
ifs
syl
vr
los
sts
hr
sl
its
ios

Left Sagittal View—Neuroimage

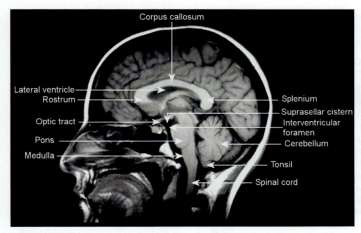

Left sagittal view of brain and brainstem.

Brain and Cranial Nerves—Inferior View

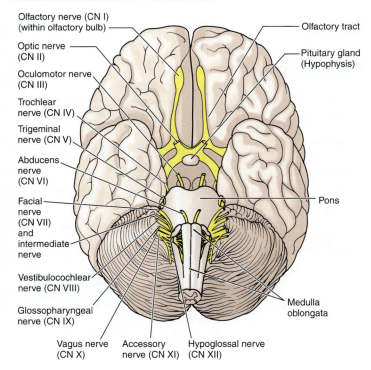

NEURO

NEURO

Brainstem Cranial Nerve—Anterior View

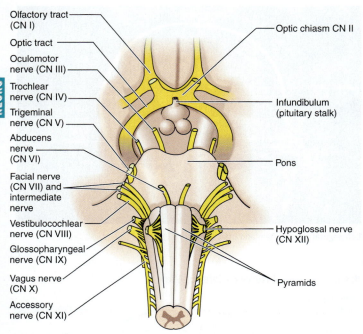

Olfactory tract (CN I)

Optic tract

Oculomotor nerve (CN III)

Trochlear nerve (CN IV)

Trigeminal nerve (CN V)

Abducens nerve (CN VI)

Facial nerve (CN VII) and intermediate nerve

Vestibulocochlear nerve (CN VIII)

Glossopharyngeal nerve (CN IX)

Vagus nerve (CN X)

Accessory nerve (CN XI)

Optic chiasm CN II

Infundibulum (pituitary stalk)

Pons

Hypoglossal nerve (CN XII)

Pyramids

Posterolateral View of Brainstem

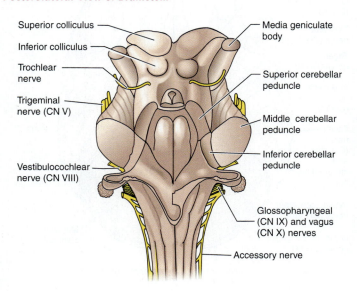

Superior colliculus

Inferior colliculus

Trochlear nerve

Trigeminal nerve (CN V)

Vestibulocochlear nerve (CN VIII)

Media geniculate body

Superior cerebellar peduncle

Middle cerebellar peduncle

Inferior cerebellar peduncle

Glossopharyngeal (CN IX) and vagus (CN X) nerves

Accessory nerve

Transverse Section Through Brain

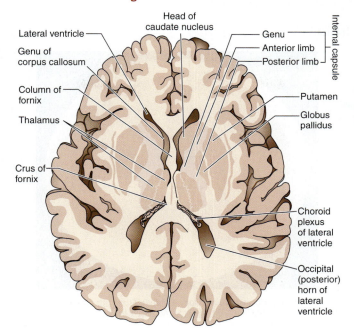

Lateral ventricle

Genu of corpus callosum

Column of fornix

Thalamus

Crus of fornix

Head of caudate nucleus

Genu
Anterior limb
Posterior limb

Internal capsule

Putamen

Globus pallidus

NEURO

Choroid plexus of lateral ventricle

Occipital (posterior) horn of lateral ventricle

Transverse Section Through Brain, Neuroimage

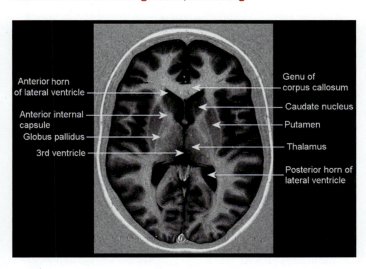

Anterior horn of lateral ventricle

Anterior internal capsule

Globus pallidus

3rd ventricle

Genu of corpus callosum

Caudate nucleus

Putamen

Thalamus

Posterior horn of lateral ventricle

Spinal Cord Cross Sections

Cervical

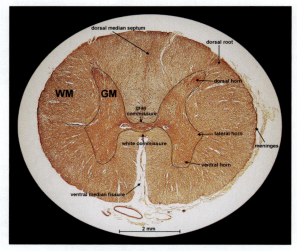

(A) Cervical spinal cord colorized histology (Rorden). From: http://www.microscopy-uk.org.uk/mag/imgapr03/HistPaper03_Fig2.jpg. Accessed April 10, 2010.

Lumbar

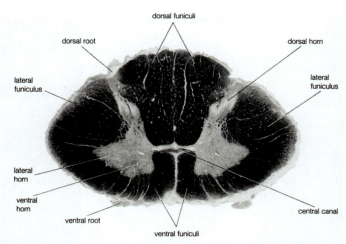

(B) Cross section of lumbar spinal cord delineating gray and white matter structures. From: http://cache-media.britannica.com/eb-media/75/2975-050-0D5D3A36.jpg. Accessed April 10, 2010.

Primary Motor/Sensory Cortex

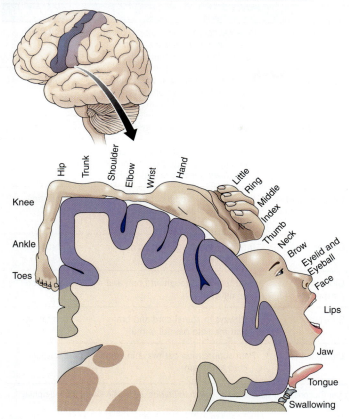

Humunculus depicting representative primary and sensory motor areas.

NEURO

■ TABLE 4.1 **Central Neurotransmitters**

Transmitter	Primary CNS Location	General Effect
Acetylcholine	Cerebral cortex (many areas); basal ganglia; limbic and thalamic regions; spinal interneurons	Excitation
Norepinephrine	Neurons originating in brainstem and hypothalamus that project throughout other areas of brain	Inhibition
Dopamine	Basal ganglia; limbic system	Inhibition
Serotonin	Neurons originating in brainstem that project upward (to hypothalamus) and downward (to spinal cord)	Inhibition
GABA = gamma-aminobutyric acid.	Interneurons throughout the spinal cord, cerebellum, basal ganglia, cerebral cortex	Inhibition
Glycine	Interneurons in spinal cord and brainstem	Inhibition
Glutamate, aspartate	Interneurons throughout brain and spinal cord	Excitation
Substance P	Pathways in spinal cord and brain that mediate painful stimuli	Excitation
Enkephalins	Pain suppression pathways in spinal cord and brain	Excitation

From: Ciccone, C: *Pharmacology in Rehabilitation,* ed. 4. FA Davis, Philadelphia, 2007, p 58.

NEURO

View of External Carotid Artery Branching

NEURO

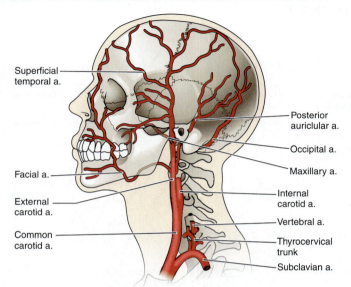

Arteries of the Head and Neck

Superficial temporal a.

Facial a.

External carotid a.

Common carotid a.

Posterior auriclular a.

Occipital a.

Maxillary a.

Internal carotid a.

Vertebral a.

Thyrocervical trunk

Subclavian a.

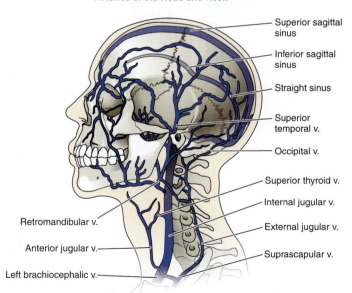

Veins of the Head and Neck

Superior sagittal sinus

Inferior sagittal sinus

Straight sinus

Superior temporal v.

Occipital v.

Superior thyroid v.

Internal jugular v.

External jugular v.

Suprascapular v.

Retromandibular v.

Anterior jugular v.

Left brachiocephalic v.

NEURO

Blood Supply to Brain and Brainstem Including Inferior View of Circle of Willis

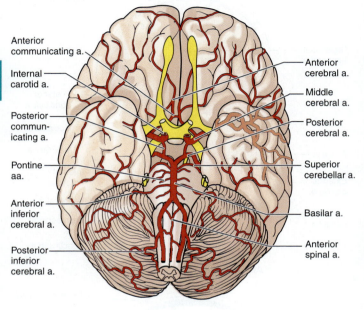

Anterior communicating a.

Internal carotid a.

Posterior communicating a.

Pontine aa.

Anterior inferior cerebral a.

Posterior inferior cerebral a.

Anterior cerebral a.

Middle cerebral a.

Posterior cerebral a.

Superior cerebellar a.

Basilar a.

Anterior spinal a.

Brainstem With Blood Supply

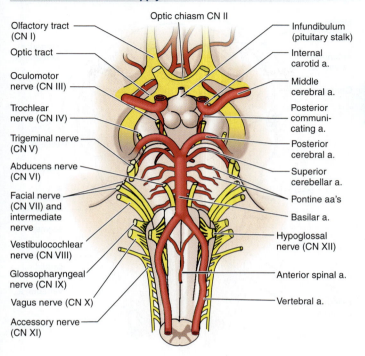

Olfactory tract (CN I)

Optic tract

Oculomotor nerve (CN III)

Trochlear nerve (CN IV)

Trigeminal nerve (CN V)

Abducens nerve (CN VI)

Facial nerve (CN VII) and intermediate nerve

Vestibulocochlear nerve (CN VIII)

Glossopharyngeal nerve (CN IX)

Vagus nerve (CN X)

Accessory nerve (CN XI)

Optic chiasm CN II

Infundibulum (pituitary stalk)

Internal carotid a.

Middle cerebral a.

Posterior communicating a.

Posterior cerebral a.

Superior cerebellar a.

Pontine aa's

Basilar a.

Hypoglossal nerve (CN XII)

Anterior spinal a.

Vertebral a.

NEURO

Orientation of Major Cerebral Vessels

NEURO

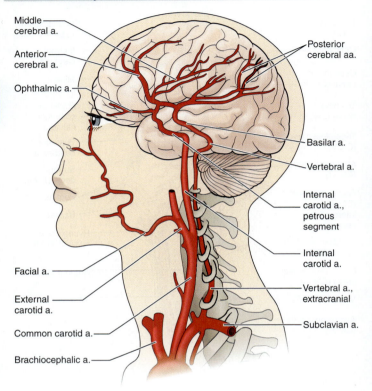

Middle cerebral a.

Anterior cerebral a.

Ophthalmic a.

Posterior cerebral aa.

Basilar a.

Vertebral a.

Internal carotid a., petrous segment

Internal carotid a.

Facial a.

External carotid a.

Vertebral a., extracranial

Common carotid a.

Subclavian a.

Brachiocephalic a.

Cutaneous Innervation: Dermatome and Peripheral Nerve Distribution—Anterior (left) and Posterior (right) View

NEURO

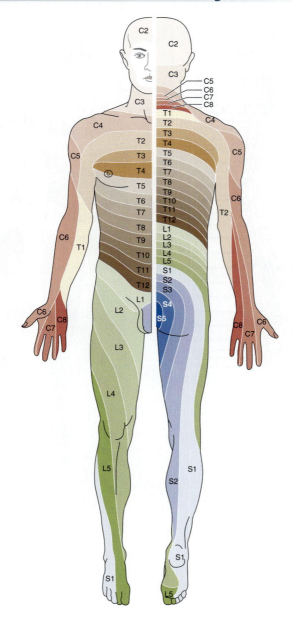

The Relationship Between the Spinal Cord and Key Anatomic/Dermatomal Landmarks

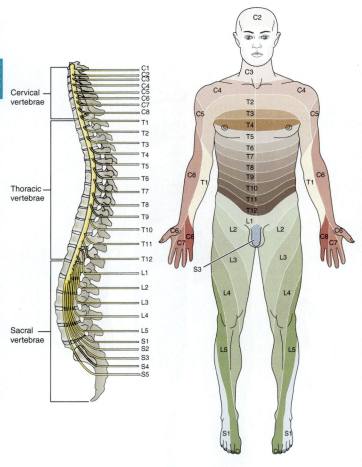

Cervical vertebrae

Thoracic vertebrae

Sacral vertebrae

Autonomic Nervous System

NEURO

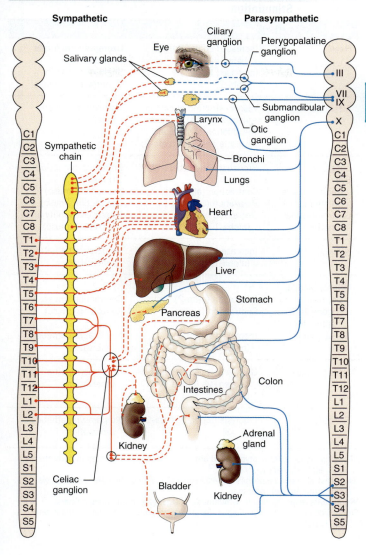

Sympathetic   **Parasympathetic**

Ciliary ganglion

Eye

Salivary glands

Pterygopalatine ganglion

III

VII
IX

Submandibular ganglion

Otic ganglion

Larynx

Sympathetic chain

Bronchi

Lungs

X

C1
C2
C3
C4
C5
C6
C7
C8

Heart

T1
T2
T3
T4
T5

Liver

T6
T7
T8
T9
T10

Stomach

Pancreas

T11
T12
L1
L2
L3
L4
L5

Intestines

Colon

S1
S2
S3
S4
S5

Kidney

Adrenal gland

Celiac ganglion

Bladder

Kidney

C1
C2
C3
C4
C5
C6
C7
C8
T1
T2
T3
T4
T5
T6
T7
T8
T9
T10
T11
T12
L1
L2
L3
L4
L5
S1
S2
S3
S4
S5

NEURO

■ TABLE 4.2 Response Of Effector Organs To Autonomic Stimulation

Organ	Sympathetic*	Parasympathetc†
Heart	Increased contractility (beta-1, -2) Increased heart rate (beta-1, -2)	Decreased heart rate (musc) Slight decrease in contractility (musc)
Arterioles	Vasoconstriction of skin and viscera (alpha-1, -2) Vasodilation of skeletal muscle and liver (beta-2)	No parasympathetic innervation
Lung	Bronchodilation (beta-2)	Bronchoconstriction (musc)
Eye		
Radial muscle	Contraction (alpha-1)	Relaxation (musc)
Ciliary muscle	Relaxation (beta-2)	Contraction (musc)
Gastrointestinal function	Decreased motility (alpha-1, -2; beta-1, -2)	Increased motility and secretion (musc)
Kidney	Increased renin secretion (alpha-1, beta-1)	No parasympathetic innervation
Urinary bladder		
Detrusor	Relaxation (beta-2)	Contraction (musc)
Trigone and sphincter	Contraction (alpha-1)	Relaxation (musc)
Sweat glands	Increased secretion (musc‡)	No parasympathetic innervation
Liver	Glycogenolysis and gluco-neogenesis (alpha-1, beta-2)	No parasympathetic innervation
Fat cells	Lipolysis (alpha-2, beta-1, -2, -3)	No parasympathetic innervation

*The primary receptor subtypes mediating each response are listed in parentheses (e.g., alpha-1, beta-2).
†Note that all organ responses to parasympathetic stimulation are mediated via muscarinic (musc) receptors.
‡Represents response due to sympathetic postganglionic cholinergic fibers.
From: Ciccone, C: *Pharmacology in Rehabilitation,* ed. 4. FA Davis, Philadelphia, 2007, p 255.

TABLE 4.3 Autonomic Receptor Locations and Responses

Receptor	Primary Location(s)	Response*
Cholinergic		
Nicotinic	Autonomic ganglia	Mediate transmission to postganglionic neuron
Muscarinic	All parasympathetic effector cells:	
	Visceral and bronchiole smooth muscle	Contraction (generally)
	Cardiac muscle	Decreased heart rate
	Exocrine glands (salivary, intestinal, lacrimal)	Increased secretion
	Sweat glands	Increased secretion
Adrenergic		
Alpha-1	Vascular smooth muscle	Contraction
	Intestinal smooth muscle	Relaxation
	Radial muscle iris	Contraction (mydriasis)
	Ureters	Increased motility
	Urinary sphincter	Contraction
	Spleen capsule	Contraction
Alpha-2	CNS inhibitory synapses	Decreased sympathetic discharge from CNS
	Presynaptic terminal at peripheral adrenergic synapses	Decreased norepinephrine release
	Gastrointestinal tract	Decreased motility and secretion
	Pancreatic islet cells	Decreased insulin secretion
Beta-1	Cardiac muscle	Increased heart rate and contractility
	Kidney	Increased renin secretion
	Fat cells	Increased lipolysis
Beta-2	Bronchiole smooth muscle	Relaxation (bronchodilation)
	Some arterioles (skeletal muscle, liver)	Vasodilation
	Gastrointestinal smooth muscle	Decreased motility
	Skeletal muscle and liver cells	Increased cellular metabolism
	Uterus	Relaxation
	Gallbladder	Relaxation

*CNS = Central nervous system.
From: Ciccone, C: *Pharmacology in Rehabilitation,* ed. 4. FA Davis, Philadelphia, 2007, p 259.

NEURO

◗ TABLE 4.4 Summary of Adrenergic Agonist/Antagonist Use According To Receptor Specificity

Primary Receptor Location: Response When Stimulated	Agonist Use(s)*	Antagonist Use(s)*
Alpha-1 Receptor Vascular smooth muscle: vasoconstriction	Hypotension Nasal congestion Paroxysmal supraventricular tachycardia	Hypertension
Alpha-2 Receptor CNS synapses (inhibitory)	Hypertension Spasticity	No significant clinical use
Beta-1 Receptor Heart: increased heart rate and force of contraction	Cardiac decompensation	Hypertension Arrhythmia Angina pectoris Heart failure Prevention of reinfarction
Beta-2 Receptor Bronchioles: bronchodilation Uterus: relaxation	Prevent bronchospasm Prevent premature labor	No signficant clinical use

*Primary clinical condition(s) that the agonists or antagonists are used to treat. See text for specific drugs in each category and a discussion of treatment rationale.
From: Ciccone, C: *Pharmacology in Rehabilitation,* ed. 4. FA Davis, Philadelphia, 2007, p 274.

Superior Sagittal Sinus and Cerebrospinal Fluid Formation

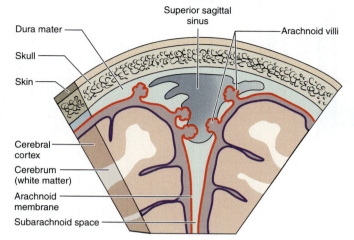

Dura mater

Skull

Skin

Superior sagittal sinus

Arachnoid villi

Cerebral cortex

Cerebrum (white matter)

Arachnoid membrane

Subarachnoid space

Sagittal view of brain and brainstem with expanded view showing location of an arachnoid villa.

Cerebrospinal Fluid Circulation Within Ventricles and Meninges

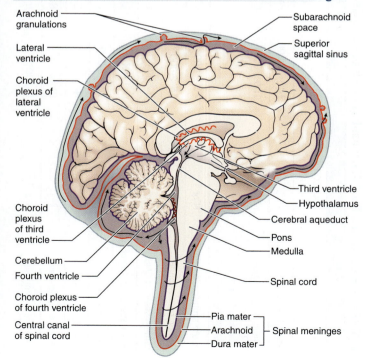

Arachnoid granulations

Lateral ventricle

Choroid plexus of lateral ventricle

Choroid plexus of third ventricle

Cerebellum

Fourth ventricle

Choroid plexus of fourth ventricle

Central canal of spinal cord

Subarachnoid space

Superior sagittal sinus

Third ventricle

Hypothalamus

Cerebral aqueduct

Pons

Medulla

Spinal cord

Pia mater
Arachnoid   Spinal meninges
Dura mater

NEURO

TABLE 4.5 Cerebrospinal Fluid Abnormalities in Various Disorders

Condition	Pressure	Wbc/µL	Predominant Cell Type	Glucose	Protein
Normal	100–200 mm H$_2$O	0–3	L	50–100 mg/dL (2.78–5.55 mmol/L)	20–45 mg/dL
Acute bacterial meningitis	←	100–10,000	PMN	→	>100 mg/dL*
Subacute meningitis (TB, *Cryptococcus* infection, sarcoidosis, leukemia, carcinoma)	N or ↑	100–700	L	→	←
Acute syphilitic meningitis	N or ↑	25–2,000	L	N	←
Paretic neurosyphilis	N or ↑	15–2,000	L	N	←
Lyme disease of CNS	N or ↑	0–500	L	N	N or ↑
Brain abscess or tumor	N or ↑	0–1,000	L	N	←
Viral infections	N or ↑	100–2,000	L	N	N or ↑
Pseudotumor cerebri	←	N	L	N	N or →
Cerebral hemorrhage	←	Bloody	RBCs	N	←
Cerebral thrombosis	N or ↑	0–100	L	N	N or ↑

NEURO

Condition	Pressure	Wbc/µL	Predominant Cell Type	Glucose	Protein
Spinal cord tumor	N	0–50	L	N	N or ↑
Guillain-Barré syndrome	N	0–100	L	N	>100 mg/dL
Lead encephalopathy	↑	0–500	L	N	↑

From: http://www.merck.com/mmpe/sec16/ch206.html#S16_CH206_T001. Accessed July 15, 2009; used with permission.

Note: Figures given for pressure, cell count, and protein are approximations; exceptions are common. Similarly, PMNs may predominate in disorders usually characterized by lymphocyte response, especially early in the course of viral infections or tuberculous meningitis. Alterations in glucose are less variable and more reliable.

L = lymphocyte; N = normal; PMN = polymorphonuclear leukocyte; ↑ = increased; ↓ = decreased.

*Up to 14% of patients may have a CSF protein level <100 mg/dL on the initial lumbar puncture.

Classification of the Cranial Nerves

Definitions

Afferent Components

general somatic afferents (GSA): Innervate receptors for touch, pain, or temperature sensibility of the skin; innervate sensory organs of muscle, joint, and tendon.

special somatic afferents (SSA): Innervate specialized receptors of ectodermal origin, specifically those for vision and vestibular and auditory sensibility.

general visceral afferents (GVA): Innervate touch, pain, or temperature receptors that are related to mucous or serous membranes, hollow organs, or glands; innervate chemoreceptors and baroreceptors.

special visceral afferents (SVA): Innervate specialized receptors found in the cranial region that are associated with visceral activity, specifically those for taste and smell.

Efferent Components

general somatic efferents (GSE): Motoneurons that innervate skeletal muscle that was not derived from the branchial arch mesoderm.

specialized visceral efferents (SVE): Motoneurons that innervate skeletal muscle that was derived from the embryonic branchial arch mesoderm, including muscles of the jaw, facial expression, pharynx, and larynx.

general visceral efferents (GVE): Motoneurons that are part of the autonomic nervous system and innervate smooth muscle, cardiac muscle, and glands.

TABLE 4.6 Functional Components of the Cranial Nerves

Number	Name	Components
I	Olfactory	SVA
II	Optic	SSA
III	Oculomotor	GSE, GVE
IV	Trochlear	GSA, GSE
V	Trigeminal	GSA, SVE
VI	Abducens	GSA, GSE
VII	Facial	GSA, GVA, GVE, SVA, SVE
VIII	Vestibulocochlear	SSA
IX	Glossopharyngeal	GSA, GVA, GVE, SVA, SVE
X	Vagus	GSA, GVA, SVA, SVE, GVE
XI	Accessory	GSA, SVE
XII	Hypoglossal	GSA, GSE

NEURO

Overview of Cranial Nerve Innervations

TABLE 4.7 Sensory Innervation

Modality	Number	Classification
Olfaction	I	SVA
Vision	II	SSA
Taste	VII, IX, X	SVA
Hearing and vestibular organs	VIII	SSA
Skin overlying face and scalp to vertex	V	GSA
Majority of mucosal membranes	V	GSA
Remainder of mucosal membranes	VII, IX, X	GVA

TABLE 4.8 Motor Innervation

Structure	Number	Classification
Muscles within orbit	III, IV, and VI	GSE
Muscles of the tongue	XII	GSE
Muscles of mastication, tensor tympani, tensor, palati (tensor veli palatini), anterior belly of digastric, mylohyoid	V	Mandibular division, SVE
Muscles of facial expression and the stapedius, stylohyoid, posterior belly of digastric	VII	SVE
Mucosal and glandular secretions including lacrimal, mucous glands, nose, palate, oral cavity; submandibular and sublingual glands	VII	GVE
Parotid gland	IX	GVE

NEURO

Sympathetic and Parasympathetic Components of the Cranial Nerves

Autonomic Nervous System Innervation of the Eye

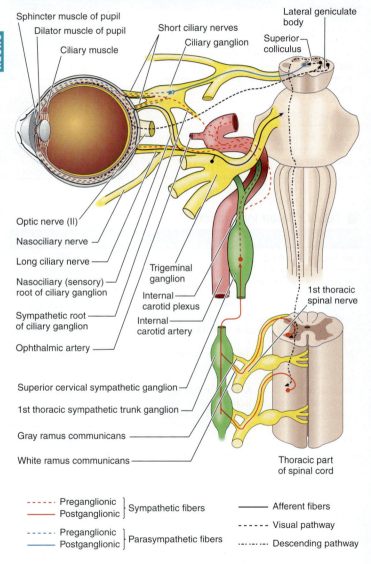

Sphincter muscle of pupil
Dilator muscle of pupil
Ciliary muscle
Short ciliary nerves
Ciliary ganglion
Lateral geniculate body
Superior colliculus

Optic nerve (II)
Nasociliary nerve
Long ciliary nerve
Nasociliary (sensory) root of ciliary ganglion
Sympathetic root of ciliary ganglion
Ophthalmic artery

Trigeminal ganglion
Internal carotid plexus
Internal carotid artery

1st thoracic spinal nerve

Superior cervical sympathetic ganglion
1st thoracic sympathetic trunk ganglion
Gray ramus communicans
White ramus communicans

Thoracic part of spinal cord

- - - - - Preganglionic
————— Postganglionic } Sympathetic fibers

- - - - - Preganglionic
————— Postganglionic } Parasympathetic fibers

————— Afferent fibers
- - - - - Visual pathway
-··-··- Descending pathway

TABLE 4.9 Parasympathetic Distribution to the Head

Cranial Nerve	Ganglion	Innervates	Course
Oculomotor	Ciliary	Sphincter pupillae and the ciliary muscles	Short ciliary nerves to the sphincter pupillae (for pupillary constriction) and to the ciliary muscle (for increased lens convexity)
Facial	Pterygopalatine	Lacrimal gland and mucosa	Via lacrimal nerve and gland and glands of nose and palate
Facial	Submandibular	Submandibular and sublingual glands and mucosa	Via chorda tympani and submaxillary ganglion and on to the submandibular and sublingual salivary glands
Glossopharyngeal	Otic	Parotid gland	Lesser petrosal nerve through the otic ganglion to the parotid gland

TABLE 4.10 Distribution of the Cranial Nerves: Major Components

Cranial Nerve	Distribution	Function
Olfactory	Olfactory mucosa	Smell
Optic	Retina	Vision
Oculomotor	Superior division: rectus superior (superior rectus) and levator palpebrae	Eye movements
	Inferior division: rectus inferior (inferior rectus) and rectus medialis (medial rectus) muscles; obliquus inferior (inferior oblique) muscle and parasympathetic accommodation fibers to the ciliary ganglion and on to the sphincter pupillae and ciliary muscles	Eye movement

(table continues on page 222)

NEURO

TABLE 4.10 Distribution of the Cranial Nerves: Major Components (continued)

Cranial Nerve	Distribution	Function
Trochlear	Obliquus superior (superior oblique) muscle	Eye movements
Trigeminal	Ophthalmic nerve: eyeball and face Maxillary nerve: upper jaw and face Mandibular nerve: muscles of mastication and to lower part of face and anterior two-thirds of tongue	Sensation of the face, scalp, eyeball, and tongue (not for taste)
Abducens	Rectus lateralis (lateral rectus) muscle	Eye movements
Facial	Muscles of face and scalp Anterior two-thirds of the tongue Submandibular, sublingual, and lacrimal glands External auditory meatus	Facial expression Taste Secretion (saliva and tears) lingual and lacrimal glands Pain and temperature of the external auditory meatus
Vestibulocochlear	Cochlear nerve Vestibular nerve	Hearing To semicircular canals, utricle, and saccule
Glossopharyngeal	Tympanic Lesser petrosal nerve Carotid Pharyngeal Muscular Tonsillar Lingual	Sensory innervation to middle ear Innervation of parotid gland (via the otic ganglion) Chemoreceptors and baroreceptors Mucosal membranes of the pharynx Innervation of stylopharyngeus muscle Sensation to the tonsils General sensation and taste to the posterior one-third of the tongue and papillae

Cranial Nerve	Distribution	Function
Vagus	Meningeal	Dura mater and posterior fossa of the skull
	Auricular	Sensation around the external acoustic meatus
	Pharyngeal	Motor nerves of the pharynx
	Superior laryngeal	Sensory innervation of the muscles and mucous membranes of the larynx
	Recurrent laryngeal (left and right)	Motor innervation to the muscles of the larynx, sensation to lower larynx, and branches to esophagus and trachea
	Cardiac	Joins cardiac plexus
	Pulmonary	Lung
	Esophageal	Esophagus and posterior pericardium
	Gastric	Stomach
	Celiac	Contributes to celiac plexus
	Hepatic	Liver
Accessory	Cranial with vagus and larynx	Muscles of pharynx and soft palate
	Spinal motor innervation to sternomastoid and trapezius	Neck movements
Hypoglossal	All muscles of the tongue except the palatoglossus	Movement of the tongue

NEURO

Visual Pathways

NEURO

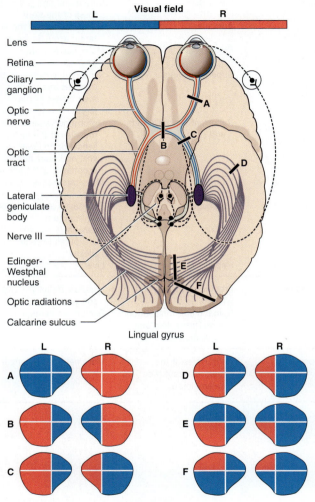

Lesions along the pathway from the eye to the visual cortex (lesions A through F) result in deficits in the visual fields, which are shown as blue areas on the corresponding visual field diagrams. The pathway through the pretectum and cranial nerve III (oculomotor), which mediates reflex constriction of the pupil in response to light, is also shown.

Cranial Nerve Testing and Additional Observations

I. Olfactory

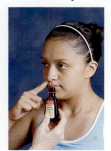

Sense of smell test.

The patient is asked to identify familiar odors (tobacco, garlic, coffee) with eyes closed.

NEURO

II. Optic field testing

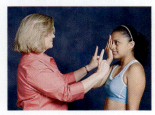

Visual acuity test.

One eye is covered as patient looks at the examiner's nose. Starting at the peripheral extent of each quadrant, the examiner moves a finger in front of the patient toward the center of vision; patient states when she or he first sees the finger, thus revealing any gross deficits.

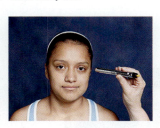

Pupillary light responses.

Additional Observations

retinal lesion: Blind spot in affected eye.

optic nerve lesion: Partial or complete blindness.

complete lesion of optic tract or of one lateral geniculate body: Blindness in opposite halves of both visual fields.

temporal lobe abnormality: Blindness in upper quadrant of both visual fields on the side opposite lesion.

parietal lobe lesion: Contralateral blindness in lower quadrants of both eyes.

occipital lobe lesion: Contralateral blindness in corresponding half of each visual field.

NEURO

III. Oculomotor

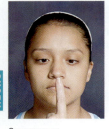

Convergence.

Examiner tests patient for an inability to elevate, depress, and adduct affected eye.

IV. Trochlear

Examiner tests patient for an inability to depress and adduct the affected eye.

V. Trigeminal

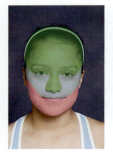

Light touch of face (forehead, cheek, and chin).

Examiner tests sensations in all areas of the patient's face bilaterally and looks for inability to sense specific stimuli or for differences in threshold in response to the same stimulus bilaterally. Corneal reflex is examined by determining if patient blinks in response to light touch of cotton to cornea. The patient's masseter and temporalis muscles are palpated in response to examiner's command to close jaw. Jaw reflex is tested by striking the middle of chin with a reflex hammer while patient's mouth is slightly open; normally there is a sudden, slight jaw closing.

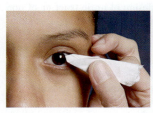

Corneal reflex.

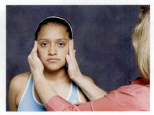

Muscles of mastication.

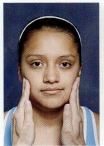
Jaw jerk reflex.

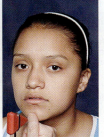
Lateral eye movement.

VI. Abducens

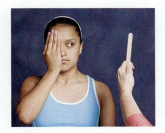

Examiner tests patient for an inability to abduct the affected eye.

Extraocular muscle innervation.

🟠 TABLE 4.11 Muscles That Move the Eye

By Movement	
Adduction	**Abduction**
Rectus medialis (medial rectus)	Obliquus inferior (inferior oblique)
Rectus superioris (superior rectus)	Obliquus superior (superior oblique)
Rectus inferior (inferior rectus)	Rectus lateralis (lateral rectus)
Medial Rotation	**Lateral Rotation**
Obliquus superior (superior oblique)	Obliquus inferior (inferior oblique)
Rectus superior (superior rectus)	Rectus inferior (inferior rectus)
Depression	**Elevation**
Obliquus superior (superior oblique)	Rectus lateralis (lateral rectus)
Rectus inferior (inferior rectus)	Rectus superior (superior rectus)
	Obliquus inferior (inferior oblique)

(table continues on page 228)

⬤ TABLE 4.11 Muscles That Move the Eye (continued)

By Muscle		
Muscle	Innervation	Function
Rectus superior (superior rectus)	Oculomotor (III)	Elevation, adduction, medial rotation
Obliquus superior (superior oblique)	Trochlear (IV)	Depression, abduction, medial rotation
Rectus inferior (inferior rectus)	Oculomotor (III)	Depression, adduction, lateral rotation
Obliquus inferior (inferior oblique)	Oculomotor (III)	Elevation, abduction, lateral rotation
Rectus medialis (medial rectus)	Oculomotor (III)	Adduction
Rectus lateralis (lateral rectus)	Abducens (VI)	Abduction

VII. Facial

Patient imitates examiner's facial expressions; patient maintains eye closure as examiner attempts to manually open eye. Sensation is tested by having patient identify taste of stimuli (sugar, salt, and so on) placed on one half of anterior tongue and with sips of water at a neutral temperature between stimuli.

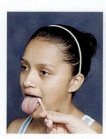

Taste of anterior two-thirds of tongue.

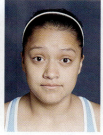

Raise eyebrows (occipito-frontalis).

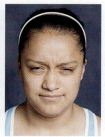

Frown (corrugators supercilli).

NEURO

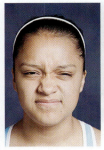

Wrinkling of nose (procerus and nasalis).

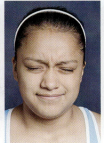

Eye close (orbicularis oculi).

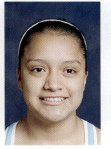

Smile and show top teeth (zygomaticus major).

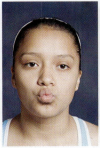

Lips purse (orbicularis oris).

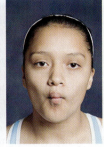

Compression of cheeks against teeth (bucchinators).

facial muscle motor loss: Involvement of supranuclear fibers supplying facial nerve leads to a motor loss in lower half of face, whereas nuclear or peripheral nerve injury leads to loss of all motor function on the side of the lesion.
facial sensory loss: Sensory loss can be caused by compromise of chorda tympani to anterior tongue.

VIII. Vestibulocochlear hearing

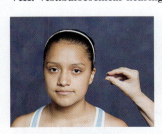

Cochlear branch-auditory acuity.

For auditory portion, examiner moves ticking watch away from ear until sound is no longer heard; both ears are tested.
lateralization: Examiner places base of tuning fork atop patient's skull while inquiring whether the sound remains central or is referred to one side.

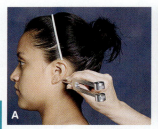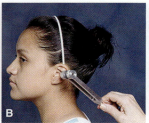

Rinne test.

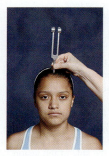

Weber test.

air and bone conduction: Examiner places tuning fork on mastoid process until patient no longer hears sound; then holds vibrating portion next to ear to determine air conduction (which is usually better than bone conduction). Deficits such as tinnitus, decreased hearing, or deafness may suggest involvement of cochlear nerve or cochlear nucleus at pontomedullary junction.

vestibular: Examiner tests for past-pointing by having the patient raise an arm and bring the index finger to the examiner's index finger; the test is performed with the patient's eyes opened and closed. With vestibular disorders the patient misses the examiner's finger by pointing to one side or the other. The patient may also have difficulty in performing the finger-to-nose test; nystagmus may also be present. Caloric testing (infiltrating one ear with cold water at 18°–20°C) should demonstrate vertigo, past-pointing, and nystagmus, whereas a patient with a defective vestibular system will not necessarily show such changes.

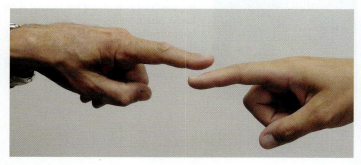

Past-pointing test.

IX. Glossopharyngeal See tests listed under the vagus nerve.

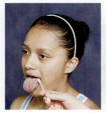

Taste in the posterior one-third of the tongue.

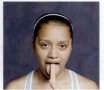

Swallowing.

X. Vagus Examiner touches side of patient's pharynx with applicator stick to elicit gag reflex and notes rise in uvula when its mucous membrane is stroked (the glossopharyngeal nerve supplies the sensory portion of this reflex). Patient's ability to swallow and to speak clearly without hoarseness as well as to demonstrate symmetrical vocal cord movements and soft palate movement suggest an intact vagus nerve to pharynx, larynx, and soft palate.

XI. Accessory Patient performs shoulder shrug against resistance (upper trapezius), resistance to lateral neck flexion with rotation (sternomastoid).

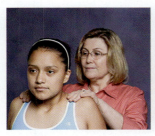

Phonation.

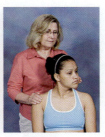

Sternomastoid muscle.

XII. Hypoglossal

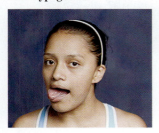

Tongue movement.

Patient protrudes tongue while examiner checks for lateral deviation, atrophy, or tremor.

NEURO

Photos from:
Fenderson, CB, and Ling, WK: Neuro Notes. FA Davis, Philadelphia, 2009, pp 22–30.

NEURO

Muscles of the Eye

TABLE 4.12 Clinical Tests for Function of Extraocular Muscles

Muscle	Movement of Eye Requested
Rectus lateralis (lateral rectus)	Outward (abduction)
Rectus medialis (medial rectus)	Inward (adduction)
Rectus superioris (superior rectus)	Elevation and adduction
Rectus inferioris (inferior rectus)	Depression and adduction
Obliquus superioris (superior oblique)	Depression and adduction
Obliquus inferioris (inferior oblique)	Elevation and adduction

The Eye and the Orbit

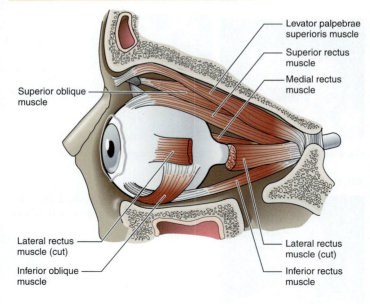

Levator palpebrae superioris muscle

Superior rectus muscle

Medial rectus muscle

Superior oblique muscle

Lateral rectus muscle (cut)

Inferior oblique muscle

Lateral rectus muscle (cut)

Inferior rectus muscle

Structures of the Eye

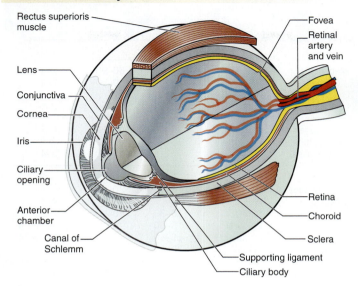

Rectus superioris muscle
Lens
Conjunctiva
Cornea
Iris
Ciliary opening
Anterior chamber
Canal of Schlemm
Fovea
Retinal artery and vein
Retina
Choroid
Sclera
Supporting ligament
Ciliary body

NEURO

Analgesia

TABLE 4.13 Opioid Analgesics

Drug	Route of Administration*	Onset of Action (min)	Time to Peak Effect (min)	Duration of Action (hr)
Strong Agonists				
Fentanyl (Sublimaze)	IM	7–15	20–30	1–2
	IV	1–2	3–5	0.5–1
Hydromorphone (Hydrostat, Dilaudid)	Oral	30	90–120	4
	IM	15	30–60	4–5
	IV	10–15	15–30	2–3
	Sub-Q	15	30–90	4
Levorphanol (Levo-Dromoran)	Oral	10–60	90–120	4–5
	IM	–	60	4–5
	IV	–	Within 20	4–5
	Sub-Q	–	60–90	4–5

(table continues on page 234)

● TABLE 4.13 Opioid Analgesics (continued)

Drug	Route of Administration*	Onset of Action (min)	Time to Peak Effect (min)	Duration of Action (hr)
Strong Agonists				
Meperidine (Demerol)	Oral	15	60–90	2–4
	IM	10–15	30–50	2–4
	IV	1	5–7	2–4
	Sub-Q	10–15	30–50	2–4
Methadone (Dolophine, Methadose)	Oral	30–60	90–120	4–6
	IM	10–20	60–120	4–5
	IV	–	15–30	3–4
Morphine (many trade names)	Oral	–	60–120	4–5
	IM	10–30	30–60	4–5
	IV	–	20	4–5
	Sub-Q	10–30	50–90	4–5
	Epidural	15–60	–	Up to 24
	Intrathecal	15–60	–	Up to 24
	Rectal	20–60	–	–
Oxymorphone (Numorphan)	IM	10–15	30–90	3–6
	IV	5–10	15–30	3–4
	Sub-Q	10–20	–	3–6
	Rectal	15–30	120	3–6
Mild-to-Moderate Agonists				
Codeine (generic)	Oral	30–45	60–120	4
	IM	10–30	30–60	4
	Sub-Q	10–30	–	4
Hydrocodone (Hycodan)	Oral	10–30	30–60	4–6
Oxycodone (OxyContin, Roxicodone)	Oral	–	60	3–4
Propoxyphene (Darvon)	Oral	15–60	120	4–6
Mixed Agonist-Antagonist				
Butorphanol (Stadol)	IM	10–30	30–60	3–4
	IV	2–3	30	2–4
Nalbuphine (Nubain)	IM	Within 15	60	3–6
	IV	2-3	30	3–4
	Sub-Q	Within 15	–	3–6

Drug	Route of Administration*	Onset of Action (min)	Time to Peak Effect (min)	Duration of Action (hr)
Mixed Agonist-Antagonist				
Pentazocine (Talwin)	Oral	15–30	60–90	3
	IM	15–20	30–60	2–3
	IV	2–3	15–30	2–3
	Sub-Q	15–20	30–60	2–3

NEURO

*IM = Intramuscular; IV = intravenous; Sub-Q = subcetaneous.
From: Ciccone, C: *Pharmacology in Rehabilitation,* ed. 4. FA Davis, Philadelphia, 2007, p 186, with permission. Originally adapted from: Gutstein, HB, and Akil, H: Opioid analgesics. In Hardman, JG, et al (eds): *The Pharmicological Basis of Therapeutics*, ed. 10. McGraw-Hill, New York, 2001.

TABLE 4.14 Opioid Receptors

Receptor Class	Primary Therapeutic Effect(s)	Other Effects
Mu (μ)	Spinal and supraspinal analgesia	Sedation; respiratory depression; constipation; inhibits neurotransmitter release (acetylcholine, dopamine); increases hormonal release (prolactin; growth hormone)
Kappa (κ)	Spinal and supraspinal analgesia	Sedation; constipation; psychotic effects
Delta (∂)	Spinal and supraspinal analgesia	Increases hormonal release (growth hormone); inhibits neurotransmitter release (dopamine)

Adapted from: Gustein, HB, and Akil, H. Opioid analgesics. In: Hardman, JG, et al (eds): *The Pharmacological Basis of Therapeutics,* ed. 10. McGraw-Hill, New York, 2001.
From: Ciccone, C: *Pharmacology in Rehabilitation,* ed. 4. FA Davis, Philadelphia, 2007, p 185, with permission.

● TABLE 4.15 Parameters for Intravenous PCA* Using Opioid Medications

Drug (Concentration)	Demand Dose	Lockout Interval (min)
Alfentanil (0.1 mg/mL)	0.1–0.2 mg	5–8
Buprenorphine (0.03 mg/mL)	0.03–0.1 mg	8–20
Fentanyl (10 µg/mL)	10–20 µg	3–10
Hydromorphone (0.2 mg/mL)	0.05–0.25 mg	5–10
Meperidine (10 mg/mL)	5–25 mg	5–10
Methadone (1 mg/mL)	0.5–2.5 mg	8–20
Morphine (1 mg/mL)	0.5–2.5 mg	5–10
Nalbuphine (1 mg/mL)	1–5 mg	5–15
Oxymorphone (0.25 mg/mL)	0.2–0.4 mg	8–10
Pentazocine (10 mg/mL)	5–30 mg	5–15
Sufentanil (0.2 µg/mL)	0.2–0.5 µg	3–10

*PCA = patient controlled analgesia.
Source: Ready p 2328, with permission.
From: Ciccone, C: *Pharmacology in Rehabilitation,* ed. 4. FA Davis, Philadelphia, 2007,
p 239, with permission. Original source: Ready, LB: Acute perioperative pain. In
Miller, RD (ed): *Anesthesia,* ed. 5. Churchill Livingston, Philadelphia, 2000.

● TABLE 4.16 Basic Features of Some Common PCA* Pumps

Feature	Abbott AMP II	Abbott LifeCare 4100 PCA Plus II	Baxter 6060	Baxter PCA II
Ambulatory use	Yes	No	Yes	No
Size (inches)	6.75 × 4.0 × 2.3	8.25 × 13.4 × 6.0	4.7 × 3.9 × 2.3	13.0 × 6.3 × 2.8
Weight (lb)	1.3	15	1.0	4.2
Power source	Wall plug in AC; 2 × 9-volt alkaline battery; NiCd rechargeable battery pack	Wall plug in AC; one 8-volt sealed lead-acid battery	2 × 9-volt alkaline or lithium batteries; external lead-acid battery pack	Four D-cell alkaline batteries; AC power kit with two rechargeable NiCd batteries

Feature	Abbott AMP II	Abbott LifeCare 4100 PCA Plus II	Baxter 6060	Baxter PCA II
Comments	Meets all basic requirements for performance, safety, and ease of use.	Performs adequately, but has a number of minor drawbacks in its ease of use and safety features.	Meets most requirements; has a mix of minor advantages and disadvantages; ease of use is only fair.	Meets most requirements and offers some advantages, but also has some drawbacks, most notably in its data logs and alarms.

*PCA = patient controlled analgesia.

Source Adapted from: Patient-controlled analgesic infusion pumps. *Health Devices* 30:168, 169, 182, 2001, with permission.

From: Ciccone, C: *Pharmacology in Rehabilitation,* ed. 4. FA Davis, Philadelphia, 2007, p 243, with permission. Original source: adapted from Patient-controlled analgesic infusion pumps. *Health Devices* 30:168, 169, 182, 2001.

Peripheral Nervous System

TABLE 4.17 Classification of Nerve Fibers

Sensory and Motor Fibers	Sensory Fibers	Largest Fiber Diameter (μm)	Fastest Conduction Velocity (m/s)	General Comments
A-α	Ia	22	120	Motor: The large α motoneurons of lamina IX, innervating extrafusal muscle fibers Sensory: The primary afferents of muscle spindles
A-α	Ib	22	120	Sensory: Golgi tendon organs, touch and pressure receptors
A-β	II	13	70	Motor: The motoneurons innervating both extrafusal and intrafusal (muscle spindle) muscle fibers Sensory: The secondary afferents of muscle spindles, touch and pressure receptors, and pacinian corpuscles (vibratory sensors)
A-γ		8	40	Motor: The small gamma motoneurons of lamina IX, innervating intrafusal fibers (muscle spindles)
A-δ	III	5	15	Sensory: Small, lightly myelinated fibers; touch, pressure, pain, and temperature
B		3	14	Motor: Small, lightly myelinated preganglionic autonomic fibers
C	IV	1	2	Motor: All postganglionic autonomic fibers (all are unmyelinated) Sensory: Unmyelinated pain and temperature fibers

From: Gilman, S, and Newman, SW: *Manter and Gatz's Essentials of Clinical Neuroanatomy and Neurophysiology*, ed. 9. FA Davis, Philadelphia, 1996, p 29, with permission.

TABLE 4.18 Relative Size and Susceptibility to Block of Types of Nerve Fibers

Fiber Type*	Function	Diameter (μm)	Myelination	Conduction Velocity (m/s)	Sensitivity to Block
Type A					
α	Proprioception, motor	12–20	Heavy	70–120	+
β	Touch, pressure	5–12	Heavy	30–70	++
γ	Muscle spindles	3–6	Heavy	15–30	++
δ	Pain, temperature	2–5	Heavy	12–30	+++
Type B					
	Preganglionic autonomic	<3	Light	3–15	++++
Type C					
Dorsal root	Pain	0.4–1.2	None	0.5–2.3	++++
Sympathetic	Postganglionic	0.3–1.3	None	0.7–2.3	++++

From: Katzung, BG: *Basic and Clinical Pharmacology*, ed. 7. Appleton & Lange, Stamford, 1998. As appearing in Ciccone, CD: *Pharmacology in Rehabilitation*, ed. 3. FA Davis, Philadelphia, 2002, p 161, with permission.
*Fiber types are classified according to the system established by Gasser, HS, and Erlanger, J: Role of fiber size in the establishment of nerve block by pressure or cocaine. *Am J Physiol* 88:581, 1929.

Pathologies of the Peripheral Nervous System

NEURO

TABLE 4.19 General Polyneuropathies: Symmetrical Generalized Neuropathies

Distal Axonopathies
Toxic: drugs, industrial and environmental chemicals Metabolic: uremia, diabetes, porphyria, endocrine Deficiencies: thiamine, pyridoxine Genetic: hereditary motor sensory neuropathy type II (HMSN II) Malignancy associated: oat-cell carcinoma, multiple myeloma

Myelinopathies
Toxic: diphtheria, buckthorn Immunologic: acute inflammatory polyneuropathy (Guillain-Barré), chronic inflammatory polyneuropathy Genetic: Refsum's disease, metachromatic leukodystrophy

Neuronopathies

Somatic Motor
Undetermined: amyotrophic lateral sclerosis Genetic: hereditary motor neuropathies

Somatic Sensory
Infectious: herpes zoster neuronitis Malignancy associated: sensory neuropathy syndrome Toxic: pyridoxine sensory neuropathy Undetermined: subacute sensory neuropathy syndrome

Autonomic
Genetic: hereditary dysautonomia (hereditary sensory neuropathy type IV [HSN IV])

TABLE 4.20 Mononeuropathy (Focal) and Multiple Mononeuropathy (Multifocal) Neuropathies

Ischemia: polyarteritis, diabetes, rheumatoid arthritis Infiltration: leukemia, lymphoma, granuloma, schwannoma, amyloid Physical injuries: severance, focal crush, compression, stretch and traction, entrapment Immunologic: brachial and lumbar plexopathy

TABLE 4.21 **Peripheral Nerve Injury Classification**

Suggested Nomenclature	Previous Nomenclature	Anatomic Lesion	Common Clinical Features
Class 1	Neuropraxia Transient Delayed reversible	Conduction block Ischemia Demyelination	A rapidly reversible loss of nerve function occurs Dysfunction of the nerve persists for a few weeks
Class 2	Axonotmesis	Axonal inter-ruption	Total loss of function occurs in the nerve until there is regener-ation of the damaged axon; wallerian de-generation occurs distal to the site of the lesion; regenerat-ing axons are guided back to their termi-nations via the intact Schwann cell tubes and other endoneural connective tissue
Class 3	Neurotmesis Partial Complete	Nerve fiber interruption Damage to Schwann cell tube and endoneural connective tissue Total nerve severance	Reinnervation may be incomplete because of a failure of the regen-erating axon to find its proper terminus Reinnervation will not occur unless the nerve is surgically repaired; neuroma formation and aberrant regener-ation are common

Based on: Schaumburg, HH, et al: *Disorders of Peripheral Nerves,* ed. 2. FA Davis, Philadelphia, 1992, p 209.

Physiological Measures

Electrodiagnosis

Purpose. From a clinical context, the purpose of electrodiagnosis is to provide information regarding the type and extent of pathophysiological changes to nerve and/or muscle. The electrodiagnostic evaluation can be considered as an extension of the neurological examination.

Types. Electrodiagnostic testing includes *Nerve Conduction Studies* and *Electromyographic (EMG) Studies* described in greater detail below.

Nerve Conduction Studies

Motor and sensory nerve conduction studies are carried out to determine disturbances of nerve function, loss of myelinated axons, or both. Routine investigations rely on recording of motor responses (referred to as the Compound Muscle Action Potential or CMAP) from relevant muscles, or of sensory responses (referred to as the Compound Sensory Action Potential or CSAP) directly from the nerve. Measurements include conduction velocity, amplitude of responses, and evaluation of the shape of the potential. Recording of the *orthodromic* or *antidromic* CMAP or CSAP may be carried out using surface or needle electrodes.

The nerve fibers studied (motor, sensory, autonomic, or mixed) should be specified. For a nerve trunk, the maximum conduction velocity is calculated from the *latency* of the evoked potential (muscle or nerve) at maximal or supramaximal intensity of stimulation at two different points. The distance between the two points (*conduction distance*) is divided by the difference between the corresponding latencies (*conduction time*). The calculated velocity represents the conduction velocity of the fastest fibers and is expressed as meters per second (m/s). As commonly used, the term *conduction velocity* refers to the maximum conduction velocity.

CLASS 1— ACUTE NERVE INJURY
(e.g., Compression)

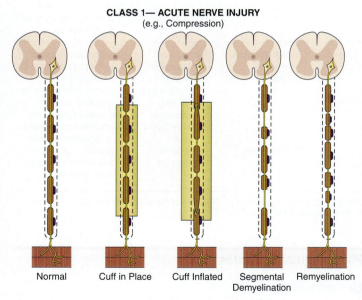

| Normal | Cuff in Place | Cuff Inflated | Segmental Demyelination | Remyelination |

Class 1 (neurapraxia) nerve injury associated with compression by a cuff. Axon movement at both edges of the cuff causes intussusception of the attached myelin across the node of Ranvier into the adjacent paranode. Affected paranodes demyelinate. Remyelination begins following cuff removal, and conduction eventually resumes. Conduction is normal in the nerve above and below the cuff since the axon has not been damaged.

CLASS 2 NERVE INJURY

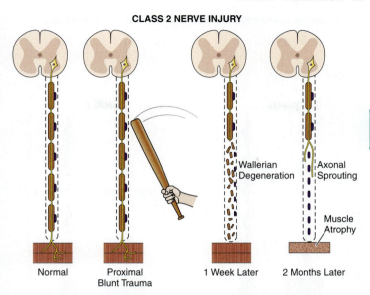

Normal   Proximal
Blunt Trauma   1 Week Later   2 Months Later

Wallerian
Degeneration

Axonal
Sprouting

Muscle
Atrophy

NEURO

Class 2 (axonotmesis) nerve injury from a crush injury to a limb. Axonal disruption occurs at the site of injury. Wallerian degeneration takes place throughout the axon distal to the injury with loss of axon, myelin, and nerve conduction. Preservation of Schwann cell tubes and other endoneurial connective tissue ensures that regenerating axons have the opportunity to reach their previous terminals and, hopefully, *re-establish functional connections.*

Degeneration and Abberant Regenreration in (Class 3) Nerve Injury

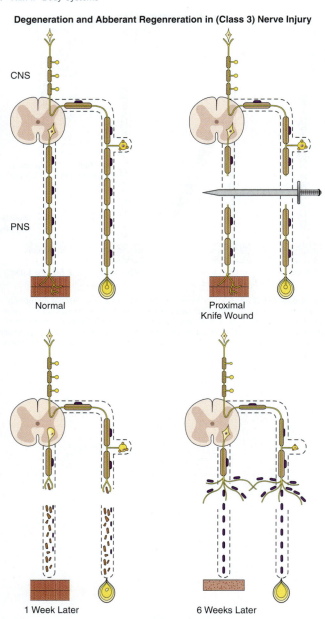

Class 3 (neurotmesis) nerve injury with severance of all neural and connective tissue elements. There is little hope of functional recovery without skilled surgery. Regenerating axons are entering inappropriate Schwann cell tubes (aberrant regeneration).

NEURO

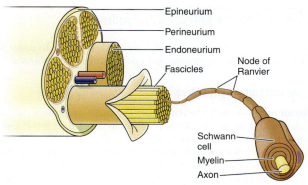

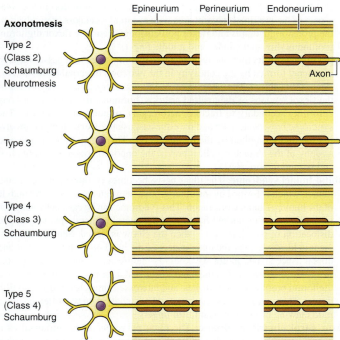

Visual representation of axontontmesis and neurotmesis using Moller "type" injury and association with Shaumberg "class" injury. Adapted from: www.utdallas.edu/~amoller/plast/2_perph_nerv.pptslide6.sept2005. Accessed July 15, 2009. Moller, AR: *Sensory Systems: Anatomy and Physiology.* Academic Press, San Diego, 2003.

Peripheral Nerve Entrapment Syndromes

The conditions presented in this section are listed alphabetically under the headings Upper Extremity Syndromes and Lower Extremity Syndromes:

Upper Extremity Syndromes

anterior interosseous nerve syndrome: The anterior interosseus nerve is compromised at or near its site of origin from the median nerve. Entrapment may occur as a result of thrombosis of the vessels that accompany the nerve, an accessory head of the flexor pollicis longus, an enlarged bicipital bursa, a tendinous origin of the deep head of the pronator muscle, or from either forearm fracture undergoing open reduction or supracondylar fractures in children. This syndrome is characterized by pain or discomfort in the volar aspect of the proximal forearm area with eventual weakness or paralysis of the pronator quadratus and flexor pollicis longus, and the flexor digitorum profundus slips to the index and middle finger.

carpal tunnel syndrome: The median nerve is compressed as it passes through the tunnel formed by the concavity in the two rows of carpal bones and the flexor retinaculum. The causes may be inflammatory, as in tenosynovitis of the flexor tendons or rheumatoid arthritis, hormonal dysfunction, or bony deformity secondary to fracture, acromegaly, or congenital stenosis. The syndrome presents as pain and paresthesias, usually worse at night, involving the digits supplied by the median nerve. There may be weakness and atrophy of the abductor pollicis brevis, the opponens pollicis, and the first and second lumbricales.

cubital tunnel syndrome: The ulnar nerve becomes entrapped at the cubital tunnel, which is formed by the ulnar groove between the medial epicondyle of the humerus and the olecranon. This syndrome can be caused by ganglion formation, arthritis, an old fracture of the lateral humeral epicondyle, and dislocation of the ulnar nerve when the elbow is flexed. Sensory involvement is localized over the ulnar aspect of the hand on both the palmar and dorsal aspects. The motor weakness is manifested in the forearm by the flexor carpi ulnaris and in the hand by the adductor pollicis, and the flexor digitorum profundus, lumbricales, and interosseus muscles (fourth and fifth digits). These weaknesses result in a radial deviation on wrist flexion and a mild clawing of the fourth and fifth fingers.

flexor carpi ulnaris syndrome: The ulnar nerve becomes entrapped as it passes under the arcuate ligament between the two heads of the flexor carpi ulnaris muscle. The symptoms are similar to those described for cubital tunnel syndrome.

posterior interosseous nerve entrapment: The posterior interosseous nerve, a branch of the radial nerve, may be entrapped as it passes through the two heads of the supinator muscle via an aponeurotic arch (arcade of Frohse). Most cases of this syndrome are found to be secondary to either thickening or narrowing of the arcade of Frohse. Predisposing factors are diabetes mellitus, leprosy, periarteritis nodosa, and heavy metal poisoning. The complete syndrome presents as pain or discomfort over the proximal or lateral aspect of the forearm. The patient radially deviates on dorsiflexion of the wrist and the fingers and thumb cannot be extended at the metacarpophalangeal (MCP) joints.

pronator teres syndrome: This syndrome occurs when the median nerve is entrapped as it passes between the two heads of the pronator teres. Symptoms are pain or discomfort over the volar proximal third of the forearm, which is aggravated when the forearm is overly pronated and the wrist flexed. Paresthesias may be present in the radial three half digits. Muscle weakness is highly variable. The flexor carpi radialis, the flexor digitorum superficialis, and the median lumbricales are often weak. The most common causes of this syndrome are the following:

1. Narrowing of the space between the two heads of the pronator
2. Direct trauma of the volar upper third of the forearm
3. Repetitive motion of the limb (forearm pronation with finger flexion)
4. An anatomic variation
5. Chronic external compression of the upper forearm

spiral groove syndrome: This syndrome results from entrapment or direct trauma to the radial nerve at the spiral groove of the humerus between the medial and lateral heads of the triceps. It usually occurs as a complication of humeral fractures or direct pressure on the nerve (Saturday night palsy). Fully manifested, its symptoms are a drop wrist with a flexed MCP joint and an adducted thumb. All muscles innervated by the radial nerve may be paralyzed, except for the triceps.

supracondylar process syndrome: The median nerve, accompanied by the brachial or ulnar artery, may become entrapped beneath the ligament of Struthers. This ligament originates from a bony process above the medial condyle and runs to the medial epicondyle of the elbow (it is present in about 1% of limbs). The patient presents with pronator teres weakness, and the radial or ulnar pulse may decrease or vanish when the arm is fully extended and supinated.

ulnar (Guyon's) tunnel syndrome: The ulnar nerve becomes entrapped as it travels through the ulnar tunnel from the forearm into the hand. This tunnel is formed by the pisohamate ligament at the wrist. Entrapment occurs usually as a result of a space-occupying lesion within the tunnel such as with rheumatoid arthritis or from the formation of ganglions. The symptoms are pain over the palmar aspect of the ulnar side of the hand and the fifth digit and the ulnar aspect of the fourth digit. Motor function shows the typical "preacher" or "benediction" hand. Atrophy of the hypothenar and interosseous muscles (especially the first dorsal interosseus) may become very noticeable.

Lower Extremity Syndromes

anterior compartment syndrome: The anterior tibial artery and veins and the deep branch of the fibular nerve are compressed as a result of increased pressure within the confines of the anterior compartment. Blood supply to the muscles within this osteofascial compartment is compromised. This syndrome may result from anterior tibial tendonitis associated with running long distances, a direct blow to the anterior aspect of the leg, or an overly tight cast to the leg. Early symptoms are intense pain in the anterior aspect of the leg with signs of vascular depletion in the foot. Muscular loss appears as an inability to dorsiflex the ankle, the toes, and the big toe. There is hypesthesia or anesthesia in the dorsal aspect of the first web space.

common fibular nerve syndrome: The common fibular nerve at the fibular head and neck is injured or entrapped as it winds around the fibula head. Some of the most common causes of this syndrome are excessive pressure from poorly applied casts or bandages, excessive pressure in bedridden patients allowed to remain in external rotation, fracture of the neck of the fibula, severe acute genu varum, and direct trauma to the nerve. In patients with a fully developed syndrome, the patient's foot appears in full plantar flexion and slight inversion as a result of weakness or paralysis in all the muscles of the anterior and lateral compartment of the leg. The patient has a steppage gait.

meralgia paresthetica: The lateral femoral cutaneous nerve is compressed as it passes into the thigh under the inguinal ligament just medial to the anterior superior iliac spine. It is brought on by trauma, postural abnormalities, occupations requiring long periods of hip flexion, obesity, and wearing of a tight belt or truss. The patient usually complains of discomfort or pain in the lateral aspect of the thigh.

piriformis syndrome: The sciatic nerve becomes entrapped as it emerges from the pelvis through the greater sciatic foramen, passing between the piriformis muscle above and the obturator internus below. The common causes of this syndrome are sustained piriformis muscle contraction and fibrotic muscle changes secondary to direct trauma, as in posterior dislocation of the hip joint. The patient has motor and sensory changes involving the posterior aspect of the thigh and the entire leg and foot. Muscle weakness of the hamstrings, gluteus maximus, ankle dorsiflexors, plantar flexors, and the intrinsics of the foot can result in a gluteus maximus lurch as well as difficulty in walking on toes or heels.

popliteal fossa entrapment: The tibial nerve is compressed as it passes through the popliteal fossa. It is usually caused by a Baker's cyst. Enlarged cysts may also compress the common peroneal and sural nerves. Other causes are proliferation of the synovial tissue in patients with rheumatoid arthritis. The patient presents with incomplete flexion of the knee joint and pain behind the knee or in the calf muscles when the foot is dorsiflexed. The gastrocnemius, tibialis posterior, flexor hallucis longus, flexor digitorum longus, and the intrinsic muscles of the foot (except for extensor digitorum brevis) are weak or paralyzed. The entire plantar surface of the foot is hypesthetic or anesthetic.

tarsal tunnel syndrome: The posterior tibial nerve or its branches are compressed as it passes under the flexor retinaculum behind the medial malleolus of the ankle joint. The most common causes of this syndrome are tenosynovitis of the flexor hallucis longus, flexor digitorum longus, or tibialis posterior caused by local trauma or systemic connective tissue diseases; venous distension or engorgement within the tunnel from chronic venous insufficiency or distortion of the canal from either developmental (pes planus, pes valgus) or traumatic deformities (fracture of the medial malleolus or fracture or dislocation of the calcaneus or talus). There is severe weakness of plantar flexion and edema in the back of the leg.

Cervical Plexus

Anatomy

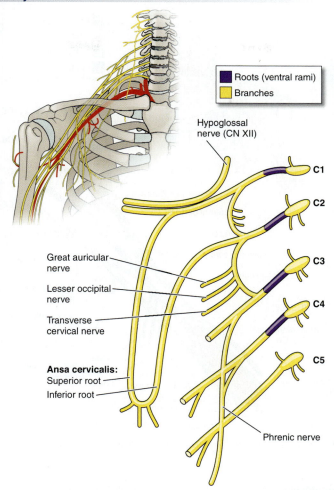

Roots (ventral rami)
Branches

Hypoglossal nerve (CN XII)

C1

C2

Great auricular nerve

Lesser occipital nerve

Transverse cervical nerve

C3

C4

C5

Ansa cervicalis:
Superior root
Inferior root

Phrenic nerve

The cervical plexus is formed by anterior primary rami of C1, C2, C3, and C4. The plexus lies almost entirely beneath the sternomastoid muscle.

Brachial Plexus

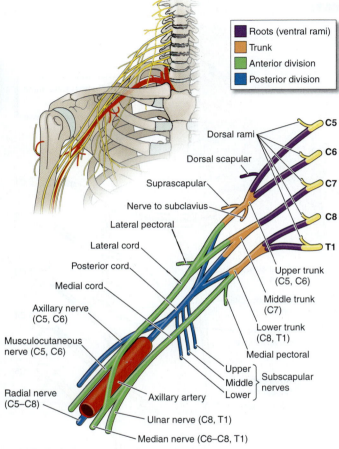

Roots (ventral rami)
Trunk
Anterior division
Posterior division

C5

Dorsal rami

C6

Dorsal scapular

C7

Suprascapular

Nerve to subclavius

C8

Lateral pectoral

T1

Lateral cord

Posterior cord

Upper trunk
(C5, C6)

Medial cord

Middle trunk
(C7)

Axillary nerve
(C5, C6)

Lower trunk
(C8, T1)

Musculocutaneous
nerve (C5, C6)

Medial pectoral

Upper

Middle } Subscapular
          nerves

Radial nerve
(C5–C8)

Lower

Axillary artery

Ulnar nerve (C8, T1)

Median nerve (C6–C8, T1)

Note that areas within posterior division give rise to nerves innervating muscles
with exterior function.

Anatomy

The brachial plexus is formed by anterior primary rami of spinal segments C5,
C6, C7, C8, and T1. The upper trunk is formed from the fibers of C5 and C6.
The middle trunk by C7, and the lower trunk by C8–T1.

The middle trunk is formed from the fibers of C7, and the lower trunk is formed from fibers of C8 and T1. The trunks divide into anterior and posterior divisions. The anterior divisions contribute to nerves that innervate flexors, and the posterior divisions contribute to nerves that innervate extensors. The anterior divisions of the middle and upper trunk form the lateral cord. The posterior divisions from all three trunks form the posterior cord. The anterior division of the lower trunk forms the medial cord. The cords are named for their relationships with the axillary artery, around which the plexus wraps.

Injuries to the Brachial Plexus

Upper Plexus Injury (Erb-Duchenne)

This is the most common injury to the brachial plexus and occurs when damage is done to the roots of C5 and C6. Common mechanisms of injury are traction injuries (as occur at birth) and compression injuries. Months or years after radiation therapy for breast cancer, upper plexus damage may become apparent. Upper plexus injuries result in paralysis of the deltoid, biceps, and brachialis; brachioradialis muscles; and sometimes the supraspinatus, infraspinatus, and subscapularis muscles. If the roots are avulsed from the spinal cord, the rhomboids, serratus anterior, levator scapulae, and the scalene muscles are also affected.

With upper plexus injuries, the arm is held limply at the patient's side, internally rotated, and adducted. The elbow is extended and the forearm is pronated in what is called the *waiter's tip* position. Biceps and brachioradialis reflexes are lost. Sensation is lost in the region of the deltoid and the radial surfaces of the forearm and hand.

Lower Plexus Injury (Klumpke)

This occurs when damage is done to the roots of C8 and T1. Forceful upward pull of the arm at birth may cause this pattern of damage. Compression of the lower part of the brachial plexus may occur due to space-occupying lesions (such as tumors) and is often due to the presence of a cervical rib. Lower plexus injuries result in paralysis of all the intrinsic hand muscles and weakness of the medial fingers and wrist flexors. Extensors of the forearm may also be weak.

A clawhand deformity is seen with lower plexus injuries; that is, the fourth and fifth digits are hyperextended at the MCP joints and flexed at the interphalangeal (IP) joints, the first phalanx is hyperextended, and the fifth finger remains abducted. Guttering of the hand may be seen due to atrophy of the intrinsic muscles. Sensation is lost in the region of the ulnar side of the arm, forearm, and hand. Lower plexus lesions are often accompanied by disturbances in the sympathetic nervous system (e.g., Horner's syndrome). Trophic changes in the arm may occur that can include edema and changes in the appearance of the skin and nails.

TABLE 4.22 Brachial Plexus Latency Determinations From Specific Nerve Root Stimulation

Plexus	Site of Stimulation	Recording Site	Range	Mean ± SD
Brachial (upper trunk and lateral cord)	C5 and C6	Biceps	4.8–6.2	5.3 ± 0.4
Brachial (posterior cord)	C6, C7, C8	Triceps	4.4–6.1	5.4 ± 0.4
Brachial (lower trunk and medial cord)	C8, T1, ulnar nerve	Abductor digiti minimi	3.7–5.5	4.7 ± 0.5

Latency Across Plexus (ms)

Based on: MacLean, IC: Nerve root stimulation to evaluate conduction across the brachial and lumbosacral plexuses. Third Annual Continuing Education Course, American Association of Electromyography and Electrodiagnosis, September 25, 1980, Philadelphia.

TABLE 4.23 Nerve Conduction Times From Erb's Point to Muscle

Muscle	n*	Distance (cm)	Latency (ms)†
Biceps	1	20	4.6 ± 0.6
	9	24	4.7 ± 0.6
	15	28	5.0 ± 0.5
	14		
Deltoid	20	155	4.3 ± 0.5
	17	18.5	4.4 ± 0.4
Triceps	16	21.5	4.5 ± 0.4
	23	26.5	4.9 ± 0.5
	16	31.5	5.3 ± 0.5
Supraspinatus	19	8.5	2.6 ± 0.3
	16	10.5	2.7 ± 0.3
Infraspinatus	20	14	3.4 ± 0.4
	15	17	3.4 ± 0.5

From: Kimura, J: *Electrodiagnosis in Diseases of Nerve and Muscle: Principles and Practice,* ed. 2. FA Davis, Philadelphia, 1989, p 119, with permission.
*Number of subjects tested to obtain values.
†Mean ± SD.

Long Thoracic Nerve and Anterior Thoracic Nerve

Long Thoracic Nerve

Long thoracic nerve, also called the external respiratory nerve of Bell, nerve to serratus anterior, or posterior thoracic nerve (a term that also includes the dorsal scapular nerve).

Origin
The long thoracic nerve arises from anterior primary rami of C5, C6, and C7.

Innervation
Motor
The long thoracic nerve innervates the serratus anterior muscle.

Cutaneous and Joint
None.

Common Injuries
Traction. Because the nerve has a long course and because it is held in place by the scaleni and slips of the serratus anterior, it is prone to stretch injuries (e.g., lifting of heavy objects); prolonged compression from lying on the lateral aspect of the trunk can lead to damage.

Surgery. Proximity to the axilla makes the nerve vulnerable during various forms of surgery (e.g., during breast surgery).

Trauma to the Base of the Neck. Forces exerted to the base of the neck damage the nerve because it is trapped against the lower cervical vertebrae.

Effects of Injuries. Instability of the scapula and winging of the scapula with medial rotation of the lower part of the scapula are common features; shoulder girdle is displaced posteriorly.

Special Tests
During a wall push-up or during protraction of the scapula, the examiner should look for winging of the scapula; slight winging of the scapula at rest can be noted, and this winging increases with shoulder flexion.

Anterior Thoracic Nerve

Anterior thoracic nerve (gives rise to the medial pectoral nerve and the lateral pectoral nerve).

Origin
The anterior thoracic nerve arises from the proximal portion of the lateral and medial cords of the brachial plexus. The fibers that form the lateral pectoral nerve are from C5, C6, and C7; the fibers that form the medial pectoral nerve are from C8 and T1.

Innervation
Motor
The lateral pectoral nerve innervates the superior and clavicular portions of the pectoralis major muscle. The medial pectoral nerve innervates pectoralis minor

muscle and the inferior part of the sternocostal portion of the pectoralis major muscle.

Cutaneous and Joint
None.

Common Injuries
Isolated injuries to these nerves are rare. Fibers that form the nerves may be damaged when there is a nerve root or brachial plexus injury.

Effects of Injuries
Depending on the extent of injury, weakness or paralysis of the pectoral muscles may result; the shoulder is held slightly posterior and may be elevated or depressed.

Special Tests
When the examiner elevates the patient's shoulders by placing his hands in the axillae, the shoulder of the affected side rises higher than that of the normal side; when the patient flexes both arms to approximately 90°, the affected arm deviates laterally.

Dorsal Scapular Nerve, Nerve to Subclavius, and Suprascapular Nerve

Course and Distribution: Posterior View

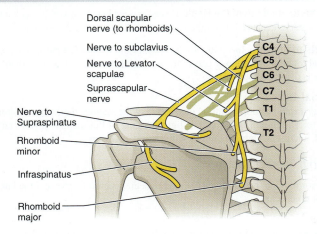

Dorsal Scapular Nerve

The dorsal scapular nerve is also called the posterior scapular nerve or the nerve to the rhomboids.

Origin
The dorsal scapular nerve arises from anterior primary rami of C5.

Innervation

Motor

The dorsal scapular nerve innervates the rhomboid minor and rhomboid major muscles and contributes innervation to the levator scapulae muscle, which also receives innervation from C3 and C4.

Cutaneous and Joint

None.

Common Injuries

Injury to the C5 root is more common than injury to the nerve.

Effects of Injuries

Depending on the extent of injury, weakness or paralysis of the rhomboid muscles and paresis of the levator scapulae may result; the inferior portion of the vertebral border of the scapula wings posteriorly.

Special Tests

When the patient is asked to brace the shoulders (i.e., stand at attention with shoulders square), the scapula of the affected shoulder is obliquely positioned with the upper vertebral border lying medially and the inferior portion lying laterally; damage to the dorsal scapular nerve can be differentiated from injury to the C5 root only by electromyographic (EMG) testing, which indicates that the lesion is isolated to the rhomboid muscles and the levator scapulae muscle.

Nerve to Subclavius

The nerve to subclavius is also called the subclavian nerve.

Origin

The subclavian nerve arises from the upper trunk of the brachial plexus from fibers originating at C5 and C6.

Innervation

Motor

The subclavian nerve innervates the subclavius muscle.

Cutaneous and Joint

None.

Common Injuries

Isolated injury to the nerve is uncommon.

Effects of Injuries

Depending on the extent of injury, weakness or paralysis of the subclavius muscle results in slight forward displacement of the lateral end of the clavicle.

Special Tests

None.

Suprascapular Nerve

Origin

The suprascapular nerve arises from the upper trunk of the brachial plexus from fibers originating at C5 and C6.

Innervation

Motor
The suprascapular nerve innervates the supraspinatus muscle and the infraspinatus muscle.

Cutaneous and Joint
There is no cutaneous distribution; the nerve supplies posterior capsule of the glenohumeral joint.

NEURO

Common Injuries
Traction and Pressure. Downward displacement on the shoulder stretches the nerve and can cause injury (e.g., as occurs with Erb's palsy or due to gymnastics).

Trauma. Wounds above the scapula will frequently affect the nerve.

Effects of Injuries
Atrophy of the supraspinatus muscle and the infraspinatus muscle are common features. There is difficulty initiating abduction and external rotation at the glenohumeral joint. When at rest, the arm may be kept slightly medially rotated.

Special Tests
To test for loss of function of the infraspinatus muscle, the examiner tests for lateral rotation; EMG testing reveals only denervation of supraspinatus and infraspinatus muscles without any denervation to other muscles innervated by C5 and C6.

Thoracodorsal Nerve and Subscapular Nerves

Thoracodorsal Nerve (Middle Subscapular)

Origin
The thoracodorsal nerve arises from the posterior cord of the brachial plexus from fibers originating at C6, C7, and C8.

Innervation

Motor
The thoracodorsal nerve innervates the latissimus dorsi muscle.

Cutaneous and Joint
None.

Common Injuries
Isolated injuries to the nerve are rare; damage is associated with injuries to the posterior cord of the brachial plexus.

Effects of Injuries
Paralysis of the latissimus dorsi muscle may result in winging of the inferior angle of the scapula and an inability to extend the arm powerfully.

Special Tests
The examiner resists shoulder extension; if the latissimus dorsi muscle is denervated, there is weakness.

Subscapular Nerves

Origin

The upper (superior) subscapular nerve and the lower (inferior) subscapular nerve arise from the posterior cord of the brachial plexus from fibers originating at C5 and C6 (the upper subscapular nerve is also called the short subscapular nerve).

Innervation
Motor
The upper subscapular nerve innervates the subscapularis muscle; the lower subscapular nerve innervates the subscapularis muscle and the teres major muscle.

Cutaneous and Joint
None.

Common Injuries
Isolated injuries to the nerves are rare; damage is associated with injuries to the posterior cord of the brachial plexus.

Effects of Injuries
Paralysis of the subscapularis muscle results in weakness of medial rotation. Paralysis of the teres major muscle does not significantly affect function.

Special Tests
The examiner resists medial rotation; there is weakness rather than loss of motion if the nerve is damaged because other medial rotators are still innervated.

Axillary Nerve

Course and Distribution: Posterior View

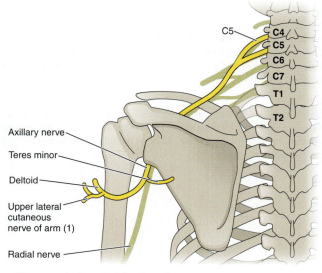

Axillary nerve
Teres minor
Deltoid
Upper lateral cutaneous nerve of arm (1)
Radial nerve

C5
C4
C5
C6
C7
T1
T2

The axillary nerve is also called the circumflex nerve.

Origin
The axillary nerve arises from the posterior cord of the brachial plexus from fibers originating at C5 and C6.

Innervation
Motor
The axillary nerve innervates the deltoid muscle (all three parts) and the teres minor muscle.

Cutaneous and Joint
Cutaneous in the area of the deltoid muscle.

Common Injuries
Fractures. Because the axillary nerve wraps around the proximal humerus, any fracture in the region of the surgical neck of the humerus may be accompanied by an axillary nerve lesion.

Dislocations. Movement of the humerus after a dislocation at the glenohumeral joint may result in an axillary nerve lesion.

Forceful Hyperextension of the Shoulder. With hyperextension of the shoulder (as might occur during a wrestling match), the axillary nerve may be compromised.

Inappropriate Use of Crutches. Pressure on the axillary region due to leaning on crutches can cause a compression injury to the axillary nerve.

Other Trauma. Contusions in the shoulder region or injuries to the scapula may be accompanied by axillary nerve lesions. Because the nerve passes between the coracoid process of the scapula and the humerus, compression of these structures often results in an entrapment syndrome.

Effects of Injuries
Paralysis of the deltoid muscle with resultant atrophy causes a change in the contour of the shoulder; the shoulder becomes flattened and loses its normal rounded shape. There is a decreased ability to abduct, flex, and extend the arm at the glenohumeral joint. Paralysis of the teres minor muscle does not significantly affect function.

Special Tests
Muscle testing of the deltoid muscle, especially in the fully abducted position, reveals severe weakness. Confirmation of denervation of the teres minor muscle can be determined only through EMG because the infraspinatus muscle is also an external rotator of the arm.

Musculocutaneous Nerve

Course and Distribution

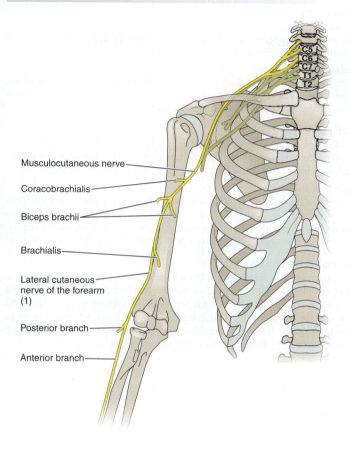

Musculocutaneous nerve

Coracobrachialis

Biceps brachii

Brachialis

Lateral cutaneous
nerve of the forearm
(1)

Posterior branch

Anterior branch

C5
C6
C7
T1
T2

Origin

The musculocutaneous nerve arises from the lateral cord of the brachial plexus from fibers originating at C5, C6, and C7.

Innervation

Motor

The musculocutaneous nerve innervates the coracobrachialis muscle, biceps brachii muscle, and most of the brachialis muscle.

Cutaneous and Joint

In the forearm, the musculocutaneous nerve gives rise to the lateral cutaneous nerve of the forearm that innervates the lateral forearm; the cutaneous division is also called the lateral antebrachial cutaneous nerve.

Common Injuries

Fractures or dislocations of the humerus can lead to lesions of the musculocutaneous nerve, as can open wounds (e.g., stab wounds). The nerve can also be entrapped by the coracobrachialis muscle or injured during surgery.

Effects of Injuries

Paralysis of the biceps brachii muscle and the brachialis muscle results in weak elbow flexion. The loss of the biceps is especially noticeable when elbow flexion is attempted with the forearm supinated. Weakness in supination occurs. Paralysis of the coracobrachialis muscle does not significantly affect function.

Special Tests

The examiner tests for the biceps brachii stretch reflex, for extreme weakness when the elbow flexors are muscle-tested with the forearm fully supinated, and for weakness when muscle-testing is performed for supination. Although EMG testing of the biceps brachii muscle, brachialis muscle, and the coracobrachialis muscle can show denervation, to determine specific nerve damage this should be accompanied by findings of impaired nerve conduction velocities.

TABLE 4.24 Values for Musculocutaneous Nerve Electrodiagnostic Testing

Age (y)	Motor Nerve Conduction Between Erb's Point and Axilla				Orthodromic Sensory Nerve Conduction Between Erb's Point and Axilla			Orthodromic Conduction Between Axilla and Elbow		
	n*	Range of Conduction Velocities (m/s)	Range of Amplitudes (µV) Axilla	Erb's Point	n*	Range of Conduction Velocities (m/s)	Range of Amplitudes (µV)	n*	Range of Conduction Velocities (m/s)	Range of Amplitudes (µV)
15–24	14	63–78	9–32	7–27	14	59–76	3.5–30	15	61–75	17–75
25–34	6	60–75	8–30	6–26	6	57–74	3–25	8	59–73	16–72
35–44	8	58–73	8–28	6–24	7	54–71	2.5–21	8	57–71	16–69
45–54	10	55–71	7–26	6–22	10	52–69	2–18	13	55–69	15–65
55–64	9	53–68	7–24	5–21	9	49–66	2–15	10	53–67	14–62
65–74	4	50–66	6–22	5–19	4	47–64	1.5–12	6	51–65	13–59

From: Trojaborg, W: Motor and sensory conduction in the musculocutaneous nerve.
J Neurol Neurosurg Psychiatry 39:890, 1976, with permission.
*Number of subjects tested to obtain values in the table.

NEURO

NEURO

TABLE 4.25 Values for Lateral and Medial (Musculo) Cutaneous Nerve

Nerve	Number of Patients Seen	Age (years) (mean)	Latency Distance (cm)	Onset (ms)*	Peak (m/s)*	Conduction Velocity (ms)*	Amplitude (μV)*
Lateral cutaneous nerve	30	20–84 (35)	12	1.8 ± 0.1	2.3 ± 0.1	65 ± 4	24.0 ± 7.2
Lateral cutaneous nerve	154	17–80 (45)	14		2.8 ± 0.2	62 ± 4	18.9 ± 9.9
Medial cutaneous nerve	155	17–80 (45)	14		27. ± 0.2	63 ± 5	11.4 ± 5.2
Medial cutaneous nerve	30	23–60 (38)	18	2.7 ± 0.2	3.3 ± 0.2	66 ± 4	15.4 ± 4.1

From: Kimura, J: *Electrodiagnosis in Diseases of Nerve and Muscle: Principles and Practice*, ed. 2. FA Davis, Philadelphia, 1989, p 122, with permission.
*Mean + SD.

Median Nerve

Course and Distribution

NEURO

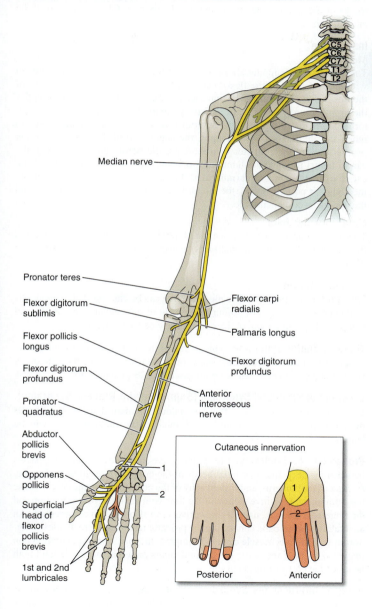

Median nerve

Pronator teres

Flexor digitorum sublimis

Flexor pollicis longus

Flexor digitorum profundus

Pronator quadratus

Abductor pollicis brevis

Opponens pollicis

Superficial head of flexor pollicis brevis

1st and 2nd lumbricales

Flexor carpi radialis

Palmaris longus

Flexor digitorum profundus

Anterior interosseous nerve

1
2

Cutaneous innervation

1

2

Posterior   Anterior

NEURO

Origin

Portions of the medial and lateral cords of the brachial plexus join together to form the median nerve. These fibers, which originated at C6, C7, C8, and T1, pass through the anterior divisions of the upper, middle, and lower trunks of the brachial plexus. Sometimes fibers from C5 also are part of the median nerve.

Innervation

Motor

The median nerve supplies all the muscles in the anterior aspect of the forearm with the exception of the flexor carpi ulnaris muscle and the medial half of the flexor digitorum profundus muscle. The main trunk of the nerve supplies the pronator teres, flexor carpi radialis, palmaris longus, and the flexor digitorum superficialis muscles; the anterior osseous nerve (a pure motor nerve) innervates the flexor pollicis longus, the lateral half of the flexor digitorum profundus, and the pronator quadratus muscle before passing through the carpal tunnel to innervate lumbricals one and two. At the level of the distal carpal ligament, a recurrent (muscular) thenar branch is given off to innervate the abductor pollicis brevis, the lateral half of the flexor pollicis brevis, and the opponens pollicis muscle.

Cutaneous and Joint

The nerve supplies the skin over the lateral (radial) side of the palm and the palmar and dorsal (terminal parts) aspects of the lateral three-and-a-half digits.

Common Injuries

Entrapment Syndromes. The median nerve can be entrapped at many points as it courses down the arm; often entrapment of the median nerve is also accompanied by entrapment of the ulnar nerve (see Ulnar Nerve).

Thoracic Outlet Syndrome. This is due to the scalenus-anticus syndrome, the presence of a cervical rib, or some other narrowing of the thoracic outlet where the median nerve can be compressed near its proximal origin.

Ligament of Struthers' Syndrome (Supracondylar Process Syndrome). This is due to the presence of an anomalous ligament that forms a fibrous tunnel near the medial condyle of humerus, the median nerve can be compressed.

Pronator Teres Syndrome. The median nerve can be compressed as it passes between the deep and superficial heads of the pronator teres muscle. Trauma, fracture of the humerus, and hypertrophy of the pronator teres muscle can cause the entrapment; repetitive motion of the limb with the forearm in pronation and the fingers flexed (e.g., using a screwdriver) can also result in compression. An anomalous fibrous band connecting the pronator teres muscle to the flexor digitorum superficialis muscle can also compress the median nerve; compression may also occur if the nerve has an anomalous path that takes it behind both heads of the pronator teres muscle.

Anterior Interosseous Syndrome. As the median nerve gives rise to the anterior interosseous nerve (just below the level of the radial tuberosity), it can be compressed by several different anomalous structures, including fibrous sheaths, and the tendinous origin of the long flexors. Thrombosis of the vessels that are in close proximity with the nerve can cause entrapment, as can the presence of an accessory head of the flexor pollicis longus muscle. Forearm fractures and supracondylar fractures in children may also result in compression.

Carpal Tunnel Syndrome. As the median nerve enters the hand, it runs beneath a wide, fibrous ligamentous band that forms the *carpal tunnel*; this is a common site of median nerve compression. In women the syndrome may, in some cases, be caused by hormonal factors that occur with pregnancy or during the menstrual cycle; in addition, hypothyroidism has been thought to cause the syndrome. Inflammatory events that occur with tenosynovitis of the flexor tendons, rheumatoid arthritis, or overuse syndromes may also cause compression at the carpal tunnel. Moreover, congenital bony deformities, deformities secondary to fractures, or acromegaly may also cause the syndrome.

Digital Nerve Entrapment Syndrome. The interdigital nerve that supplies the skin of the second and third digits and half of the fourth digit may be compressed against the edge of the deep transverse metacarpal ligament. This syndrome appears to be caused by trauma (such as phalangeal fractures), tumors, or inflammation of the MCP joints.

Trauma

In addition to causing compression syndromes, trauma may lead to direct injuries to the median nerve.

Humeral Fractures. These fractures may lead to disruption of the median nerve above the elbow. This is especially true of supracondylar fractures.

Lacerations of the Wrist. The superficial course of the median nerve at the wrist makes it vulnerable to damage from accidental lacerations (that occur with falls on sharp objects) or lacerations associated with suicide attempts.

Carpal Bone Injuries. Because the median nerve courses directly over the carpal bones, trauma to these bones often results in damage to the nerve. This damage may occur with fractures or dislocations or from direct trauma at the time the carpal bone was injured.

Effects of Injuries

The deficits associated with damage to the median nerve depend on the severity of the injury and the site of the lesion. To determine specific deficits for each syndrome and type of injury, the course of the nerve must be considered and the resultant loss of motor and sensory function distal to the site determined (see the listing of peripheral nerve entrapment syndromes for descriptions of the symptoms of some of the more common syndromes). Pain is a common feature of the entrapment syndromes; however, sensory effects can also include hypesthesia, paresthesia, and even complete sensory loss.

General Motor Defects With Median Nerve Lesions

Loss of opposition of the thumb, loss of ability to make a fist, and atrophy of the thenar eminence are common general motor defects.

Common deformities seen with median nerve lesions include the following:

Simian (ape) hand: occurs because of denervation and resultant atrophy of muscles in the thenar eminence. Opposition is lost. As a result of the atrophy and paralysis, the hand flattens.

Benediction sign: occurs because of paralysis to the flexors of the middle and ring fingers. When a person with a median nerve injury attempts to make a fist, these fingers do not fully flex, and they remain in a position similar to that used when clergy make a benediction.

Special Tests

Depending on the severity and site of the lesion, many different tests can be used to ascertain median nerve damage. General muscle and sensory testing can be used to indicate the level of the lesion by determining which portion of the nerve is damaged.

Motor

If, as part of general paralysis or weakness of all muscles innervated by the median nerve, muscles above the elbow are affected (e.g., flexor carpi radialis muscle and other long flexors), the main portion of the nerve must be injured. If the long flexors (those muscles first innervated by the nerve) are spared but there is isolated paralysis of the flexor pollicis longus muscle, the lateral half of the flexor digitorum profundus muscle, and the pronator quadratus muscle, damage to the anterior interosseous nerve is indicated. If paralysis or paresis is isolated to the abductor pollicis brevis, lateral half of the flexor pollicis brevis, and the opponens pollicis muscles, then damage to the thenar branch is indicated.

Cutaneous and Joint

Total sensory loss of the tip of the index finger and decreased sensation on the lateral (radial) side of the palm and the lateral three-and-a-half digits over their palmar aspects indicate interruption of the nerve at a level above the lower third of the forearm. Lesions distal to the origin of the palmar cutaneous branch (which arises proximal to the level of the wrist) result in preserved sensation of the more proximal portions of the dorsal surface of the hand, but loss of sensation in the most distal distribution of the median nerve (e.g., loss of sensation in the distal portion of the second and third fingers and some loss in the distal fourth finger).

Specific Tests

Adson's maneuver (test for thoracic outlet syndrome).

The patient turns the head to the side of the suspected lesion, extends the neck fully, and takes and holds a deep breath while the examiner checks for a decreased radial pulse (in some patients the effect may be more noticeable if the patient turns the head away from the side of the suspected lesion). If the thoracic outlet is compromised, this maneuver further narrows the outlet and indicates whether the median nerve is likely to be compressed at this level.

Tests for Compression by Ligament of Struthers (Supracondylar Process Syndrome). The examiner checks for decrease or absence of radial and/or ulnar pulses when the forearm is fully extended and supinated. The presence of weakness and EMG abnormalities of the pronator teres muscle indicates possible compression due to a ligament of Struthers (this muscle is usually not affected by the pronator teres syndrome); nerve conduction testing can also be used to determine blockage across the antecubital fossa.

Tests for Pronator Teres Syndrome. Test for a pattern of weakness in the flexor carpi radialis muscle, flexor digitorum superficialis muscle, thenar muscles, and lumbricals one and two. Nerve conduction velocity testing indicates a slowing of velocity across the elbow, and there will be a diminished evoked response (see test for ligament of Struthers). The EMG shows denervation in affected muscles. Electrodiagnostic testing for pronator teres syndrome is usually not considered positive based on findings of abnormalities in the pronator teres because this muscle is usually spared in this syndrome. Phalen's sign and testing for normal conduction latencies are used to rule out carpal tunnel syndrome (see appropriate tests).

Tests for Anterior Interosseous Syndrome. The patient is asked to make an "OK" sign (an *O* between the thumb and index finger) using the first two digits. The shape is observed. If there is damage to the interosseous nerve, a triangle (the "pinch sign") rather than a circle will be formed. Routine nerve conduction studies of the median nerve are normal with this syndrome, but slowed conduction velocities of the anterior interosseous nerve may be discerned by recording compound muscle action potentials from the pronator quadratus muscle after stimulation of the nerve at the elbow; EMG shows denervation in the flexor pollicis longus, flexor digitorum profundus (first and second fingers), and pronator quadratus muscles.

Tests for Carpal Tunnel Syndrome. The examiner taps the patient's wrist over the carpal tunnel; if pain is felt in the cutaneous distribution of the median nerve (Tinel's sign), carpal tunnel syndrome is likely. The examiner can use Phalen's test by forcefully flexing the patient's wrist and holding it in that position for a minute; in this way the carpal tunnel is compressed and pain in the distribution of the median nerve is felt if carpal tunnel syndrome is present. In carpal tunnel syndrome, conduction abnormalities of sensory and motor fibers are usually seen in the wrist-to-palm segment of the median nerve with the distal segment of the nerve remaining relatively normal; EMG may be normal, or, in severe cases, signs of denervation may be seen in the median nerve-innervated lumbricals.

Observable Signs. Look for the benediction sign or the appearance of a simian hand.

NEURO

NEURO

■ **TABLE 4.26 Values for Electrodiagnostic Testing: Median Nerve[a]**

Site of Stimulation	Amplitude[b] Motor (mV) Sensory (V)	Latency[c] to Recording Site (ms)	Difference Between Right and Left (ms)	Conduction Time Between Two Points (ms)	Conduction Velocity (m/s)
Motor Fibers					
Palm	6.9 ± 3.2 (3.5)[d]	1.86 ± 0.28 (2.4)[e]	0.19 ± 0.17 (0.5)[e]		
Wrist	7.0 ± 3.0 (3.5)	3.49 ± 0.34 (4.2)	0.24 ± 0.22 (0.7)	1.65 ± 0.25 (2.2)[e]	48.8 ± 5.3 (38)[f]
Elbow	7.0 ± 2.7 (3.5)	7.39 ± 0.69 (8.8)	0.31 ± 0.24 (0.8)	3.92 ± 0.49 (4.9)	57.7 ± 4.9 (48)
Axilla	7.2 ± 2.9 (3.5)	9.81 ± 0.89 (11.6)	0.42 ± 0.33 (1.1)	2.42 ± 0.39 (3.2)	63.5 ± 6.2 (51)
Sensory Fibers					
Digit	39.0 ± 16.8 (20)	1.37 ± 0.24 (1.9)	0.15 ± 0.11 (0.4)	1.37 ± 0.24 (1.9)	58.8 ± 5.8 (47)
Palm	38.5 ± 15.6 (19)	2.84 ± 0.34 (3.5)	0.18 ± 0.14 (0.5)	1.48 ± 0.18 (1.8)	56.2 ± 5.8 (44)
Wrist	32.0 ± 15.5 (16)	6.46 ± 0.71 (7.9)	0.29 ± 0.21 (0.7)	3.61 ± 0.48 (4.6)	61.9 ± 4.2 (53)

From: Kimura, J: *Electrodiagnosis in Diseases of Nerve and Muscle: Principles and Practice*, ed. 2. FA Davis, Philadelphia. 1989, p 107, with permission.

[a]Mean ± standard deviation (SD) in 122 nerves from 61 patients, 11–74 years of age (average, 40), with no apparent disease of the peripheral nerves.

[b]Amplitude of the evoked response, measured from the baseline to the negative peak.

[c]Latency, measured to the onset of the evoked response, with the cathode at the origin of the thenar nerve in the palm.

[d]Lower limits of normal, based on the distribution of the normative data.

[e]Upper limits of normal, calculated as the mean + 2 SD.

[f]Lower limits of normal, calculated as the mean − 2 SD.

Ulnar Nerve

Course and Distribution

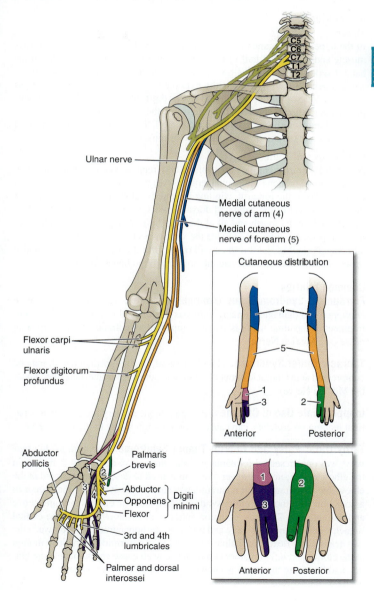

NEURO

Ulnar nerve

Medial cutaneous
nerve of arm (4)

Medial cutaneous
nerve of forearm (5)

Cutaneous distribution

Flexor carpi
ulnaris

Flexor digitorum
profundus

Abductor
pollicis

Palmaris
brevis

Abductor
Opponens   Digiti
Flexor   minimi

3rd and 4th
lumbricales

Palmer and dorsal
interossei

Anterior

Posterior

Origin

The medial cord of the brachial plexus gives rise to the ulnar nerve. Fibers originate in C8 and T1 and pass through the lower trunk of the brachial plexus and the anterior division before joining the medial cord.

Innervation

Motor

In the upper arm a branch of the ulnar nerve supplies the flexor carpi ulnaris muscle and the medial half of the flexor digitorum profundus muscle. In the hand a superficial branch is given off to supply the palmaris brevis muscle, while a deep branch innervates the hypothenar muscles, the opponens digiti minimi, abductor digiti minimi, and flexor digiti minimi muscles. After supplying innervation to the hypothenar muscles, the deep branch supplies interossei, third and fourth lumbricals, adductor pollicis muscle, and the deep head (or medial half) of the flexor pollicis brevis muscle.

Cutaneous and Joint

An articular branch is given off in the elbow region, where it innervates that joint. A dorsal branch (a pure cutaneous nerve) is given off in the forearm and continues down the forearm, winding around the ulna to supply the skin over the dorsal aspect of the hand and dorsal aspects of the medial one-and-a-half fingers (half of the fourth and all of the fifth digit). A superficial branch arises near the pisiform bone to innervate the volar aspects of the medial one-and-a-half fingers (half of the fourth and all of the fifth digit); a palmar branch also arises near the wrist to innervate the proximal hypothenar region.

Common Injuries

Entrapment Syndromes and Mononeuropathies. The ulnar nerve can be entrapped and damaged at many points as it courses down the arm. Often entrapment of the ulnar nerve is also accompanied by entrapment of the median nerve (see Median Nerve).

Thoracic Outlet Syndrome. The ulnar nerve, like the median nerve, may be compressed at the thoracic outlet (see thoracic outlet syndrome, described under the Median Nerve).

Inappropriate Use of Crutches. Pressure on the axillary region, due to a patient leaning on crutches, can cause a compression injury to the ulnar nerve.

Tardy Ulnar Palsy and Cubital Tunnel Syndrome. The term *tardy ulnar palsy* was once reserved for damage to the ulnar nerve secondary to trauma in the elbow region; now, however, the term is used to describe entrapment at the elbow due to traumatic and nontraumatic causes. This syndrome may occur in association with thoracic outlet syndrome (see thoracic outlet syndrome above and on page 31). The most common entrapment at the elbow is in the cubital tunnel, where the nerve is large and underlies the aponeurotic band between the two heads of the flexor carpi ulnaris muscle. Joint deformities, repetitive motion at the elbow, and inflammatory conditions may all cause entrapment at the tunnel, and trauma to the elbow is known to lead to ulnar nerve damage.

Anomalous Anatomic Features at the Elbow. A ligament of Struthers, if present, may cause compression of the ulnar nerve similar to the way such a ligament affects the median nerve (see ligament of Struthers syndrome under the Median Nerve). The presence of an anomalous anconeus muscle (an epitrochleoanconeus muscle) can compress the ulnar nerve near the elbow; a hypertrophied flexor carpi ulnaris muscle may also press on the ulnar nerve.

Compression at Guyon's Canal (Ulnar Tunnel). The ulnar nerve can be entrapped as it crosses from the forearm into the hand through Guyon's canal (the ulnar tunnel). The tunnel is formed by the pisohamate ligament superficially, and the base of the tunnel is formed by the pisiform and the hamate bones; space-occupying lesions within the tunnel of the type that can occur with rheumatoid arthritis and ganglia can cause damage to the ulnar nerve. Persons who engage in activities that can traumatize the hypothenar region (e.g., persons who engage in karate or who have jobs requiring them to use the hypothenar portion of their hands to press or bang) are also at risk.

Bicycle Rider's Syndrome. Prolonged bicycle riding causes compression of the ulnar nerve in the hypothenar region; a similar compression injury may occur from pressing the hypothenar region on a crutch.

Digital Nerve Entrapment Syndrome. The digital nerves that supply the skin of the fifth digits and half of the fourth digit may be compressed against the edge of the deep transverse metacarpal ligament; this syndrome appears to be caused by trauma (such as phalangeal fractures), tumors, or inflammation of the MCP joints.

Effects of Injuries

The deficits associated with damage to the ulnar nerve depend on the severity of the injury to the nerve and the site of the lesion. To determine specific deficits for each syndrome and type of injury, the course of the nerve must be considered and the resultant loss of motor and sensory function distal to the site determined (see Peripheral Nerve Entrapment Syndromes for descriptions of the symptoms of some of the more common syndromes). Pain is a common feature of the entrapment syndromes; however, sensory effects can also include hypesthesia, paresthesia, and even complete sensory loss.

Motor Deficits at the Hand. Clawhand occurs with lesions to the ulnar nerve due to the unopposed action of the radial nerve–innervated extensor digitorum communis muscle in the fourth and fifth digits. The first phalanx is hyperextended and the distal two phalanges are flexed while the fifth finger remains abducted; there is an inability to abduct or adduct the fingers because of a loss of the interossei muscles. Flexion at the DIP joints of the fourth and fifth digits is lost because of denervation of the medial half of the flexor digitorum profundus muscle. Denervation of the adductor pollicis muscle results in weakened opposition of the thumb, and there is also a total loss of opposition by the fifth finger and an inability to abduct the little finger.

Motor Deficits at the Wrist. Resisted palmar flexion of the wrist results in deviation of the wrist to the radial side because of denervation of the flexor carpi ulnaris muscle.

Special Tests
Adson's Maneuver (Test for Thoracic Outlet Syndrome). The patient turns head to the side of the suspected lesion, extends neck fully, and takes and holds a deep breath while the examiner checks for a decreased radial pulse (in some patients the effect may be more noticeable if the patient turns head away from the side of the suspected lesion). If the thoracic outlet is compromised, this maneuver further narrows the outlet and indicates whether the ulnar nerve is likely to be compressed at this level.

Tests for Compression by Ligament of Struthers (Supracondylar Process Syndrome). The examiner checks for decrease or absence of radial and/or ulnar pulses when the forearm is fully extended and supinated.

Froment's Sign. The patient is asked to grasp a piece of paper between thumb and index finger; because of paralysis of the adductor pollicis muscle, the patient flexes the thumb. This flexion becomes more pronounced when the examiner pulls the paper away.

Observable Signs. Guttering occurs between the fingers because of atrophy of the intrinsic muscles. There is flattening of the hypothenar eminence due to atrophy of the palmaris brevis muscle and the muscles of the fifth digit.

TABLE 4.27 Values for Electrodiagnostic Testing[a]: Ulnar Nerve

Site of Stimulation	Amplitude[b] Motor (mV) Sensory (V)	Latency[c] to Recording Site (ms)	Difference Between Right and Left (ms)	Conduction Time Between Two Points (ms)	Conduction Velocity(m/s)
Motor Fibers					
Wrist	5.7 ± 2.0 (2.8)[d]	2.59 ± 0.39 (3.4)[e]	0.28 ± 0.27 (0.8)[e]		
Below elbow	5.5 ± 2.0 (2.7)	6.10 ± 0.69 (7.5)	0.29 ± 0.27 (0.8)	3.51 ± 0.51 (4.5)[e]	58.7 ± 5.1 (49)[f]
Above elbow	5.5 ± 1.9 (2.7)	8.04 ± 0.76 (9.6)	0.34 ± 0.28 (0.9)	1.94 ± 0.37 (2.7)	61.0 ± 5.5 (50)
Axilla	5.6 ± 2.1 (2.7)	9.90 ± 0.91 (11.7)	0.45 ± 0.39 (1.2)	1.88 ± 0.35 (2.6)	66.5 ± 6.3 (54)
Sensory Fibers					
Digit Wrist	35.0 ± 14.7 (18)	2.54 ± 0.29 (3.1)	0.18 ± 0.13 (0.4)	2.54 ± 0.29 (3.1)	54.8 ± 5.3 (44)
Below elbow	28.8 ± 12.2 (15)	5.67 ± 0.59 (6.9)	0.26 ± 0.21 (0.5)	3.22 ± 0.42 (4.1)	64.7 ± 5.4 (53)
Above elbow	28.3 ± 11.8 (14)	7.46 ± 0.64 (8.7)	0.28 ± 0.27 (0.8)	1.79 ± 0.30 (2.4)	66.7 ± 6.4 (54)

From: Kimura, J: *Electrodiagnosis in Diseases of Nerve and Muscle: Principles and Practice*, ed. 2. FA Davis, Philadelphia, 1989, p 114, with permission.

[a]Mean ± standard deviation (SD) in 130 nerves from 65 patients, 13–74 years of age (average, 39), with no apparent disease of the peripheral nerves.

[b]Amplitude of the evoked response, measured from the baseline to the negative peak.

[c]Latency, measured to the onset of the evoked response, with the cathode 3 cm above the distal crease in the wrist.

[d]Lower limits of normal, based on the distribution of the normative data.

[e]Upper limits of normal, calculated as the mean + 2 SD.

[f]Lower limits of normal, calculated as the mean − 2 SD.

NEURO

NEURO

Radial Nerve

Course and Distribution

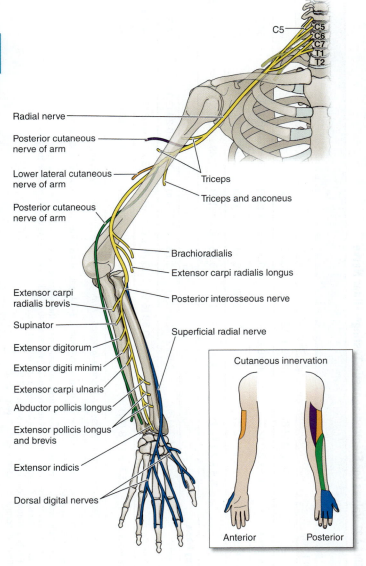

C5

C5
C6
C7
T1
T2

Radial nerve

Posterior cutaneous
nerve of arm

Lower lateral cutaneous
nerve of arm

Posterior cutaneous
nerve of arm

Triceps

Triceps and anconeus

Brachioradialis

Extensor carpi radialis longus

Extensor carpi
radialis brevis

Posterior interosseous nerve

Supinator

Extensor digitorum

Superficial radial nerve

Extensor digiti minimi

Extensor carpi ulnaris

Abductor pollicis longus

Extensor pollicis longus
and brevis

Extensor indicis

Dorsal digital nerves

Cutaneous innervation

Anterior

Posterior

Origin

The radial nerve arises from the posterior cord of the brachial plexus. Fibers originating in C5, C6, C7, C8, and T1 pass through the posterior divisions of the upper, middle, and lower trunks to contribute to the radial nerve.

Innervation

Motor

After traveling in the posterior compartment of the arm, the radial nerve travels in the cubital fossa anterior to the lateral epicondyle of the humerus; at this point it gives rise to lateral muscular branches that innervate the brachioradialis, and the extensor carpi radialis longus muscles. A deep branch (posterior interosseous nerve) continues on to innervate the triceps, anconeus, extensor carpi radialis brevis, supinator, extensor digitorum, extensor digiti minimi, extensor carpi ulnaris, abductor pollicis longus, extensor pollicis longus, extensor pollicis brevis, and extensor indicis muscles.

Cutaneous and Joint

After leaving the brachial plexus, the radial nerve courses deep to the axillary artery and winds around the upper arm in the spiral groove, where it gives off the posterior (antebrachial) cutaneous nerve, which innervates the medial posterior portion of the arm. A lower lateral cutaneous nerve innervates the medial portion of the arm on the anterior and posterior surfaces. The radial nerve continues on in the arm and at the level of the epicondyle gives off the superficial radial nerve (a sensory nerve), which supplies the dorsum of the hand on the radial side via dorsal digital nerves. The posterior interosseous nerve innervates joint structures of the wrist and the carpal bones.

Common Injuries

Entrapment Syndromes and Mononeuropathies. The radial nerve is especially vulnerable to compression because of its location in the brachial plexus and its proximity to the humerus.

Saturday Night Palsies. Pressure on the nerve at the spiral groove causes damage to the radial nerve. When a person is drunk and falls asleep with an arm against a hard object, this is called *Saturday night palsy*; the result is denervation of all muscles innervated by the radial nerve except the triceps muscle.

Inappropriate Use of Crutches. Pressure on the nerve at the spiral groove causes damage to the radial nerve. This may occur when patients lean on their crutches.

Sequelae to Fractures. During the repair of humeral fractures, newly formed callus may compress the radial nerve.

Compression at the Arcade of Frohse (Posterior Interosseous Nerve Entrapment). The posterior interosseous branch of the radial nerve passes through a fibrous arch (the arcade of Frohse) at the level of the spinator muscle, and it may be compressed at this site.

Tennis Elbow. Compression of a branch of the radial nerve at the lateral epicondyle of the humerus may give rise to pain at the elbow. This form of tennis elbow may also involve entrapment of the deep branch of the nerve.

NEURO

Trauma

Because the radial nerve runs superfically during part of its course and because it lies against the rigid spiral groove of the humerus, the nerve is very vulnerable to trauma. Shoulder dislocations, humeral fractures, and radial neck fractures can all cause damage to the radial nerve. The location of the radial nerve also makes it highly vulnerable to gunshot and stab wounds.

Effects of Injuries

The deficits associated with damage to the radial nerve depend on the severity of the injury to the nerve and the site of the lesion. To determine specific deficits for each syndrome and type of injury, the course of the nerve must be considered and the resultant loss of motor and sensory function distal to the site determined.

General Motor Defects With Radial Nerve Lesions. A lesion of the radial nerve above the innervation of the triceps muscle is possible, but quite rare; most lesions to the radial nerve affect all muscles innervated by the radial nerve except the triceps. The general findings with such lesions are an inability to extend the MCP joints, the wrist, and the thumb (tenodesis action may allow passive extension); inability to supinate unless the biceps muscle is used; weakness in palmar abduction of the thumb, although opposition is preserved; and paralysis of the brachioradialis muscle resulting in weakness of elbow flexors.

Special Tests

Palm-to-Palm Test (Wrist Drop). When separating hands that have been placed palm to palm, the hand of the affected side drops at the wrist. Wrist drop during functional activities is also an observable sign of radial nerve injury.

Impaired Gripping. Patients have trouble gripping objects because of their inability to extend their wrists.

⬤ **TABLE 4.28 Values for Electrodiagnostic Testing: Radial Nerve**

Conduction	n*	Conduction Velocity (m/s) or Conduction Time (ms)†	Amplitude: Motor (mV) Sensory (V)†	Distance (cm)†
Motor				
Axilla–elbow	8	69 ± 5.6	11 ± 7.0	15.7 ± 3.3
Elbow–forearm	10	62 ± 5.1	13 ± 8.2	18.1 ± 1.5
Forearm–muscle	10	2.4 ± 0.5	14 ± 8.8	6.2 ± 0.9

Conduction	n*	Conduction Velocity (m/s) or Conduction Time (ms)†	Amplitude: Motor (mV) Sensory (V)†	Distance (cm)†
Sensory				
Axilla–elbow	16	71 ± 5.2	4 ± 1.4	18.0 ± 0.7
Elbow–wrist	20	69 ± 5.7	5 ± 2.6	20.0 ± 0.5
Wrist–thumb	23	58 ± 6.0	13 ± 7.5	13.8 ± 0.4

Adapted from: Trojaborg, W, and Sindrup, EH: Motor and sensory conduction in different segments of the radial nerve in normal subjects. *J Neurol Neurosurg Psychiatry* 32:354–359, 1969, with permission.
*Number of subjects tested to obtain values in the table.
†Mean ± SD.

Lumbar Plexus

The lumbar plexus is formed from the anterior primary rami of L1, L2, and L3, with a contribution from L4. There is often a contribution from T12 (the subcostal nerve). The lower part of the plexus gives off the lumbosacral trunk, which contributes to the sacral plexus.

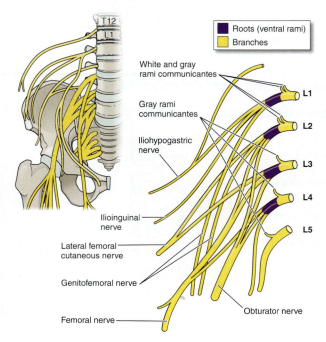

Anatomy

The lumbar plexus lies within the psoas major muscle and is composed of the anterior primary rami of L1, L2, and L3, with a contribution from L4. A contribution from T12 (the subcostal nerve) is quite common. Fibers from L4 contribute to the lumbosacral trunk, which forms part of the sacral plexus.

Injuries to the Lumbar Plexus

True lesions of the lumbar plexus are rare because the plexus lies deep within the abdomen. Damage to the plexus is often accompanied by fatal injuries. Fractures, dislocations, and space-occupying lesions (such as tumors), however, may occasionally damage the plexus. Stereotypical patterns of damage to the lumbar plexus are essentially nonexistent, although structures giving rise to the plexus may be associated with cauda equina lesions or spinal cord injuries.

NEURO

🟠 **TABLE 4.29 Lumbar Plexus Latency Determinations From Specific Nerve Root Stimulation**

	Latency Across Plexus (ms)			
Plexus	**Site of Stimulation**	**Recording Site**	**Range**	**Mean ± SD**
Lumbar	L2–L4 femoral nerve	Vastus medialis	2.0–4.4	3.4 ± 0.6

Based on: MacLean, IC. Nerve root stimulation to evaluate conduction across the brachial and lumbosacral plexuses. Third Annual Continuing Education Course, American Association of Electromyography and Electrodiagnosis, September 25, 1980, Philadelphia.

Ilio-Inguinal Nerve and Genitofemoral Nerve

Course and Distribution

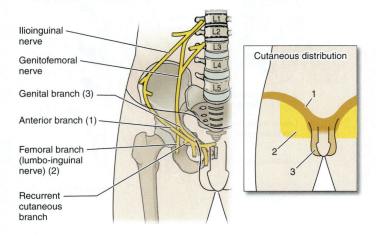

Ilio-Inguinal Nerve

Origin
The ilio-inguinal nerve is formed by fibers from L1, L2, L3, and L4. Although it is part of the lumbar plexus, it is functionally similar to the thoracic nerve because it innervates a segmental region.

Innervation
Motor
The nerve gives off segmental innervation to the obliquus internus abdominis and the transversus abdominis muscles.

Cutaneous and Joint
A cutaneous branch arises in the medial portion of the inguinal canal. An anterior branch innervates the anterior abdominal wall that overlies the pubic symphysis, the base and dorsum of the penis and the upper part of the scrotum in the male or the mons pubis and the labium majus in the female, and the thigh medial to the femoral triangle. A lateral recurrent branch innervates the skin over the thigh adjacent to the inguinal ligament.

Common Injuries
The nerve is rarely damaged; however, if it is injured, the deficit is manifest in a segmental pattern of loss. Damage may occur during surgery.

Effects of Injuries
Segmental deficits are of little clinical importance; however, some patients with ilio-inguinal neuropathies report pain in the groin, especially when they stand.

Special Tests
If an examiner applies pressure just medial to the anterior superior iliac spine (ASIS) and this causes pain to radiate into the crural region, there is evidence of an ilio-inguinal neuropathy.

Genitofemoral Nerve

The genitofemoral nerve is also called the genitocrural nerve.

Origin
Fibers from the roots of L1 and L2 unite to form the genitofemoral nerve. The nerve branches to form the lumboinguinal (femoral) branch and genital (external spermatic) branch.

Innervation
Motor
The genital (external spermatic) nerve innervates the cremasteric muscle.

Cutaneous and Joint
The genital (external spermatic) nerve innervates the skin of the inner aspect of the upper thigh and in males the scrotum and in females the labium; the lumboinguinal (femoral branch) nerve innervates the skin over the femoral triangle.

NEURO

Common Injuries

Trauma to the groin may result in injury to the genitofemoral nerve; the nerve is sometimes injured during surgery or damaged by adhesions after surgery.

Effects of Injuries

With lesions, pain may be felt in the inguinal region; there is a loss of sensation over the femoral triangle, and in males the cremasteric reflex is absent.

Special Tests

To test the nerve in males the examiner strokes the inner aspect of the thigh, and the testicle elevates if the genitofemoral nerve is intact.

NEURO

Lateral Cutaneous Nerve of the Thigh and Obturator Nerve

Course and Distribution

Anterior View

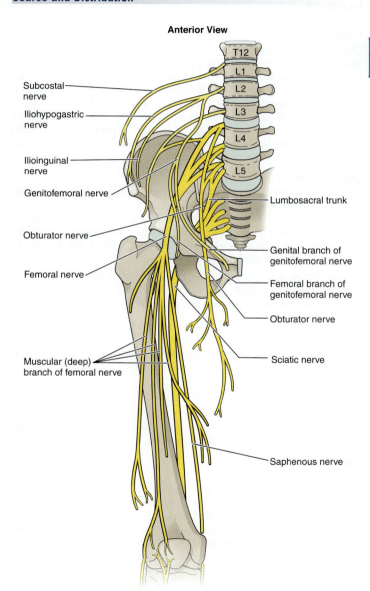

Subcostal nerve

Iliohypogastric nerve

Ilioinguinal nerve

Genitofemoral nerve

Obturator nerve

Femoral nerve

Muscular (deep) branch of femoral nerve

T12
L1
L2
L3
L4
L5

Lumbosacral trunk

Genital branch of genitofemoral nerve

Femoral branch of genitofemoral nerve

Obturator nerve

Sciatic nerve

Saphenous nerve

Lateral Cutaneous Nerve of the Thigh

Origin
The nerve is formed by contributions from L2 and L3.

Innervation
Motor
None.

Cutaneous and Joint
After being formed by fibers from L2 and L3, the nerve penetrates the psoas major muscle, crosses the iliacus muscle, and then descends downward to pass below the inguinal ligament. The nerve moves from a position deep to the fascia lata to become superficial to the fascia lata; at a level about 10 cm below the ASIS, anterior and posterior branches are formed. The anterior branch innervates the anterior aspect of the thigh to the level of the knee; the posterior branch supplies the lateral two thirds of the upper thigh and the lateral aspect of the buttocks below the greater trochanter.

Common Injuries
In the region where the lateral cutaneous nerve passes through the inguinal ligament, it is prone to entrapment; the resultant syndrome is called *meralgia paresthetica*. The exact mechanism resulting in compression at the inguinal ligament may vary between persons, although trauma, prolonged hip flexion, obesity, increased abdominal pressures, postural abnormalities, and the use of a tight belt or corset are often implicated.

Effects of Injuries
Meralgia paresthetica results in a sensory disturbance in the lateral aspect of the thigh; patients may report burning, pain, numbness, paresthesia, or even anesthesia.

Special Tests
Sensory nerve conduction studies are used to determine if there is slowing across the suspected site of compression.

Obturator Nerve

Origin
Fibers from the anterior primary rami of L3 and L4 give rise to the obturator nerve. Sometimes there are also fibers from L2.

Innervation
Motor
The obturator nerve passes through the psoas major muscle, emerging at the inner border of that muscle to descend posterior to the common iliac vessels. After passing through the obturator foramen, an anterior (superficial) branch and a posterior (deep) branch are given off. The anterior branch supplies the adductor longus, adductor brevis, and gracilis muscles; the posterior branch supplies the obturator externus, part of the adductor magnus, and the adductor brevis muscles.

Cutaneous and Joint

The anterior branch gives rise to a cutaneous branch that innervates the medial aspect of the thigh and the hip joint.

Common Injuries

The obturator nerve may be damaged during labor or from the pressure caused by a gravid uterus. Pelvic fractures may also result in obturator nerve damage, as may surgical procedures designed to correct obturator hernias.

Effects of Injuries

Weakness of adduction, internal rotation, and external rotation of the thigh are seen with damage to the obturator nerve. With injuries to the nerve, pain in the groin may be felt to radiate along the medial aspect of the thigh.

Special Tests

The primary symptom of obturator nerve damage is the pain that radiates along the medial thigh. The pain may be greatest in the region of the knee.

Femoral Nerve

Course and Distribution

NEURO

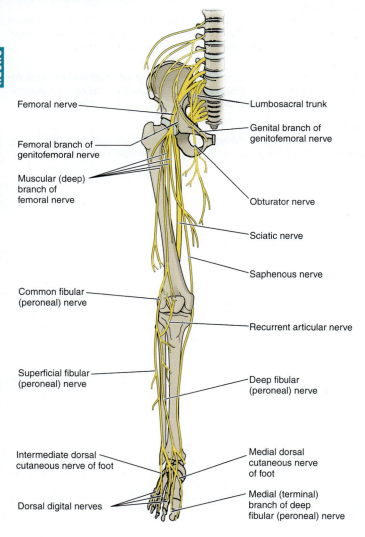

Femoral nerve

Lumbosacral trunk

Genital branch of genitofemoral nerve

Femoral branch of genitofemoral nerve

Muscular (deep) branch of femoral nerve

Obturator nerve

Sciatic nerve

Saphenous nerve

Common fibular (peroneal) nerve

Recurrent articular nerve

Superficial fibular (peroneal) nerve

Deep fibular (peroneal) nerve

Intermediate dorsal cutaneous nerve of foot

Medial dorsal cutaneous nerve of foot

Dorsal digital nerves

Medial (terminal) branch of deep fibular (peroneal) nerve

Origin

Fibers from the anterior primary rami of L2, L3, and L4 give rise to the femoral nerve.

Innervation

Motor

The femoral nerve passes through the psoas major muscle and emerges from the lateral border before passing below the inguinal ligament and giving off a branch to innervate the iliacus muscle. After passing beneath the inguinal ligament to reach the thigh, the nerve innervates the pectineus, sartorius, and quadriceps femoris muscles.

Cutaneous and Joint

Below the inguinal ligament, the femoral nerve gives rise to sensory nerves; the anterior femoral cutaneous nerve supplies the anterior portion of the thigh while the saphenous nerve descends downward. The saphenous nerve, along with the femoral vessels, passes under the sartorius muscle (in the subsartorial canal); the saphenous nerve gives off an infrapatellar branch that supplies sensory innervation to the medial aspect of the knee. The main branch of the saphenous nerve continues down the leg to supply sensory innervation to the medial side of the leg and foot.

Common Injuries

The femoral nerve is vulnerable to compression as it passes through the pelvis; damage may be caused by tumors of the vertebrae, psoas abscesses, retroperitoneal lymphadenopathies, hematomas, and fractures of the pelvis and upper femur. Direct trauma to the nerve may occur with proximal femoral fractures or during cardiac catherization. Femoral neuropathies may also be caused by vascular compromise and secondary to diabetes. The saphenous portion of the femoral nerve may be compressed as it exits the subsartorial canal (in Hunter's canal); the compression may be due to obstructive vascular disease that causes the femoral artery to press on the nerve.

Effects of Injuries

The deficits associated with damage to the femoral nerve depend on the severity of the injury to the nerve and the site of the lesion. To determine specific deficits for each type of injury, the course of the nerve must be considered and the resultant loss of motor and sensory function distal to the site determined.

General Motor Deficits. If the lesion is above the innervation of the iliacus muscle, there is weakness in hip flexion. The nerve to the quadriceps muscle is the most often injured branch of the femoral nerve. Loss of innervation of the quadriceps results in difficulty in walking because of an inability to keep the knee from buckling; walking down stairs is especially difficult with paralysis of the quadriceps muscle.

General Sensory Deficits. Sensory disturbances of the anterior thigh and medial side of leg and foot occur with lesions to the sensory portions of the femoral nerve. With saphenous nerve injuries, pain is felt in the medial aspect of the knee; this pain often radiates distally to the medial side of the foot.

Special Tests

Denervation of the quadriceps muscle results in weakness often requiring the patient to use a hand to steady the thigh; there is loss of the quadriceps reflex. With painful lesions to the saphenous nerve, the pain becomes worse with exercise and especially with stair climbing.

TABLE 4.30 Values for Diagnostic Testing: Femoral Nerve

Stimulation Point	Recording Site	n*	Age	Onset Latency (ms)†	Conduction Velocity (m/s)†
Just below inguinal ligament	14 cm from stimulus point	42	8–79	3.7 ± 0.45	70 ± 5.5 between the two recording sites
	30 cm from stimulus point	42	8–79	6.0 ± 0.60	

Based on: Gassel, MM: A study of femoral nerve conduction time. *Arch Neurol* 9:607, 1963.
*Number of subjects tested to obtain values in the table.
†Mean ± SD.

Saphenous Nerve

TABLE 4.31 Values for Diagnostic Testing: Saphenous Nerve

Method	Age (yr)	n*	Inguinal Ligament—Knee Amplitude (µV)	Inguinal Ligament—Knee Conduction Velocity (m/s)	n*	Knee—Medial Malleolus Amplitude (µV)†	Knee—Medial Malleolus Conduction Velocity (m/s)†
Orthodromic	17–38	33	4.2 ± 2.3	59.6 ± 2.3	10	4.8 ± 2.4	52.3 ± 2.3
Orthodromic	<40	28	5.5 ± 2.6	58.9 ± 3.2	22	2.1 ± 1.1	51.2 ± 4.7
	>40	41	5.1 ± 2.7	57.9 ± 4.0	32	1.7 ± 0.8	50.2 ± 5.0
Antidromic	20–79			Peak latency of 3.6 ± 1.4 for 14 cm	80	9.0 ± 3.4	41.7 ± 3.4
Orthodromic	18–56	71					54.8 ± 1.9

From: Kimura, J: Electrodiagnosis in Diseases of Nerve and Muscle: Principles and Practice, ed. 2. FA Davis, Philadelphia, 1989, p 134, with permission.
*Number of subjects tested to obtain values in the table.
†Mean ± SD.

NEURO

Sacral Plexus

The sacral plexus is formed by the lumbosacral trunk, which comes from the lumbar plexus (L4), and the anterior primary rami of L5, S1, S2, and S3. Contributions may also come from S4.

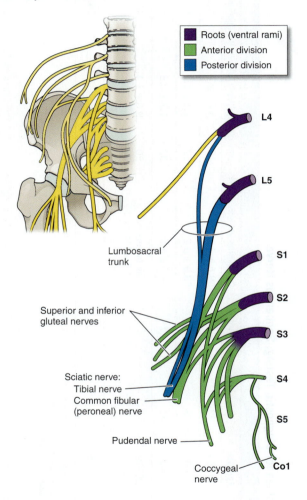

Roots (ventral rami)
Anterior division
Posterior division

L4

L5

Lumbosacral trunk

S1

S2

Superior and inferior gluteal nerves

S3

Sciatic nerve:
Tibial nerve
Common fibular (peroneal) nerve

S4

S5

Pudendal nerve

Coccygeal nerve

Co1

Anatomy

The lumbosacral trunk from the lumbar plexus joins with fibers from the anterior primary rami of L4, L5, S1, S2, and S3 to form the sacral plexus. There may also be contributions from S4. The plexus lies in front of the sacroiliac joint.

Injuries to the Sacral Plexus

Injuries to the sacral plexus are quite rare, although damage to roots of the lumbar region occurs relatively frequently with disk disease. Fractures, dislocations, and space-occupying lesions (such as tumors), however, may occasionally cause damage to the plexus.

● **TABLE 4.32 Sacral Plexus Latency Determinations From Specific Nerve Root Stimulation**

Plexus	Site of Stimulation	Recording Site	Range	Mean ± SD
Sacral	L5 and S1 sciatic nerve	Abductor hallucis	2.5–4.9	3.9 ± 0.7

Latency Across Plexus(ms)

Sciatic Nerve, Tibial Nerve, Sural Nerve, and Common Fibular Nerve: Posterior View

Course and Distribution

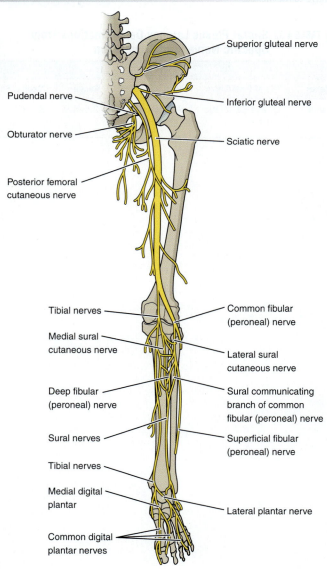

- Superior gluteal nerve
- Inferior gluteal nerve
- Sciatic nerve
- Pudendal nerve
- Obturator nerve
- Posterior femoral cutaneous nerve
- Tibial nerves
- Medial sural cutaneous nerve
- Deep fibular (peroneal) nerve
- Sural nerves
- Tibial nerves
- Medial digital plantar
- Common digital plantar nerves
- Common fibular (peroneal) nerve
- Lateral sural cutaneous nerve
- Sural communicating branch of common fibular (peroneal) nerve
- Superficial fibular (peroneal) nerve
- Lateral plantar nerve

NEURO

Sciatic Nerve

Origin
The sciatic nerve is derived from fibers originating in the anterior primary rami of L4, L5, S1, S2, and S3.

Innervation
Motor
The sciatic nerve initially travels as one bundle but is actually made up of divisible units that give rise to the tibial nerve and the common fibular nerve. The sciatic nerve leaves the pelvis via the greater sciatic foramen and courses under the gluteus maximus muscle to pass between the greater trochanter and the ischial tuberosity. In the thigh the nerve descends between the adductor magnus and the hamstring muscles. Rami from the tibial portion of the nerve innervate the long head of the biceps femoris, semitendinosus, semimembranosus, and adductor magnus muscles; in the thigh, rami of the peroneal portion innervate the short head of the biceps femoris muscle. Above the popliteal fossa the nerve divides, giving rise to the tibial and common fibular nerves.

Cutaneous and Joint
The sciatic nerve has no direct cutaneous innervation; the tibial and fibular nerves, which are derived from the sciatic nerve, provide cutaneous innervation to the lateral leg and foot.

Common Injuries
Intramuscular injections improperly given in the buttock region may injure the sciatic nerve. Fractures of the pelvis and femur may result in damage to the sciatic nerve. Wounds (stab and gunshot) are common causes of damage to the sciatic nerve, and it is often affected by tumors originating in the genitourinary tract or rectum. Compression of the nerve may also be due to pressure from a gravid uterus or from an abscess in the pelvic floor. A Baker's popliteal cyst may compress the lower portion of the sciatic nerve. Prolonged squatting can cause damage to the sciatic nerve owing to pressure on the nerve as it passes between ischial tuberosity and the greater trochanter or as it passes between the adductor magnus and the hamstring muscles.

Piriformis syndrome may occur when the nerve is compressed between the piriformis and the obturator internus muscles as it exits the pelvis in the greater sciatic foramen. Sustained contractions of the piriformis muscle and fibrotic changes in the piriformis muscle secondary to trauma have been implicated in causing piriformis syndrome.

Effects of Injuries
The deficits associated with damage to the sciatic nerve depend on the severity of the injury to the nerve and the site of the lesion. To determine specific deficits for each type of injury, the course of the nerve must be considered and the resultant loss of motor and sensory function distal to the site determined. Lesions to the sciatic nerve are always accompanied by loss of function of the common fibular nerve, the tibial nerve, or both.

General Motor Deficits. With loss of the sciatic nerve, there is loss of voluntary flexion at the knee due to denervation of the hamstring muscles. Paralysis of all the muscles of the leg and foot leads to a steppage gait and an inability to run; footdrop is noticeable. With piriformis syndrome, there can be weakness of the hamstrings and all the muscles innervated by the peroneal and tibial nerve derivates.

General Sensory Deficits. With lesions of the sciatic nerve, there is a loss of sensation on the lateral side of the leg and the foot; with piriformis syndrome, pain and/or diminished sensation may be felt on the posterior aspect of the leg and the plantar surface of the foot.

Special Tests

Loss of the Achilles reflex and the plantar reflex is seen with lesions of the sciatic nerve; there is an inability to stand on the toes or heels. If the nerve is damaged, placing the sciatic nerve on stretch by straight leg raising may evoke Lasègue's sign (pain along the distribution of the sciatic nerve). With sciatic nerve damage, joint position sense is lost for the foot and toes.

Tibial Nerve

Origin

The tibial nerve arises from the sciatic nerve above the level of the popliteal fossa. It contains fibers from the anterior primary rami of L4, L5, S1, S2, and S3.

Innervation
Motor

The tibial nerve passes through the popliteal fossa and down the back of the leg and gives off branches that innervate both heads of the gastrocnemius, plantaris, soleus, popliteus, and the tibialis posterior muscles. The portion of nerve below the popliteal fossa was called the *posterior tibial nerve* but is now considered part of the tibial nerve. Below the popliteal fossa, the tibial nerve innervates the flexor digitorum longus and flexor hallucis longus muscles. After the tibial nerve passes the level of the heel, it divides into two terminal branches—the medial plantar nerve and the lateral plantar nerve.

The medial plantar nerve innervates the flexor digitorum brevis, abductor hallucis, flexor hallucis brevis, and the first lumbrical muscles, and the lateral plantar nerve, which innervates the quadratus plantae, abductor digiti minimi, flexor digiti minimi brevis, opponens digit minimi, the plantar and dorsal interossei, and the second, third, and fourth lumbrical muscles.

Cutaneous and Joint

In the region of the popliteal fossa, the sural nerve, a cutaneous division of the tibial nerve, branches off and descends down the lateral leg; the sural nerve supplies innervation to the posterolateral leg and gives rise to the lateral calcaneal nerve at the level of the heel. The lateral calcaneal nerve innervates the posterolateral heel area; as the tibial nerve reaches the heel, it gives rise to the medial calcaneal nerve, which innervates the posteromedial heel area.

After the tibial nerve passes the level of the heel, it divides into two branches—the medial plantar nerve and the lateral plantar nerve. Digital branches from the medial plantar nerve innervate the medial plantar surface of the foot and the plantar surfaces of the medial three-and-a-half digits; digital branches from the lateral plantar nerve innervate the lateral portion of the plantar surface of the foot and the plantar surfaces of the lateral one-and-a-half toes.

NEURO

Common Injuries

Damage to the sciatic nerve usually involves portions that form the tibial nerve. Isolated damage to the tibial nerve is usually due to an injury in or below the popliteal space; this region is particularly vulnerable to trauma. The tibial nerve is often compressed by the flexor retinaculum (the tarsal tunnel) as it passes behind and beneath the medial malleolus; this is called *tarsal tunnel syndrome* and is thought to occur as a result of trauma, tenosynovitis, or venous stasis of the posterior tibial vein.

The digital branches of the medial and lateral plantar nerves may be compressed under the metatarsal heads, giving rise to Morton's neuroma, a painful condition of the foot. Symptoms similar to those seen with Morton's neuroma are caused by other mechanical problems, such as irritation by ligaments placed on stretch due to the wearing of high-heeled shoes; hallux valgus, rheumatoid arthritis, congenital malformations, or trauma may also cause pain.

Effects of Injuries

The deficits associated with damage to the tibial nerve depend on the severity of the injury to the nerve and the site of the lesion. To determine specific deficits for each type of injury, the course of the nerve must be considered and the resultant loss of motor and sensory function distal to the site determined. With damage to the tibial nerve, there is an inability to plantar flex, adduct, and invert the foot and an inability to flex, abduct, and adduct the toes; patients are unable to stand on their toes and find walking fatiguing and even painful.

Tarsal tunnel syndrome results in pain and/or sensory loss on the plantar surface of the foot. This pain may be most severe after prolonged walking or standing; pain may be restricted to the area of the medial foot and the great toe.

Special Tests

With lesions of the tibial nerve, the Achilles reflex is lost. To test for tarsal tunnel syndrome, the examiner taps the medial malleolus just above the margin of the flexor retinaculum; paresthesias felt in the foot are indicative of tarsal tunnel syndrome.

NEURO

NEURO

TABLE 4.33 Values for Diagnostic Testing[a]: Tibial Nerve

Site of Stimulation	Amplitude[b] (mV)	Latency to Recording Site (ms)	Difference Between Two Sides (ms)	Conduction Time Between Two Points (ms)	Conduction Velocity (m/s)
Ankle	5.8 ± 1.9 (2.9)[d]	3.96 ± 1.00 6.0)[e]	0.66 ± 0.57 (1.8)[e]	8.09 ± 1.09 (10.3)[e]	48.5 ± 3.6 (41)[f]
Knee	5.1 ± 2.2 (2.5)	12.05 ± 1.53 (15.1)	0.79 ± 0.61 (2.0)		

From: Kimura, J: *Electrodiagnosis in Diseases of Nerve and Muscle: Principles and Practice*, ed. 2. FA Davis, Philadelphia, 1989, p 123, with permission.

[a]Mean ± standard deviation (SD) in 118 nerves from 59 patients, 11–78 years of age (average, 39), with no apparent disease of the peripheral nerves.
[b]Amplitude of the evoked response, measured from the baseline to the negative peak.
[c]Latency, measured to the onset of the evoked response, with a standard distance of 10 cm between the cathode and the recording electrode.
[d]Lower limits of normal, based on the distribution of the normative data.
[e]Upper limits of normal, calculated as the mean + 2 SD.
[f]Lower limits of normal, calculated as the mean − 2 SD.

TABLE 4.34 Latency Comparison Between Fibular and Tibial Nerves in the Same Limb*

Site of Stimulation	Fibular	Tibial Nerve (ms)	Difference (ms)
Ankle	3.89 ± 0.87 (5.6)[†]	4.12 ± 1.06 (6.2)[†]	0.77 ± 0.65 (2.1)[†]
Knee	12.46 ± 1.38 (15.2)	12.13 ± 1.48 (15.1)	0.88 ± 0.71 (2.3)

From: Kimura, J: *Electrodiagnosis in Diseases of Nerve and Muscle: Principles and Practice*, ed. 2. FA Davis, Philadelphia, 1989, p 124, with permission.

*Mean ± standard deviation (SD) in 104 nerves from 52 patients, 17–86 years of age (average, 41), with no apparent disease of the peripheral nerve.
[†]Upper limits of normal, calculated as the mean + 2 SD.

Sural Nerve

TABLE 4.35 Values for Diagnostic Testing: Sural Nerve

Stimulation Point	Recording Site	n*	Age (yr)	Amplitude (V)†	Latency (ms)†	Conduction Velocity (m/s)†
Foot	High ankle	40	13–41	6.3 (1.9–17)		44.0 ± 4.7
Lower third of leg	Lateral malleolus	38 62	1–15 Over 15	23.1 ± 4.42 3.7 ± 3.8	1.46 ± 0.43 2.27 ± 0.43 (Peak)	52.1 ± 5.1 46.2 ± 3.3
15 cm above lateral malleolus	Dorsal aspect of foot	71	15–30 40–65			51.2 ± 4.5 48.3 ± 5.3
14 cm above lateral malleolus	Lateral malleolus	101	13–66		3.50 ± 0.25 (Peak)	40.1
Lower third of leg	Lateral malleolus	80	20–79	18.9 ± 6.7	3.7 ± 0.3 (Peak)	41.0 ± 2.5
Distal 10 cm		102				33.9 ± 3.25
Middle 10 cm	Lateral malleolus	102				51.0 ± 3.8
Proximal 10 cm		102				51.6 ± 3.8
14 cm above lateral malleolus	Lateral malleolus	52	10–40 41–84	20.9 ± 8.0 17.2 ± 6.7	2.7 ± 0.3 2.8 ± 0.3 (Onset)	52.5 ± 5.6 51.1 ± 5.9

From: Kimura, J: *Electrodiagnosis in Diseases of Nerve and Muscle: Principles and Practice*, ed. 2. FA Davis, Philadelphia, 1989, p 131, with permission.
*Number of subjects tested to obtain values in the table.
†Mean ± SD.

Common Fibular (Lateral Popliteal) Nerve

Origin

The common fibular nerve arises from the sciatic nerve above the level of the popliteal fossa. It contains fibers from the anterior primary rami of L4, L5, S1, and S2.

Innervation

Motor

The common fibular nerve arises from the sciatic nerve at the upper part of the popliteal fossa, descends along the posterior border of the biceps femoris muscle, and courses around the head of the fibula to the anterior compartment of the leg. Below the head of the fibula, it divides to form the deep fibular nerve, which innervates the tibialis anterior, extensor digitorum longus, extensor hallucis longus, peroneus tertius, and extensor digitorum brevis muscles, and the superficial fibular nerve, which innervates the peroneus longus and the peroneus brevis muscles.

Cutaneous and Joint

At the level of the popliteal fossa, the common fibular nerve gives off the superior and inferior articular branches that innervate the knee joint. The lateral cutaneous nerve exits the common fibular nerve above the head of the fibula (see figure on page 300 with superficial fibular nerve); this branch innervates the lateral upper leg. Branches of the superficial fibular nerve innervate the anterior portion of the leg, with the exception of the space between the great toe and the first toe, which is innervated by the deep fibular nerve; the deep fibular nerve also supplies the ankle joint, the inferior tibiofibular joint, and the joints of the toes.

Common Injuries

Damage to the sciatic nerve usually involves portions that form the common fibular nerve. Because of the superficial course of the common fibular nerve as it crosses by the head of the fibula, the nerve is more likely to be damaged than are either of its major branches. As a result of the firm attachment of the nerve to the fibular head, there is an additional predisposing factor to injury because the nerve cannot easily move when compressed.

Habitual sitting in a cross-legged position or prolonged squatting may compress the common fibular nerve at the neck of the fibula; the nerve may also be injured at this site during sleep or anesthesia. Improper application of elastic bandages and plaster casts can damage the nerve near the fibula. Persons who are bedridden and allowed to maintain their legs in excessive external rotation are also prone to compression injuries of the common fibular nerve.

Effects of Injuries

Complete lesions to the common fibular nerve result in paralysis of the muscles of the anterior and lateral compartments of the leg; the subject cannot dorsiflex or evert the foot. Patients exhibit a steppage gait (e.g., to compensate for lack of dorsiflexion they use excessive hip flexion), and at heel strike the lateral border of the foot contacts the ground before the heel. Footdrop deformities commonly develop in patients who have lesions of the common fibular nerve;

sensation is lost in the lateral portion of the leg and in the dorsum of the foot with this lesion. Pain is a rare component of common fibular injuries; when pain is present, it is quite mild.

Special Tests

Lesions to the common fibular nerve can be differentiated from spinal root and sciatic nerve lesions because the Achilles reflex is preserved with the common fibular nerve lesion and there is also normal inversion of the foot. Lesions of the common fibular nerve are relatively apparent because of the pattern of motor loss and the footdrop that is not accompanied by symptoms of sciatic nerve damage.

NEURO

TABLE 4.36 Values for Diagnostic Testing[a]: Common Fibular Nerve

Site of Stimulation	Amplitude[b] (mV)	Latency[c] to Recording Site (ms)	Difference Between Right and Left (ms)	Conduction Time Between Two Points (ms)	Conduction Velocity (m/s)
Ankle	5.1 ± 2.3 (2.5)[d]	3.77 ± 0.86 (5.5)[e]	0.62 ± 0.61 (1.8)[e]	7.01 ± 0.89 (8.8)[e]	48.3 ± 3.9 (40)[f]
Below knee	5.1 ± 2.0 (2.5)	10.79 ± 1.06 (12.9)	0.65 ± 0.65 (2.0)	1.72 ± 0.40 (2.5)	52.0 ± 6.2 (40)
Above knee	5.1 ± 1.9 (2.5)	12.51 ± 1.17 (14.9)	0.65 ± 0.60 (1.9)		

From: Kimura, J: *Electrodiagnosis in Diseases of Nerve and Muscle: Principles and Practice*, ed. 2. FA Davis, Philadelphia, 1989, p 126, with permission.

[a]Mean ± standard deviation (SD) in 120 nerves from 60 patients, 16–86 years of age (average, 41), with no apparent disease of the peripheral nerves.

[b]Amplitude of the evoked response, measured from the baseline to the negative peak.

[c]Latency, measured to the onset of the evoked response, with a standard distance of 7 cm between the cathode and the recording electrode.

[d]Lower limits of normal, based on the distribution of the normative data.

[e]Upper limits of normal, calculated as the mean + 2 SD.

[f]Lower limits of normal, calculated as the mean − 2 SD.

Deep Fibular Nerve

Course and Distribution
Muscles innervated by nerves are listed in italics.

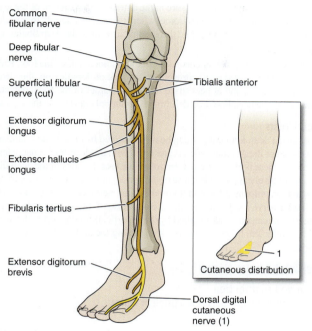

The deep fibular nerve arises from the common fibular nerve just below the head of the fibula. The fibers originated in L4, L5, and S1.

Origin
The deep fibular nerve arises from the common fibular nerve just below the head of the fibula. The fibers originated in L4, L5, and S1.

Innervation
Motor
The deep fibular nerve arises below the neck of the fibula and then courses anteriorly down the leg along the interosseous membrane. As the nerve passes down the leg, it innervates the tibialis anterior, extensor digitorum longus, extensor hallucis longus, peroneus tertius, and extensor digitorum muscles.

Cutaneous and Joint
At the level of the foot, the deep fibular nerve gives rise to a dorsal cutaneous branch that innervates the space between the great toe and the first toe; the deep fibular nerve also supplies the ankle joint, the inferior tibiofibular joint, and the joints of the toes.

Common Injuries

Isolated injuries to the deep fibular nerve are less likely than are injuries to the common fibular nerve. With complete common fibular nerve lesions, there is loss of innervation to all structures innervated by the deep fibular nerve (see common fibular nerve); lesions of the deep fibular nerve, however, can occur in the region of the fibular neck. Increased pressure in the anterior compartment of the leg can lead to anterior compartment syndrome, where the vascular supply to muscles of the anterior leg is compromised and there is impairment of the deep fibular nerve.

Effects of Injuries

After injury to the deep fibular nerve, the patient cannot dorsiflex the foot. Patients exhibit a steppage gait (i.e., to compensate for lack of dorsiflexion, they use excessive hip flexion), and at heel strike the lateral border of the foot contacts the ground before the heel. Footdrop deformities commonly develop in these patients.

Special Tests

Lesions to the deep fibular nerve can be differentiated from root and sciatic nerve lesions because the Achilles reflex is preserved with the deep fibular nerve lesions and because there is also normal inversion of the foot. Lesions of the deep fibular nerve are relatively apparent because of the pattern of motor loss and the footdrop that is not accompanied by symptoms of sciatic nerve damage. Lesions of the deep fibular nerve can be differentiated from those of the common fibular nerve because the cutaneous area supplied by the superficial fibular nerve (the anterior leg) is not affected, but the space between the big toe and the first toe may lose sensation.

Superficial Fibular Nerve

Course and Distribution

Muscles innervated by nerves are listed in italics.

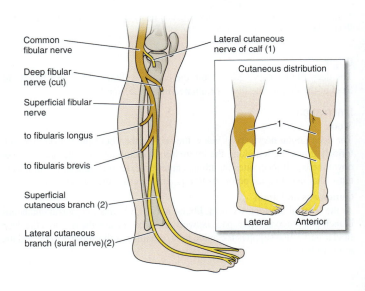

Origin

The superficial fibular nerve is formed by the continuation of the common fibular nerve in the lateral crural compartment after the deep fibular nerve has branched off below the level of the fibular neck. The fibers originated in the L4, L5, and S1 roots.

Innervation

Motor

As the superficial fibular nerve passes down the leg, it innervates the peroneus longus and the peroneus brevis muscles.

Cutaneous and Joint

Above the ankle, medial and lateral cutaneous branches arise from the superficial fibular nerve. These branches innervate the anterior portion of the leg and foot with the exception of the space between the great toe and the first toe, which is innervated by the deep fibular nerve.

Common Injuries

Isolated injuries to the superficial fibular nerve are very rare and are much less likely than injuries to the common fibular nerve. With complete common fibular nerve lesions, there is loss of innervation to all structures innervated by the superficial fibular nerve (see common fibular nerve).

Effects of Injuries

With complete lesions of the superficial fibular nerve, there is an inability to evert the foot. Dorsiflexion is preserved but is always accompanied by inversion. Sensory loss is most notable on the medial part of the dorsum of the foot.

Special Tests

The loss of eversion, preservation of inversion and dorsiflexion, and the pattern of sensory loss on the dorsum of the foot are indicative of the rare isolated lesion to the superficial fibular nerve.

NEURO

NEURO

TABLE 4.37 Values for Diagnostic Testing: Deep Fibular Nerve

Stimulation Point	Recording Site	n*	Age (years)	Amplitude (V)†	Latency (ms)†	Conduction Velocity (m/s)†
5 cm above, 2 cm medial to lateral malleolus	Dorsum of foot	50	1–15	13.0 ± 4.6	1.22 ± 0.40 (Peak)	53.1 ± 5.3 (Distal segment)
		50	Over 15	13.9 ± 4.0	2.24 ± 0.49 (Peak)	47.3 ± 3.4 (Distal segment)
Anterior edge of fibula, 12 cm above the active electrode	Medial border of lateral malleolus	50	3–60	20.5 ± 6.1	2.9 ± 0.3 (Peak)	65.7 ± 3.7 (Proximal segment)
Anterolateral aspect of leg, 14 cm above the active electrode	Medial border of lateral malleolus	80		18.3	2.8 ± 0.3 (Onset)	51.2 ± 5.7 (Proximal segment)

From: Kimura, J: *Electrodiagnosis in Diseases of Nerve and Muscle: Principles and Practice*, ed. 2. FA Davis, Philadelphia, 1989, p 129, with permission.
*Number of subjects tested to obtain values in the table.
†Mean ± SD.

Electromyographic (EMG) Studies

Activity Patterns

The aim of the clinical EMG study is to determine whether muscle weakness is due to a neurogenic disorder or to myopathy. The clinical EMG study uses needle electrode recordings to discern pathology. Because EMG findings in individual muscles may be nonspecific, several of the following tests in clinically involved muscles and unaffected muscles are typically assessed:

- **activity at rest:** denervation activity–fibrillation potentials, positive sharp waves; presence of fasciculations; complex repetitive discharges; myotonic activity; and neuromyotonia.
- **voluntary minimal effort:** the duration, amplitude, and shape of motor unit potentials (MUPs); and incidence of polyphasic potentials.
- **voluntary maximal effort:** the amplitude and interference pattern of the electrical activity; and turns and amplitude ratios.

Due to the large variability of MUP duration and amplitude in various muscles, and to the effect of age, it is recommended to measure 20–30 MUPs from as many as 10 different insertion sites in the muscle to obtain a representative sample. The findings should be compared to age-matched control data for the muscle examined. The following specific and nonspecific criteria are considered when making a diagnosis for neurogenic disease or myopathy:

TABLE 4.38 EMG Criteria for Neuromuscular Disease (from concentric needle)

	Specific Criteria	Nonspecific Criteria
Criteria for Myopathy Activity at rest	—	Fibrillation activity and positive sharp waves
Voluntary minimal effort	Decrease in duration MUP (>20% shortened)	Increased incidence of polyphasic potentials (>12%)
Voluntary maximal effort	Full recruitment pattern in a weak and wasted muscle Decreased amplitude of full recruitment pattern	Reduced recruitment pattern
Criteria for Peripheral Nerve and Root Disease Activity at rest	—	Fibrillation activity and positive sharp waves (4–10 sites)

(table continues on page 304)

TABLE 4.38 EMG Criteria for Neuromuscular Disease (from concentric needle) (continued)

	Specific Criteria	Nonspecific Criteria
Voluntary minimal effort	Increase in duration MUP (>20% prolonged) Increase in amplitude	Increased incidence of polyphasic potentials (>12%)
Voluntary maximal effort	Discrete activity; Increased amplitude	Reduced recruitment pattern
Criteria of Anterior Horn Cell Disease Activity at rest	Fasciculations (malignant, intervals of >3 sec)	Fasciculations (benign, intervals <1 sec)
Voluntary minimal effort	Increase in amplitude (>500% increased)	Increase in amplitude of individual Mumps (200%)
Voluntary maximal effort	Increased amplitude (>6 mV)	—

From: Krarup, C: Pitfalls in electrodiagnosis. *J Neurol* 246:1115–1126, 1999, with permission.

Electromyographic Patterns for Normal, Neurogenic, and Myogenic Lesions

Examples of EMG activity for various diseases and lesions are provided in the figure on page 305. *Insertional activity* refers to electrical activity recorded when the needle is inserted or moved within the muscle. *Spontaneous activity* refers to the electrical activity recorded after the cessation of insertional activity in resting muscle. The *motor unit potential* is the compound electrical wave formed by the depolarization of the muscle fibers belonging to a motor unit. The *interference pattern* is the electrical activity recorded from a muscle during maximal voluntary effort.

Lesion / EMG steps	Normal	Neurogenic Lesion		Myogenic Lesion		
		Motoneuron	CNS	Myopathy	Myotonia	Polymyositis
1 Insertional activity	Normal	Increased	Normal	Normal	Myotonic discharge	Increased
2 Spontaneous activity		Fibrillation / Positive wave			Myotonic discharge	Fibrillation / Positive wave
3 Monitor unit potential	0.5-1.0 mV / 5-10 ms	Large unit / Limited recruitment	Normal	Small unit / Early recruitment	Myotonic discharge	Small unit / Early recruitment
4 Interference pattern	Full	Reduced / Fast firing rate	Reduced / Slow firing rate	Full amplitude / Low	Full amplitude / Low	Full amplitude / Low

Electrodes Used for Clinical EMG Studies

Although surface electrodes are easily applied, and the response is reproducible, the shape of the potentials cannot be studied in detail and therefore needle electrodes are used. Needles record from a much smaller detection area than surface electrodes and therefore multiple insertions are required to adequately sample from the muscle. The different types of needle electrodes used in clinical EMG studies are shown schematically in the figure on page 306. The number of fibers that contribute to the potential depends on the surface recording area of the EMG electrode, with macro-electrode > monopolar electrode > concentric needle > bifilar needle > single-fiber electrode.

NEURO

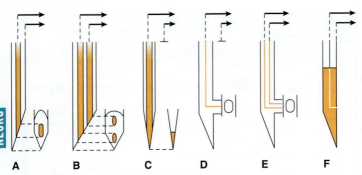

Schematic illustration of standard or coaxial bipolar (A), concentric bipolar
(B), monopolar (C), single fiber needles (D and E), and Macro EMG (F). Dimensions
vary, but the diameters of the outside cannulas shown resemble 26-gauge hypodermic
needles (460 μm) for A, D, and E; a 23-gauge needle (640 μm) for B; and a 28-gauge
needle (360 μm) for C and F. The exposed-tip areas measure 150×300 μm, with
spacing between wires of 200 μm center to center for B; 0.14 sq mm for C; and
25 μm in diameter for D, E, and F. A flat-skin electrode completes the circuit with
unipolar electrodes shown in C and D. For Macro EMG (F), a 10-mm side port is
located behind the tip, exposing a 25-g diameter platinum wire. Macro EMG recording
is made on one channel from the side port electrode with the cannula as reference
(ordinary single-fiber EMG recording), and other channel potentials are recorded
between the cannula and a remote subcutaneous concentric needle electrode as
reference, placed at least 30 cm away. Contribution from all muscle fibers in a motor
unit is extracted using *spike-triggered averaging* from the two channels.

TABLE 4.39 Types of Electrodiagnostic Waveforms

Waveform	Definition	Description/Interpretation
A wave	Compound action potential evoked from a muscle by submaximal electric stimuli to the nerve.	The amplitude of the A wave is similar to that of the F wave, but the latency is more constant. Due to normal or pathological axonal branching.
Auditory evoked potentials (AEPs) *See Brainstem auditory evoked potentials.*	Electric waveforms of biological origin elicited in response to sound stimuli.	Classified by their latency as short-latency brainstem AEPs (BAEPs) with a latency of up to 10 ms, middle-latency AEPs with a latency of 10–50 ms, and long-latency AEPs with a latency of over 50 ms.
Blink responses (somatosensory-evoked blink response [SBRI])	Compound muscle action potentials evoked from orbicularis oculi muscles as a result of brief electrical stimulation of a peripheral nerve or the skin of the body or limbs.	Early (R1) and Late (R2) components of the waveform are identified. It was first reported in patients with Miller–Fisher syndrome and in patients with various neurological disorders such as Parkinson's disease and hemifacial spasm.
Brainstem auditory evoked potentials (BAEPs or BAERs, BERs)	Electric waveforms of biological origin elicited in response to sound stimuli.	Normal BAEP consists of a sequence of up to seven waves, named I to VII, which occur during the first 10 ms after the onset of the stimulus and have positive polarity at the vertex of the head.
Complex repetitive discharge (synchronized fibrillation)	Polyphasic or serrated action potentials that may begin spontaneously or after a needle movement.	Have a uniform frequency, shape, and amplitude, with abrupt onset, cessation, or change in configuration. Amplitude ranges from 100 µV to 1 mV, and frequency of discharge from 5 to 100 Hz. Nonspecific abnormality. Sounds like "motorboat or motorcycle."

(table continues on page 308)

NEURO

NEURO

TABLE 4.39 Types of Electrodiagnostic Waveforms (continued)

Waveform	Definition	Description/Interpretation
Cramp discharge	Involuntary repetitive firing of motor unit action potentials at a high frequency (up to 150 Hz) in a large area of muscles.	Usually associated with painful muscle contraction. Both the discharge frequency and the number of motor unit action potentials firing increase gradually during development and both subside gradually with cessation.
End-plate activity	Spontaneous electric activity recorded with a needle electrode close to muscle end-plates.	May be either of two forms: *Monophasic:* Low-amplitude (10–20 μV), short-duration (0.5–1 ms), monophasic (negative) potentials that occur in a dense, steady pattern and are restricted to a localized area of the muscle. These nonpropagated potentials are probably miniature end-plate potentials recorded extracellularly. *Biphasic:* Moderate-amplitude (100–300 μV), short-duration (2–4 ms), biphasic (negative-positive) spike potentials that occur irregularly in short bursts with a high frequency (50–100 Hz), restricted to a localized area within the muscle. These propagated potentials are generated by muscle fibers excited by activity in nerve terminals.
F wave (F reflex or F response)	A compound action potential evoked intermittently from a muscle by a supramaximal electric stimulus to the nerve.	The F wave has a smaller amplitude (1%–5% of the M wave), variable configuration and a longer, more variable latency. The F wave can be found in many muscles of the upper and lower extremities, and the latency is longer with more distal sites of stimulation. The F wave is due to antidromic activation of motor neurons.

Waveform	Definition	Description/Interpretation
Fasciculation potential	The electric potential often associated with a visible fasciculation (twitching) that has the configuration of a motor unit action potential but that occurs spontaneously.	Most commonly occur sporadically and are termed "single fasciculation potentials." Occasionally, they occur as a grouped discharge and are termed a "brief repetitive discharge." May be benign or pathological.
Fibrillation potential	An action potential associated with a spontaneously contracting (fibrillating) muscle fiber. It is the action potential of a single muscle fiber.	May occur spontaneously or after movement of the needle electrode; they usually fire at a constant rate, although a small proportion fire irregularly. Typically seen as biphasic spikes of short duration (usually less than 5 ms) with an initial positive phase (peak-to-peak amplitude <1 mV) and a firing rate of 1–50 Hz that often decreases just before cessation of an individual discharge. Detectable 2 to 3 weeks after denervation; consistent with axonal degeneration; may be seen with myopathy. Sounds like "rain on a tin roof."
H wave (H response or Hoffmann reflex)	A compound muscle action potential having a consistent latency evoked regularly, when present, from a muscle by an electric stimulus to the nerve.	Regularly found only in a limited group of physiological extensors, particularly the calf muscles. The H wave has a smaller amplitude, a longer latency, and a lower optimal stimulus intensity than the M wave of the same muscle. The H wave is thought to be due to a spinal reflex, the Hoffmann reflex, with electric stimulation of afferent fibers in the mixed nerve to the muscle and activation of motor neurons to the muscle through a monosynaptic connection in the spinal cord.

(table continues on page 310)

NEURO

TABLE 4.39 Types of Electrodiagnostic Waveforms (continued)

Waveform	Definition	Description/Interpretation
Insertion activity	Electric activity caused by insertion or movement of a needle electrode.	The amount of the activity may be described as normal, reduced, increased (prolonged), with a description of the waveform and repetitive rate.
Jitter (single fiber electromyographic jitter)	The variability with consecutive discharges of the interpotential interval between two muscle fiber action potentials belonging to the same motor unit.	Usually expressed quantitatively as the mean value of the difference between the interpotential intervals of successive discharges (the mean consecutive difference, MCD).
M wave (M response)	A compound action potential evoked from a muscle by a single electric stimulus to its motor nerve.	By convention, the M wave elicited by supramaximal stimulation is used for motor nerve conduction studies. The configuration of the M wave (usually biphasic) is quite stable with repeated stimuli at slow rates (1–15 Hz). The latency (motor latency), baseline-to-peak amplitude, and duration are specified.
Macro motor unit action potential (macro MUAP)	The average electric activity of that part of an anatomic motor unit that is within the recording range of a macro-EMG electrode. See EMG electrodes.	Characterized by its consistent appearance when the small recording surface of the macro-EMG electrode is positioned to record action potentials from one muscle fiber.
Motor unit action potential (MUAP)	Action potential reflecting the electric activity of a single anatomic motor unit.	The compound action potential of those muscle fibers within the recording range of an electrode.

NEURO

Waveform	Definition	Description/Interpretation
Myokymic potentials (grouped fasciculations)	Spontaneous, rhythmic bursts of grouped motor unit potentials.	The EMG bursts (30–60 Hz) are followed by a period of silence and a subsequent repetition of identical discharges. The spontaneous activities are not altered by voluntary activation of the muscles. Myokymia is a form of involuntary muscular movement (continuous rippling movement beneath skin) often associated with chronic nerve injury. The electrical discharges arise from peripheral regenerating nerves.
Myotonic discharge (myotonic potential)	High-frequency repetitive discharges seen in myotonia and evoked by insertion of a needle electrode, percussion of a muscle, or stimulation of a muscle or its motor nerve.	Repetitive discharge at rates of 20–80 Hz are of two types: (1) biphasic (positive-negative) spike potentials less than 5 ms in duration resembling fibrillation potentials; (2) positive waves of 5–20 ms in duration resembling positive sharp waves. Represents delayed relaxation of muscle fibers. The amplitude and frequency of the potentials must both wax and wane and be identified as myotonic discharges (sound of a "dive bomber").
Neuromyotonic discharge	Bursts of motor unit action potentials which originate in the motor axons firing at high rates (150–300 Hz) for a few seconds, and which often start and stop abruptly.	The amplitude of the response typically wanes. Discharges may occur spontaneously or be initiated by needle movement, voluntary effort and ischemia, or percussion of a nerve.
Polyphasic action potential	An action potential having five or more phases.	

(table continues on page 312)

NEURO

■ **TABLE 4.39 Types of Electrodiagnostic Waveforms** (continued)

Waveform	Definition	Description/Interpretation
Positive sharp waves (positive waves)	A biphasic, positive-negative action potential recurring in a uniform, regular pattern (1–50 Hz); spontaneous or initiated by needle movement.	Recorded from the damaged areas of fibrillating muscle fibers when the potential arises from an area immediately adjacent to the needle electrode. The discharge frequency may decrease slightly just before cessation of discharge. The initial positive deflection is rapid (<1 ms), its duration is usually less than 5 ms, and the amplitude is up to 1 mV. The negative phase is of low amplitude, with a duration of 10–100 ms. Sounds like "ticking of a clock."
Satellite potential	A small action potential separated from the main MUAP by an isoelectric interval and firing in a time-locked relationship to the main action potential.	These potentials usually follow, but may precede, the main action potential.
Sensory nerve action potential (SNAP)	A *compound nerve action potential* evoked from afferent fibers where the recording electrodes detect activity only in a sensory nerve or in a sensory branch of a mixed nerve; or if the electric stimulus is applied to a sensory nerve or a dorsal nerve root, or an adequate stimulus is applied synchronously to sensory receptors.	The amplitude, latency, duration, and configuration should be noted and compared to established norms.

Waveform	Definition	Description/Interpretation
Serrated action potential (complex or pseudopolyphasic action potential)	Complex repetitive polyphasic discharge that has uniform frequency, shape, and amplitude, with abrupt onset, cessation, or change in configuration. May begin spontaneously or after needle movement.	Amplitudes range form 100 uV to 1 mV and frequency of discharge from 5–100 Hz.
Short-latency somatosensory evoked potential (SSEP)	The short-latency portion of the somatosensory evoked potential waveform.	Normally occurs within 25 ms after stimulation of the median nerve in the upper extremity at the wrist, 40 ms after stimulation of the common peroneal nerve in the lower extremity at the knee, and 50 ms after stimulation of the posterior tibial nerve in the lower extremity at the ankle.
Somatosensory evoked potentials (SEPs) or spinal evoked potential	Electric waveforms of biologic origin elicited by electric stimulation or physiological activation of peripheral sensory fibers.	The normal SEP is a complex waveform with several components that are specified by polarity and average peak latency. *See short-latency somatosensory evoked potentials.*
T wave	A *compound action potential* evoked from a muscle by rapid stretch of its tendon, as part of the muscle stretch reflex.	Abnormal latency and amplitude values of the T wave are used to assess segmental functional disturbances in various myelopathies.
Visual evoked potentials (VEPs) or visual evoked responses (VERs)	Electric waveforms of biologic origin recorded over the cerebrum and elicited by light stimuli.	Classified by stimulus rate as transient or steady state VEPs, and can be further divided by presentation mode.

Adapted from: Nomenclature Committee of the American Association of Electrodiagnostic Medicine (formerly American Association of Electromyography and Electrodiagnosis): AAEE's Glossary of Terms in Clinical Electromyography. *Muscle & Nerve* 10:G1–G20, 1987, and with permission. Approval for inclusion of the glossary in this book in no way implies review or endorsement by the AAEM of material contained in the book.

AAEE Glossary of Terms Used in Electrodiagnosis

antidromic: Propagation of an impulse in the direction opposite to physiological conduction; e.g., conduction along motor nerve fibers away from the muscle and conduction along sensory fibers away from the spinal cord. Contrast with *orthodromic.*

collision: When used with reference to nerve conduction studies, the interaction of two action potentials propagated toward each other from opposite directions on the same nerve fiber so that the refractory periods of the two potentials prevent propagation past each other.

decrementing response: A reproducible decline in the amplitude and/or area of the *M wave* of successive responses to *repetitive nerve stimulation.* The rate of stimulation and the total number of stimuli should be specified. Decrementing responses with disorders of neuromuscular transmission are most reliably seen with slow rates (2–5 Hz) of nerve stimulation. A decrementing response with repetitive nerve stimulation commonly occurs in disorders of neuromuscular transmission but can also be seen in some neuropathies, myopathies, and motor neuron disease.

electroneurography (ENG): The recording and study of the action potentials of peripheral nerves. Synonymous with *nerve conduction studies.*

fasciculation: Rhythmic, visible twitching of a muscle with weak voluntary or postural contraction that appears on EMG as spontaneous discharges (*fasciculation potentials—see Table 4.39*) of all or part of a motor unit when the subject is at rest. The phenomenon occurs in neuromuscular disorders in which the motor unit territory is enlarged and the tissue covering the muscle is thin.

fiber density: (1) Anatomically, fiber density is a measure of the number of muscle or nerve fibers per unit area. (2) In *single fiber electromyography*, the fiber density is the mean number of *muscle fiber action potentials* fulfilling amplitude and rise time criteria belonging to one motor unit within the recording area of the *single fiber needle electrode* encountered during a systematic search in the weakly, voluntarily contracted muscle.

jitter: Normal EMG variability measured using single fiber recording techniques in the interval between two action potentials of successive discharges in the same single muscle fiber in the same motor unit

macroelectromyography (macro-EMG): General term referring to the technique and conditions that approximate recording of all *muscle fiber action potentials* arising from the same motor unit.

microneurography: The technique of recording peripheral nerve action potentials in man by means of intraneural electrodes.

midlatency SEP: That portion of the waveforms of a *somatosensory evoked potential* normally occurring within 25–100 ms after stimulation of a nerve in the upper extremity at the wrist, within 40–100 ms after stimulation of a nerve in the lower extremity at the knee, and within 50–100 ms after stimulation of a nerve in the lower extremity at the ankle.

motor latency: Interval between the onset of a stimulus and the onset of the resultant *compound muscle action potential (M wave).* The term may be qualified as "proximal motor latency" or "distal motor latency," depending on the relative position of the stimulus.

motor point: The point over a muscle where a contraction of a muscle may be elicited by a minimal-intensity, short-duration electric stimulus. The motor point corresponds anatomically to the location of the terminal portion of the motor nerve fibers (end-plate zone).

myokymia: Continuous quivering or undulating movement of surface and overlying skin and mucous membrane associated with spontaneous, repetitive discharge of *motor unit potentials.* See *myokymic discharge* and *fasciculation.*

myokymic discharge (grouped fasciculations): Grouped *motor unit action potentials* that fire repetitively and may be associated with clinical myokymia.

myotonia: The clinical observation of delayed relaxation of muscle after voluntary contraction or percussion. The delayed relaxation may be electrically silent, or accompanied by propagated electric activity, such as *myotonic discharge* or *complex repetitive discharge (see Table 4.39).*

myotonic discharge: High frequency repetitive discharges of motor unit action potentials.

orthodromic: Propagation of an impulse in the direction the same as physiological conduction, for instance, conduction along motor nerve fibers toward the muscle and conduction along sensory nerve fibers toward the spinal cord. Contrast with *antidromic.*

scanning EMG: A technique by which an electromyographic electrode is advanced in defined steps through muscle, while a separate *SFEMG* electrode is used to trigger both the oscilloscope sweep and the advancement device. This recording technique provides temporal and spatial information about the motor unit. Distinct maxima in the recorded activity are considered to be generated by muscle fibers innervated by a common branch of the axon.

single fiber electromyography (SFEMG): General term referring to the technique and conditions that permit recording of a single *muscle fiber action potential.* See *jitter.*

spontaneous activity: Electric activity recorded from muscle or nerve at rest after insertion activity has subsided and when there is no voluntary contraction or external stimulus.

strength-duration curve: Graphic presentation of the relationship between the intensity (Y axis) and various durations (X axis) of the threshold electric stimulus for a muscle with the stimulating cathode positioned over the *motor point.* The *rheobase* is the intensity of an electric current of infinite duration necessary to produce a minimal visible twitch of a muscle when applied to the motor point. In clinical practice, a duration of 300 ms is used to determine the rheobase. The *chronaxie* is the time required for an electric current twice the *rheobase* to elicit the first visible muscle twitch.

waning discharge: General term referring to a *repetitive discharge* that gradually decreases in frequency or amplitude before cessation. Contrast with *myotonic discharge.*

Adapted from:

Nomenclature Committee of the American Association of Electrodiagnostic Medicine (formerly American Association of Electromyography and Electrodiagnosis): AAEE's Glossary of Terms in Clinical Electromyography. Muscle & Nerve 10:G1–G20, 1987, with permission. Approval for inclusion of the glossary in this book in no way implies review or endorsement by the AAEM of material contained in the book.

Electroencephalography

The Electroencephalogram. The electroencephalogram (EEG) is a record of the spontaneous firing of post-synaptic potentials of neurons recorded from multiple electrodes attached to the human scalp. Most EEG signals originate in the brain's cerebral cortex. The recorded signals are transmitted to an EEG system composed of amplifiers, filters, and paper chart or computer monitor.

Diagnostic Use of EEGs. A routine *clinical EEG* is completed in 20 to 40 minutes. The following list summarizes the different diagnostic applications for clinical EEGs:

- distinguish epileptic seizures from psychogenic non-epileptic seizures, syncope (fainting), subcortical movement disorders, and migraine variants
- differentiate "organic" encephalopathy or delirium from primary psychiatric syndromes such as catatonia
- adjunct test for brain death
- prognosis for patients in coma
- management of anti-epileptic medication

Sometimes it is necessary to continuously monitor the EEG of a patient for multiple hours or for one or more days. *Continuous EEG monitoring* may take place as a hospital admission with time-synchronized video and audio recording, or by means of a portable ambulatory recording system. The following list summarizes the different diagnostic applications of continuous EEG monitoring:

- to distinguish epileptic seizures from other types of spells
- to characterize seizures for the purposes of treatment
- to localize the region of brain from which a seizure originates for workup of possible seizure surgery
- to monitor the depth of anesthesia
- as an indirect indicator of cerebral perfusion in carotid endarterectomy
- in the intensive care units for brain function monitoring (e.g., to monitor the effect of sedative/anesthesia in patients in medically induced coma)

EEG Recording and Electrode Placement

In standard clinical practice, 19 to 25 recording electrodes are placed uniformly over the scalp (e.g., the *International 10–20 System*). In addition, one or two reference electrodes (often placed on ear lobes) and a ground electrode (often placed on the nose to provide amplifiers with reference voltages) are required. In *referential recordings*, potentials between each recording electrode and a fixed reference are measured over time. In *bipolar recordings*, potential differences between adjacent scalp electrodes are measured to record tangential electric fields (or current densities). The different ways of combining electrode pairs to measure potential differences on the head is referred to as the *electrode montage*.

Note: The 10–20 system has been extended by the American Clinical Neurophysiology Society (https://www.acns.org/) to create a standard for higher spatial resolution using 75 electrodes.

Conventional Orientation & EEG Reference Sites (Superior View of Head)

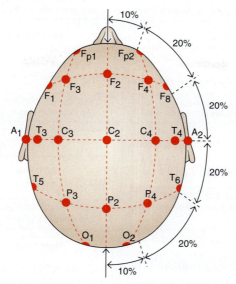

Conventional orientation of EEG reference sites (superior view of head).

NEURO

Electroencephalogram Signal Patterns

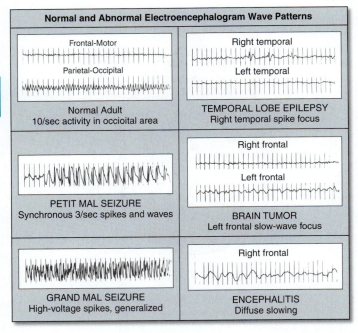

Normal and Abnormal Electroencephalogram Wave Patterns	
Frontal-Motor Parietal-Occipital **Normal Adult** 10/sec activity in occioital area	Right temporal Left temporal **TEMPORAL LOBE EPILEPSY** Right temporal spike focus
PETIT MAL SEIZURE Synchronous 3/sec spikes and waves	Right frontal Left frontal **BRAIN TUMOR** Left frontal slow-wave focus
GRAND MAL SEIZURE High-voltage spikes, generalized	Right frontal **ENCEPHALITIS** Diffuse slowing

Representative normal and abnormal EEG patterns for a variety of disorders. Related technologies.

Derivatives of the EEG technique include *evoked potentials (EPs)*, which involves averaging the EEG activity time-locked to the presentation of a stimulus (visual, somatosensory, or auditory stimuli—e.g., repeated light flashes, auditory tones, finger pressure, or mild electric shocks). *Event-related potentials (ERPs)* refer to averaged EEG responses that are time-locked to more complex processing of stimuli; this technique is used in cognitive science, cognitive psychology, and psychophysiological research. Steady state *visually evoked potentials (SSVEPs)* use a continuous sinusoidally modulated flickering light, typically superimposed in front of a TV monitor displaying a cognitive task. The brain response in a narrow frequency band containing the stimulus frequency is measured.

Assessment

Reflex Testing

🔵 TABLE 4.40 Muscle Stretch (Deep Tendon) Reflexes (listed in cephalad to caudal order)

NEURO

Reflex	
Jaw (maxillary) 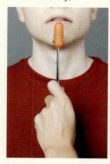	Stimulus: Tap mandible in half-open position. Response: Closure of jaw Segmental Level and Nerve: Pons (trigeminal nerve)
Biceps 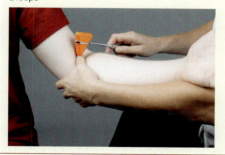	Stimulus: Tap biceps tendon. Response: Contraction of biceps Segmental Level and Nerve: C5 and C6 (musculocutaneous nerve)
Brachioradialis (periosteoradial) 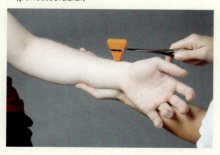	Stimulus: Tap styloid process of radius (insertion of brachioradialis). Response: Flexion of elbow and pronation of forearm Segmental Level and Nerve: C5 and C6 (musculocutaneous nerve)

(table continues on page 320)

NEURO

● TABLE 4.40 Muscle Stretch (Deep Tendon) Reflexes (listed in cephalad to caudal order) (continued)

Reflex

Triceps

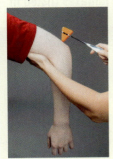

Stimulus: Tap triceps tendon.
Response: Extension of elbow
Segmental Level and Nerve: C6–C8 (radial nerve)

Wrist flexion

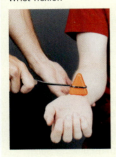

Stimulus: Tap wrist flexor tendons.
Response: Flexion of wrist
Segmental Level and Nerve: C6–C8 (median nerve)

Patellar

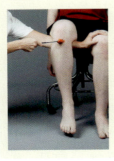

Stimulus: Tap patellar tendon.
Response: Extension of leg at knee
Segmental Level and Nerve: L2–L4 (femoral nerve)

Reflex	
Tendocalcaneus	

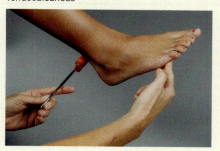

Stimulus: Tap Achilles tendon.
Response: Plantar flexion at ankle
Segmental Level and Nerve: S1 and S2 (tibial nerve)

NEURO

Grading of Muscle Stretch (Deep Tendon) Reflexes

0	Areflexia
+	Hyporeflexia
1 to 3	Average
3+ to 4+	Hyperreflexia

TABLE 4.41 Modified Ashworth Scale for Grading Spasticity

Grade	Description
0	No increase in muscle tone
1	Slight increase in muscle tone, manifested by a catch and release or by minimal resistance at the end of the ROM when the affected part(s) is moved in flexion or extension
1 +	Slight increase in muscle tone, manifested by a catch, followed by minimal resistance throughout the remainder (less than half) of the ROM
2	More marked increase in muscle tone through most of the ROM, but affected part(s) easily moved
3	Considerable increase in muscle tone, passive movement difficult
4	Affected part(s) rigid in flexion or extension

Based on: Ashworth, B: Preliminary trial of carisoprodol in multiple sclerosis. *Practitioner* 192:540, 1964.
ROM = range of motion.

● TABLE 4.42 **Antispasticity Drugs**

Drug	Oral Dosage	Comments
Baclofen (Lioresal)	Adult: 5 mg tid initially; increase by 5 mg at 3-day intervals as required; maximum recommended dosage is 80 mg/day. Children: No specific pediatric dosage is listed; the adult dose must be decreased according to the size and age of the child.	More effective in treating spasticity resulting from spinal cord lesions (versus cerebral lesions).
Dantrolene sodium (Dantrium)	Adult: 25 mg/day initially; increase up to 100 mg 2, 3, or 4 times per day as needed; maximum recommended dose is 400 mg/day. Children (older than 5 yr of age): initially, 0.5 mg/kg body weight bid; increase total daily dosage by 0.5 mg/kg every 4-7 days as needed, and give total daily amount in 4 divided dosages; maximum recommended dose is 400 mg/d.	Exerts an effect directly on the muscle cell; may cause generalized weakness in all skeletal musculature.
Diazepam (Valium)	Adult: 2–10 mg tid or qid. Children (older than 6 mo of age): 1.0–2.5 mg tid or qid (in both adults and children, begin at lower end of dosage range and increase gradually as tolerated and needed).	Produces sedation at dosages that decrease spasticity.
Gabapentin (Neurontin)	Adult:* initially, 300 mg tid. Can be gradually increased up to 3,600 mg/day based on desired response. Children* (3–12 yr of age): Initially, 10–15 mg/kg body weight in 3 divided dosages; increase over 3 days until desired effect or a maximum of 50 mg/kg/day.	Developed originally as an anticonvulsant; may also be helpful as an adjunct to other drugs in treating spasticity associated with spinal cord injury and multiple sclerosis.
Tizanidine (Zanaflex)	Adult: 8 mg every 6–8 h as needed. Children: The safety and efficacy of this drug in treating spasticity in children have not been established.	May reduce in spinal cord disorders while producing fewer side effects and less generalized muscle weakness than other agents (oral baclofen, diazepam).

bid = twice a day; qid = four times a day; tid = three times a day.
From: Ciccone, C: *Pharmacology in Rehabilitation,* ed. 4. FA Davis, Philadelphia, 2007, p 167, with permission.

NEURO

TABLE 4.43 Drugs Commonly Used to Treat Skeletal Muscle Spasms

Drug	Usual Adult Oral Dosage (mg)	Onset of Action (min)	Duration of Action (hr)
Carisoprodol (Soma, Vanadom)	350 tid and bedtime	30	4–6
Chlorphenesin carbamate (Maolate)	Initially: 800 tid; reduce to 400 qid or less	–	–
Chlorzoxazone (Paraflex, Parafon Forte, others)	250–750 tid or qid	Within 60	3–4
Cyclobenzaprine (Flexeril)	10 tid	Within 60	12–24
Diazepam (Valium)	2–10 tid or qid	15–45	Variable
Metaxalone (Skelaxin)	800 tid or qid	60	4–6
Methocarbamol (Carbacot, Robaxin, Skelex)	1,000 qid or 1,500 tid	Within 30	24
Orphenadrine citrate (Antiflex, Norflex, others)	100 bid	Within 60	12

From: Ciccone, C: *Pharmacology in Rehabilitation,* ed. 4. FA Davis, Philadelphia, 2007, p 165, with permission.

TABLE 4.44 Common Superficial Reflexes Tested (listed in cephalad to caudal order)

Reflex

Light reflex

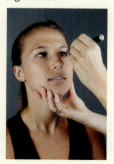

Stimulus: Examiner projects light on the retina.
Response: Constriction of pupil
Segmental Level: Mesencephalon

(table continues on page 324)

● TABLE 4.44   Common Superficial Reflexes Tested (listed in cephalad to caudal order) (continued)

Reflex	
Consensual light	Stimulus: Examiner projects light into the eye opposite the one being evaluated. Response: Constriction of the pupil in the eye not receiving the light Segmental Level: Commissural pathways in the pretectal area, as well as the same pathways used in the light reflex
Accommodation	Stimulus: Examiner asks the patient to look at a nearby object. Response: Convergence of eyes with constriction of the pupils Segmental Level: Occipital cortex (if light reflexes exist) and mesencephalon (afferent: optic nerve; efferent: oculomotor nerve)
Blink reflex (of Descartes)	Stimulus: Unexpected movement of object near and toward eyes Response: Closure of the eyes Segmental Level: Mesencephalon and occipital cortex (afferent: optic nerve; efferent: facial nerve)
Corneal (conjunctival) 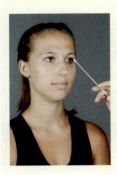	Stimulus: Touching cornea with hair or cotton wisp Response: Contraction of orbicularis oculi (closing the eye) Segmental Level: Pons (afferent: trigeminal nerve; efferent: facial nerve)

Reflex

Nasal (sneeze)

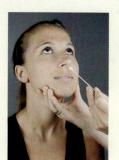

Stimulus: Lightly touching nasal mucosa with cotton wisp
Response: Sneezing
Segmental Level: Pons and medulla (afferent: trigeminal nerve; efferent: trigeminal nerve, facial, glossopharyngeal, and vagus nerves)

Pharyngeal (gag)

Stimulus: Touching posterior wall of pharynx
Response: Contraction of pharynx
Segmental Level: Medulla (afferent: glossopharyngeal nerve; efferent: vagus nerve)

Palatal (uvular)

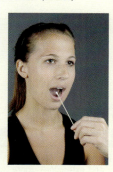

Stimulus: Touching soft palate
Response: Elevation of palate
Segmental Level: Medulla (afferent: glossopharyngeal nerve; efferent: vagus nerve)

Abdominal

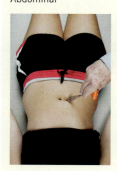

Stimulus: Stroking beneath costal margins and above the inguinal ligament
Response: Contraction of the abdominal muscles in the stimulated quadrant
Segmental Level: T8–T12 (depending on the quadrant stimulated)

(table continues on page 326)

TABLE 4.44 **Common Superficial Reflexes Tested (listed in cephalad to caudal order)** (continued)

Reflex	
Plantar	

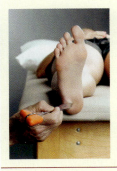

Stimulus: Stroking sole of foot
Response: Plantar flexion of toes (children may also retract foot)
Segmental Level: S1 and S2 (tibial nerve)

| Superficial anal | Stimulus: Pricking perineum
Response: Contraction of rectal sphincters
Segmental Level: S5 and coccygeal (pudendal nerves) |

Based on: Waxman, SG, and deGroot, J: *Correlative Neuroanatomy,* ed. 22. Appleton & Lange, Norwalk, CT, 1996.

Major Pathological Reflexes

TABLE 4.45 **Pathological Reflexes—Upper Motor Neuron**

Reflex	Stimulus	Response
Clonus	Examiner rapidly extends the wrist or dorsiflexes ankle.	Rapid reciprocal flexion and extension—more than three beats is considered positive.
Hoffmann's sign (upper extremity)	Examiner snaps the nail of the middle finger.	Flexion of first finger and thumb.
Babinski's sign (lower extremity)	Examiner strokes the outer edge of sole of foot.	Extension of the great toe, flexion of small toes, and spreading of small toes.

Coordination Tests

● TABLE 4.46 Coordination Tests (in alphabetical order*)

Test	Description
Alternate heel to knee; heel to toe	From a supine position, the patient is asked to touch his knee and big toe alternately with the heel of the opposite extremity.
Alternate nose to finger	The patient alternately touches the tip of his nose and the tip of the therapist's finger with the index finger. The position of the therapist's finger may be altered during testing to assess ability to change distance, direction, and force of movement.
Drawing a circle	The patient draws an imaginary circle in the air with either upper or lower extremity (a table or the floor also may be used). This also may be done using a figure-eight pattern. This test may be performed in the supine position for lower extremity assessment.
Finger to finger	Both shoulders are abducted to 90° with the elbows extended. The patient is asked to bring both hands toward the midline and approximate the index fingers from opposing hands.
Finger to nose	The shoulder is abducted to 90° with the elbow extended. The patient is asked to bring the tip of the index finger to the tip of the nose. Alterations may be made in the initial starting position to assess performance from different planes of motion.
Finger opposition	The patient touches the tip of the thumb to the tip of each finger in sequence. Speed may be gradually increased.
Finger to therapist's finger	The patient and therapist sit opposite each other. The therapist's index finger is held in front of the patient. The patient is asked to touch the tip of the index finger to the therapist's index finger. The position of the therapist's finger may be altered during testing to assess ability to change distance, direction, and force of movement.
Fixation or position holding	Upper extremity: The patient holds arms horizontally in front.
	Lower extremity: The patient is asked to hold the knee in an extended position.

(table continues on page 328)

● TABLE 4.46 Coordination Tests (in alphabetical order*) (continued)

Test	Description
Heel on shin	From the supine position, patient slides the heel of one foot up and down the shin of the opposite lower extremity.
Mass grasp	An alternation is made between opening and closing fist (from finger flexion to full extension). Speed may be gradually increased.
Pointing and past-pointing	The patient and therapist are opposite each other, either sitting or standing. Both patient and therapist bring shoulders to a horizontal position of 90° of flexion with elbows extended. Index fingers are touching, or the patient's finger may rest lightly on the therapist's. The patient is asked to fully flex the shoulder (fingers will be pointing toward ceiling) and then return to the horizontal position such that index fingers will again approximate. Both arms should be tested, either separately or simultaneously. A normal response consists of an accurate return to the starting position. In an abnormal response, there is typically a "past-pointing," or movement beyond the target. Several variations to this test include movements in other directions such as toward 90° of shoulder abduction or toward 0° of shoulder flexion (finger will point toward floor). Following each movement, the patient is asked to return to the initial horizontal starting position.
Pronation/ supination	With elbows flexed to 90° and held close to body, the patient alternately turns his palms up and down. This test also may be performed with shoulders flexed to 90° and elbows extended. Speed may be gradually increased. The ability to reverse movements between opposing muscle groups can be assessed at many joints. Examples include active alternation between flexion and extension of the knee, ankle, elbow, fingers, and so forth.
Rebound test	The patient is positioned with the elbow flexed. The therapist applies sufficient manual resistance to produce an isometric contraction of biceps. Resistance is suddenly released. Normally, the opposing muscle group (triceps) will contract and "check" movement of the limb. Many other muscle groups can be tested for this phenomenon, such as the shoulder abductors or flexors, and elbow extensors.

NEURO

Test	Description
Tapping (foot)	The patient is asked to "tap" the ball of one foot on the floor without raising the knee; heel maintains contact with floor.
Tapping (hand)	With the elbow flexed and the forearm pronated, the patient is asked to "tap" his hand on the knee.
Toe to examiner's finger	From a supine position, the patient is instructed to touch his great toe to the examiner's finger. The position of finger may be altered during testing to assess ability to change distance, direction, and force of movement.

From: O'Sullivan, SB, and Schmitz, TJ: *Physical Rehabilitation: Assessment and Treatment,* ed. 3. FA Davis, Philadelphia, 1994, p 102, with permission.
*Tests should be performed first with eyes open and then with eyes closed. Abnormal responses include a gradual deviation from the "holding" position and/or a diminished quality of response with vision occluded. Unless otherwise indicated, tests are performed with the patient in a sitting position.

TABLE 4.47 Tests for Common Disturbances That Affect Coordination (in alphabetical order)

Deficit	Sample Test
Asthenia	Fixation or position holding (upper and lower extremity) Application of manual resistance to assess muscle strength
Bradykinesia	Walking, observation of arm swing Walking, alterations in speed and direction Request that a movement or gait activity be stopped abruptly Observation of functional activities
Disturbances of gait	Walk along a straight line Walk sideways, backward March in place Alter speed of ambulatory activities Walk in a circle
Disturbances of posture	Fixation or position holding (upper and lower extremity) Displacement of balance unexpectedly in sitting or standing Standing, alterations in base of support Standing, one foot directly in front of the other Standing on one foot

(table continues on page 330)

NEURO

NEURO

TABLE 4.47 Tests for Common Disturbances That Affect Coordination (in alphabetical order) (continued)

Deficit	Sample Test
Dysdiadochokinesia	Finger to nose Alternate nose to finger Pronation/supination Knee flexion/extension Walking with alternations in speed
Dysmetria	Pointing and past-pointing Drawing a circle or figure eight Heel on shin Placing feet on floor markers while walking
Hypotonia	Passive movement Deep tendon reflexes
Movement decomposition	Finger to nose Finger to therapist's finger Alternate heel to knee Toe to examiner's finger
Rigidity	Passive movement Observation during functional activities Observation of resting posture(s)
Tremor (intention)	Observation during functional activities (tremor will typically increase as target is approached or when the patient attempts to hold a position) Alternate nose to finger Finger to finger Finger to therapist's finger Toe to examiner's finger
Tremor (postural)	Observation of normal standing posture
Tremor (resting)	Observation of patient at rest Observation during functional activities (tremor will diminish significantly or disappear)

Neuropsychological Tests Listed by Function Tested

Abstraction and Executive Functioning

Category Test: A measure of abstract reasoning, problem solving, and executive functioning. Patients must compare stimuli for similarities and differences to discover an abstract rule governing success or failure. The test also incorporates a memory trial. The test is not timed but takes under 45 min.

Delis-Kaplan Executive Function System: A comprehensive battery of tests measuring executive functioning, problem solving, and reasoning ability. Incorporates a process-oriented approach that attempts to delineate factors responsible for impairment. Entire battery takes approximately 2 hr, but individual tests can be administered alone and most are under 15 min.

Wisconsin Card Sorting Test: A measure of abstract reasoning, problem solving, and executive functioning using a sorting task. A highly sensitive measure of frontal lobe functioning and of the presence of brain damage. The test is not timed but takes under 1 hr.

Affective State, Adaptive Behavior, and Community Integration

Beck Anxiety Inventory: A self-report, multiple-choice instrument for measuring the presence and severity of anxiety-related symptoms. The test is not timed but takes under 15 min.

Beck Depression Inventory–II: A self-report, multiple-choice instrument for measuring the presence and severity of depression-related symptoms. The test is not timed but takes under 15 min.

Clinical Assessment Scales for the Elderly: A self- or other-report questionnaire for diagnosing psychiatric disorders in adults aged 55 to 90. Includes scales measuring Anxiety, Cognitive Competence, Depression, Fear of Aging, Obsessive-Compulsiveness, Paranoia, Psychoticism, Somatization, Mania, Substance Abuse, and validity of responses. The test takes 20 to 40 min to complete.

Community Integration Questionnaire: A 15-item questionnaire, often completed by interviewing a patient or proxy, that measures integration into the community following traumatic brain injury. The test takes 15 min.

Frontal Systems Behavior Scale: A self- and other-report questionnaire measuring three frontal lobe-related behavioral syndromes: apathy, disinhibition, and executive dysfunction. It asks responders to rate both current and past (pre-onset of frontal damage) behavior in order to quantify change since onset. The test takes 10 min.

Geriatric Depression Scale: A self-report questionnaire for measuring the presence and severity of depression-related symptoms in the elderly. Does not include items that may reflect change in function due to aging that may be confused with depression. The test is not timed but takes under 15 min.

Independent Living Scales: An individually administered assessment that quantifies adults' ability to care for themselves and their property. Scales measure memory, money management, management of home and transportation, health and safety, and social adjustment, with items measuring both knowledge and actual application of skills during the assessment. The test takes under 1 hr.

Minnesota Multiphasic Personality Inventory–2 Restructured Format (MMPI–2-RF): The most widely used standardized and normed measure of personality and emotional disorders. It uses a true-false response format. It includes several validity scales useful for determining patients' response biases, scales covering the major psychiatric disorders, and a broad range of personality variables. The test is not timed but takes between 90 min and 2 hr.

Vineland Adaptive Behavior Scales: A standardized and normed instrument assessing personal and social skills. Separate forms can be administered as an interview or questionnaire or can be completed by an observer (e.g., a teacher). Administration time varies with the form used, but the test takes under 90 min.

NEURO

Attention

Connors Continuous Performance Test—2: A computer-administered assessment of sustained attention over time. Provides information on distractibility, impulsivity, inattention, and vigilance. The test takes 14 min.

Paced Auditory Serial Addition Test: An assessment of sustained attention and speed of information processing using a serial addition task presented on audiotape. The test takes under 20 min.

Trail Making Tests A and B: A timed, paper-and-pencil test of the ability to follow a sequence (Part A) and to alternate between two sequences (Part B). Because the test requires a broad range of skills including visual scanning, mental concentration, and drawing, it is sensitive to damage in many areas of the brain. Parts A and B together take under 10 min.

Composite Batteries

Dementia Rating Scale–2: A brief measure of attention, initiation, perseveration, constructional ability, abstract conceptualization, and memory. The test is suitable for patients with severe impairment who might be untestable by other means. Useful in the diagnosis of dementia. The test is not timed but takes under 1 hr.

Halstead-Reitan Battery (HRB): A battery comprised of the Sensory Perceptual Examination, use of a hand dynamometer, Category Test, Tactual Performance Test, Seashore Rhythm Test, Speech Sounds Perception Test, Finger Tapping Test, Grooved Pegboard Test, Aphasia Screening Test, and several additional tests. The battery is designed to detect, lateralize, localize, and measure the severity of brain damage. It is often supplemented with additional tests of memory, intellectual functioning, and personality. Depending on the tests included, it takes from 3–8 hr (could be longer).

Neuropsychological Assessment Battery (NAB): A comprehensive, modularly organized assessment battery covering the areas of attention, language, memory, spatial perception, and executive function. Screening items are also included that allow the examiner to determine which modules must be administered. The battery is normed on a sample matching the U.S. population based on census data. Administration time varies based on number of modules administered, but can take several hours.

Intellectual and Achievement

Wechsler Abbreviated Scale of Intelligence (WASI): A shortened version of the Wechsler Adult Intelligence Scale–III that yields estimated IQ scores based on tests of vocabulary, verbal abstracting ability, design construction, and perception of logical sequences. An updated version (WASI-2) is under development. The test takes under 30 min.

Wechsler Adult Intelligence Scale–IV (WAIS–IV): The most widely used standardized and normed measure of intellectual functioning, incorporating verbal and performance subscales. Subtests examine attention, general information, vocabulary, numerical reasoning, verbal abstracting, pictorial reasoning, puzzle construction, and other intelligence-related abilities. This test takes under 90 min.

Wechsler Individual Achievement Test (WIAT): An individually administered measure of basic academic achievement in the areas of arithmetic, reading, spelling, etc. The test takes under 2 hr.

Wechsler Test of Adult Reading (WTAR): A test of written word pronunciation that uses reading and demographic data to yield a prediction of intellectual test scores prior to the onset of a neurological condition. Scores can be compared with current intellectual test scores to determine if there has been a statistically significant decline in intellectual performance. The test takes under 10 min.

Woodcock Johnson III Tests of Achievement: A comprehensive, standardized, and normed battery of tests providing a thorough assessment of academic achievement.

NEURO

Language

Aphasia Screening Test: A test that screens for aphasia and associated disorders. Items assess speech comprehension, oral expression, speech repetition, naming, oral reading, reading comprehension, writing, written and oral calculation, and constructional (drawing) ability. The test is not timed but takes under 15 min.

Boston Diagnostic Aphasia Examination: This examination provides a thorough and comprehensive assessment of oral and written language disorder. It includes subtests measuring fluency, comprehension, naming, repetition, oral reading, reading comprehension, and written and oral spelling. It also includes supplementary tests in many areas permitting for a more refined assessment. The test may take over 1 hr.

Boston Naming Test: A test of confrontation naming using pictures of objects. Names vary from high frequency to low frequency words, and phonemic and semantic cues are provided. The test is not timed but takes under 15 min.

Controlled Oral Word Association Test: An assessment of word fluency using three trials in which words beginning with a target letter are named within a defined period. The test takes 3 min.

Speech Sounds Perception Test: An assessment of ability to identify nonsense syllables that match those presented via audiotape. The test is used for detecting brain damage and subtle language deficits. The test takes from 15–20 min.

Token Test: An assessment of language comprehension using increasingly long and complex commands relating to manipulation of tokens of varying colors, sizes, and shapes. The test is not timed but takes under 30 min.

Western Aphasia Battery–2: A comprehensive assessment of oral and written language disorders, with items measuring fluency, naming, repetition, comprehension, reading, writing, and spelling. The test also includes items that assess praxis, calculations, and constructional abilities. The test is not timed but takes under 30 min.

Memory

Autobiographical Memory Interview: A standardized test of retrograde amnesia using information and events from a patient's own life. The test is not timed but takes under 30 min.

Brief Visuospatial Memory Test Revised: An assessment of ability to learn and retain visuospatial information (geometric figures). It includes three learning trials, delayed recall and recognition trials, and a copy trial that distinguishes drawing from memory impairments. Six equivalent alternate forms are available, permitting serial assessment in order to measure recovery over time or pre- and post-rehabilitation. The test takes under 1 hr.

California Verbal Learning Test–2: An assessment of ability to learn and retain verbal information using mock shopping lists. It permits a sophisticated process-oriented analysis of memory performance that delineates factors responsible for a given level of impairment. An equivalent alternate form is available for serial assessment, as well as a short form for testing more cognitively compromised patients who cannot take the full version. The test takes under 1 hr, including a 20-min delayed recall interval.

Rivermead Behavioural Memory Test: An assessment of ability to learn and retain new information using everyday memory content, including names, faces, an appointment, prose, and a route. Incorporating everyday content, the test potentially gives greater ecologic validity than other instruments. It is available in four parallel forms. The test takes under 30 min.

Rey-Osterreith Complex Figure Test: A measure of memory for a complex design that requires the design to first be drawn in full view and then from memory after varying intervals of time since exposure. A delayed recognition trial is also included. The test takes under 45 min.

Wechsler Memory Scale–IV: A widely used comprehensive battery of tests assessing the ability to learn and retain new information. The battery includes lists, paired associate, prose, and design learning tasks. It also incorporates measures of attention. The test takes under 1 hr.

Motor

Finger Tapping Test: Patients tap a key with their index finger as rapidly as possible while a counter records the number of taps. The test is administered to each hand separately to assess motor speed and coordination. The test takes under 10 min.

Grooved Pegboard Test: Patients attempt to rapidly insert ridged pegs into variously oriented slots. The test is administered to each hand separately to assess fine motor coordination and speed. The test takes under 10 min.

Hand Dynamometer: A dynamometer-based test that quantifies strength of grip in each hand in kilograms. Several trials are administered, alternating hands, and an average is obtained for each hand. The test takes under 10 min.

Perception

Behavioral Inattention Test: A comprehensive assessment of neglect syndromes using items that require line crossing, letter cancellation, star cancellation, figure copying, line bisection, drawing, picture scanning, telephone dialing, reading, telling and setting time on a clock, coin sorting, writing, map navigation, and card sorting. The test is not timed but takes under 1 hr.

Benton Facial Recognition Test: An assessment of ability to match and discriminate faces. The test is not timed but takes under 30 min.

Benton Judgment of Line Orientation Test: An assessment of ability to judge the orientation of lines in space. The test is not timed but takes under 30 min.

Ishihara Test for Color Blindness: A test that detects the most common forms of congenital and acquired color blindness. The test is not timed but takes under 10 min.

Line Bisection Test: A test that detects the presence of a neglect syndrome using lines of various lengths and in various positions on a page, which patients attempt to bisect. The test is not timed but takes under 10 min.

Seashore Rhythm Test: An assessment of auditory perception using pairs of rhythmic beats, presented by audiotape, which patients must judge as the same or different. The test takes from 15–20 min.

Sensory-Perceptual Examination: A standardization of procedures from neurological examinations. The test includes confrontation testing of visual fields, unilateral and bilateral simultaneous stimulation perception, detection of fingers touched, detection of numbers traced on fingers, discrimination of coins, and visual recognition of tactually presented shapes. The test is not timed but takes under 20 min.

Tactual Performance Test: An assessment of tactile perception and memory using variously shaped blocks that blindfolded patients attempt to fit into slots on a board. Each hand is tested separately and then together. Patients then attempt to draw shapes from memory in their correct spatial position. The test takes approximately 40 min.

Test of Visual Neglect: A test that detects neglect syndromes by requiring patients to make hatch marks through lines placed in what appear to be random positions on a page. The test is not timed but takes under 10 min.

Visual Object and Space Perception Battery: A battery that includes tests that assess various aspects of visual and spatial perception including discrimination of forms, identification of incomplete letters, identification of objects depicted as rotated silhouettes, dot counting, determination of the position of points in space, and estimation of quantity. The test is not timed but takes under 30 min.

NEURO

TABLE 4.48 Common Gait Deviations Seen in Patients With Hemiplegia

Stance Phase	
Derivation	**Cause**
Ankle and Foot Equinus gait	Excessive activity of the gastrocnemius muscle. Plantar flexion contracture.
Varus foot	Excessive activity of the tibialis anterior, tibialis posterior, or toe flexor muscles causes the foot to come down on the lateral surface at heel strike.
Painful short steps	Contraction of the toe flexors causes excessive pressure on the toes and results in the patient taking short steps to minimize stance time and rollover.
Excessive flexion	Flexion contracture. Excessive dorsiflexion. Poor position sense. Weak knee quadriceps.

(table continues on page 336)

TABLE 4.48 Common Gait Deviations Seen in Patients With Hemiplegia (continued)

Stance Phase	
Derivation	**Cause**
Ankle and Foot Hyperextension	Plantar flexion contracture. Poor position sense. Excessive activity of the quadriceps muscles. Compensatory locking of the knee to adjust for weak knee extensors (patient leans forward to mechanically lock the knee).
Lateral (Trendelenburg or gluteus medius) limb	Weak hip abductors.
Scissoring	Excessive activity of the adductors.
Improper positioning of the hip	Weakness of hip girdle. Poor position sense.
Trunk and Pelvis Flexed trunk	Compensation for weak knee flexors (the patient brings center of gravity forward). Weak hip extensors.
Improper positioning	Poor position sense.
Lack of pelvic rotation	Weakness and lack of control of pelvic girdle muscle.
Swing Phase	
Ankle and Foot Equinus gait	Excessive activity of the gastrocnemius. Plantar flexion contracture. Weak dorsiflexors.
Varus foot	Excessive activity of the tibialis anterior. Weakness of peroneals and toe extensors.
Equinovarus	Excessive activity of the triceps surae.
Excessive dorsiflexion	Part of powerful flexor synergy pattern.

Based on: O'Sullivan, SB, and Schmitz, TJ: *Physical Rehabilitation: Assessment and Treatment,* ed. 3. FA Davis, Philadelphia, 1994, p 342.

Disorders of the Central Nervous System

Non-Progressive Disorders of the Brain

Global Disorders of the Brain
Traumatic Brain Injury
Types of traumatic brain injury

1. Intracranial hemorrhages
   a. **Epidural hematoma** occurs from impact loading to the skull with associated laceration of the dural arteries or veins, often by fractured bones and sometimes by diploic veins in the skull's marrow. More often, a tear in the middle meningeal artery causes this type of hematoma. When hematoma occurs from laceration of an artery, blood collection can cause rapid neurological deterioration.
   b. **Subdural hematoma** tends to occur in patients with injuries to the cortical veins or pial artery in severe TBI. The associated mortality rate is high, approximately 60% to 80%.
   c. **Intracerebral hemorrhages** occur within the cerebral parenchyma secondary to lacerations or to contusion of the brain, with injury to larger, deeper cerebral vessels occurring with extensive cortical contusion.
   d. **Intraventricular hemorrhage** tends to occur in the presence of very severe TBI and is, therefore, associated with an unfavorable prognosis.
   e. **Subarachnoid hemorrhage** may occur in cases of TBI in a manner other than secondary to ruptured aneurysms, being caused instead by lacerations of the superficial microvessels in the subarachnoid space. If not associated with another brain pathology, this type of hemorrhage could be benign. Traumatic subarachnoid hemorrhage may lead to a communicating

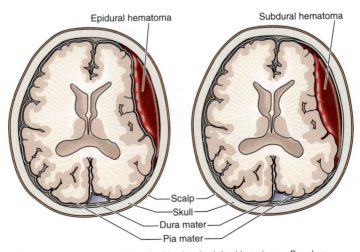

Epidural hematoma   Subdural hematoma

Scalp
Skull
Dura mater
Pia mater

Intracranial hemorrhages: Location of epidural and subdural hematomas. Based on: Woo, BH, and Nesathurai, S (eds): *The Rehabilitation of People With Traumatic Brain Injury*. Boston Medical Center, Boston, MA, 2000.

hydrocephalus if blood products obstruct the arachnoid villi or in the event of a non-communicating hydrocephalus secondary to a blood clot obstructing the third or fourth ventricle.

2. Coup and contrecoup contusions
   a. A combination of vascular and tissue damage leads to cerebral contusion.
   b. Coup contusions occur at the area of direct impact to the skull and occur because of the creation of negative pressure when the skull, distorted at the site of impact, returns to its normal shape.
   c. Contrecoup contusions are similar to coup contusions but are located opposite the site of direct impact. Cavitation in the brain, from negative pressure due to translational acceleration impacts from inertial loading, may cause contrecoup contusions as the skull and dura matter start to accelerate before the brain on initial impact.
   d. The amount of energy dissipated at the site of direct impact determines whether the ensuing contusion is of the coup or contrecoup type. Most of the energy of impact from a small, hard object tends to dissipate at the impact site, leading to a coup contusion. In contrast, impact from a larger object causes less injury at the impact site, because energy is dissipated at the beginning or end of the head motion, leading to a contrecoup contusion.

NEURO

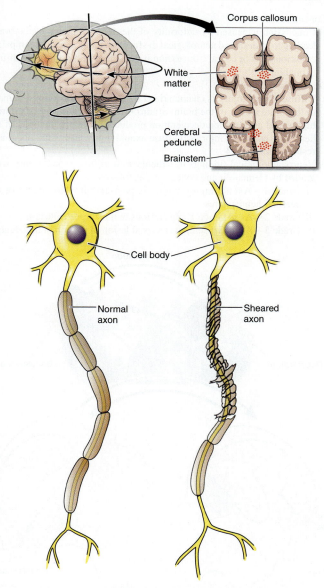

Potential mechanism of injury (upper left) and common sites of diffuse axonal injury (upper right). Adapted from: Woo, BH, and Nesathurai, S (eds): *The Rehabilitation of People With Traumatic Brain Injury*. Boston Medical Center, Boston, MA, 2000.

3. Concussions
   a. Concussion is caused by deformity of the deep structures of the brain, leading to widespread neurological dysfunction that can result in impaired consciousness or coma. Concussion is considered a mild form of diffuse axonal injury.
4. Diffuse axonal injury
   a. Diffuse axonal injury is characterized by extensive, generalized damage to the white matter of the brain. Strains of the tentorium and falx during high-speed acceleration/deceleration produced by lateral motions of the head may cause the injuries. Diffuse axonal injury also could occur as a result of ischemia.
   b. Neuropathological findings in patients with diffuse axonal injury were graded by Gennarelli and colleagues, as follows:
      i. Grade 1—Axonal injury mainly in parasagittal white matter of the cerebral hemispheres
      ii. Grade 2—As in Grade 1, plus lesions in the corpus callosum
      iii. Grade 3—As in Grade 2, plus a focal lesion in the cerebral peduncle

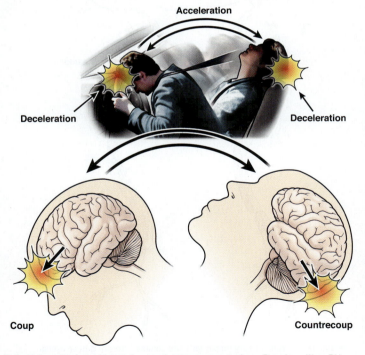

Potential mechanism of injury for coup/contrecoup contusions. Based on: Woo, BH, and Nesathurai, S (eds): *The Rehabilitation of People With Traumatic Brain Injury.* Boston Medical Center, Boston, MA, 2000.

5. Penetrating head injuries
   a. Gunshot wounds and missile/non-missile projectiles cause many penetrating head injuries. The energy dissipated on entry is equal to ½ mass × velocity squared. Therefore, high-velocity missiles tend to cause the most profound damage.

TBI and Functional Capability

Consciousness

Five abnormal states of consciousness can result from a TBI:

- **Stupor**—the patient is unresponsive but can be aroused briefly by a strong stimulus, such as sharp pain.
- **Coma**—the patient is totally unconscious, unresponsive, unaware, and unarousable. Patients in a coma do not respond to external stimuli, such as pain or light, and do not have sleep-wake cycles. Coma results from widespread and diffuse trauma to the brain, including the cerebral hemispheres of the upper brain and the lower brain or brainstem. Coma generally is of short duration, lasting a few days to a few weeks. After this time, some patients gradually come out of the coma, some progress to a vegetative state, and others die.
- **Vegetative state**—the patient is unconscious and unaware of his/her surroundings, but continues to have a sleep-wake cycle and can have periods of alertness. Unlike coma, where the patient's eyes are closed, patients in a vegetative state often open their eyes and may move, groan, or show reflex responses. A vegetative state can result from diffuse injury to the cerebral hemispheres of the brain without damage to the lower brain and brainstem. Anoxia, or lack of oxygen to the brain, which is a common complication of cardiac arrest, can also bring about a vegetative state. Many patients emerge from a vegetative state within a few weeks, but those who do not recover within 30 days are said to be in a:
  - **Persistent vegetative state (PVS)**—the chances of recovery depend on the extent of injury to the brain and the patient's age, with younger patients having a better chance of recovery than older patients. Generally adults have a 50% chance and children a 60% chance of recovering consciousness from a PVS within the first 6 months. After a year, the chances that a PVS patient will regain consciousness are very low and most patients who do recover consciousness experience significant disability. The longer a patient is in a PVS, the more severe the resulting disabilities will be. Rehabilitation can contribute to recovery, but many patients never progress to the point of being able to take care of themselves.
- **Locked-in syndrome**—patient is aware and awake, but cannot move or communicate due to complete paralysis of the body.

Severity

1. TBI defined by the Head Injury Interdisciplinary Special Interest Group of the American Congress of Rehabilitation Medicine
   - Mild head injury is defined as "a traumatically induced physiological disruption of brain function, as manifested by one of the following:
     - Any period of loss of consciousness (LOC),
     - Any loss of memory for events immediately before or after the accident,
     - Any alteration in mental state at the time of the accident,
     - Focal neurological deficits, which may or may not be transient."

NEURO

- The other criteria for defining mild TBI include the following:
  - Glasgow Coma Scale—GCS (see Section III, Outcome Instruments) score greater than 12
  - No abnormalities on computed tomography (CT) scan
  - No operative lesions
  - Length of hospital stay less than 48 hours
- The following criteria define moderate TBI:
  - Length of stay at least 48 hours
  - GCS score of 9 to 12 or higher
  - Operative intracranial lesion
  - Abnormal CT scan findings

Adapted from:

O'Sullivan, SB, & Schmitz, TJ: Physical Rehabilitation, ed. 5. FA Davis, Philadelphia, 2005.

Other TBI scales (located in Section III, Outcome Instruments) include the following:

Glasgow Coma Scale—defines the severity of a TBI within 48 hours of injury

Rancho Los Amigos Scale of Cognitive Functioning—describes the severity of deficit in cognitive functioning

Disability Rating Scale (DRS)—describes functioning after TBI across impairment, disability, and handicap categories from coma to community re-entry.

References:

Dawodu, ST, et al: Traumatic Brain Injury (TBI)—Definition, Epidemiology, Pathophysiology. http://emedicine.medscape.com/article/326510-overview. Accessed July 2009.

Woo, BH, and Nesathurai, S (eds): The Rehabilitation of People With Traumatic Brain Injury. Boston Medical Center, Boston, MA, 2000

Santa Clara Valley Medical Center. The Center for Outcome Measurement in Brain Injury. 2006. http://www.tbims.org/combi/. Accessed July 2009.

Pangilinan, PH, et al: Classification and Complications of Traumatic Brain Injury: Multimedia. http://emedicine.medscape.com/article/326643-overview. Accessed July 2009.

Traumatic Brain Injury: Hope Through Research. National Institute of Neurological Disorders and Stroke. http://www.ninds.nih.gov/disorders/tbi/detail_tbi.htm. Accessed July 2009.

Seizure and Epilepsy

Definitions and Characterization

epilepsy: A chronic disorder characterized by recurrent unprovoked seizures.
- An epileptic seizure refers to transient occurrence of signs and or symptoms due to abnormal, excessive, or synchronous neuronal activity in the brain.
- The epileptic seizure may be characterized by sensory, motor, or autonomic phenomena with or without loss of consciousness.
- All persons with epilepsy have seizures, but all those who have seizures do not have epilepsy. Seizures occurring in a setting of an acute illness or medical condition like high fever, hypoglycemia, and so on are classified as acute symptomatic seizures.

seizure: A paroxysmal event that mimics an epileptic seizure but does not involve abnormal, rhythmic discharges of cortical neurons. Common types of seizures include the following:

- Partial
  - Begin focally in a restricted area of the cortex
  - The symptoms could be simple (motor and sensory phenomenon) or complex (automatisms and/or unawareness)
  - Partial seizures can spread to other areas and evolve into generalized tonic-clonic seizures
- Generalized
  - Arise diffusely in both hemispheres, with bilateral non-focal onset, usually with impairment of consciousness at the beginning
  - The seizures may manifest with absences, tonic-clinic seizures, myoclonic jerks, or akinetic or atonic attacks

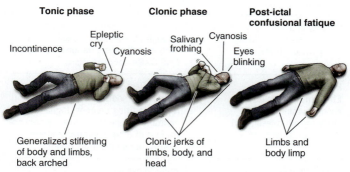

Tonic phase

Incontinence
Epleptic cry
Cyanosis

Generalized stiffening of body and limbs, back arched

Clonic phase

Salivary frothing
Cyanosis
Eyes blinking

Clonic jerks of limbs, body, and head

Post-ictal confusional fatique

Limbs and body limp

Characteristics of seizure phases in a generalized tonic-clonic seizure. From: Epilepsy Foundation: Epilepsy Classroom, developed by UCB, Inc. An Introduction to Epilepsy, 2008. http://www.epilepsyclassroom.com. Accessed July 2009.

🔶 **TABLE 4.49 Disorders Commonly Mistaken for Aphasia**

Disorders of speech production
Dysarthria
Aphemia (verbal apraxia)
Mutism
Auditory disorders
Peripheral hearing loss
Pure word deafness
Cortical deafness
Defects in arousal and attention
Global confusional state
Narcolepsy
Psychiatric disorders
Schizophrenia
Conversion disorder and other somatoform disorders
Uncooperative patient

🔵 TABLE 4.50 Chemical Classification and Action of Antiepileptic Agents

Chemical Class	Possible Mechanism of Action
Barbiturates Amobarbital (Amytal)* Mephobarbital (Mebaral) Pentobarbital (Nembutal)* Phenobarbital (Solfoton, others) Primidone (Mysoline) Secobarbital (Seconal)*	Potentiate inhibitory effects of GABA: may also decrease excitatory effects of glutamae
Benzodiazepines Clonazepam (Klonopin) Clorazepate (Tranxene) Diazepam (Valium) Lorazepam (Ativan)	Potentiate inhibitory effects of GABA
Carboxylic acids Valproic acid (Depakene, Depakote, others)	Unclear; may hyperpolarize membrane through an effect on potassium channels; higher concentrations increase CNS GABA concentrations
Hydantoins Ethotoin (Peganone) Fosphenytoin (Cerebyx)* Mephenytoin (Mesantoin) Phenytoin (Dilantin)	Primary effect is to stabilize membrane by blocking sodium channels in repetitive-firing neurons; higher concentrations may also influence concentrations of other neurotransmitters (GABA, norepinephrine, others)
Iminostilbenes Carbamazepine (Tegretol) Oxcarbazepine (Trileptal)	Similar to hydantoins
Succinimides Ethosuximide (Zarontin) Methsuximide (Celontin)	Affect calcium channels; appear to inhibit spontaneous firing in thalamic neurons by limiting calcium entry

*GABA = gamma-aminobutyric acid.
*Parental use only (IV injection).
From: Ciccone, C: *Pharmacology in Rehabilitation,* ed. 4. FA Davis, Philadelphia, 2007, p 108.

TABLE 4.51 Common Methods of Treating Specific Seizures

Seizure Type	First-line Drugs	Alternative Agents
Partial seizures	Carbamazepine Phenytoin Lamotrigine Valproic acid Oxcarbazepine	Gabapentin Topiramate Levetiracetam Zonisamide Tiagabine Primidone, phenobarbital Felbamate
Generalized seizures		
Absence	Valproic acid, ethosuximide	Lamotrigine
Myoclonic	Valproic acid, clonazepam	Lamotrigine, topiramate, felbamate
Tonic-clonic	Phenytoin, carbamazepine, valproic acid	Lamotrigine, topiramate, phenobarbital, primi- done, oxcarbazepine

From: Gidal, BE, et al. Epilepsy. In DiPiro, JT, et al. (eds): *Pharmacotherapy: A Pathophysiologic Approach,* 5 ed. McGraw-Hill; New York; 2002; p1036.
From: Ciccone, C: *Pharmacology in Rehabilitation,* ed. 4. FA Davis, Philadelphia, 2007, p 111.

NEURO

NEURO

TABLE 4.52 Dosages of Common Antiepileptic Drugs*

Drug	Adult				Child		
	Initial Dose (mg)	Increment** (mg)	Maintenance (mg/day)		Initial Dose (mg/kg/day)	Maintenance (mg/kg/day)	
Carbamazepine	200 bid	200 q wk	600–1,800		10 qd	10–35 (<6 yr)	
Ethosuximide	250 qd	250 q 3–7 days	750		15	15–40	
Felbamate	600–1,200 qd	600–1,200 q 1–2 wk	2,400–3,600		15	15–45	
Gabapentin	300 qd	300 q 3–7 days	1,200–3,600		10	25–50	
Lamotrigine	25 qd	25 q 2 wk	400		0.15–0.5	5	
Levetiracetam	500 bid	500 q wk	2,000–4,000		20	40–100	
Oxcarbazepine	300 qd	300 q wk	900–2,400		8–10	30–46	
Phenobarbital	30–60 qd	30 q 1–2 wk	60–120		3	3–6	
Phenytoin	200 qd	100 q 5–7 days	200–300		4	4–8	

Drug	Adult				Child		
	Initial Dose (mg)	Increment** (mg)	Maintenance (mg/day)		Initial Dose (mg/kg/day)	Maintenance (mg/kg/day)	
Primidone	125–250 qd	250 q 1–2 wk	500–750		10	10–25	
Tiagabine	4 qd	4–8 q wk	6–32		0.1	0.4	
Topiramate	25 qd	25 q 1–2 wk	100–400		3	3–9	
Valproic acid	250 qd	250 q 3–7 days	750–3,000		15	15–45	
Zonisamide	100 qd	100 q 2 wk	200–400		4	4–12	

From: Ranta, A, and Fountain, NB: Seizures and epilepsy in adolescents and adults. In Rakel, RE. and Bope, ET (eds): *Conn's Current Therapy 2005.* Elsevier/Saunders; New York; 2005, p 1026.

bid = twice a day; qd = every day.

* Dosages reflect monotherapy. Dosages may very if combining the drug with other antiseizure agents, or other drugs that affect liver enzyme function.

** Increments reflect the rate that dosage can typically be increased when trying to find the appropriate therapeutic dose.

From: Ciccone, C: *Pharmacology in Rehabilitation*, ed. 4. FA Davis, Philadelphia, 2007, p 112.

TABLE 4.53 Distinguishing Between a Psychogenic Episode and an Epileptic Seizure

Features	Psychogenic Episode	Epilepsy
Age and gender	Usually young, more common in women	Any age
Precipitating factor	Emotional disturbance	Lack of sleep, poor drug compliance
Occurrence in sleep	No	Yes
Duration	Minutes to hours	Seconds to minutes
Movements	Vocalization, pelvic thrusting, bizarre flinging of limbs	Tonic or tonic-clonic jerks
Eyes	Forcibly closed, resistance to opening	Open
Injuries including tongue	Infrequent bite	Frequent
Post-ictal confusion, headache, sleep	Uncommon	Common
Pattern of attacks	Variable	Stereotyped
EEG/video EEG	Normal	Usually abnormal

TABLE 4.54 Distinguishing Between Syncope and Seizure

Features	Syncope	Seizures
Precipitating factors	Common	Rare
Occurrence	Awake, mostly when upright	Awake or asleep
Premonition (nausea, sweating, light-headedness)	Common	Uncommon
Onset	Less abrupt	Abrupt
Jerking of limbs	Occasional	Frequent
Incontinence	Rare	Common

Features	Syncope	Seizures
Post-ictal recovery	Rapid	Slow
Post-ictal confusion	Uncommon	Common
EEG	Usually normal	May be abnormal

Classification of Seizures

1) Generalized seizures
   a) Tonic-clonic (in any combination)
   b) Absence
      i) Typical
      ii) Atypical
      iii) Absence with special features
        (1) Myoclonic absence
        (2) Myoclonia
   c) Myoclonic
      i) Myoclonic
      ii) Myoclonic atonic
      iii) Myoclonic tonic
   d) Clonic
   e) Tonic
   f) Atonic
   g) Epileptic spasms
2) Focal seizures

Descriptors of Focal Seizures

1) According to severity
   a) Without impairment of consciousness/responsiveness
      i) With observable motor or autonomic components
      ii) Involving subjective sensory or psychic phenomena only
   b) With impairment of consciousness/responsiveness
   c) Becoming secondarily generalized
2) According to putative site of origin
   a) With frontal lobe semiology
   b) With temporal lobe semiology
   c) With parietal lobe semiology
   d) With occipital lobe semiology
   e) With multi-lobar semiology
   f) Without localizing features
3) According to elemental sequence of clinical features

Electroclinical Syndromes and Other Epilepsies

1) Electroclinical syndromes
   a) Neonatal period
      i) Benign familial neonatal seizures (BFNS)
      ii) Early myoclonic encephalopathy (EME)
      iii) Ojhtahara syndrome
   b) Infancy
      i) Migrating partial seizures of infancy
      ii) West syndrome
      iii) Myoclonic epilepsy in infancy (MEI)
      iv) Benign infantile seizures
      v) Dravet syndrome
      vi) Myoclonic encephalopathy in non-progressive disorders
   c) Childhood
      i) Febrile seizures plus (FS+); can start in infancy
      ii) Early onset benign childhood occipita epilepsy (Panayiotopoulos type)
      iii) Epilepsy with myoclonic astatic seizures
      iv) Benign childhood epilepsy with centrotemporal spikes (BCECTS)
      v) Autosomal-dominant nocturnal frontal lobe epilepsy (ADNFLE)
      vi) Late onset childhood occipital epilepsy (Gastaut type)
      vii) Epilepsy with myoclonic absences
      viii) Lennox-Gastaut syndrome
      ix) Epileptic encephalopathy with continuous spike-and-wave during sleep (CSWS); including Landau-Kleffner syndrome (LKS)
      x) Childhood absence epilepsy (CAE)
   d) Adolescent-adult
      i) Juvenile absence epilepsy (JAE)
      ii) Juvenile myoclonic epilepsy (JME)
      iii) Progressive myoclonus epilepsies (PME)
      iv) Autosomal dominant partial epilepsy with auditory features (ADPEAF)
      v) Other familial temporal lobe epilepsies
      vi) Epilepsy with generalized tonic-clonic seizures alone
   e) Less specific age relationship
      i) Familial focal epilepsy with variable foci (childhood to adult)
      ii) Reflex epilepsies
2) Distinctive constellations
   a) Masial temporal lobe epilepsy with hippocampal sclerosis (MTLE with HS)
   b) Rasmussen syndrome
   c) Gelastic seizures with hypothalamic hamartoma
3) Epilepsies attributed to structural-metabolic causes (by cause)
   a) Malformations of cortical development
   b) Tuberous sclerosis complex
   c) Tumors
   d) Infections
   e) Trauma
   f) Perinatal insults
   g) Stroke

4) Epilepsies of unknown cause
5) Conditions with epileptic seizures that are traditionally not diagnosed as a form of epilepsy
   a) Benign neonatal seizures (BNS)
   b) Febrile seizures (FS)

References:

Report of the International League Against Epilepsy Commission on Classification and Terminology: Update and Recommendations, 2009; Anne T. Berg, Chair.
Guidelines for the Management of Epilepsy in India; Indian Epilepsy Association, 18th Annual International Epilepsy Congress Trust, 2008.
Epilepsy Foundation: The Epilepsy Classroom. http://www.epilepsyclassroom.com. Accessed July 2009.

Focal Disorders of the Brain

Stroke

Definition

- Defined as the abrupt loss of neurological function caused by an interruption of blood flow to the brain
- Term used interchangeably with cerebrovascular accident (CVA)
- Neurological deficits must persist for at least 24 hours following initial onset of symptoms

Types of Stroke

- **Hemorrhagic:** occurs when blood vessels within the brain rupture, causing leaking of blood around the brain and adjacent structures
- **Ischemic:** occurs when a clot blocks or impairs the flow of blood to the brain, depriving the brain of essential nutrients and oxygen (most common type of stroke, accounting for approximately 80% of all strokes)
- **Acute Ischemic Cerebrovascular Syndrome/Transient Ischemic Attack (TIA):** occurs in the presence of thrombolitic disease and is the result of transient ischemia in the brain and surrounding tissues. A TIA is different than a small stroke. The symptoms of TIAs do not last as long as a stroke and do not show changes on CT or MRI scans. (Small strokes do show changes on such tests.)
  - *Thrombotic*: caused by hypertension and atherosclerotic plaques. Plaques usually form in the first major branching of cerebral arteries and may be present for years without ever becoming symptomatic.
  - *Embolic*: The embolus that causes a stroke may come from an internal carotid thrombus, from the heart, or from an atheromatous plaque of the carotid sinus. With embolic infarctions, collateral blood supply is not established because of the speed of the obstruction formation, so there is less survival of the tissue distal to the area of embolic infarct compared to a thrombotic infarct.

⬤ TABLE 4.55 Early Warning Signs of Stroke

Sudden numbness or weakness of the face, arm, or leg, especially on one
side of the body
Sudden confusion, trouble speaking or understanding
Sudden trouble seeing in one or both eyes
Sudden trouble walking, dizziness, loss of balance, or coordination
Sudden, severe headaches, with no known cause
Other important but less common stroke symptoms include the following:
Sudden nausea, fever, and vomiting distinguished from a viral illness by
the speed of onset (minutes or hours vs. several days)
Brief loss of consciousness or a period of decreased consciousness (fainting,
confusion, convulsions, or coma)

⬤ TABLE 4.56 Risk Factors Associated With Stroke

Modifiable Risk Factors	Non-Modifiable Risk Factors
Heart disease	Age (>55)
Hypertension	Gender (females > males)
Diabetes	Race (African Americans have
Hypercholesterolemia	highest incidence)
Atrial fibrillation (5 times	Family history
increased risk)	
Previous TIAs	
Obesity	
Smoking	
Lack of exercise	
Poor diet	
Excessive alcohol consumption	

Classification of Strokes by Arterial Involvement

⬤ TABLE 4.57 Clinical Manifestations of Anterior Cerebral Artery Syndrome

Signs and Symptoms	Structures Involved
Contralateral hemiparesis involving mainly the LE (UE is more likely spared)	Primary motor area, medial aspect of cortex, internal capsule
Contralateral hemisensory loss involving mainly the LE (UE is more likely spared)	Primary sensory area, medial aspect of cortex
Urinary incontinence	Posteromedial aspect of superior frontal gyrus

Signs and Symptoms	Structures Involved
Problems with imitation and bimanual tasks, apraxia	Corpus callosum
Abulia (akinetic mutism), slowness, delay, lack of spontaneity, motor inaction	Uncertain localization
Contralateral grasp reflex, sucking reflex; can be asymptomatic if circle of Willis is competent	Uncertain localization

LE = Lower Extremity
UE = Upper Extremity
From: O'Sullivan, SB, and Schmitz, TJ: *Physical Rehabilitation,* ed. 5. F.A. Davis, Philadelphia, 2005.

TABLE 4.58 Clinical Manifestations of Middle Cerebral Artery Syndrome

Signs and Symptoms	Structures Involved
Contralateral hemiparesis involving mainly the UE and face (LE is more likely spared)	Primary motor cortex and internal capsule
Contralateral hemisensory loss involving mainly the UE and face (LE is more likely spared)	Primary sensory cortex and internal capsule
Motor speech impairment: Broca's or nonfluent aphasia with limited vocabulary and slow, hesitant speech	Broca's cortical area (third frontal convolution) in the dominant hemisphere, typically the left hemisphere
Receptive speech impairment: Wernicke's or fluent aphasia with impaired auditory comprehension and fluent speech with normal rate and melody	Wernicke's cortical area (posterior portion of the temporal gyrus) in the dominant hemisphere, typically the left
Global aphasia: nonfluent speech with poor comprehension	Both third frontal convolution and posterior portion of the superior temporal gyrus
Perceptual deficits: unilateral neglect, depth perception, spatial relations, agnosia	Parietal sensory association cortex in the nondominant hemisphere, typically the right
Limb-kinetic apraxia	Premotor or parietal cortex

(table continues on page 354)

TABLE 4.58　Clinical Manifestations of Middle Cerebral Artery Syndrome (continued)

Signs and Symptoms	Structures Involved
Contralateral homonymous hemianopsia	Optic radiation in internal capsule
Loss of conjugate gaze to the opposite side	Frontal eye fields or their descending tracts
Ataxia of contralateral limb(s) (sensory ataxia)	Parietal lobe
Pure motor hemiplegia (lacunar stroke)	Upper portion of posterior limb of internal capsule

From: O'Sullivan, SB, and Schmitz, TJ: *Physical Rehabilitation*, ed. 5. FA Davis, Philadelphia, 2005.

TABLE 4.59　Clinical Manifestations of Posterior Cerebral Artery Syndrome

Signs and Symptoms	Structures Involved
Peripheral territory	
Contralateral homonymous hemianopsia	Primary visual cortex or optic radiation
Bilateral homonymous hemianopsia with some degree of macular sparing	Calcarine cortex (macular sparing is due to the occipital pole receiving collateral blood supply from MCA)
Visual agnosia	Left occipital lobe
Prosopagnosia (difficulty naming people on sight)	Visual association cortex
Dyslexia (difficulty reading) without agraphia (difficulty writing), color naming (anomia), color discriminating problems	Dominant calcarine lesion and posterior part of corpus callosum
Memory deficit	Lesion of inferomedial portions of temporal lobe bilaterally or on the dominant side only
Topographic disorientation	Nondominant primary visual area, usually bilaterally
Central territory	

Signs and Symptoms	Structures Involved
Peripheral territory	
Central post-stroke (thalamic pain) Spontaneous pain and dysesthesias; sensory impairments (all modalities)	Ventral posterolateral nucleus of thalamus
Involuntary movements; choreo-athetosis, intention tremor, hemiballismus	Subthalamic nucleus or its pallidal connections
Contralateral hemiplegia	Cerebral peduncle of midbrain
Weber's syndrome Oculomotor nerve palsy and contralateral hemiplegia	Third nerve and cerebral peduncle of midbrain
Paresis of vertical eye movements, slight miosis and ptosis, and sluggish papillary light response	Supranuclear fibers to third cranial nerve

From: O'Sullivan, SB, and Schmitz, TJ: *Physical Rehabilitation,* ed. 5. FA Davis, Philadelphia, 2005.

TABLE 4.60 Clinical Manifestations of Vertebrobasilar Artery Syndrome

Medial Medullary Syndrome	
Signs and Symptoms	**Structures Involved**
	Occlusion vertebral artery, medullary branch
Ipsilateral to lesion Paralysis with atrophy of half the tongue with deviation to the paralyzed side when tongue is protruded	CN XII, hypoglossal, or nucleus
Contralateral to the lesion Paralysis of UE and LE	Corticospinal tract
Impaired tactile and proprioceptive sense	Medial lemniscus

(table continues on page 356)

NEURO

TABLE 4.60 Clinical Manifestations of Vertebrobasilar Artery Syndrome (continued)

Lateral Medullary (Wallenburg's) Syndrome	
Signs and Symptoms	**Structures Involved**
	Occlusion of posterior inferior cerebellar artery or vertebral artery
Ipsilateral to lesion Decreased pain and temperature sensation in face	Descending tract and nucleus of CNV, trigeminal
Cerebellar ataxia: gait and limbs ataxia	Cerebellum or inferior cerebellar peduncles
Vertigo, nausea, vomiting	Vestibular nuclei and connections
Nystagmus	Vestibular nuclei and connections
Horner's syndrome: miosis, ptosis, decreased sweating	Descending sympathetic tract
Dysphagia and dysphonia: paralysis of palatal and laryngeal muscles, diminished gag reflex	CN IX, glossopharyngeal, and CN X, vagus, or nuclei
Sensory impairment of ipsilateral UE, trunk, or LE	Cuneate and gracile nuclei
Contralateral to lesion Impaired pain and thermal sense over 50% of body, sometimes face	Spinal lemniscus-spinothalamic tract
Complete Basilar Artery Syndrome (locked-in syndrome)	
Signs and Symptoms	**Structures Involved**
	Basilar artery, ventral pons
Tetraplegia (quadriplegia)	Corticospinal tracts bilaterally
Bilateral cranial nerve palsy: upward gaze is spared	Long tracts to cranial nerve nuclei bilaterally
Coma	Reticular activating system
Cognition is spared	

Medial Inferior Pontine Syndrome	
Signs and Symptoms	**Structures involved**
	Occlusion of paramedian branch of basilar artery
Ipsilateral to lesion Paralysis of conjugate gaze to side of lesion (preservation of convergence)	Pontine center for lateral gaze paramedian pentine reticular formation (PPRF)
Nystagmus	Vestibular nuclei and connections
Ataxia of limbs and gait	Middle cerebellar peduncle
Diplopia on lateral gaze	CN VI, abducens, or nucleus
Contralateral to lesion Paresis of face, UE, and LE	Corticobulbar and corticospinal tract in lower pons
Impaired tactile and proprioceptive sense over 50% of body	Medial lemniscus

Lateral Inferior Pontine Syndrome	
Signs and Symptoms	**Structures Involved**
	Occlusion of anterior inferior cerebellar artery, a branch of the basilar artery
Ipsilateral to the lesion Horizontal and vertical nystagmus, vertigo, nausea, vomiting	CN VIII, vestibular, or nucleus
Facial paralysis	CN VII, facial, or nucleus
Paralysis of conjugate gaze to side of lesion	Pontine center for lateral gaze (PPRF)
Deafness, tinnitus	CN VIII, cochlear, or nucleus
Impaired sensation over face	Main sensory nucleus and descending tract of fifth nerve
Contralateral to the lesion Impaired pain and thermal sense over half the body (may include face)	Spinothalamic tract

(table continues on page 358)

TABLE 4.60 Clinical Manifestations of Vertebrobasilar Artery Syndrome (continued)

Medial Midpontine Syndrome	
Signs and Symptoms	**Structures Involved**
	Occlusion of paramedian branch of the mid-basilar artery
Ipsilateral to the lesion Ataxia of limbs and gait (more prominent in bilateral involvement)	Middle cerebellar peduncle
Contralateral to lesion Paralysis of face, UE, and LE	Corticobulbar and corticospinal tract
Deviation of eyes	PPRF

Lateral Midpontine Syndrome	
Signs and Symptoms	**Structures Involved**
	Occlusion of short circumferential artery
Ipsilateral to lesion Ataxia of limbs	Middle cerebellar peduncle
Paralysis of muscles of mastication	Motor fibers or nucleus of CN V, trigeminal
Impaired sensation over side of face	Sensory fibers or nucleus of CN V, trigeminal

Medial Superior Pontine Syndrome	
Signs and Symptoms	**Structures Involved**
	Occlusion of paramedian branches of upper basilar artery
Cerebellar ataxia	Superior or middle cerebellar peduncle
Internuclear ophthalmoplegia	Medial longitudinal fasciculus
Contralateral to lesion Paralysis of face, UE, and LE	Corticobulbar and corticospinal tract

Lateral Superior Pontine Syndrome

Signs and Symptoms	Structures Involved
	Occlusion of superior cerebellar artery, a branch of the basilar artery
Ipsilateral to lesion ...of limbs and gait, Cere... lesion fa...	Middle and superior cerebellar peduncles, superior surface of cerebellum, dentate nucleus
...a, vomiting	Vestibular nuclei
...gmus	Vestibular nuclei
...gate gaze (ipsilateral)	Uncertain
...etic nystagmus	Uncertain
...rome: miosis, ptosis, ... sweating on opposite side	Descending sympathetic fibers
...alateral to lesion ...aired pain and thermal sense of face, ...limbs, and trunk	Spinothalamic tract
Impaired touch, vibration, and position sense, more in LE than UE (tendency to incongruity of pain and touch deficits)	Medial lemniscus (lateral portion)

CN: Cranial Nerve
UE: Upper Extremity
LE: Lower Extremity
From: O'Sullivan, SB, & and Schmitz, T.J.: (2005). Physical Rehabilitation, ed. 5. Philadelphia: F.A. Davis, Philadelphia, 2005.

TABLE 4.61 Hemispheric Differences Commonly Seen Following Stroke

Right Brain Injury	Left Brain Injury
Left-side hemiplegia/paresis	Right-side hemiplegia/paresis
Left-side hemisensory loss	Right-side hemisensory loss
Visual-perceptual impairments: Left-side unilateral neglect Agnosia Visuospatial impairments Disturbances of body image and body Scheme	Speech and language impairments: dominant hemisphere/ right-handed individuals) Nonfluent (Broca's) aphasia Fluent (Wernicke's) aphasia Global aphasia

(table continues on page 360)

TABLE 4.61 Hemispheric Differences Commonly Seen Following Stroke (continued)

Right Brain Injury	Left Brain Injury
Difficulty sustaining a movement	Difficulty planning and sequencing movements, apraxia (most common: ideational or ideomotor)
Quick, impulsive behavioral style	Slow, cautious behavior
Difficulty grasping the overall organization or pattern, problem-solving and synthesizing facts	Disorganized problem-solving
Often unaware of impairments Poor judgment Inability to self-correct; increased safety risk	Often very aware of impairments Anxious about poor performance
Rigidity of thought Difficulty with abstract reasoning	Difficulty with processing delays
Difficulty with perception of emotions, expression of negative emotions	Difficulty with expression of positive emotions
Difficulty processing visual cues	Difficulty processing verbal cues, verbal commands
Memory impairments, typically related to spatial-perceptual information	Memory impairments, typically related to language

Dysfunction of either hemisphere depending on lesion location:
Visual field deficits
Emotional abnormalities: lability, apathy, irritability, low frustration levels, depression
Cognitive deficits: confusion, short attention span, loss of memory, executive functions

From: O'Sullivan, SB, and Schmitz, TJ: *Physical Rehabilitation,* ed. 5. FA Davis, Philadelphia, 2005.

References:

O'Sullivan, SB, and Schmitz, TJ: Physical Rehabilitation, ed. 5. FA Davis, Philadelphia, 2005.
Umphred, DA: Neurological Rehabilitation, ed. 5. Mosby, St. Louis, MO, 2007.

Nonprogressive Disorders of the Spinal Cord

Traumatic Spinal Cord Injury

TABLE 4.62   Functional Expectations for Individuals With AIS A and AIS B Spinal Cord Injuries*

Most distal nerve root segments innervated and key muscles	Available movements	Functional capabilities (assistive equipment may be required)	Equipment and assistance required.

C1, C2, C3
Face and neck muscles (cranial innervation)
	Talking
	Mastication
	Sipping
	Blowing
		1. Bed skills
		ADL
		  a. Total dependence in ADLs
		  b. Activation of light switches, page turners, call buttons, electrical appliances, and speaker phones
			Respirator dependent; may use phrenic nerve stimulator during the day.
			Full-time attendant required.
			Environmental control units.

		2. Wheelchair skills	Indpendent with powered wheelchair (typical components include an electrically controlled seating system, a seat belt and trunk support); a portable ventilator is typically attached; microswitch or sip-and-puff controls may be used.
		3. Transfers	Dependent

(table continues on page 362)

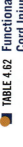

NEURO

TABLE 4.62 Functional Expectations for Individuals With AIS A and AIS B Spinal Cord Injuries* (continued)

C4 Diaphragm Trapezius	Respiration Scapular elevation	Dependent
	1. Bed skills ADLs a. Limited self-feeding	Mobile arm supports (possibly with powered elbow orthosis), powered flexor hinge hand splint. Adapted eating equipment (long straws, built-up handles on utensils, plate guards, and so forth). Plexiglas lapboard.
	b. Typing	Computer keyboard using head or mouth stick or sip-and-puff controls; another option is a rubber-tipped stick held in hand by a splint (in combination with mobile arm supports and powered splints).
	c. Page turning	Head or mouth stick. Environmental control unit for powered page turner.
	d. Activation of light switches, call buttons, electrical appliances, and speaker phone	Environmental control units.
	2. Wheelchair skills	Independent with power wheelchair with mouth, chin, breath, or sip-and-puff controls.

	a. Pressure relief	Power tilt-in-space
	b. Transfers and bed mobility	Dependent
	3. Skin inspection	Dependent.
	4. Cough with glossopharangeal breathing	Dependent.
	5. Recreation. a. Table games such as cards or checkers b. Painting and drawing	Head or mouth stick. Built-up playing pieces. Full-time attendant required.
C5 Biceps brachialis Brachioradialis Deltoid Infraspinatus Rhomboid (major and minor) Supinator Elbow flexion and supination Shoulder external rotation Shoulder abduction to 90° Limited shoulder flexion	1. Bed skills ADLs: a. Able to accomplish all activities of a C4 quadriplegic with less adaptive equipment and more skill b. Self-feeding	Some assistance is required in setting up individual with necessary equipment; individual can then accomplish activity independently. Mobile arm supports. Adapted utensils and splinting.
	b. Typing	Computer keyboard. Hand splints. Adapted typing sticks. Some individuals may require mobile arm supports or slings.

(table continues on page 364)

NEURO

NEURO

TABLE 4.62 Functional Expectations for Individuals With AIS A and AIS B Spinal Cord Injuries* (continued)

c. Page turning	Same as above.
d. Limited upper extremity dressing	Assistance required. Hand splints. Adapted equipment (wash mitt, adapted toothbrush, and so forth).
e. Limited self-care (i.e., washing, brushing teeth, and grooming)	
2. Wheelchairs skills	Independent with anual wheelchair with plastic-coated hand-rim projections. Power wheelchair with joystick or adapted upper extremity controls.
3. Transfer activities	Dependent. Overhead swivel bar. Sliding board.
4. Skin inspection Pressure relief	Dependent. Independent with power tilt-in-space wheelchair.
5. Cough with manual pressure to diaphragm	Assistance required.
6. Driving	Van with hand controls. Part-time attendant required.

NEURO

C6 Extensor carpi radialis Infraspinatus Latissimus dorsi Pectoralis major (clavicular portion) Pronator teres Serratus anterior Teres minor	Shoulder flexion, extension, internal rotation, and adduction Scapular abduction and upward rotation Forearm pronation Wrist extension (tenodesis grasp)	1. Bed skills ADLs a. Self-feeding b. Dressing c. Self-care	Some assistance to independent with use of side rails on bed or overhead triangle Universal cuff. Intertwine utensils in fingers. Adapted utensils. Utilizes momentum, button hooks, zipper pulls, or other clothing adaptations; dependent on momentum to extend limbs. Cannot tie shoes. Flexor hinge splint. Universal cuff. Adaptive equipment.
		2. Wheelchair skills	Independent with manual wheelchair with projection or friction surface hand rims; power wheelchair may be required for long distances and community mobility.
		3. Transfer activities	Independent with sliding board on level surfaces.
		4. Skin inspection and pressure relief	Independent.
		5. Bowel and bladder care	Can be independent with equipment depending on bowel and bladder routine.

(table continues on page 366)

NEURO

TABLE 4.62 Functional Expectations for Individuals With AIS A and AIS B Spinal Cord Injuries* (continued)

	6. Cough with application of pressure to abdomen	Independent.
	7. Driving	Automobile with hand controls and U-shaped cuff attached to steering wheel. Usually requires assistance in getting wheelchair into car.
	8. Wheelchair sports	Limited participation.
	Meal preparation	Can be independent with occasional light meals with adaptive equipment.
C7 Extensor pollicis longus and brevis Extrinsic finger extensors Flexor carpi radialis Triceps	Elbow extension Wrist flexion Finger extension	1. Bed skills ADLs a. Self-feeding b. Dressing c. Self-care	Independent. Independent. Button hook may be required. Shower chair. Hand-held shower nozzle. Adapted handles on bathroom items may be required.
	2. Wheelchair skills	Independent with manual wheelchair with friction surface hand rims.
	3. Transfers	Independent (with or without sliding board).

NEURO

	4. Bowel and bladder care	Independent with appropriate equipment (digital stimulator, suppositories, raised toilet seat, urinary drainage device, and so forth).
	5. Manual cough	Independent.
	6. Housekeeping	Light kitchen activities. Requires wheelchair-accessible kitchen and living environment. Adapted kitchen tools.
	7. Driving	Automobile with hand controls. Able to get wheelchair in and out of car.
C8–T1 Extrinsic finger flexors Flexor carpi ulnaris Flexor pollicis longus and brevis Intrinsic finger flexors	Full innervation of upper extremity muscles including fine coordination and strong grasp	1. Bed skills ADLs	Independent in all self-care and personal hygiene. Some adaptive equipment may be required (e.g., tub seat, grab bars, and so forth).
	2. Wheelchair skills	Independent with manual wheelchair with standard hand rims.

(table continues on page 368)

TABLE 4.62 Functional Expectations for Individuals With AIS A and AIS B Spinal Cord Injuries* (continued)

	3. Housekeeping	Independent in light housekeeping and meal preparation. Some adaptive equipment may be required (e.g., reachers). Requires a wheelchair-accessible living environment.
	4. Driving	Automobile with hand controls.
	5. Employment	Able to work in a building free of architectural barriers.
T4–T6 Top half of intercostals Long muscles of back (sacrospinalis and semi-spinalis)	Improved trunk control Increased respiratory reserve Pectoral girdle stabilized for lifting objects	
	1. Bed skills ADL	Independent. Independent in all areas.
	2. Wheelchair skills a. Curb climbing in wheelchair b. Wheelchair sports	Independent with manual wheelchair. Able to negotiate curbs using a "wheelie" technique. Full participation.
	3. Transfers	Independent.

		2. Physiological standing (not practical for functional ambulation)	Standing table or frame. Bilateral knee-ankle orthoses (KAKOs) with spinal attachment. Some individuals may be able to ambulate for short distances with assistance.
		3. Housekeeping	Independent with routine activities. Requires a wheelchair-accessible living environment.
T9–T12 Lower abdominals All intercostals	Improved trunk control Increased endurance	1. Household ambulation	Bilateral Knee Ankle Foot Orthotics (KAFOs) and crutches or walker (high energy consumption for ambulation).
		2. Wheelchair skills	Wheelchair used for energy conservation.
L2, L3, L4 Gracilis Iliopsoas Quadratus lumborum Rectus femoris Sartorius	Hip flexion Hip adduction Knee extension	1. Functional ambulation 2. Wheelchair skills	Bilateral KAFOs and crutches. Wheelchair used for convenience and energy conservation.
L4, L5 Extensor digitorum	Strong hip flexion Strong knee extension	1. Functional ambulation	Bilateral KAFOs and crutches or canes.

(table continues on page 370)

NEURO

TABLE 4.62 Functional Expectations for Individuals With AIS A and AIS B Spinal Cord Injuries* (continued)

Low back muscles	Weak knee flexion	Wheelchair used for convenience and energy conservation.
Medial hamstrings (weak)	Improved trunk control	
Tibialis posterior	2. Wheelchair skills.	
Quadriceps		
Tibialis anterior		

Modified from: O'Sullivan, SB, and Schmitz, TJ: *Physical Rehabilitation*, ed. 5. FA Davis, Philadelphia, 2007, pp 961–964.

*This table presents general functional expectations for individuals with injuries classified as AIS A or AIS B at various lesion levels. Each progressively lower segment includes the muscles from the previous levels. Although the key muscles listed frequently receive innervation from several nerve root segments, they are listed here at the neurological levels where they add to functional outcomes. Motor function varies among individuals with injuries classified as AIS C and AIS D due to differences in the degree of damage to the various spinal pathways.

ADLs = activities of daily living.

Progressive Disorders of the Brain and Spinal Cord

Global Progressive Disorders

Hyrodrocephalus

Classification of Chronic Hydrocephalus

Hydrocephalus, or "water in the head," is caused by excess cerebral spinal fluid (CSF) in the intracranial cavity. In the normal brain, a balance between CSF production and CSF resorption maintains CSF pressure (Pcsf) in the range of 6–20 cm H_2O. Disorders of CSF circulation arise when this equilibrium is disrupted, either by obstructing normal CSF flow patterns or by perturbing the production/resorption balance.

From:

Irani, DN: Cerebrospinal Fluid in Diseases of the Nervous System. Saunders, Philadelphia, 2008. Ebook through MD consult. http://www.mdconsult.com. Accessed December 7, 2009.

Possible Etiologies

1. Communicating hydrocephalus: communication between the ventricles and lumbar CSF. The CSF flow over the surface of the brain is obstructed, or there is a failure of absorption of the CSF.
   a. Impaired CSF reabsorption in the arachnoid granulations.
      i. Causes include: meningitis or infection, cerebral hemorrhage, or carcinomatous meningitis.
   b. Obstruction of flow in the subarachnoid space.
   c. Excess CSF production (rare): *Choroid plexus papillomas* are rare ventricular tumors that can produce excessive volumes of CSF
2. Non-communicating hydrocephalus.
   a. Obstruction of flow within the ventricular system.
      i. Common sites include:
         1. Lateral ventricle obstruction by tumors, including basal ganglia gliomas, and thalamic gliomas.
         2. Third ventricle obstruction, caused by colloid cysts or other tumors of the third ventricle.
         3. Obstruction of the aqueduct of Sylvius, either by congenital stenosis or secondary to lesions such as pineal tumors.
         4. Fourth ventricular obstruction caused by posterior fossa tumors, such as medulloblastomas, ependymomas, and acoustic neuromas.
         5. Basal cisterns, often as a result of congenital developmental abnormalities, such as those associated with spina bifida.

From:

Chapter 63: Hydrocephalus, in Schapira, AH: Neurology and Clinical Neuroscience. Copyright © 2008 Mosby, An Imprint of Elsevier. Ebook through MD consult. http://www.mdconsult.com. Accessed December 7, 2009.

NEURO

TABLE 4.63   Signs and Symptoms of Acute Adult Hydrocephalus

The major presenting features of acute onset hydrocephalus are symptoms and signs of raised intracranial pressure (ICP). The most important feature is *deterioration of conscious state.*
Other features that may be seen include the following:
Headache
Vomiting
Papilledema
Sixth nerve palsy
Impairment of upward gaze, caused by compression of the rostral tectum by the enlarged third ventricle

From: Hydrocephalus. In Schapira, AH: *Neurology and Clinical Neuroscience.* Copyright © 2008 Mosby, An Imprint of Elsevier. E-book through MD consult. http://www.mdconsult.com. Accessed December 7, 2009.

Normal Pressure Hydrocephalus

Normal pressure hydrocephalus (NPH) is so named because a lumbar puncture typically demonstrates a CSF pressure within the normal range. Neurological impairment in NPH is probably a result of progressive impairment of the periventricular microcirculation. NPH (http://www.mdconsult.com.proxy.library.emory.edu/book/player/linkTo?type=bookPage&isbn=978-0-323-03354-1&eid=4-u1.0-B978-0-323-03354-1..50067-5—bib43&appID=MDC) is characterized by the triad of the following:

1. Gait disturbance
2. Urinary incontinence
3. Cognitive changes that may occasionally progress to a subcortical-type dementia

Gait impairment and postural instability are usually the first symptoms of NPH and are also the most responsive to shunting. The gait abnormalities, described as "frontal gait disorder," are not specific; slower velocity, shorter and more varying strides, reduced ground clearance and ankle dorsiflexion during the swing phase, and increased base of gait (step width) are all seen. There may be postural instability with frequent falls, gait ignition failure, or freezing (typically unresponsive to levodopa). Pyramidal signs, including extensor plantar responses, may be seen in the lower limbs.

TABLE 4.64   Description of Idiopathic Normal-Pressure Hydrocephalus (NPH) Classification: Probable, Possible, and Unlikely Categories

Probable NPH

I. History:
   Reported symptoms should be corroborated by an informant familiar with the patient's premorbid and current condition, and must include:
   A. Insidious onset (versus acute)
   B. Origin after age 40 yr
   C. A minimum duration of at least 3 to 6 mo

Probable NPH

 D. No evidence of an antecedent event such as head trauma, intracerebral hemorrhage, meningitis, or other known causes of secondary hydrocephalus

 E. Progression over time

 F. No other neurological, psychiatric, or medical conditions that are sufficient to explain the presenting symptoms

II. Brain imaging

A brain imaging study (CT or MRI) performed after onset of symptoms must show evidence of:

 A. Ventricular enlargement not entirely attributable to cerebral atrophy or congenital enlargement (Evan's index >0.3 or comparable measure)

 B. No macroscopic obstruction to CSF flow

 C. At least one of the following supportive features:

  1. Enlargement of the temporal horns of the lateral ventricles not entirely attributable to hippocampus atrophy

  2. Callosal angle of 40 degrees or more

  3. Evidence of altered brain water content, including periventricular signal changes on CT and MRI not attributable to microvascular ischemic changes or demyelination

  4. An aqueductal or fourth ventricular flow void on MRI

III. Clinical

Findings of gait/balance disturbance must be present, plus at least one other area of impairment in cognition, urinary symptoms, or both.

 A. With respect to gait/balance, at least two of the following should be present and not be entirely attributable to other conditions:

  1. Decreased step height

  2. Decreased step length

  3. Decreased cadence (speed of walking)

  4. Increased trunk sway during walking

  5. Widened standing base

  6. Toes turned outward on walking

  7. Retropulsion (spontaneous or provoked)

  8. En bloc turning (turning requiring three or more steps for 180 degrees)

  9. Impaired walking balance, as evidenced by two or more corrections out of eight steps on tandem gait testing

 B. With respect to cognition, there must be documented impairment (adjusted for age and educational attainment) and/or decrease in performance on a cognitive screening instrument (such as the Monumental State examination), or evidence of at least two of the following on examination that is not fully attributable to other conditions:

  1. Psychomotor slowing (increased response latency)

  2. Decreased fine motor speed

  3. Decreased fine motor accuracy

  4. Difficulty dividing or maintaining attention

  5. Impaired recall, especially for recent events

  6. Executive dysfunction, such as impairment in multistep procedures, working memory, formulation of abstractions/similarities, insight

  7. Behavioral or personality changes

(table continues on page 374)

TABLE 4.64 **Description of Idiopathic Normal-Pressure Hydrocephalus (NPH) Classification: Probable, Possible, and Unlikely Categories** (continued)

NEURO

Probable NPH

C. To document symptoms in the domain of urinary continence, either one of the following should be present:
  1. Episodic or persistent urinary incontinence not attributable to primary urological disorders
  2. Persistent urinary incontinence
  3. Urinary and fecal incontinence
     Or any two of the following should be present:
  1. Urinary urgency as defined by frequent perception of a pressing need to void
  2. Urinary frequency as defined by more than six voiding episodes in an average 12-hour period despite normal fluid intake
  3. Nocturia as defined by the need to urinate more than two times in an average night

IV. Physiological
  A. CSF opening pressure in the range of 5–18 mm Hg (or 70–245 mm H_2O) as determined by a lumbar puncture or a comparable procedure.
  B. Appropriately measured pressures that are significantly higher or lower than this range are not consistent with a probable NPH diagnosis.

Possible NPH

I. History
  A. Reported symptoms may:
  B. Have a subacute or indeterminate mode of onset
  C. Begin at any age after childhood
  D. May have less than 3 mo or indeterminate duration
  E. May follow events such as mild head trauma, remote history of intracerebral hemorrhage, or childhood and adolescent meningitis or other conditions that in the judgment of the clinician are not likely to be causally related
  F. Coexist with other neurological, psychiatric, or general medical disorders but in the judgment of the clinician not be entirely attributable to these conditions
  G. Be nonprogressive or not clearly progressive

II. Brain imaging
  A. Ventricular enlargement consistent with hydrocephalus but associated with any of the following:
  B. Evidence of cerebral atrophy of sufficient severity to potentially explain ventricular size
  C. Structural lesions that may influence ventricular size

III. Clinical
  A. Symptoms of either:
  B. Incontinence and/or cognitive impairment in the absence of an observable gait or balance disturbance
  C. Gait disturbance or dementia alone

Possible NPH

IV. Physiological
  A. Opening pressure measurement not available or pressure outside the range required for probable NPH

Unlikely NPH

  I. No evidence of ventriculomegaly
 II. Signs of increased intracranial pressure such as papilledema
III. No component of the clinical triad of INPH is present
IV. Symptoms explained by other causes (e.g., spinal stenosis)

Adapted from: Belkin, N, et al: Diagnosing idiopathic normal-pressure hydrocephalus. *Neurosurgery* 57:S2-4–S2-16, 2005.

TABLE 4.65 Comparison of Cognitive Deficits in Alzheimer's Disease and Idiopathic Normal-Pressure Hydrocephalus

Cognitive Skills	Alzheimer's Disease	Idiopathic Normal-Pressure Hydrocephalus
Impaired	Memory Learning Orientation Attention concentration Executive functions Writing	Psychomotor slowing Fine motor speed Fine motor accuracy
Borderline	Motor and psychomotor skills Visuospatial skills Language Reading	Auditory memory (immediate and delayed) Attention concentration Executive function Behavioral or personality changes

Shunting Procedures for Hydrocephalus

1. *External Drainage:* An external ventricular drain used for urgent treatment of acute hydrocephalus associated with rapid deterioration of consciousness (ventricular hemorrhage, acute infection, or a cerebral mass lesion). ICP may be monitored.
2. *Internal Drainage:* All shunts consist of a proximal catheter inserted in a CSF space (either the ventricle or the lumbar subarachnoid space), a passive valve mechanism (differential pressure valve), and a distal catheter that carries CSF to some extracerebral site for resorption. The peritoneal cavity, the jugular vein, or the intrapleural space are the most common distal sites currently being used.

From:

Hydrocephalus: Treatment, in Schapira, AH: Neurology and Clinical Neuroscience. Copyright © 2008 Mosby, An Imprint of Elsevier. Ebook through MD consult. http://www. mdconsult.com. Accessed December 7, 2009.

Complications

Although they are engineered for long-term use, all shunts can malfunction over time, including obstruction, disconnection, or valve failure. Malfunction is the most common complication of shunts in both adults and children. Shunt obstruction is the most common form of malfunction, a process that usually occurs somewhere within the shunt catheters and less frequently in the valve itself.

Shunt obstruction in children is more likely to be a life-threatening emergency than it is in adults, mainly because children are more commonly shunted for obstructive hydrocephalus

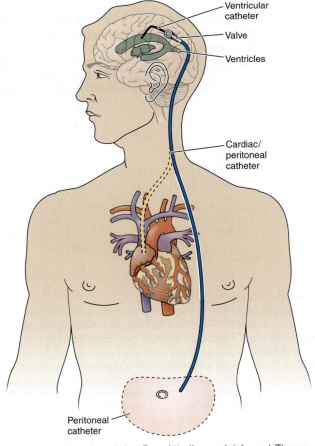

Ventricular catheter

Valve

Ventricles

Cardiac/ peritoneal catheter

Peritoneal catheter

Shunting procedure for hydrocephalus. From: http://www.nph-info.co.uk/Therapy Awareness/Treatment/1183101062590.htm#image1. Accessed August 2009.

Multiple Sclerosis

Pathophysiology

Multiple sclerosis (MS) is believed to be an autoimmune disease in which the nerve-insulating myelin is attacked by the body's own immune system. Communication between the brain and parts of the body become disrupted. Triggers may be linked to environmental causes or perhaps a virus. Initial symptoms are often blurred or double vision, red-green color distortion, or even blindness in one eye.

NEURO

🟠 **TABLE 4.66 Common Symptoms in Multiple Sclerosis**

Motor symptoms: Weakness or paralysis, fatigue, spasticity, incoordination, intention tremor, impaired balance, gait disturbances.	*Sensory symptoms:* Hypoesthesia, numbness, paresthesias.
	Cardiovascular dysautonomia.
Visual symptoms: Blurred or double vision, diminished acuity/ loss of vision, scotoma, nystagmus.	*Pain:* Dysesthesias, optic or trigeminal neuritis, Lhermitte's sign, chronic pain.
Cognitive symptoms: Memory or recall problems, decreased attention/concentration, diminished abstract reasoning, diminished problem solving/ judgment, diminished speed of processing, diminished visual-spatial abilities.	*Speech and swallowing:* Dysarthria, diminished verbal fluency, dysphonia, dysphagia.
Bowel symptoms: Constipation, diarrhea, incontinence.	*Bladder symptoms:* Urinary urgency/ frequency, nocturia, incontinence, urinary hesitancy, dribbling.
Emotional symptoms: Depression, pseudobulbaar affect, anxiety.	*Sexual symptoms:* Impotence, decreased libido, decreased vaginal lubrication, impaired ability to achieve orgasm.

Adapted from: O'Sullian, SB, and Schmitz, TJ: *Physical Rehabilitation,* ed. 5. FA Davis, Philadelphia, 2005, pp 777–780.

Diagnostic Criteria

● TABLE 4.67 The 2005 Revisions to the McDonald Diagnostic Criteria for MS

Clinical Presentation	Additional Data Needed For MS Diagnosis
• 2 or more attacks • Objective clinical evidence of 2 or more lesions	• None
• 2 or more attacks • Objective clinical evidence of 1 lesion	• Dissemination in space, demonstrated by: → MRI or → 2 or more MRI detected lesions consistent with MS plus positive CSF *OR* → Await further clinical attack implicating a different site
• 1 attack • Objective clinical evidence of 2 or more lesions	• Dissemination in time, demonstrated by: → MRI *OR* → Second clinical attack
• 1 attack • Objective clinical evidence of 1 lesion (monosymptomatic presentation, clinically isolated syndrome)	• Dissemination in space, demonstrated by: → MRI *OR* → 2 or more MRI-detected lesions consistent with MS plus positive CSF AND • Dissemination in time, demonstrated by: → MRI *OR* → Second clinical attack
• Insidious neurological progression suggestive of MS	• One year of disease progression (retrospective or prospectively determined) AND • Two out of three of the following: 1) Positive brain MRI (9T2 lesions or 4 or more T2 lesions with positive visual-evoked potentials) 2) Positive spinal cord MRI (two or more focal T2 lesions) 3) Positive CSF

From: Polman, et al: Diagnostic criteria for multiple sclerosis: 2005 revisions to the "McDonald" criteria. *Ann Neurol* 58:840–846, 2005.

There are four possible disease courses:

Relapsing-remitting MS (RRMS)

RRMS is the most common form of the disease. It is characterized by clearly defined acute attacks with full recovery (left) or with residual deficit upon recovery (right). Periods between disease relapses are characterized by a lack of disease progression. Approximately 85% of people with MS begin with a *relapsing-remitting* course.

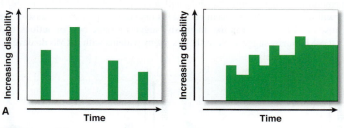

Relapsing-remitting.

Primary progressive MS (PPMS)

PPMS is characterized by progression of disability from onset, without plateaus or remissions (left) or with occasional plateaus and temporary minor improvements (right). A person with PPMS, by definition, does not experience acute attacks. Of people with MS are diagnosed, only 10% have PPMS. In addition, the diagnostic criteria for PPMS are less secure than those for RRMS so that often the diagnosis is only made long after the onset of neurological symptoms and at a time when the person is already living with significant disability.

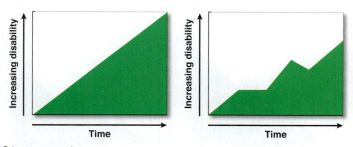

Primary-progressive.

NEURO

Secondary-progressive MS (SPMS)

SPMS begins with an initial relapsing-remitting disease course, followed by
    progression of disability (left) that may include occasional relapses and
    minor remissions and plateaus (right). Typically, secondary-progressive dis-
    ease is characterized by: less recovery following attacks, persistently
    worsening functioning during *and between* attacks, and/or fewer and fewer
    attacks (or none at all) accompanied by progressive disability. According
    to some natural history studies, of the 85% who start with relapsing-
    remitting disease, more than 50% will develop SPMS within 10 years; 90%
    within 25 years. More recent natural history studies (perhaps because of the
    use of MRI to assist in the diagnosis) suggest a more benign outlook that
    these numbers suggest. Nevertheless, many patients with RRMS do develop
    SPMS ultimately.

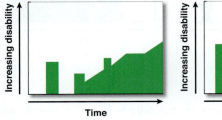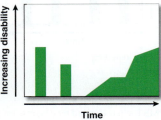

Secondary-progressive.

Progressive-relapsing MS (PRMS)

PRMS, which is the least common disease course, shows progression of dis-
    ability from onset but with clear acute relapses, with (left) or without (right)
    full recovery. Approximately 5% of people with MS appear to have PRMS
    at diagnosis. Not infrequently a patient may be initially diagnosed as having
    PPMS and then will experience an acute attack, thereby establishing the di-
    agnosis of PRMS.

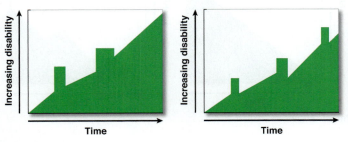

Progressive-relapsing.

Assessment of Disease Progression

Disease progression is evaluated in four ways:

1) *Radiographically*—by looking for new lesions, gadolinium-enhanced lesions, or an increased amount of disease on MRI
2) *Electrophysiologically*—by measuring changes in the sensory-evoked potentials
3) *Neurologically*—by measuring changes in function on the neurological examination
4) *Functionally*—by assessing the person's physical and cognitive abilities

NEURO

From:

National Multiple Sclerosis Society. http://www.nationalmssociety.org/. Accessed July 15, 2009.
National Institute of Neurological Disorders and Stroke. Multiple sclerosis information page.
http://www.ninds.nih.gov/disorders/multiple_sclerosis/multiple_sclerosis.htm. Accessed
August 1, 2009.

Considerations for Rehabilitation

Despite the inability of rehabilitation to alter the actual disease course, improvements in mobility, activities of daily living, quality of life, prevention of complications, reduction in health-care utilization, and gains in safety and independence may be attained at all stages of the disease through carefully planned programs of exercise, functional training, and activities specific to the needs of the individual.

1. The physician should consider referral of individuals with MS for assessment by rehabilitation professionals (including rehabilitation physician, occupational, physical, speech and language therapists) when there is an abrupt or gradual worsening of function or increase in impairment that has a significant impact on the individual's mobility, safety, independence, and/or quality of life.
2. Patients who present with any functional limitation should have an initial evaluation and appropriate management.
3. Assessment for rehabilitation services should be considered early in the disease when behavioral and lifestyle changes may be easier to implement.
4. The complex interaction of motor, sensory, cognitive, functional, and affective impairments in an unpredictable, progressive, and fluctuating disease such as MS, requires periodic reassessment, monitoring, and rehabilitative interventions.
5. The frequency, intensity, and setting of the rehabilitative intervention must be based on individual needs. Some complex needs are best met in an interdisciplinary, inpatient setting, while other needs are best met at home or in outpatient settings. The health-care team should determine the most appropriate setting. Whenever possible, patients should be seen by rehabilitation therapists who are familiar with neurological degenerative disorders.

6. Research and professional experience support the use of rehabilitative interventions (including exercise, functional training, equipment prescription, provision of assistive technology, orthotics prescription, teaching of compensatory strategies, caregiver/family support and education, counseling, and referral to community resources) in concert with other medical interventions for the following impairments in MS:

 a. Mobility impairments (i.e., impaired strength, gait, balance, range of motion, coordination, tone, and endurance)

 b. Fatigue

 c. Pain

 d. Dysphagia

 e. Bladder/bowel dysfunction

 f. Decreased independence in activities of daily living (ADLs)

 g. Impaired communication

 h. Diminished quality of life (often caused by inability to work, engage in leisure activities, and/or pursue usual life roles)

 i. Depression and other affective disorders

 j. Cognitive dysfunction

7. Appropriate assessments and outcome measures must be applied periodically to establish and revise goals, identify the need for treatment modification, and measure the results of the intervention.

8. Known complications of MS, such as contractures, disuse atrophy, decubiti, risk of falls, and increased dependence may be reduced or prevented by specific rehabilitative interventions.

9. In a fluctuating and progressive disease, maintenance of function, optimal participation, and quality of life are essential outcomes.

10. Maintenance therapy includes rehabilitation interventions designed to preserve current status of ADLs, safety, mobility, and quality of life, and to reduce the rate of deterioration and development of complications.

11. A thorough assessment for wheelchairs, positioning devices, other durable medical equipment (DME), and environmental modification by rehabilitation professionals is recommended and will result in the use of the most appropriate equipment.

12. Regular and systematic communication between the referring health-care provider and rehabilitation professionals will facilitate comprehensive, quality care.

13. Third-party payers should cover appropriate and individualized restorative and maintenance rehabilitation services for people with MS.

From:

http://www.nationalmssociety.org. *Accessed October 3, 2009.*

🔴 TABLE 4.68 Common Symptoms of Weakness and Fatigue in MS

Common symptoms of weakness and fatigue in MS caused by impaired nerve
  conduction in the central nervous system can be exacerbated by a variety
  of factors:
  An elevated core body temperature (from overheating, overexertion, or
    infection with fever)
  Certain medications, such as those used to treat spasticity and pain
  Obesity
  Disrupted sleep (caused by bladder urgency, periodic limb movements,
    spasticity, and pain, among other factors)
  Affective disorders such as depression
  Stress
  Other medical conditions, such as anemia
Other "invisible" symptoms are cause for frustration in patients, including
  impairments of sensation, vision, cognition, bowel and bladder, and sexual
  function

From: Clinical changes that may impact therapy interventions in individuals with
  MS. In Provance, PG: *Physical Therapy in Multiple Sclerosis Rehabilitation.*
  http://www.nationalmssociety.org. Accessed October 10, 2009.

🔴 TABLE 4.69 Purpose of Disease-Modifying Medications in MS

Reduce the frequency and severity of clinical attacks (also called relapses or
  exacerbations), which are defined as the sudden worsening of an MS
  symptom or symptoms, or the appearance of new symptoms, which lasts at
  least 24 hr and is separated from a previous exacerbation by at least 1 mo.
Reduce the accumulation of lesions (damaged or active disease areas) within
  the brain and spinal cord as seen on MRI (magnetic resonance imaging).
Appear to slow down the accumulation of disability.

From: http://www.nationalmssociety.org/DMD. Accessed November 22, 2009.

NEURO

■ TABLE 4.70 Medications Approved by the U.S. Food and Drug Administration in Treating Relapsing Forms of MS (October 2009)

Drug	Indication	Frequency/Route of Delivery/ Usual Dose	Common Side Effects
Immunomodulating Drugs			
Avonex interferon beta-1a	For the treatment of relapsing forms of MS, and for a first clinical episode if MRI features consistent with MS are also present.	Once a week; intramuscular injection; 30 mcg.	Flu-like symptoms following injection, which lessen over time for many. *Less common:* depression, mild anemia, liver abnormalities, allergic reactions, heart problems.
Betaseron interferon beta-1b	For the treatment of relapsing forms of MS and secondary progressive MS with relapses; and for patients who have experienced a first clinical episode and have MRI features consistent with MS.	Every other day; subcutaneous injection; 250 mcg.	Flu-like symptoms following injection, which lessen over time for many. Injection site reactions, about 5% of which need medical attention. *Less common:* allergic reactions, depression, liver abnormalities, low white blood cell counts.
Copaxone glatiramer acetate	For the treatment of relapsing-remitting MS; and for patients who have experienced a first clinical episode and have MRI features consistent with MS.	Every day; subcutaneous injection; 20 mg (20,000 mcg).	Injection site reactions. Less common: vasodilation (dilation of blood vessels); chest pain; a reaction immediately after injection, which includes anxiety, chest pain, palpitations, shortness of breath, and flushing. This lasts 15–30 min, passes without treatment, and has no known long-term effects.

Drug	Indication	Frequency/Route of Delivery/ Usual Dose	Common Side Effects
Extavia interferon beta-1b	For the treatment of relapsing forms of MS and secondary-progressive MS with relapses; and for patients who have experienced a first clinical episode and have MRI features consistent with MS.	Every other day; subcutaneous injection; 250 mcg.	Flu-like symptoms following injection, which lessen over time for many. Injection site reactions, about 5% of which need medical attention. *Less common:* allergic reactions, depression, liver abnormalities, low white blood cell counts.
Rebif interferon beta-1a	For the treatment of relapsing forms of MS.	Three times a week; subcutaneous injection; 44 mcg.	Flu-like symptoms following injection, which lessen over time for many. Injection site reactions. *Less common:* Liver abnormalities, depression, allergic reactions, and low red or white blood cell counts.
Tysabri natalizumab	For the treatment of relapsing forms of MS as a monotherapy (not used in combination with any other disease-modifying medication). Generally recommended for patients who have had inadequate response to, or are unable to tolerate, another disease-modifying medication.	Every 4 wk by IV infusion in a registered infusion facility; 300 mg.	Headache, fatigue, urinary tract infections, depression, lower respiratory tract infections, joint pain, and chest discomfort. *Less common:* allergic or hypersensitivity reactions within 2 hr of infusion (dizziness, fever, rash, itching, nausea, flushing, low blood pressure, difficulty breathing, chest pain), liver abnormalities. Patients must be monitored for PML.

(table continues on page 386)

TABLE 4.70 Medications Approved by the U.S. Food and Drug Administration in Treating Relapsing Forms of MS (October 2009) (continued)

Drug	Indication	Frequency/Route of Delivery/ Usual Dose	Common Side Effects
Immunosuppressant Drug			
Novantrone Mitoxantrone; as of 2006, available as a generic drug	For treatment of worsening relapsing-remitting MS and for progressive-relapsing or secondary-progressive MS.	Four times a year by IV infusion in a medical facility. Lifetime cumulative dose limit of approximately 8–12 doses over 2–3 yr (140 mg/m^2).	Blue-green urine 24 hr after administration; infections, bone marrow suppression (fatigue, bruising, low blood cell counts), nausea, hair thinning, bladder infections, mouth sores. Patients must be monitored for serious liver and heart damage.

PML: Progressive Multifocal Leukoencephalopathy

From: http://www.nationalmssociety.org/DMD. Accessed November 22, 2009.

Amyotrophic Lateral Sclerosis

Pathophysiology

Amyotrophic lateral sclerosis (ALS), sometimes called Lou Gehrig's disease, is a rapidly progressive, fatal neurological disease characterized by the gradual degeneration and death of the motor neurons responsible for controlling voluntary muscles. Both the upper motor neurons and the lower motor neurons degenerate. Unable to function, muscles gradually atrophy, and twitch *(fasciculations)*. The ability of the brain to start and control voluntary movement is progressively lost.

Eventually, all muscles under voluntary control are affected, and patients lose their strength and the ability to move their arms, legs, and body. When muscles in the diaphragm and chest wall fail, patients lose the ability to breathe without ventilatory support. Most people with ALS die from respiratory failure, usually within 3 to 5 years from the onset of symptoms. However, about 10% of ALS patients survive for 10 or more years.

> *From:*
>
> *National Institute of Neurological Disorders and Stroke. Amyotrophic Lateral Sclerosis. www.ninds.nih.gov/disorders/amyotrophiclateralsclerosis/amyotrophiclateralsclerosis.htm Accessed August 2, 2009.*

ALS Signs and Symptoms

- Initial symptoms of muscle weakness in one or more of the following: hands, arms, legs or the muscles of speech, swallowing, or breathing
- Fasciculation and cramping of muscles, especially those in the hands and feet
- Impairment of the use of the arms and legs
- "THICK speech" and difficulty in projecting the voice
- In more advanced stages, shortness of breath, difficulty in breathing and swallowing

Classifications of ALS

1) Sporadic—the most common form of ALS in the United States—90% to 95% of all cases.
2) Familial—occurring more than once in a family lineage (genetic dominant inheritance); accounts for a very small number of cases in the United States—5% to 10% of all cases.
3) Guamanian— an extremely high incidence of ALS was observed in Guam and the Trust Territories of the Pacific in the 1950s.

> *From:*
>
> *Amyotrophic Lateral Sclerosis Association. http://www.alsa.org. Accessed July 17, 2009*

Revised Diagnostic Criteria

The diagnosis of ALS requires the following:

(A) Presence of:
    (A:1) evidence of lower motor neuron (LMN) degeneration by clinical, electrophysiological, or neuropathological examination,

(A:2) evidence of upper motor neuron (UMN) degeneration by clinical examination, and

(A:3) progressive spread of symptoms or signs within a region or to other regions, as determined by history or examination,

together with:

(B) Absence of

(B:1) electrophysiological or pathological evidence of other disease processes that might explain the signs of LMN and/or UMN degeneration, and

(B:2) neuroimaging evidence of other disease processes that might explain the observed clinical and electrophysiological signs.

NEURO

From:

Brooks, BR , et al: World Federation of Neurology Research Group on Motor Neuron Diseases. El Escorial revisited: Revised criteria for the diagnosis of amyotrophic lateral sclerosis. ALS and other motor neuron disorders 1:293–299, 2000.

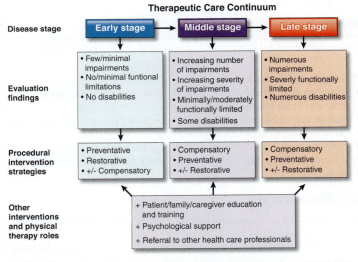

Framework for the rehabilitation of patients with ALS. From: Framework for Rehabilitation for Individuals with ALS. In O'Sullivan, SB, and Schmitz, TJ: *Physical Rehabilitation*, ed. 5. FA Davis, Philadelphia, 2005, p 831.

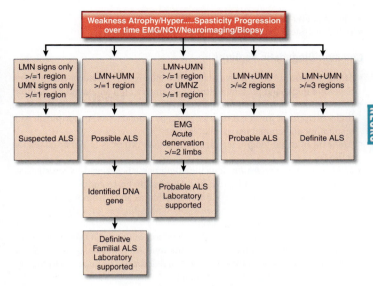

El Escorial Criteria for the Diagnosis of ALS. From: El Escorial Criteria for the Diagnosis of ALS. In O'Sullivan, SB, and Schmitz, TJ: *Physical Rehabilitation,* ed. 5. FA Davis, Philadelphia, 2005, p 825.

Guillain-Barré/Acute Inflammatory Demyelinating Polyradiculoneuropathy

Pathophysiology

- Most common form of the demyelinating polyradiculoneuropathy diseases
- Affects nerve roots of peripheral nerves leading to motor neuropathy and flaccid paralysis
- Spinal roots and peripheral nerves are infiltrated with macrophages and T-lymphocytes following a systemic trigger
- Macrophages strip the myelin sheaths from the nerves leading to impaired salutatory propagation of an action potential
- Delayed salutatory propagation of an action potential leads to
  - slowed conduction velocities
  - dys-synchrony of conduction
  - impaired conduction of higher frequency impulses
  - partial or complete conduction blocks

Etiology

- Autoimmune disease of unknown origin
- May be triggered by a viral or bacterial infection

- The infection changes the nature of nervous system cells
- Immune system treats altered cells as foreign

Common Diagnostic Features

- *Motor weakness*: progressive symptoms and signs of motor weakness that develop rapidly and present relatively symmetrical in an ascending fashion
- *Progression of weakness*: from distal to proximal and self-limiting to distal limbs of upper or lower extremities that may extend to full quadriplegia with respiratory and cranial nerve involvement
- *Areflexia* of distal tendon reflexes, which may progress to proximal tendon reflexes
- *Mild sensory symptoms or signs* including paresthesias and hyperesthesias, often with a stocking-and-glove-like distribution presentation
- *Autonomic dysfunction* (tachycardia arrhythmias and vasomotor symptoms)
- *Absence of fever at onset of symptoms* with a history of a flu-like illness within the last 2 weeks is common
- *Muscular aching pain* typically described as similar to DOMS with a symmetrical distribution, affecting large bulk muscles (gluteals, quadriceps, and hamstrings), often exacerbated at night, and described as intense burning, hypersensitivity to touch or air movement
- Abnormal nerve conduction velocities are typical

Differential Diagnosis

- Hysteria, brainstem CVA, botulism, chronic inflammatory demyelinating polyneuropathy (CIDP), tick paralysis, poliomyelitis, spinal cord lesion, vitamin B_{12} deficiency, transverse myelitis, West Nile virus, or periodic paralysis syndrome

Prognosis

- Recovery typically begins approximately 2 to 4 weeks after plateau of disease process
- Some patients have a fulminating course of progress with maximal paralysis within 1 to 2 days of onset, reaching the nadir, or point of greatest severity
  - 50%: within 1 week
  - 70%: within 2 weeks
  - 80%: within 3 weeks

  In some cases, the process of progressive weakness continues for 1 to 2 months.

- Recovery period may occur in a few weeks or it may take years
  - 30% of those with GBS have residual weakness after 3 years
  - Approximately 3% may suffer a relapse of muscle weakness and impaired sensory integrity many years after the initial attack
- Most common long-term deficits are weakness of anterior tibialis musculature and occasional residual weakness of hand and foot intrinsics, quadriceps, and gluteal musculature
- Muscle strength returns in a descending pattern, opposite of the pattern noted during disease onset

Medical Intervention

- Plasmapheresis (plasma exchange)
  - Whole blood is removed from the body and processed so that the white and red blood cells are separated from the plasma
  - Blood cells are returned to the patient without the plasma, which the body quickly replaces

Rehabilitation Intervention

- Maintain the patient's musculoskeletal system in an optimal state
- Prevent overwork
- Pace recovery process to obtain maximal function as reinnervation occurs
- Exercise routines must avoid fatigue and provide frequent rest periods for muscles with a strength grade less than 3+/5
- Muscle strength return in a descending pattern, opposite of the pattern noted during disease onset

References:

Goodman, C, Fuller, K, and Boissonnault, W: Pathology: Implications for the Physical Therapist, ed. 2. Saunders, Philadelphia, 2003.

Guillain-Barré syndrome. http://www.ninds.nig.gov/disorders/gbs.htm. 2009.

O'Sullivan, SB, & Schmitz, TJ: Physical Rehabilitation, ed. 5. Philadelphia: FA Davis, Philadelphia, 2005.

Umphred, DA: Neurological Rehabilitation, ed. 5. St. Mosby, Louis, MO, 2007.

Focal Progressive Disorders

Basal Ganglia-Related Disorders

Major Movement Disorders of the Basal Ganglia

1. *Hypokinetic disorders:* characterized by impaired initiation of movement (akinesia) and by a reduced amplitude and velocity of movement (bradykinesia).
   a. The best example is Parkinson's disease. It results from overactivity in the indirect pathway of the basal ganglia.
2. *Hyperkinetic disorders:* characterized by excessive motor activity, resulting in involuntary movements (dyskinesias) and decreased muscle tone (hypotonia).
   a. Exemplified by Huntington's disease and hemiballismus. It results from underactivity in the indirect pathway of the basal ganglia.
   b. Involuntary movements include the following:
      i. *Athetosis:* slow, writhing movements of the extremities.
      ii. *Chorea:* jerky, random movements of the limbs and orofacial structures.
      iii. *Ballismus:* violent, large amplitude, proximal limb movements.
      iv. *Dystonia:* sustained abnormal postures with cocontraction of agonist/antagonist muscles.

From:

Delong, M: The basal ganglia. In: Kandel, ER, Schwartz, JH, and Jessell, TM (eds): Principles of Neural Science, ed. 4. Elsevier, New York, 2000, pp 861–862.

Parkinson's Disease

Pathophysiology

Parkinson's disease (PD) results from the loss of dopamine-producing brain cells in the substantia nigra of the basal ganglia. Symptoms will appear when approximately 80% of the dopaminergic cells are damaged.

From:

National Parkinson Foundation. *http://www.parkinson.org.* Accessed August 1, 2009.

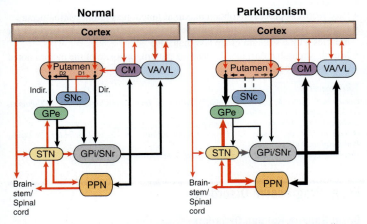

Parkinsonism-related changes in overall activity (rate model) in the basal ganglia–thalamocortical motor circuit. Black arrows indicate inhibitory connections and red arrows indicate excitatory connections. The thickness of the arrows corresponds to their presumed activity. *Abbreviations:* CM, centromedian nucleus of thalamus; CMA, cingulate motor area; Dir., direct pathway; D1 and D2, dopamine receptor subtypes; GPe, external segment of the globus pallidus; GPi, internal segment of the globus pallidus; Indir., indirect pathway; M1, primary motor cortex; Pf, parafascicular nucleus of the thalamus; PMC, premotor cortex; PPN, pedunculopontine nucleus; SMA, supplementary motor area; SNc, substantia nigra pars compacta; SNr, substantia nigra pars reticulata; STN, subthalamic nucleus; VA, ventral anterior nucleus of thalamus; VL, ventrolateral nucleus of thalamus. From: Galvan A, and Wichmann T: Pathophysiology of parkinsonism. *Clin Neurophysiol* 119:1459–1474, 2008; used with permission.

Cardinal Features of PD: "Trap"

1) Resting tremor
2) Rigidity
3) Akinesia/bradykinesia
4) Postural instability

TABLE 4.71 Clinical Motor and Nonmotor Features of Parkinson's Disease

Motor Features	Nonmotor Features
Resting Tremor • 70% of patients • Often manifests as supination-pronation tremor in hands (i.e., "pill-rolling") • Can also involve lips, chin, jaw, and legs	**Psychiatric Disorders** • Depression in up to 40% of patients • Anxiety in ~30% of patients
Bradykinesia • 80% to 90% of patients • Slowness of movement • Most disabling symptom of PD	**Cognitive Disorders** • Mild cognitive impairment (bradyphenia) • Dementia in 15% to 40% of patients
Rigidity • >90% of patients • Resistance to passive movement of flexor and extensor muscles • Characterized as "cogwheel" (resistance fluctuates in intensity usually due to superimposed tremor) or "lead pipe" (continuous resistance)	**Sleep Abnormalities** • Insomnia • Affects >70% of patients • Daytime somnolence • REM sleep behavior disorder
	Autonomic Dysfunction • Dysphagia and choking • Hypersalivation • Impaired gastrointestinal motility • Constipation • Orthostatic hypotension
Postural Instability • Usually last symptom to occur • Indicative of progression to advanced stages of disease • Frequent cause of falls and injuries	**Sensory** • Olfactory dysfunction (i.e., anosmia) • Pain
	Miscellaneous • Fatigue • Weight loss

From: Hou, JG, and Lai, EC: Overview of Parkinson's disease: Clinical features, diagnosis, and management. In Trail, M, Protas, EJ, and Lai, EC (eds): *Neurorehabilitation in Parkinson's Disease: An Evidence-Based Treatment Model.* Slack, Thorofare, NJ, 2008, pp 15–16.

Primary Parkinson's Disease

- A commonly accepted diagnostic criteria is the finding of at least *two cardinal symptoms* in the absence of other apparent causes of parkinsonism.
- Initial symptoms typically *asymmetrical.*
- A *positive response to levodopa* can be used as a diagnostic indicator of likely primary PD.

Clinical Subtypes

1) *Tremor-predominant:* initial symptoms present as a unilateral, pill-rolling tremor at rest. The tremor disappears (or attenuates) during finger-to-nose coordination testing.
2) *Postural Instability, Gait Dysfunction:* initial symptoms present with postural instability with resultant gait abnormalities, no tremor.

Neurological Examination

- Patients cannot perform rapidly alternating or rapid successive movements well.
- Sensation and strength are usually normal.
- Reflexes are normal but may be difficult to elicit because of marked tremor or rigidity.
- Patients cannot suppress eye closure when the frontal muscle is tapped between the eyes (glabellar reflex; if persistent, called Myerson's sign).
- Differentiate slowness of movement caused by rigidity (velocity-independent resistance to passive movement) from spasticity (velocity-dependent resistance to passive movement).

From:

Hou, JG, and Lai, EC. Overview of Parkinson's disease: Clinical features, diagnosis, and management. In Trail, M, Protas, EJ, and Lai, EC (eds): Neurorehabilitation in Parkinson's Disease: An Evidence-Based Treatment Model. Slack, Thorofare, NJ, 2008, pp 6, 15.
Eidelberg, D, and Pourfar, M: Parkinson's disease. In The Merck Manuals: Online Medical Library. http://www.merck.com/mmpe/sec16/ch221/ch221g.html#tb_221-004. Accessed August 12, 2009.

Parkinsonism

To differentiate Parkinson's disease from secondary parkinsonism, clinicians note whether levodopa results in dramatic improvement, suggesting Parkinson's disease. Causes of parkinsonism can be identified by the following:

- A thorough history, including occupational, drug, and family history
- Neurological deficits characteristic of disorders other than Parkinson's disease (such as neurodegenerative disorders)
- Neuroimaging when indicated

TABLE 4.72 Some Causes of Parkinsonism

Cause	Comments
Neurodegenerative Disorders	
Amyotrophic lateral sclerosis-parkinsonism-dementia complex of Guam	Responds poorly to antiparkinsonian drugs
Corticobasal ganglionic degeneration	Begins asymmetrically, usually after age 60 Causes cortical and basal ganglia signs, often with apraxia, dystonia, myoclonus, and alien limb syndrome (movement of a limb that seems independent of the patient's conscious control) Causes immobility after about 5 yr and death after about 10 yr Responds poorly to antiparkinsonian drugs
Dementia (e.g., Alzheimer's disease, chromosome 17–linked frontotemporal dementias, diffuse Lewy body dementia)	Parkinsonism often preceded by dementia with prominent memory loss
Multiple system atrophy	May include prominent autonomic dysfunction May have predominantly cerebellar features Often causes early falls and balance problems Responds poorly to antiparkinsonian drugs
Progressive supranuclear palsy	First manifests with gait and balance problems Causes progressive ophthalmoparesis starting with downward gaze Responds poorly to antiparkinsonian drugs
Spinocerebellar ataxia 3	Responds poorly to antiparkinsonian drugs
Other Disorders	
Cerebrovascular disease	Manifests with rigidity and bradykinesia or akinesia (akinetic-rigid syndrome) that predominantly involves the lower extremities, with prominent gait disturbance Rarely responds to antiparkinsonian drugs
Brain tumors near the basal ganglia	Manifests with hemiparkinsonism (i.e., restricted to one side of the body)

(table continues on page 396)

NEURO

TABLE 4.72 **Some Causes of Parkinsonism** (continued)

Cause	Comments
Repeated traumatic brain injury	Often causes dementia (described as punch-drunk)
Hydrocephalus	Usually, normal-pressure hydrocephalus; rarely, obstructive hydrocephalus
Hypoparathyroidism	Causes calcification of the basal ganglia; may cause chorea and athetosis
Viral (e.g., West Nile) encephalitis, infectious or postinfectious autoimmune	Can cause parkinsonism transiently during the acute phase or, rarely, permanently (e.g., postencephalitic parkinsonism after the epidemic of encephalitis lethargica in 1915–1926) In postencephalitic parkinsonism: Forced, sustained deviation of the head and eyes (oculogyric crises); other dystonias; autonomic instability; depression; and personality changes
Drugs Antipsychotics	Can cause reversible* parkinsonism
Meperidine (trade name Demerol): analog (MPTP)†	Can cause sudden, irreversible parkinsonism Occurs in IV drug users
Methyldopa (trade name Aldomet)	Can cause reversible* parkinsonism May be dose-dependent or related to the patient's susceptibility (risk factors include older age and female sex)
Metoclopramide (trade name Reglan)	Same as for methyldopa (Aldomet)
Reserpine (trade name Serpasil)	Same as for methyldopa (Aldomet)
Lithium (trade names Eskalith, Lithobid, Lithonate), long-term use	Same as for methyldopa (Aldomet)
Toxins Carbon monoxide	Can cause irreversible parkinsonism
Methanol	As contaminated moonshine, can cause hemorrhagic necrosis of the basal ganglia

NEURO

Cause	Comments
Manganese	Can cause parkinsonism with dystonia and cognitive changes when toxicity is chronic Usually occupation-related

*When drugs are withdrawn, symptoms usually resolve within a few weeks, although they may persist for months.
†MPTP results from unsuccessful attempts to produce meperidine for illicit use. MPTP = N-methyl-1,2,3,4-tetrahydropyridine.
From: Eidelberg, D, and Pourfar, M: Parkinson's disease. In *The Merck Manuals: Online Medical Library.* http://www.merck.com/mmpe/sec16/ch221/ch221g.html#tb_221-004. Accessed August 12, 2009.

NEURO

TABLE 4.73 Modified Hoehn and Yahr Classification of Disability in PD

STAGE 0	No signs of disease.
STAGE 1	Unilateral disease with minimal or absent disability.
STAGE 1.5	Unilateral plus axial involvement.
STAGE 2	Bilateral disease, without impairment of balance.
STAGE 2.5	Mild bilateral disease, with recovery on pull test.
STAGE 3	Mild to moderate bilateral disease; some postural instability with impaired righting reflexes; physically independent.
STAGE 4	Severe disability; still able to walk or stand unassisted. Requires help with some activities of daily living.
STAGE 5	Wheelchair bound or bedridden unless aided.

From: Hoen, MM, and Yahr, MD: Parkinsonism: Onset, progression, and mortality. *Neurology* 57(10 suppl 3):S11–S26, 2001.

TABLE 4.74 Overview of Drug Therapy in Parkinson's Disease

Drug	Mechanism of Acion	Special Comments
Levodopa	Resolves dopamine deficiency by being converted to dopamine after crossing blood-brain barrier.	Still the best drug for resolving parkinsonian symptoms; long-term use limited by side effects and decreased efficacy.
Dopamine agonists Bromocriptine Cabergoline Pergolide Premipexole Ropinirole	Directly stimulates dopamine receptors in basal ganglia.	May produce fewer side effects (dyskinesias, fluctuations in response) than levodopa; preliminary evidence suggests that early use may also delay the progression of Parkinson's disease.

(table continues on page 398)

◖ TABLE 4.74 Overview of Drug Therapy in Parkinson's Disease (continued)

Drug	Mechanism of Acion	Special Comments
Anticholinergics	Inhibit excessive acetylcholine influence caused by dopamine deficiency.	Use in Parkinson's disease limited by frequent side effects.
Amantadine	Unclear; may inhibit the effects of excitatory amino acids in the basal ganglia.	May be used alone during early/mild stages or added to drug regimen when levodopa loses effectiveness.
Selegiline	Inhibits the enzyme that breaks down dopamine in the basal ganglia; enables dopamine to remain active for longer periods of time.	May improve symptoms, especially in early stages of Parkinson's disease; ability to produce long-term benefits unclear.
COMT inhibitors Entacapone Tolcapone	Help prevent breakdown of dopamine in peripheral tissues; allows more levodopa to reach the brain.	Useful as an adjunct to levodopa/carbidopa administration; may improve and prolong effects of levodopa.

COMT: catechol-O-methyltransferase.
From: Ciccone, C: *Pharmacology in Rehabilitation,* ed. 4. FA Davis, Philadelphia, 2007, p 122.

Special Considerations for Rehabilitation

1. Coordinate therapy session with peak dose effects of Parkinson medications and low fatigue levels.
    a. Levodopa therapy: peak dose usually occurs ~ 1 hour after taking medication.
2. Monitor blood pressure in patients receiving anti-Parkinson medications, as most drugs cause orthostatic hypotension. This may lead to an increase in falls.
3. Using physical and occupational therapy interventions to maintain motor function can diminish the patient's need for anti-Parkinson drugs.

From:

Ciccone, CD: Pharmacological management of Parkinson disease. In Pharmacology in Rehabilitation, ed. 4. FA Davis, Philadelphia, 2007, p 130.

TABLE 4.75 Proactive Physical Management Plan for Parkinson's Disease Based on Hoehn & Yahr Staging

NEURO

Hoehn & Yahr (H&Y) Stages 0–3

Health Promotion

Objective:	Examples of Means:
• Posture	• Frequent correction
• Endurance	• Walking, swimming, biking
• Muscle strength	• Resisted exercise (community gyms)
• Joint flexibility	• Regular stretching, yoga
• Balance	• Balance ball, tai chi, dancing
• Knowledge	• Education, resource material, lay conferences
• Oral care	• Brushing, regular checks, dental hygiene
• Voice and articulation	• Choir, voice training (acting lessons)
• Vital capacity	• Choir, swimming

H & Y Stages 2–4

Functional Maintenance
"Nipping problems in the bud."

Objective:	Examples of Means:
• Focal problems	• Focused exercise, modalities
• Functional "tricks"	• Cueing (laser pointer, auditory cues)
• Maintaining function	• ADL reviews, occupational therapy
• Functional profiles	• % of day "off" versus "on," fatigue
• Caregiver support	• Practical tips to facilitate function
• Oral care	• Brushing, regular checks, dental hygiene
• Diet and swallowing	• Nutritionist, speech language pathologist
• Speech	• Speech language pathologist

H & Y Stages 4–5

Functional Adaptation

Objective:	Examples of Means:
• Adapt transfers	• Sit to stand, rolling in bed
• Adaptive equipment	• Wheeled walkers, grab bars
• Home adaptation	• Shower seat, chair lift
• Management of complications	• Skin, chest, nutrition
• Caregiver support	• Problem solving, respite, support groups

From: Turnbull, GI, and Millar, J: A proactive physical management model of Parkinson's Disease. *Top Geriatr Rehabil* 22(2):162–171, 2006.

One of the most debilitating motor problems associated with PD is wearing off and presence of levodopa induced dyskinesias (LID) and freezing. Nearly 50% of people with PD may develop these complications. There are a number of drug regimens and other procedures (e.g., deep brain stimulation [DBS]) that have evolved to specifically address reducing motor fluctuations and dyskinesia.

Huntington's Disease

Pathophysiology

Huntington's disease (HD) is a hereditary, progressive neurodegenerative disorder characterized by the development of emotional, behavioral, and psychiatric abnormalities; loss of previously acquired intellectual or cognitive functioning; and movement abnormalities (motor disturbances). Although symptoms typically become evident during the fourth or fifth decades of life, the age at onset is variable and ranges from early childhood to late adulthood (e.g., 70s or 80s). Also known as Huntington's chorea, the disorder is named for the American physician who initially described the condition in 1872.

HD is transmitted within families as an autosomal dominant trait. The disorder occurs as the result of abnormally long sequences or "repeats" of coded instructions within a gene on chromosome 4 (4p16.3). The progressive loss of nervous system function associated with HD results from loss of neurons in certain areas of the brain, including the basal ganglia and cerebral cortex.

From:

Worldwide Education and Awareness for Movement Disorders. We Move. Huntington's disease. http://www.wemove.org/hd/. Accessed August 3, 2009.

Postmortem changes in HD brains include neuronal loss and gliosis in the cortex and the striatum, particularly the caudate nucleus. Progressive motor dysfunction, dementia, dysphagia, and incontinence eventually lead to institutionalization and death from aspiration, infection, and poor nutrition. On the average, duration of illness from onset to death is about 15 years for adult HD, but it is about 4 to 5 years shorter for the juvenile variant.

From:

Huntington disease: Clinical aspects. In Fahn, S, and Jankovic, J: Principles and Practice of Movement Disorders. Churchill Livingstone, 2007. E-book through MD consult. http://www. mdconsult.com. Accessed December 7, 2009.

● TABLE 4.76 Classic Signs of Huntington's Disease

Chorea: involuntary, rapid, irregular, jerky movements that may affect the face, arms, legs, or trunk.
Dementia: gradual loss of thought processing and acquired intellectual abilities.
Disorientation: There may be impairment of memory, abstract thinking, and judgment; improper perceptions of time, place, or identity.
Personality disintegration: increased agitation and personality changes.

Worldwide Education and Awareness for Movement Disorders. We Move. Huntington's disease. http://www.wemove.org/hd/. Accessed August 3, 2009.

TABLE 4.77 Characteristics of Huntington's Disease

Features	Adult Onset	Juvenile Onset
Age at onset	35–40	<15
Inheritance	Autosomal dominant	AD (usually from the father)
Initial features	Personality changes, chorea	Personality changes, rigidity, bradykinesia, dystonia
Late features	Dementia, dysarthria, abnormal eye movements, dystonia, rigidity	Dementia, dysarthria, abnormal eye movements, tremor, seizures, ataxia, myoclonus
Duration	15–30 yr	5–20 yr

From: Huntington disease: Clinical aspects. In Fahn, S, and Jankovic, J: *Principles and Practice of Movement Disorders*. Churchill Livingstone, 2007. E-book through MD consult. http://www.mdconsult.com. Accessed December 7, 2009.

Treatment

Non-Pharmacological Management

- Physical and occupational therapy for trouble walking, unsteadiness, falls, clumsiness, home environment assessments.
- Speech therapy for difficulties of speech, treat/prevent aspiration.
- Psychological support for irritability, depression, paranoia, memory loss, intellectual decline.
- Adequate nutrition to minimize weight loss.
- Caregiver support: life-planning, disability benefits, household help, home equipment, supervised smoking, child care, day care, institutional care, hospice.

Pharmacological Management

- Anxiolytics: benzodiazepines, propranolol, clonidine
- Antidepressants: tricyclics (nortriptyline, amitriptyline, imipramine); SSRIs (fluoxetine, sertraline, fluvoxamine, paroxetine, venlafaxine, citalopram)
- DA receptor–blocking drugs or DA-depleting drugs for severe chorea, psychosis: quetiapine, olanzapine, ziprasidone, clozapine, fluphenazine, risperidone, haloperidol, tetrabenazine (TBZ)
- Glutamate release inhibitors and receptor blockers (remacemide, riluzole)
- Mitochondrial electron transport enhancers and free radical scavengers (CoQ10, nicotinamide, creatine)
- Caspase and iNOS inhibitors (minocycline, ethyl eicosapentaenoate or ethyl-EPA, LAX-101)
- Histone deacetylase inhibitors
- Trophic factors

Modified from:

Huntington Disease: Clinical Aspects. In Fahn, S, and Jankovic, J: Principles and Practice of Movement Disorders. Churchill Livingstone, 2007. E-book through MD consult. http://www. mdconsult.com. Accessed December 7, 2009.

Brain Tumors

Symptoms

Depends on the location, size, and rate of tumor growth:

- 68% progressive neurological deficit, typically involving motor weakness (45%)
- 54% headache
- 26% seizures

Primary brain tumors can be benign or malignant. Benign brain tumors do not contain cancer cells and usually have an obvious border or edge. Due to location in the brain, benign brain tumors can impact cognition and be life threatening. Although benign tumors rarely grow back after removal, they can become malignant. Malignant tumors (also called brain cancer) contain cancer cells. They are likely to grow rapidly and invade nearby healthy brain tissue.

Tumor Grades

Grade I:
- Slow-growing cells
- Almost normal appearance under a microscope
- Least malignant
- Usually associated with long-term survival

Grade II:
- Relatively slow-growing cells
- Slightly abnormal appearance under a microscope
- Can invade adjacent normal tissue
- Can recur as a higher grade tumor

Grade III:
- Actively reproducing abnormal cells
- Abnormal appearance under a microscope
- Infiltrate adjacent normal brain tissues
- Tumor tends to recur, often at a higher grade

Grade IV:
- Abnormal cells that reproduce rapidly
- Very abnormal appearance under a microscope
- Form new blood vessels to maintain rapid growth
- Areas of dead cells in center

Treatments—Depending on the Histological Type, Location, and Size of the Tumor

Surgical
- Stereotactic localization
- Laser microsurgery
- Ultrasonic aspiration

Radiation
- External radiation therapy
  - Intensity-modulated radiation therapy
  - Proton beam radiation therapy
  - Stereotactic radiation therapy
- Internal radiation therapy (implant or brachytherapy)

Chemotherapy
- Intravenous (by mouth or vein)
- Implanted wafers

Medications
- Steroids
- Anticonvulsants

Rehabilitation
- Cognitive rehabilitation
- Speech therapy
- Physical therapy
- Occupational therapy

Brain Tumor Statistics and Incidence

The following are the most common primary brain tumors by age group:

- 0–4: Embryonal/primitive neuroectodermal tumors/medulloblastomas (incidence rate of 1.06 per 100,000 people) followed by pilocytic astrocytomas (0.99)
- 5–9: pilocytic astrocytomas (1.01 per 100,000) followed by embryonal/primitive/medulloblastomas (0.73)
- 10–14: pilocytic astrocytomas (0.83 per 100,000) followed by malignant gliomas (0.44)
- 15–19: pilocytic astrocytomas (0.63 per 100,000) followed by pituitary tumors (0.60)
- 20–34: pituitary (1.16 per 100,000) followed by meningioma tumors (0.91)
- 35–44: meningiomas (3.32 per 100,000) followed by pituitary tumors (1.56)
- 45–54: meningiomas (6.87 per 100,000) followed by glioblastoma (3.70)
- 55–64: meningiomas (10.91 per 100,000) followed by glioblastoma (8.09)
- 65–74: meningiomas (17.61 per 100,000) followed by glioblastoma (12.47)
- 74 to 84: meningiomas (24.42 per 100,000) followed by glioblastoma (14.13)
- > 85: meningiomas (29.53 per 100,000) followed by glioblastoma (7.63)

From:

Anderson, SW, and Ryken, TC: Intracranial tumors. In J. E. Morgan, JE, and Ricker, JH (eds): *Textbook of Clinical Neuropsychology.* Taylor & Francis, New York, 2008, pp 578–587.

Louis, DN, et al: The 2007 WHO Classification of Tumours of the Central Nervous System. Acta Neuropathol 114:97–109, 2007.

American Brain Tumor Association: A Primer on Brain Tumors. http://www.abta.org. Accessed July 2009.

National Cancer Institute: What You Need to Know About Brain Tumors. http://www.cancer.gov. Accessed July 2009.

Head, neck, and brain tumor embolization. Am J Neuroradiol 22:S14–S15, September 2001. © 2001 American Society of Neuroradiology.

Incontinence

Urinary incontinence (UI) is defined as any involuntary leakage of urine. The related condition for defecation is known as *fecal incontinence*.

Innervation of the Urinary Bladder and Rectum

Peripheral Nervous System for Voluntary Control

pudendal nerve (S2, S3, S4): Supplies the voluntary muscles of the external and urethral sphincters, which provide a means for voluntary control over these orifices. Sensory fibers to the mucosa of the anal canal and to the urethra are also supplied.

Autonomic Nervous System

sympathetic fibers: Reach the rectum by both the inferior mesenteric and the inferior hypogastric plexuses, and the urinary bladder through the inferior hypogastric plexus. Preganglionic fibers originate from the upper lumbar area. The afferents associated with the sympathetic system are associated with painful sensations (e.g., overdistension) from the bladder and rectum. The sympathetic efferents cause contraction of the internal anal and vesical sphincters, with relaxation of the muscular walls of these organs.

parasympathetic fibers: Reach the rectum and urinary bladder from the inferior hypogastric plexus. Preganglionic fibers enter this plexus by the pelvic splanchnic nerves. The afferents associated with the parasympathetic system carry information regarding normal sensations of bladder and rectal distension. The parasympathetic efferents supply the urinary bladder and the rectal muscle for micturition and defecation.

Urinary Incontinence

Continence and micturition require a balance between urethral closure and detrusor muscle activity. Urine normally remains in the bladder because urethral pressure normally exceeds bladder pressure. Continence is maintained despite increases in intra-abdominal pressure (e.g., from coughing and sneezing) because any increase in intraabdominal pressure is transmitted to both urethra and bladder equally, leaving the pressure differential unchanged. Normal voiding is the result of changes in the pressure differential: urethral pressure falls and bladder pressure rises.

NEURO

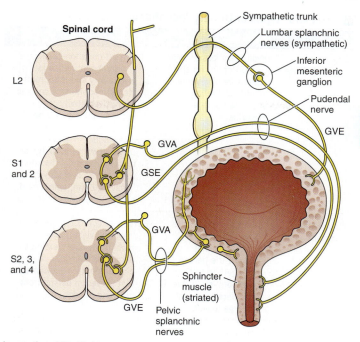

Innervation of the bladder.

TABLE 4.78 **Types of Urinary Incontinence**

Type	Description	Cause
Stress incontinence (SUI)	The loss of small amounts of urine associated with coughing, laughing, sneezing, exercising or other movements that increase intra-abdominal pressure and thus increase pressure on the bladder.	Insufficient strength of the pelvic floor muscles. Stress incontinence following a prostatectomy is the most common form of incontinence in men. In women, physical changes resulting from pregnancy, childbirth, menopause, and high-level involvement in sports can contribute to stress incontinence.

(table continues on page 406)

TABLE 4.78 **Types of Urinary Incontinence** (continued)

Type	Description	Cause
Urge incontinence	Involuntary loss of urine occurring for no apparent reason while suddenly feeling the need or urge to urinate.	The most common cause of urge incontinence is involuntary and inappropriate detrusor muscle contractions. Overactivity of detrusor muscle may be related to local infections and bladder irritation *(idiopathic overactivity)*, or from neurological disorders *(neurogenic overactivity)* involving brain, spinal cord, nerves to bladder, or muscle.
Functional incontinence	Loss of urine due to a physical or mental limitations that prevent the person from getting to the bathroom in sufficient time once they feel the urge to void.	States of confusion, dementia, impaired vision, poor mobility, lack of dexterity, depression, anxiety, or environmental conditions that prevent a person from reaching a toilet.
Overflow incontinence	Chronic leaking or dribbling of urine following micturition.	More common in men. Weak bladder muscles, resulting in incomplete emptying of the bladder (urinary retention); overfilling of bladder due to autonomic neuropathy (from diabetes or MS); restriction of urinary flow due to blockage by tumors, kidney stones, or benign prostatic hyperplasia (BPH); or spinal cord and other neurological disorders.
Other		Bedwetting (enuresis) during sleep—normal in young children; structural incontinence (rare; such as extopic ureter or vaginal fistulas); mixed urinary incontinence disorders in elderly females.

The Neurogenic Bladder

Classification of Neurogenic Bladders

The term *neurogenic bladder* refers to many disorders and does not connote a specific diagnosis or single etiology. The following classification system is followed by a simpler description of functional bladder types.

Sensorimotor Neuron Lesion
1. Lesions above the conus medullaris spinal reflex center (commonly called *upper motor neuron lesions*)
   a. Complete
   b. Incomplete
2. Lower motor neuron lesions (below the conus medullaris)
   a. Complete
   b. Incomplete
3. Mixed lesions
   a. Complete
   b. Incomplete

Sensory Neuron Lesions
1. Complete
2. Incomplete

Motor Neuron Lesions
1. Complete
2. Incomplete

Functional Bladder Types

atonic bladder (also called the flaccid, denervated, afferent, or hypotonic bladder): This type of bladder is caused by lesions to the parasympathetic pathways to and from the bladder, which result in loss of the afferent or the efferent limb of the reflex arc from the detrusor muscle. An atonic bladder may also be the result of destruction to the last few segments of the spinal cord (S3) in the conus medullaris (as in fractures of the spine at the thoracolumbar junction). Cystometrograms are flat, and there is retention with overflow. Abdominal straining may empty the bladder more. Cystograms may differ slightly according to the lesion site. The external sphincter is usually tonically active for the denervated bladder, whereas for lesions of the sacral portion of the cord, the external sphincter is usually flaccid.

spastic bladder (also called the reflex or efferent neurogenic bladder): This type of bladder is caused by lesions of the higher pathways to and from the cortex, with preservation of the spinal sacral segments and their innervation. The spastic bladder is commonly associated with disorders of the pyramidal tracts, as in gunshot wounds, multiple sclerosis, whiplash injuries, or transverse myelitis. The cystometrogram is "jumpy," showing many uninhibited contractions without the patient feeling the need to void. Bladder capacity is reduced, and the residual urine further decreases the true capacity. Incontinence, dribbling, and residual urine are often present with this type of bladder, even with training and medication.

Fecal Incontinence

Fecal continence is primarily dependent on two mechanisms, (i) the reflex action of the external anal sphincter initiated by contraction of the rectum, and (ii) the reservoir capability of the colon independent of sphincteric action *(reservoir continence)*.

Effects of Spinal Cord Lesions on the Bowel

spinal shock: Fecal retention and paralysis of peristalsis is the immediate effect of spinal cord transection at any level. After the phase of spinal shock, one of the following conditions may occur, depending on the type of lesion.

Automatic Reflex Activity

For lesions above the thoracolumbar junction:

1. Peristalsis, bowel sounds, anal and bulbocavernosus reflexes return after spinal shock.
2. Intermittent automatic reflex defecation occurs following the return of reflex activity and peristalsis.
3. Greatly increased tone of the external anal sphincter (during the stage of hyperreflexia) results in increased resistance to the expulsive function of sigmoid and rectum.

For lesions above T6, hyperreflexive abdominal muscles may interfere with the propulsive activity of the various compartments of the intestinal tract.

Autonomous Function

For lesions resulting in destruction of the lumbosacral or spinal roots, there is the following:

1. Lower motor neuron type paralysis (flaccid, denervation) with loss of normal response of sigmoid and rectum to distension.
2. Loss of tone (reflexes) of the external sphincter.
3. Impaired function of the levator ani.
4. Progressive accumulation of feces leading to impaction and fecal incontinence. The patient is usually dependent on digital evacuation aided by increased intra-abdominal pressure, suppositories, and enemas.

Disorders of Balance and Vestibular Function

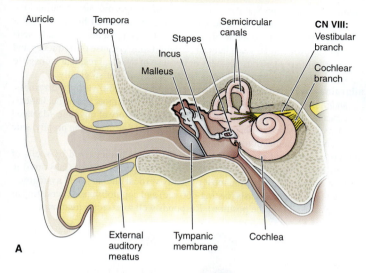

NEURO

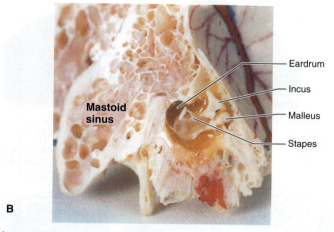

Inner ear anatomy and histological section.

Vestibular Diagnoses

Meniere's syndrome: Spontaneous episodes of vertigo, unilateral hearing loss, tinnitus, and a sense of ear fullness lasting 30 min to 24 hr. In the earlier stages, patients are completely normal between episodes. Typically self-limiting over 8 to 10 years but can be debilitating because of frequency and severity of spontaneous episodes or because of eventual residual damage to vestibular and auditory systems. Treated medically or surgically.

migraine-equivalent events: Characterized by episodic vertigo, dizziness, and/or nystagmus lasting minutes to hours with or without headache. Patients typically have history of migraine and/or family history of migraine. Managed by reducing stresses, changing diet, limiting caffeine, and using prophylactic or abortive medications.

benign paroxysmal positional vertigo (BPPV): Characterized by spells of vertigo and concomitant nystagmus when the person's head (labyrinth) in is in a dependent position, most typically vertical and torsional nystagmus. Two forms: canalithiasis (lasting <60 sec) and cupulolithiasis (persisting as long as head is in the position). Responds well to exercise treatment.

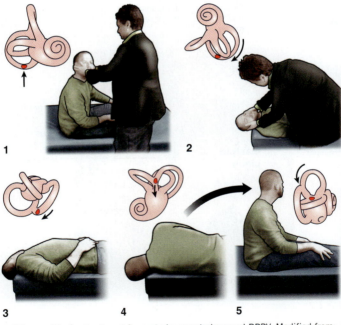

Canalith repositioning treatment for posterior or anterior canal BPPV. Modified from: Herdman, SJ, Hall, CD, Schubert, MC, Das, VE, Tusa, RJ. Recovery of dynamic visual acuity in bilateral vestibular hypofunction. *Arch Otolaryngol Head Neck Surg.* 133L:383–389, 2007.

benign vertigo of childhood: Episodic vertigo with imbalance that is reminiscent of BPPV but is actually a migraine event (with or without headache). Managed medically and/or with psychological support for stress reduction.

vestibular neuronitis: Inflammation of vestibular nerve, most commonly from herpes simplex. Acutely causes vertigo, nystagmus, disequilibrium, oscillopsia, and nausea. Lasts 48 to 72 hr but residual problems can cause imbalance and visual blurring.

labyrinthitis: Inflammation of the labyrinth. Distinguished from neuronitis by loss of hearing as well as acute vertigo, nystagmus, disequilibrium, oscillopsia, and nausea. Lasts 48 to 72 hr but residual problems can cause imbalance and visual blurring. Hearing loss is typically permanent.

Ramsey Hunt syndrome: Combined unilateral vestibular, facial, and auditory nerve damage from herpes zoster.

bilateral vestibular hypofunction: Decreased or lost vestibular function bilaterally can occur as a progressive loss (not to be confused with age-related decline in vestibular function), sequential loss (separate occurrences of vestibular neuronitis or labyrinthitis), or iatrogenically (as a consequence of medical or surgical intervention). The most common iatrogenic cause is the use of the gentamicin (see Medications). Vertigo typically not part of the presentation except in sequential bilateral loss.

perilymphatic fistula: Abnormal communication between endolymph and perilymph spaces. Usually caused by barotrauma or head trauma; aggravated by sneezing or straining. Signs and symptoms include vertigo and hearing loss. Managed by bed rest or surgical repair.

superior canal dehiscence: Vertigo and oscillopsia associated with loud sounds or to changes in intracranial or middle ear pressure. The underlying cause is the absence of a portion of the bony wall of superior semicircular canal. Managed surgically.

Mal de Debarquement (MDD): Sensation of rocking or swaying as if on a boat persisting for several months. Often noted to have begun after a cruise. Typically decreases when person is in a moving car. Medical management has the best success; vestibular exercises are not beneficial. Patients may respond to low doses of anti-anxiety medications.

motion sensitivity: Intense feeling of dizziness and nausea that can be accompanied by diaphoresis. Can be induced by movement of the environment or by sensory mismatch. Common in people with history of migraine.

Vestibular Definitions

Alexander's law: Nystagmus increases when the patient looks in the direction of the quick component and decreases when the patient looks in the direction of slow component.

disequilibrium: The sense of being off-balance.

dizziness: Generic term for sensation, meaning, e.g., off-balance, lightheaded, swimming, floating, rocking, or vertigo.

gain: Output/input; relationship of eye velocity (output) to head velocity (input).

jerk nystagmus: Nystagmus with a slow component and a quick component; nystagmus is named by the direction of the quick component with respect to the patient's head.

nystagmus: Irregular, involuntary eye movement; can be pendular or jerk.

oscillopsia: Visual blurring; when occurring during head movement it is a symptom of a reduced vestibulo-ocular reflex. Can also occur with acute nystagmus.

pendular nystagmus: Nystagmus in which velocity of eye movement is the same in both directions.

vertigo: An illusion of movement; typically spinning but can also be a sensation of being pushed or shoved. Vertigo occurs when there is an asymmetry in vestibular function.

vestibular nystagmus: Direction-fixed jerk nystagmus that follows Alexander's law; sign of asymmetry of the resting state of the peripheral vestibular system; quick component is toward the more active side.

vestibulo-ocular reflex: Maintains gaze stability (eye position in space) so a person can see clearly during head movements; vestibular information about head velocity generates an eye movement that is equal but opposite the head movement keeping the eyes steady in space.

Vestibular Examination

Bedside Tests

head impulse test or head thrust test: Test of the vestibulo-ocular reflex. Patient's head is held firmly with both hands on the side of their head. Head is tilted forward 30° so that horizontal semicircular canals are level in the horizontal plane. Patient instructed to look at your nose (A). Move the patient's head slowly horizontally being sure the patient is relaxed. The Head Impulse Test is an unpredictable, rapid, small amplitude head movement in one direction with the position held at the end of the movement. Observe for the patient's ability to maintain visual fixation. In a normal response, the eyes stay looking at the target (see B, below). If the eyes come off the target, the patient will make a corrective saccade to re-fixate your nose. Direction of head movement that caused a corrective saccade is the side of the deficit. If the patient makes corrective saccades with near target fixation, repeat this procedure with the patient visually fixating a distant target. Test must be positive (cause corrective saccades) with both near and distant targets.

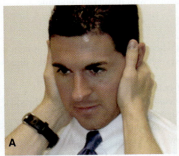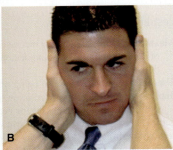

Head impulse test or head thrust test hand positioning.

dynamic visual acuity (DVA): Measurement of the functional deficit occurring with vestibular hypofunction. Difference between visual acuity with the head stationary and visual acuity during head movements performed at 2 Hz. Acuity is measured using an ETDRS (used in the Early Treatment Diabetic Retinopathy Study) visual acuity chart. DVA is considered abnormal if acuity degrades by three or more lines.

Dix-Hallpike test: Patient sits on the examination table and turns his/her head 45° horizontally (A). The head and trunk are quickly brought straight back "en bloc" so that the head is hanging over the edge of the examination table by 20° (B). Presence of nystagmus is sought and the patient is asked if they have vertigo. Not shown, the patient then slowly returns to a sitting position with the head still turned 45° and presence of nystagmus is sought again. This test then is repeated with the head turned 45° in the other direction.

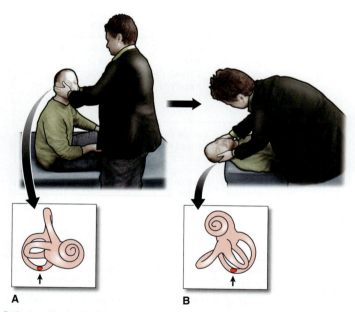

A **B**

Patient positioning for Dix-Hallpike test. For the side-lying test, an alternative to the Dix-Hallpike test, and the roll test, see Herdman, S: *Vestibular Rehabilitation*, ed. 3. FA Davis, Philadelphia, 2007.

TABLE 4.79 Management of Benign Paroxysmal Positional Vertigo

Semicircular canal	Posterior or inferior	Anterior or superior	Horizontal or or lateral	Unknown
Provoking maneuvers	Dix-Hallpike	Dix-Hallpike	Roll test although may occur during Dix-Hallpike	May have occurred before coming to clinic
Nystagmus	Upbeating and torsional toward affected side	Downbeating and torsional toward affected side	Geotropic and brief if canalithiasis Apogeotropic and persistent if cupulolithiasis	Not observable
Optimal treatment	Canalith repositioning treatment (aka Eply maneuver)	Canalith repositioning treatment	270° bar b que roll or the Appiani exercise	Brandt-Daroff
Precautions	May convert to AC or HC BPPV during treatment	Can be confused with central nystagmus which is often downbeating, especially if persistent	Causes greater nausea, vomiting, and imbalance	May not be BPPV

Note: Most common cause of vertigo from a peripheral vestibular problem. Incidence increases with increasing age. Can recur, especially if caused by head trauma. Treatments are effective 85% to 95% after one treatment. Poor management would be repeatedly treating for BPPV when the patient has a central problem.

Treatment of the Most Common Form of BPPV

Movements are performed actively with the therapist guiding the movement, not forcing the movement. During CRT (see figure, page 410) the patient is first moved into the Hallpike-Dix position toward the side of the affected ear (shown for left) and stays in that position for 30 to 60 sec or for twice the duration of the nystagmus (A to B). Then, the head is slowly rotated through moderate extension toward the unaffected side and kept in the new position for 30 sec or for twice the duration of the nystagmus (C). Then the patient is rolled into a side-lying position with the head turned 45° down (toward the floor) Again, the patient stays in that position for about 30 sec or for twice the duration of the original nystagmus (D). Keeping the head deviated toward the unaffected side and the head pitched down, the patient then slowly sits up (E). Restrictions concerning head position or lying down after the treatment are not necessary although you might want the patient to sit quietly for 20 minutes before leaving the clinic.

Filled arrows indicate location of free-floating debris in the posterior semicircular canal. Note that the movement of the patient's head will gradually shift the debris away from the cupula and into the common crus.

NEURO

🔵 **TABLE 4.80 Expected Test Results in Patients With Unilateral Vestibular Loss (UVL)**

Test Results	Acute (first 2 wk) UVL	Compensated UVL
Spontaneous nystagmus (Recovers in <10 days, not affected by exercises)	Spontaneous and gaze evoked in light and dark	Still present in dark
VOR (Does not recover, not affected by exercises)	Abnormal with both slow and rapid head thrusts	Abnormal with rapid head thrusts toward side of lesion
Imbalance—especially while walking; improved with exercises	Present with all walking: slow, cautious gait	Essentially only with rapid turns toward affected side
Oscillopsia with head movement; improves with exercises	May or may not be significant complaint	Little or no complaints, may be affected by depression, poor coping
Dizziness with head movement; improves with exercises	Major complaint	Little or no complaints; affected by depression, poor coping
Confidence in balance; improves with exercises	ABC score <80%	ABC score >80%
Anxiety	Commonly present; depends on individual	Should decrease w/ return to activities
Depression	May or may not be present	If situational, should decrease
Walking speed; improves with exercises	~50% slow for age	Only 14.6% abnormally slow for age

(table continues on page 416)

TABLE 4.80 Expected Test Results in Patients With Unilateral Vestibular Loss (UVL) (continued)

Test Results	Acute (first 2 wk) UVL	Compensated UVL
Risk for falling; improves with exercises	DGI score ≤19 indicating risk for falling	67% no longer at risk; 22% improved but still at risk; 11% no improvement;
Vision during head movements; improves with exercises	Abnormal for age	78% improve significantly with majority to within normal for age
Participation in normal societal interactions	Disability scores range from bothersome (1) to out of work or on long-term disability (5)	Disability scores shift to 0–2 except for those out of work for >1 year or are on long-term disability
Performance of basic ADLs	Most can perform independently	Can perform independently
Driving	Unsafe	Safe although some may modify or limit driving
Romberg	Often, but not always positive	Negative
Sharpened Romberg	Cannot perform	Normal with eyes open; cannot perform with eyes closed
CSTIB—foam, eyes closed	Most cannot maintain balance on foam with eyes open	Normal with eyes open; most will be normal with eyes closed
Gait Improves with exercises	Wide-based, slow cadence, decreased rotation, may need help for a few days	Normal except for very rapid turns toward affected side
Turn head while walking	Cannot keep balance	Normal; some may slow cadence

NEURO

V

CARDIOVASCULAR

Anatomy

Heart

Anterior View

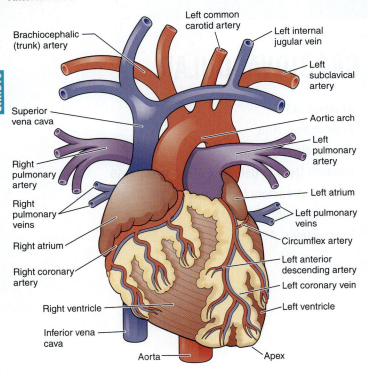

Brachiocephalic (trunk) artery

Left common carotid artery

Left internal jugular vein

Left subclavian artery

Superior vena cava

Aortic arch

Left pulmonary artery

Right pulmonary artery

Right pulmonary veins

Left atrium

Left pulmonary veins

Right atrium

Circumflex artery

Right coronary artery

Left anterior descending artery

Left coronary vein

Right ventricle

Left ventricle

Inferior vena cava

Aorta

Apex

CARDIO

Posterior View

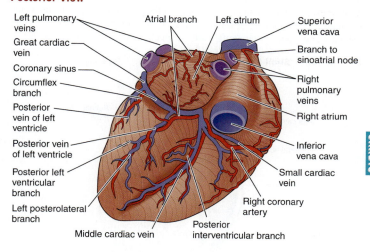

Left pulmonary veins

Great cardiac vein

Coronary sinus

Circumflex branch

Posterior vein of left ventricle

Posterior vein of left ventricle

Posterior left ventricular branch

Left posterolateral branch

Middle cardiac vein

Atrial branch

Left atrium

Posterior interventricular branch

Superior vena cava

Branch to sinoatrial node

Right pulmonary veins

Right atrium

Inferior vena cava

Small cardiac vein

Right coronary artery

CARDIO

Blood Supply to the Heart

There is considerable variation in the arterial venous branches to the myocardium. The table below lists the most common distributions.

Coronary artery dominance is a term used to describe which artery descends posteriorly from the crux to the apex of the myocardium. The right coronary artery is dominant and branches into the *posterior descending branch* in approximately two-thirds of humans; this is called *right dominance*. In these persons

⬤ TABLE 5.1 Arterial Blood Supply to the Heart

Artery	Area Supplied
Circumflex artery	Inferior wall of left ventricle (when not supplied by right coronary artery) Left atrium Sinoatrial (SA) node (in approximately 40% of humans)
Right coronary artery (RCA)	Right atrium Right ventricle Inferior wall of left ventricle (in most humans) Atrioventricular (AV) node Bundle of His Sinoatrial (SA) node (in approximately 60% of humans)
Left anterior descending (LAD) artery	Left ventricle Interventricular septum Right ventricle Inferior areas of the apex Inferior areas of both ventricles

the right coronary artery supplies part of the left ventricle and ventricular septum. In the remaining third of humans, a branch of the circumflex is dominant, which is called *left dominance*, or dominance is from branches from both the right coronary artery and the circumflex artery, which is called a *balanced pattern*.

Conduction System of the Heart

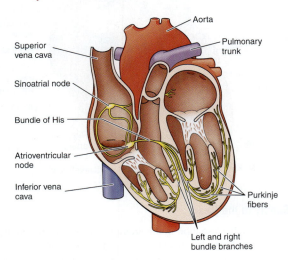

- Aorta
- Superior vena cava
- Pulmonary trunk
- Sinoatrial node
- Bundle of His
- Atrioventricular node
- Inferior vena cava
- Purkinje fibers
- Left and right bundle branches

Arteries

For circulation of the brain, see pages 205-208 in Section IV, Neuromuscular.

Branches of the Aorta

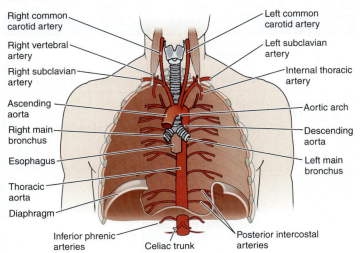

- Right common carotid artery
- Right vertebral artery
- Right subclavian artery
- Ascending aorta
- Right main bronchus
- Esophagus
- Thoracic aorta
- Diaphragm
- Left common carotid artery
- Left subclavian artery
- Internal thoracic artery
- Aortic arch
- Descending aorta
- Left main bronchus
- Inferior phrenic arteries
- Celiac trunk
- Posterior intercostal arteries

CARDIO

TABLE 5.2 Branches of the Aorta

Location	Name	Status
	Thorax	
Ascending aorta	Right and left coronary arteries	One pair
Aortic arch	Brachiocephalic trunk	Unpaired
	Right subclavian	
	Right common carotid	
	Left common carotid	Unpaired
	Left subclavian	Unpaired
Descending aorta	Visceral branches	Unpaired
	Esophageal	
	Left upper and lower bronchial	
	Right bronchial	
	Pericardial	
	Mediastinal	Paired
	Parietal branches	
	Posterior intercostal (T3–T11)	
	Subcostal (T12)	
	Superior phrenic	
Abdominal	**Visceral Branches**	
	Celiac	Unpaired
	Superior mesenteric	
	Inferior mesenteric	
	Glandular/visceral branches	Paired
	Suprarenal	
	Renal	
	Testicular (ovarian)	
	Parietal branches	
	Inferior phrenic	Paired
	Lumbar (L1–L4)	Paired
	Median sacral	Unpaired

CARDIO

Arteries of the Body

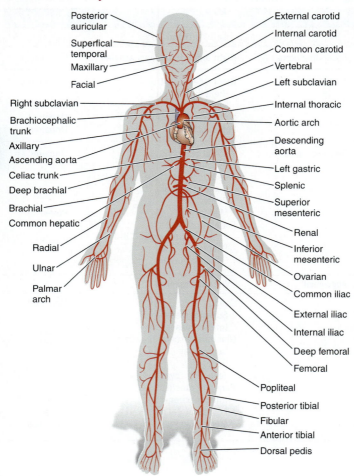

CARDIO

Posterior auricular
Superfical temporal
Maxillary
Facial
Right subclavian
Brachiocephalic trunk
Axillary
Ascending aorta
Celiac trunk
Deep brachial
Brachial
Common hepatic
Radial
Ulnar
Palmar arch

External carotid
Internal carotid
Common carotid
Vertebral
Left subclavian
Internal thoracic
Aortic arch
Descending aorta
Left gastric
Splenic
Superior mesenteric
Renal
Inferior mesenteric
Ovarian
Common iliac
External iliac
Internal iliac
Deep femoral
Femoral
Popliteal
Posterior tibial
Fibular
Anterior tibial
Dorsal pedis

TABLE 5.3 Arteries of the Pelvis and Perineum

Parent Vessel		
Primary Branch	**Secondary Branches**	**Area Supplied**
Internal Iliac (visceral)		
Umbilical	Superior vesical	Bladder
	Ductus deferens	Ductus deferens
	Middle vesical	Fundus of bladder, seminal vesicles
Inferior vesicular		Bladder
Middle rectal		Rectal
Uterine	Vaginal	Uterus, Vagina
Internal Iliac (anterior parietal)		
Obturator	Iliac	Iliacus muscle
	Vesical	Bladder
	Pubic	
	Anterior	Obturator externus, pectineus, gracilis, and adductor muscles
	Posterior	Hip joint, buttocks
Internal pudendal (Listings here are for the male; in the female the artery is smaller and supplies homologous structures.)	Muscular	Levator ani, obturator , internus, piriformis, coccygeus, and gluteus maximus muscles and other lateral rotators
	Inferior rectal	Muscles and integument of the anal region
	Perineal	Bulbospongiosus, ischiocavernosus, scrotum
	Artery of the bulb the penis	Bulb of the penis
	Urethral	Urethra
	Deep artery of the penis	Erectile tissue
	Dorsal artery of the penis	Glans, prepuce
Internal Iliac (posterior parietal)		
Iliolumbar	Lumbar	Psoas major and quadratus lumborum muscles
	Iliac	Iliacus and gluteal and abdominal muscles
Lateral sacral	Superior	Skin and muscles on the dorsum of the sacrum
	Inferior	Skin and muscles on dorsum of the sacrum
Superior gluteal	Superficial	Gluteus maximus, skin over the dorsal sacrum
	Deep	Gluteal muscles, hip joint

(table continues on page 424)

CARDIO

TABLE 5.3 **Arteries of the Pelvis and Perineum** (continued)

Parent Vessel		
Primary Branch	**Secondary Branches**	**Area Supplied**
Internal Iliac (posterior parietal)		
Inferior gluteal	Muscular	Gluteus maximus, lateral rotator muscles, upper part of hamstring muscles
	Coccygeal	Gluteus maximus and skin over the coccyx
	Artery of sciatic nerve	Artery that runs in the sciatic nerve and supplies that nerve
	Articular	Capsule of the hip joint
	Cutaneous	Skin of buttock and posterior thigh
External Iliac		
Inferior epigastric	Cremasteric (in males)	Cremaster muscle
	Artery of the round ligament (in females)	Round ligament
	Pubic	
	Muscular	Abdominal muscles
	Deep iliac circumflex	

TABLE 5.4 **Arteries of the Trunk**

Parent Vessel		
Primary Branch	**Secondary Branches**	**Area Supplied**
Thoracic Aorta (visceral)		
Pericardial		Pericardium, pleura, diaphragm
Bronchial		Bronchial tubes, areolar tissue of lung, bronchial lymph nodes
Esophageal		
Mediastinal		Lymph nodes, vessels, nerve and loose areolar tissue in the posterior mediastinum
Thoracic Aorta (parietal)		
Posterior intercostal	Dorsal branch	Muscles of the back, dorsal ramus of the spinal nerve
	Collateral intercostal	

Parent Vessel		
Primary Branch	**Secondary Branches**	**Area Supplied**
Thoracic Aorta (parietal)		
	Muscular	Intercostal, pectoral, and serratus anterior muscles
	Lateral cutaneous	Skin and superficial fascia overlying the intercostal space
	Mammary	Breasts
Subcostal		
Superior phrenic		Dorsal part of the upper surface of the diaphragm
Abdominal Aorta (visceral)		
Celiac	Left gastric	Cardiac portion of the stomach, lower esophagus, stomach
	Common hepatic (branches listed below)	
	Gastroduodenal	Pylorus, pancreas, duodenum
	Right gastric	Pylorus, stomach
	Right hepatic	Liver and via the cystic artery to the gallbladder
	Left hepatic	Capsule of the liver, caudate lobe of the liver
	Middle hepatic	Quadrate lobe of liver
Splenic (lienal)	Pancreatic	Pancreas
	Leftgastroepiploic	Stomach
	Short gastrics	Fundus and cardia of stomach
	Splenic	Spleen
Superior mesenteric	Inferior pancreaticoduodenal	Pancreas, duodenum
	Intestinal (jejunal and ileal)	Small intestine
	Ileocolic	Ascending colon, cecum, appendix, termination of ileum
	Right colic	Ascending colon
	Middle colic	Transverse colon
Inferior Mesenteric		
	Left colic	Descending colon, left part of transverse colon
	Sigmoid	Caudal part of descending colon, sigmoid colon
	Superior rectal	Rectum

(table continues on page 426)

CARDIO

TABLE 5.4 **Arteries of the Trunk** (continued)

Parent Vessel		
Primary Branch	**Secondary Branches**	**Area Supplied**
Inferior Mesenteric		
Middle suprarenal Renal Testicular (ovarian)		Suprarenal glands Kidneys Epididymis (ovaries, round ligament, skin of inguinal region, labia majora)
Abdominal Aorta (parietal)		
Inferior phrenic	Medial branch Lateral branch	Inferior vena cava, esophagus
Lumbar Middle sacral		Muscles and skin of the back
Abdominal Aorta (terminal branch)		
Common iliacs (see Table 5.3, Arteries of the Pelvis and Perineum)		

Arteries of the Upper Extremity

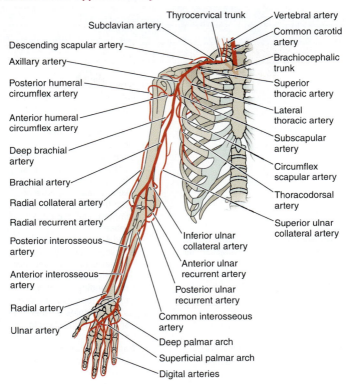

CARDIO

Thyrocervical trunk
Subclavian artery
Descending scapular artery
Axillary artery
Posterior humeral circumflex artery
Anterior humeral circumflex artery
Deep brachial artery
Brachial artery
Radial collateral artery
Radial recurrent artery
Posterior interosseous artery
Anterior interosseous artery
Radial artery
Ulnar artery

Vertebral artery
Common carotid artery
Brachiocephalic trunk
Superior thoracic artery
Lateral thoracic artery
Subscapular artery
Circumflex scapular artery
Thoracodorsal artery
Superior ulnar collateral artery
Inferior ulnar collateral artery
Anterior ulnar recurrent artery
Posterior ulnar recurrent artery
Common interosseous artery
Deep palmar arch
Superficial palmar arch
Digital arteries

TABLE 5.5 Arteries of the Head and Upper Extremity

Parent Vessel		
Primary Branch	Secondary Branches	Area Supplied
Subclavian		
Vertebral	Spinal	Periosteum and bodies of vertebrae
	Muscular	Deep muscles of neck
	Meningeal	Fax cerebelli
	Posterior spinal	
	Anterior spinal	Pia mater and spinal cord
	Posterior inferior cerebellar	Medulla and choroid plexus of fourth ventricle, inferior surface of the cerebellum to the lateral border

(table continues on page 428

TABLE 5.5 Arteries of the Head and Upper Extremity (continued)

Parent Vessel		
Primary Branch	**Secondary Branches**	**Area Supplied**
Subclavian		
	Basilar	Pons and midbrain
		Internal ear
		Lateral aspect of the pons, anterolateral and antero-medial parts of the inferior surface of the cerebellum
		Superior surface of the cerebellum, midbrain, pineal body, anterior medullary velum, tela choroidea of the third ventricle
		Temporal and occipital lobes
Thyrocervical trunk	Inferior thyroid	Inferior part of thyroid gland
	Suprascapular	Supraspinatus and infraspinatus muscles and sternocleidomastoid and surrounding muscles, skin of anterior superior chest, and structures of the shoulder joint, clavicle, and scapulae
	Transverse cervical	Trapezius, levator scapulae and deep cervical muscles, rhomboid and serratus posterior superior, subscapularis, supraspinatus, and infraspinatus muscles
Internal thoracic	Pericardiophrenic	Pleura and pericardium
	Mediastinal	Lymph nodes and areolar tissue in the anterior mediastinum
	Thymic	Thymus
	Sternal	Transversus thoracis muscle and posterior surface of the sternum
	Anterior intercostals	Intercostal muscles
	Musculophrenic	Diaphragm, abdominal muscles
	Superior epigastric	Abdominal muscles and overlying skin

CARDIO

Parent Vessel		
Primary Branch	Secondary Branches	Area Supplied
Subclavian		
Costocervical trunk	Highest (supreme) intercostal	
	Deep cervical	Semispinalis capitis, cervicis and adjacent muscles
	Descending scapular	
Axillary		
Highest thoracic		Pectoral muscles
Thoracoacromial		
	Pectoral	Pectoral muscles and breast
	Acromial	Deltoid muscle
	Clavicular	
	Deltoid	Pectoralis major and deltoid muscle
	Suprascapular	Sternoclavicular joint and subclavius muscles
Lateral thoracic		Serratus anterior, pectoral, and subscapularis, and axillary lymph nodes
Subscapular	Scapular circumflex	Infraspinatus, teres major and minor muscles, long head of the triceps and deltoid muscles
	Thoracodorsal	Subscapularis, latissimus dorsi, serratus anterior, and intercostal muscles
Posterior humeral circumflex		Deltoid muscle and shoulder joint
Anterior humeral circumflex		Head of humerus and shoulder joint
Brachial		
Deep brachial		
	Radial collateral	
	Middle collateral	
	Deltoid (ascending)	Brachialis and deltoid muscles
	Nutrient	Humerus
Principal nutrient of the humerus		Humerus
Superior ulnar collateral		
Inferior ulnar collateral		
Muscular		Coracobrachialis, biceps brachii, and brachialis muscles

(table continues on page 430)

CARDIO

TABLE 5.5 **Arteries of the Head and Upper Extremity** (continued)

Parent Vessel		
Primary Branch	**Secondary Branches**	**Area Supplied**
Radial		
Radial recurrent		Supinator, brachioradialis and brachialis muscles, elbow joint
Muscular		Brachioradialis and pronator teres muscles
Palmar carpal		Carpal bones
Superficial palmar		Muscles of the thenar eminence
Dorsal carpal		Fingers
First dorsal metacarpal		Thumb and index finger
Princeps pollicis		Skin and subcutaneous tissue of the thumb
Radial indicis		Ulnar aspect of the index finger
Deep palmar arch		
Palmar metacarpal		
Perforating		
Recurrent		Intercarpal articulations
Ulnar		
Anterior ulnar recurrent		Brachialis and pronator teres muscles
Posterior ulnar recurrent		Elbow joint and muscles near the elbow joint
Common interosseus	Palmar (anterior) interosseous	Flexor digitorum profundus and flexor pollicis longus muscles, radius and ulna
	Dorsal (posterior) interosseous	Superficial and deep muscles of the posterior compartment of the forearm
Muscular		Superficial and deep flexors of the finger and muscles on the ulnar aspect of the forearm
Palmar carpal		
Dorsal carpal		Ulnar aspect of dorsal surface of the little finger
Deep palmar		
Superficial palmar arch		
Common palmar digital		Soft parts on the dorsum of the middle and distal phalanges
	Proper palmar digital	

CARDIO

Arteries of the Lower Extremity

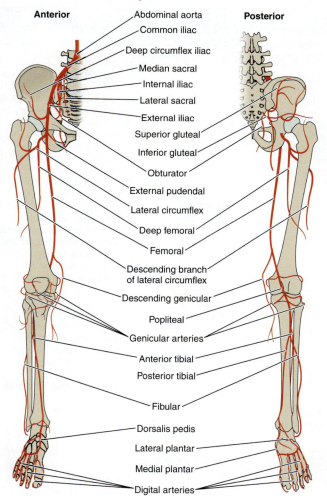

Anterior

Posterior

Abdominal aorta

Common iliac

Deep circumflex iliac

Median sacral

Internal iliac

Lateral sacral

External iliac

Superior gluteal

Inferior gluteal

Obturator

External pudendal

Lateral circumflex

Deep femoral

Femoral

Descending branch
of lateral circumflex

Descending genicular

Popliteal

Genicular arteries

Anterior tibial

Posterior tibial

Fibular

Dorsalis pedis

Lateral plantar

Medial plantar

Digital arteries

CARDIO

TABLE 5.6 Arteries of the Lower Extremity

Parent Vessel		
Primary Branch	**Secondary Branches**	**Area Supplied**
Femoral		
Superficial epigastric		Superficial subinguinal lymph nodes
Superficial iliac circumflex		Skin of the groin and superficial subinguinal lymph nodes
Superficial external pudendal		Skin of the lower part of the abdomen, scrotum, and penis (labia majora in female)
Deep external pudendal		Skin of the scrotum (labia majora in female)
Muscular		Sartorius, vastus medialis, adductor muscles
Deep femoral	Medial femoral circumflex	Ascending to adductor muscles, gracilis and obturator externus muscles; transverse to the adductor magnus and brevis muscles; acetabular branch to the fat in the acetabular fossa
	Lateral femoral circumflex	
	Perforating	First perforating to adductor brevis and magnus muscles, biceps femoris and gluteus maximus muscles; second perforating to posterior femoral muscles
	Muscular	Adductor muscles, hamstring muscles
Descending genicular	Saphenous	Skin on the upper and medial leg
	Articular branch	Knee joint
Popliteal		
Superior muscular		Lower parts of the adductor magnus and hamstring muscles
Sural		Gastrocnemius, soleus, and plantaris muscles
Cutaneous		Skin on the back of the leg
Superior genicular	Medial superior genicular	Vastus medialis muscle, femur, knee joint
	Lateral superior genicular (superficial and deep branches)	Vastus lateralis muscle, femur, knee joint
Middle genicular		Ligaments and synovial membrane of the knee joint

CARDIO

Parent Vessel		
Primary Branch	**Secondary Branches**	**Area Supplied**
Popliteal		
Inferior genicular	Medial inferior genicular Lateral inferior genicular	Popliteus muscle, upper end of tibia, knee joint
Anterior Tibial		
Posterior tibial recurrent		Popliteus muscle
Anterior tibial recurrent		
Muscular		Muscles along the vessel
Anterior medial malleolar		
Anterior lateral malleolar		Lateral aspect of the ankle
Dorsalis Pedis		
Lateral tarsal	Arcuate, anterior lateral malleolar, lateral plantar, peroneal	Extensor digitorum brevis muscle
Medial tarsal		
Arcuate		
First dorsal metatarsal		Medial border of the great toe
Deep plantar		
Posterior Tibial		
Circumflex fibular		Soleus and peroneal muscles
Peroneal	Muscular	Soleus, tibialis posterior, flexor hallucis longus, and peroneal muscles
	Nutrient (fibular)	Fibular
	Perforating	Tarsal bones
	Communicating	
	Lateral malleolar	
	Lateral calcaneal	
Nutrient (tibial)		Tibialis posterior muscle, tibia
Muscular		Soleus and deep muscles along the back of the leg
Medial malleolar		
Communicating		
Medial calcaneal		Muscles on the tibial side of the sole of the foot
Medial plantar		
Lateral plantar	Perforating	Digits

Veins

Veins of the Body

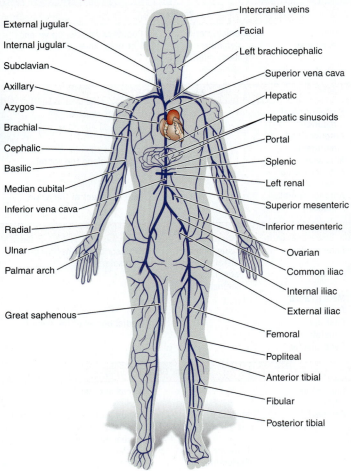

External jugular
Internal jugular
Subclavian
Axillary
Azygos
Brachial
Cephalic
Basilic
Median cubital
Inferior vena cava
Radial
Ulnar
Palmar arch
Great saphenous

Intercranial veins
Facial
Left brachiocephalic
Superior vena cava
Hepatic
Hepatic sinusoids
Portal
Splenic
Left renal
Superior mesenteric
Inferior mesenteric
Ovarian
Common iliac
Internal iliac
External iliac
Femoral
Popliteal
Anterior tibial
Fibular
Posterior tibial

CARDIO

Veins of the Upper Extremity

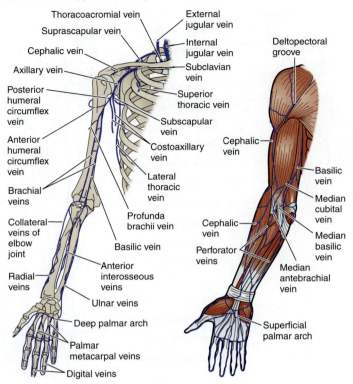

CARDIO

Veins of the Lower Extremity

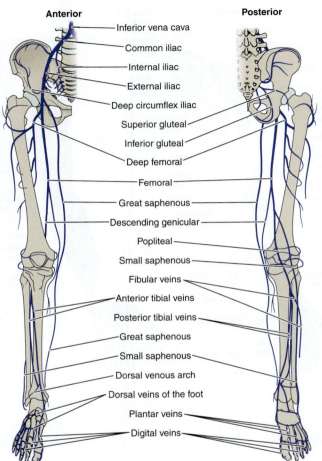

Anterior

Posterior

- Inferior vena cava
- Common iliac
- Internal iliac
- External iliac
- Deep circumflex iliac
- Superior gluteal
- Inferior gluteal
- Deep femoral
- Femoral
- Great saphenous
- Descending genicular
- Popliteal
- Small saphenous
- Fibular veins
- Anterior tibial veins
- Posterior tibial veins
- Great saphenous
- Small saphenous
- Dorsal venous arch
- Dorsal veins of the foot
- Plantar veins
- Digital veins

CARDIO

TABLE 5.7 Venous Drainage From the Lungs

Vein	Primary Tributary	Area Drained
Right pulmonary veins (2)	Right superior pulmonary	Right superior and middle lobes
	Apical segmental	Apex and anterior segments
	Posterior segmental	Posterior middle and superior lobes
	Anterior segmental	Right superior lobe
	Right middle lobe	Middle lobe
	Right inferior pulmonary	Right inferior hilum
	Superior segmental	Medial middle lobe
	Common basal	Anterior basal, lateral basal, and posterior basal segments
Left pulmonary veins (2)	Left superior pulmonary	Apicoposterior, anteriorsegments
	Apicoposterior segmental	Apicoposterior segments
	Posterior segmental	Intrasegmental and intersegmental areas
	Lingular division	Superior and inferior lingular segments
	Left inferior pulmonary	Intrasegmental and intersegmental areas
	Superior basal	Anterior basal segments
	Inferior basal	Posterior and lateral basal segments

TABLE 5.8 Venous Drainage of the Heart

Vein	Primary Tributary	Area Drained
Coronary sinus	Great cardiac	Left atrium, both ventricles
	Small cardiac	Posterior right atrium and ventricles
	Middle cardiac	Both ventricles
	Posterior vein of left ventricle	Left ventricle
	Oblique vein of left atrium	Left atrium
Anterior cardiac		Anterior right ventricle
Small cardiac (thebesian)		Both atria

CARDIO

CARDIO

🔵 TABLE 5.9 Venous Drainage of the Face—Deep

Vein	Primary Tributary	Area Drained
Maxillary	Confluence of veins of pterygoid plexus	Cavernous sinus
Pterygoid plexus	Veins accompanying maxillary artery	Muscles of mastication

🔵 TABLE 5.10 Venous Drainage of the Face—Superficial

Vein	Primary Tributary	Area Drained
Facial	Angular, which is formed by the following:	
	Frontal	Anterior scalp
	Supraorbital	Forehead
	Deep facial	Muscles of facial expression
	Superficial temporal	Vertex and side of head
	Posterior auricular	Back of ear
	Occipital	Superior sagittal and transverse sinuses
	Retromandibular	Parotid gland and masseter

🔵 TABLE 5.11 Venous Drainage of the Cranium—the Brain

Vein	Primary Tributary	Area Drained
External cerebral	Superior cerebral (8–12 veins)	Superior, lateral, and medial surfaces of hemisphere and opens into the superior sagittal sinus
	Middle cerebral	Lateral hemispheric surfaces into cavernous and sphenoparietal sinuses
	Inferior cerebral	Inferior hemispheric surfaces into superior sagittal sinus
Internal cerebral	Great cerebral (Galen's) Internal cerebral, which is formed by the following:	Interior of hemispheres into inferior sagittal sinus
	Thalamostriate	Corpus striatum, thalamus
	Choroid	Choroid plexus, hippocampus, fornix, corpus callosum
	Basal	Insula, corpus striatum
Cerebellar	Superior cerebellar	Superior vermis into the straight sinus
	Inferior cerebellar	Lower cerebellum into transverse, occipital, and superior petrosal sinuses

TABLE 5.12 Venous Drainage of the Cranium—Sinuses of the Dura Mater

Vein	Primary Tributary	Area Drained
Posterior superior sinuses	Superior sagittal sinus	Superior cerebral veins, dura mater
	Inferior sagittal sinus	Falx cerebri and medial surfaces of the hemispheres
	Straight sinus	Inferior sagittal sinus, great cerebral vein
	Transverse sinuses	Right drains superior sagittal and the left straight sinuses; also receives blood from the superior petrosal sinuses
	Sigmoid sinuses	Transverse sinuses
	Occipital sinus	Posterior internal vertebral venous plexus into the confluence of sinuses
	Confluence of sinuses	Superior sagittal, straight, occipital, and both transverse sinuses
Anterior inferior sinuses	Cavernous sinus	Superior and inferior ophthalmic veins, some cerebral veins, sphenoparietal sinus
	Superior ophthalmic vein	Corresponding branches of ophthalmic artery
	Inferior ophthalmic vein	Muscles of eye movements
	Intercavernous sinuses	Connects the two cavernous sinuses across the midline
	Superior petrosal sinus	Cerebellar and inferior cerebral veins, veins from tympanic cavity; connects cavernous and transverse sinuses
	Inferior petrosal sinus	Internal auditory veins, veins from medulla, pons, and inferior surface of cerebellum; drains into the internal jugular bulb
	Basilar plexus	Connects inferior petrosal sinuses

CARDIO

TABLE 5.13 **Venous Drainage of the Cranium—Diploic and Emissary Veins**

Vein	Primary Tributary	Area Drained
Diploic	Frontal	Communicates with supraorbital vein and superior sagittal sinus
	Anterior temporal	Temporal communicates with the sphenoparietal sinus and the deep temporal veins
	Posterior temporal	Transverse sinus
	Occipital	Occipital vein, transverse sinus, or confluence of sinuses
Emissary	Mastoid	Connects transverse sinus with the posterior auricular or occipital veins
	Parietal	Connects superior sagittal sinus with veins of the scalp
	Rete hypoglossal canal	Joins transverse sinus with vertebral vein and deep veins of the neck
	Rete foramen ovalis	Connects cavernous sinus with pterygoid plexus through foramen ovale
	Internal carotid plexus	Connects cavernous sinus and internal jugular vein via carotid canal
	Vein of foramen cecum	Connects superior sagittal sinus with veins of nasal cavity

TABLE 5.14 **Venous Drainage of the Neck**

Vein	Primary Tributary	Area Drained
External jugular	Posterior external jugular	Skin and superficial muscles in cranium and posterior neck
	Anterior jugular	Inferior thyroid veins by way of jugular venous arch, internal jugular
	Transverse cervical	Trapezius and surrounding muscles
	Suprascapular	Supraspinatus, and feeds into the external jugular near the subclavian
Internal jugular	Inferior petrosal sinus	Internal auditory veins and veins of brain stem
	Lingual	Tongue
	Pharyngeal	Pharynx and vein of pterygoid canal
	Superior thyroid	Thyroid gland and receives superior laryngeal and cricothyroid veins
	Middle thyroid	Inferior thyroid gland
Vertebral	Anterior vertebral	Upper cervical vertebrae
	Accessory vertebral	Cervical vertebrae
	Deep cervical	Suboccipital muscles and cervical vertebrae

CARDIO

⬤ TABLE 5.15 Venous Drainage of the Thorax

Vein	Primary Tributary	Area Drained
Azygos	Posterior inter-costals	Dorsal spinal musculature and thoracic vertebrae
	Subcostal	Musculature about the 12th rib and thoracic vertebrae
	Hemiazygos	Four or five intercostal veins, left subcostal vein, some esophageal and mediastinal veins
	Accessory hemiazygos	Intercostal veins on the left side
	Bronchial	Bronchi of lungs
Brachiocephalic	Right brachiocephalic	Right vertebral, internal thoracic, inferior thyroid, and first intercostal veins
	Left brachiocephalic	Same as right brachiocephalic, except that it drains left side
Internal thoracic		Drainage corresponds to arterial blood supply of internal thoracic
Inferior thyroid		Lower portion of thyroid gland and receives esophageal, tracheal, and inferior laryngeal veins
Highest intercostal		Upper two or three intercostal spaces; Right drains into azygos and left into brachiocephalic
Veins of vertebral column	External vertebral venous plexus	Mostly cervical vertebrae and connects with vertebral, occipital, and deep cervical veins
	Internal vertebral venous plexus	Posterior aspects of vertebrae, including ligaments and arches and connects with vertebral veins, occipital sinus, and basilar plexus
	Basivertebral	Foramina of dorsal vertebral bodies and communicates with anterior external vertebral plexuses
	Intervertebral	Internal and external vertebral plexuses and ends in vertebral, intercostal, lumbar, and lateral sacral veins
	Veins of spinal cord	Spinal cord into vertebral veins

CARDIO

⬤ TABLE 5.16 Venous Drainage of the Abdomen

Vein	Primary Tributary	Area Drained
Inferior vena cava	Lumbar	Posterior wall muscles, vertebral plexuses, and into azygos system via ascending lumbar veins
	Testicular (in males)	Epididymis, testis, spermatic cord; right testicular enters the inferior vena cava and left into the renal vein
	Ovarian (in females)	Ovaries, broad ligament; right enters the inferior vena cava and left into the renal vein
	Renal	Kidneys and receives left testicular (or ovarian), inferior phrenic, and suprarenal veins
	Suprarenal	Suprarenal glands
	Inferior phrenic	Undersurface of diaphragm and ending in renal or suprarenal vein on left and inferior vena cava on right
	Hepatic	Liver

⬤ TABLE 5.17 Venous Drainage of the Liver—Portal Venous Drainage

Vein	Primary Tributary	Area Drained
Portal	Lienal (splenic)	Spleen and entering superior mesenteric vein to form the portal vein
	Branches: Short gastric	Greater curvature of the stomach
	Left gastroepiploic	Stomach and greater omentum
	Pancreatic	Body and tail of pancreas
	Inferior mesenteric	Rectum, sigmoid and descending colon and receives sigmoid, and inferior rectal veins
	Superior mesenteric	Small intestine, cecum, ascending and transverse colon
	Branches: Right gastroepiploic	Stomach and greater omentum
	Pancreaticoduodenal	Pancreas and duodenum
	Coronary	Stomach and its lesser curvature, lesser omentum ending in portal vein
	Pyloric	Pyloric portion of lesser curvature of stomach and ending in portal vein
	Cystic	Gallbladder ending in right branch of portal vein
	Paraumbilical	Ligamentum teres of liver and connecting veins of anterior abdominal wall to portal, internal, and common iliac veins

🔶 TABLE 5.18   Venous Drainage of the Pelvis and Perineum

Vein	Primary Tributary	Area Drained
Common iliac	Iliolumbar	Posterior pelvis and lumbar vertebrae
	Lateral sacral	Anterior sacrum
	Middle sacral	Additional sacral drainage to left common iliac vein
Internal iliac	Superior gluteal	Buttocks
	Inferior gluteal	Posterior thigh and buttocks
	Internal pudendal	Penis, urethral bulb
	Obturator	Adductor region of the thigh
	Lateral sacral	Anterior surface of sacrum
	Middle rectal	Rectal plexus, bladder, prostate, seminal vesicle, and levator ani
	Inferior rectal	Lower rectum draining into the internal pudendal vein
	Dorsal vein of penis	Superficial vein drains preputce and skin while deep vein drains glans penis, corpora cavernosa
	Vesical	Bladder and base of prostate
	Uterine	Uterus
	Vaginal	Vagina

🔶 TABLE 5.19   Venous Drainage of the Lower Extremity—Boundary of Abdomen and Lower Extremity

Vein	Primary Tributary	Area Drained
External iliac	Inferior epigastric	Internal surface of lower abdominal wall
	Deep iliac circumflex	Deep tissue around anterior superior iliac spine and inner pelvic brim
	Superficial external pudendal	Superficial lower abdomen, scrotum, and labia and upper thigh

CARDIO

◆ TABLE 5.20　Venous Drainage of the Lower Extremity—Superficial

Vein	Primary Tributary	Area Drained
Great saphenous		Medial aspect of leg from ankle upward across medial knee and thigh to enter femoral vein at femoral ring
	Accessory saphenous	Medial and posterior thigh
Small saphenous		Lateral to Achilles tendon up posterior leg to popliteal vein
Dorsal digital		Clefts between toes
Intercapitular		From short common digital veins to produce dorsal venous arch
Plantar cutaneous venous arch		Sole of the foot

◆ TABLE 5.21　Venous Drainage of the Lower Extremity—Deep

Vein	Primary Tributary	Area Drained
Plantar digital		Plantar surface of toes of foot to drain into plantar metatarsal veins
Plantar metatarsal		Along metatarsal bones to ankle and contributing to deep plantar venous arch
Medial plantar		Medial aspect of sole of foot and upward to form posterior tibial vein
Lateral plantar		Lateral aspect of sole of foot and upward to form posterior tibial vein
Posterior tibial		Medial portion of deep muscles of leg and draining into popliteal vein
Peroneal		Venous plexus of heel along lateral leg to drain into posterior tibial vein
Anterior tibial		Anterior compartment of leg to drain into popliteal vein

Vein	Primary Tributary	Area Drained
Popliteal		Posteromedial muscles of thigh to become femoral vein
Femoral		Anterior compartment of thigh to drain into external iliac
Femoral profunda		Deep muscles of anterior, anteromedial, and antero-lateral thigh to drain into femoral vein

CARDIO

TABLE 5.22 Venous Drainage of the Upper Extremity—Superficial

Vein	Primary Tributary	Area Drained
Palmar digital		Palmar surface of digits and connected to dorsal digital veins by oblique intercapit-ular veins
Dorsal digital venous network		Tissues of fingers and along fingers dorsally to back of hand
Medial antebrachial		Superficial veins of hand up forearm to basilic vein below elbow
Basilic		Back of hand to anterior surface of arm above elbow to upper third of arm, draining into brachial vein
Accessory cephalic		Ulnar side of dorsal venous network to cephalic at elbow
Cephalic		Drainage of hand, forearm, and arm by extending up lateral aspect of arm to axillary vein near clavicle

◖ TABLE 5.23 Venous Drainage of the Upper Extremity—Deep

Vein	Primary Tributary	Area Drained
Superficial and deep palmar venous arches		Fingers
Palmar and dorsal metacarpal		Metacarpals
Brachial		From the elbow on each side of forearm, draining deep tissues to form the axillary in the arm
Axillary		Axillary and clavicular join to drain into subclavian vein
Subclavian		Drains external jugular and anterior jugular and enters the internal jugular vein, along with thoracic duct on left and right lymphatic duct on right

Lymphatic System

Lymphatic System (Anterior View)

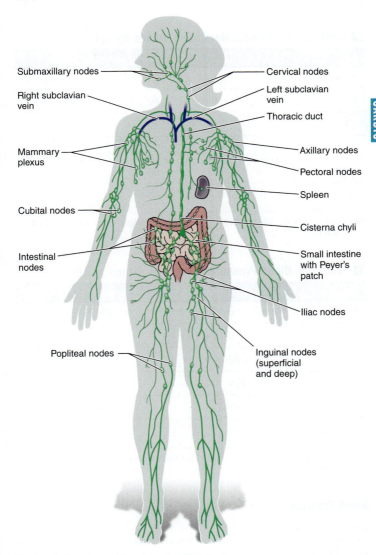

The lymphatic system, with major nodes illustrated.

Examination

Vital Signs

TABLE 5.24 Heart Rate Normative Values by Age

Age	Heart Rate (beats/min)
Newborn	70–190
3 yr	80–125
10 yr	70–110
16 yr	55–100
Adult	60–90
Older adult	60–90

Data from: O'Sullivan, SB, and Schmitz, TJ: *Physical Rehabilitation,* ed. 5. FA Davis, Philadelphia, 2007, p 82.

TABLE 5.25 Blood Pressure Normative Values by Age

Age	Systolic (mm Hg)	Diastolic (mm Hg)
Newborn	50–52	25–30
3 yr	78–114	46–78
10 yr	90–120	56–84
16 yr	104–120	60–84
Adult	95–119	60–79
Older adult	90–140	60–90

Data from: O'Sullivan, SB, and Schmitz, TJ: *Physical Rehabilitation,* ed. 5. FA Davis, Philadelphia, 2007, p 82.

Blood Pressure

Systole
Systole is the period of cardiac contraction and represents the highest pressure exerted by the blood against the arterial walls.

Diastole
Diastole is the period of cardiac relaxation, or cardiac filling, and represents the highest pressure exerted by the blood against the arterial walls.

Pulse Pressure

The mathematical difference between systolic and diastolic blood pressure.

Mean Arterial Pressure

The average pressure during each cycle of the heartbeat. Equal to the cardiac output multiplied by the vascular resistance. Generally estimated as (systolic blood pressure $\times$ $\frac{1}{3}$) + (diastolic blood pressure $\times$ $\frac{2}{3}$).

Procedure for Measuring Blood Pressure

The cuff is placed 1 to 2 inches above the antecubital fossa and inflated until no radial pulse is palpable; then the brachial artery is auscultated over the fossa during deflation of the cuff. The sounds heard vary in intensity and quality during deflation and are called *Korotkoff's sounds*. Five phases of Korotkoff's sounds are described.

phase 1: First sounds that are heard, clear tapping sounds that increase in intensity. Systolic blood pressure is when rhythmic tapping is first heard.

phase 2: The clear tapping sound of phase 1 is replaced with a softer muffled sound or murmur.

phase 3: A less clear but louder and crisper tapping sound replaces the muffled sound of phase 2.

phase 4: Tapping of phase 3 changes to muffled, soft blowing sound. This is sometimes called the *first diastolic pressure*.

phase 5: Disappearance of all sounds. Diastolic blood pressure generally measured as this phase if only two values are recorded. If three pressures are recorded, phase 5 is the *second diastolic pressure*.

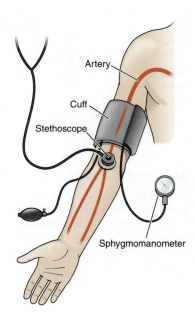

Placement of the blood pressure cuff and stethoscope for monitoring brachial artery pressure.

Cardiac Auscultation

auscultation: Listening to the intensity and quality of heart sounds as they vary over the surface of the chest. Four primary areas are identified over which to auscultate the cardiac valves.

⬤ **TABLE 5.26 Areas to Auscultate for the Cardiac Valves**

Valve	Area to Auscultate
Aortic	Second right intercostal space at right sternal border (base of heart)
Pulmonic	Second left intercostal space at left sternal border
Tricuspid	Fourth left intercostal space along lower left sternal border
Mitral	Fifth left intercostal space at midclavicular line (apical area)

Cardiac Auscultation

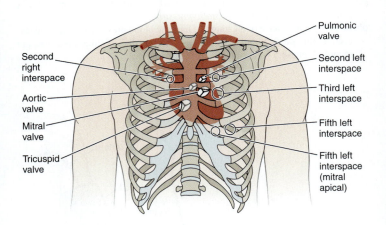

Basic Heart Sounds

The four basic heart sounds are termed S_1, S_2, S_3, and S_4.

S_1 and S_2: Often referred to as "lub-dub," respectively, with S_1 being the first sound after the longest pause between pairs of beats.

S_1: Occurs at the onset of systole when the mitral and tricuspid valves close and should be loudest when auscultated over the apex of the heart (left lower sternal border).

S$_2$: Attributed to closure of the aortic and pulmonic valves and should be loudest over the base of heart (left upper sternal border). Systole is the period between S$_1$ and S$_2$, and diastole is the period between S$_2$ and the next S$_1$.

splitting of S$_1$ or S$_2$: Occurs when valves close asynchronously and may be a normal or pathologic finding.

A$_2$ and P$_2$: When splitting is heard, S$_2$ is referred to as A$_2$ and P$_2$.

M$_1$ and T$_1$: When splitting is heard, S$_1$ is referred to as M$_1$ and T$_1$.

S$_3$: Is difficult or impossible to hear without a stethoscope. It is associated with ventricular filling and occurs soon after S$_2$. A normal or physiologic S$_3$ is often found in young people. When S$_3$ is heard in older individuals with heart disease, it may indicate congestive failure and is called a *ventricular gallop*.

S$_4$: Is difficult or impossible to hear without a stethoscope. It is associated with ventricular filling as well as atrial contraction and occurs just before S$_1$. An audible S$_4$ is generally pathologic and may indicate hypertensive cardio-vascular disease, coronary artery disease, postmyocardial infarction, aortic stenosis, or cardiomyopathy.

summation gallop: May be present with severe myocardial disease. It is a long heart sound that occurs when S$_3$ and S$_4$ blend together.

ventricular gallop: See S$_3$.

Extra Heart Sounds

Described as *snaps, clicks, rubs,* and *murmurs*. Snaps and clicks are usually considered valvular sounds and thus are S$_3$ or S$_4$ subtypes. Murmurs are caused by disturbances in the normal blood flow through the cardiac chambers and are usually classified based on their duration (timing), intensity, quality, pitch, location, and radiation. The following criteria are used for classification:

timing: During systole, diastole, or both. A murmur may be described as lasting an entire time period (holosystolic or pansystolic) or during a portion of a time period (early diastolic).

intensity: The following system is used for evaluating the intensity of extra sounds:

    grade 1: Softest audible murmur

    grade 2: Murmur of medium intensity

    grade 3: Loud murmur without thrill

    grade 4: Murmur with thrill

    grade 5: Loudest murmur that cannot be heard with stethoscope off the chest

    grade 6: Audible with stethoscope off the chest

quality: This describes the tone of the murmur, such as harsh, musical, blowing, rumbling. A crescendo murmur increases in intensity, a decrescendo murmur falls, and a crescendo-decrescendo murmur rises and then falls.

pitch: High, medium, or low pitched.

location: Area of the precordium in which the murmur is heard: aortic, pulmonic, tricuspid, mitral.

radiation: This describes when the sound of the murmur is transmitted to other regions of the body, such as across the chest, into the axilla or neck, or down the left sternal border.

The Cardiac Cycle

The events of the cardiac cycle are depicted below, showing changes in left atrial pressure, left ventricular pressure, aortic pressure, ventricular volume, the electrocardiogram (ECG), and the phonocardiogram.

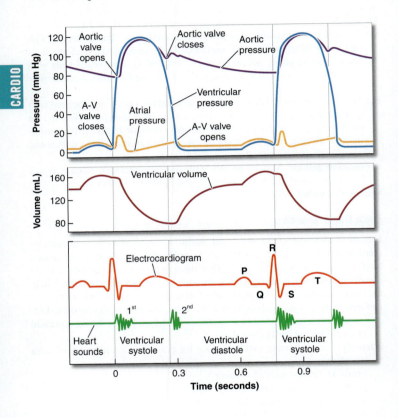

Electrocardiograms (ECG)

Electrocardiographic Waves, Segments, and Intervals

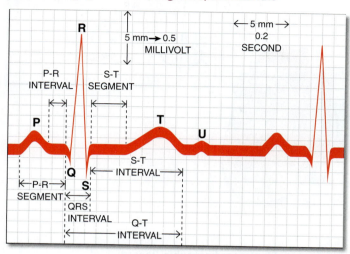

CARDIO

🟠 TABLE 5.27 Normal Ranges of Electrocardiographic Components

	Duration	Amplitude
P wave	<0.10 sec	1–3 mm
PR interval	0.12–0.20 sec	Isoelectric after the P-wave deflection
QRS	0.06–0.10 sec	25–30 mm (maximum)
ST segment	0.12 sec	$-1/2$ to +1 mm
T wave	0.16 sec	5–10 mm

Electrocardiographic Recording of Myocardial Activity

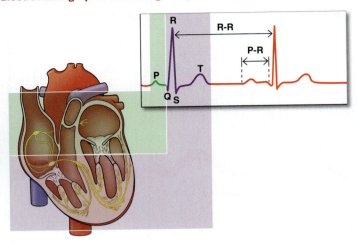

CARDIO

TABLE 5.28 Electrocardiographic Recording of Myocardial Activity

Electrocardiographic Component	Myocardial Event
P wave	Atrial depolarization
QRS complex	Ventricular depolarization
T wave	Ventricular repolarization

Interpreting the Electrocardiogram

Steps to Follow When Interpreting an Electrocardiogram Rhythm Strip

1. Calculate the rate.
2. Examine the rhythm and determine if regular or irregular.
3. Identify P waves.
4. Evaluate PR interval for duration and relationship of P wave to QRS complex.
5. Evaluate QRS complex for shape and duration.
6. Identify extra waves or complexes.
7. Determine clinical significance of a dysrhythmia.

Abbreviations Used in Electrocardiographic Interpretations

APC (APB)	Atrial premature contraction (beat)
CHB	Complete heart block

JPC (JPB)	Junctional premature contraction (beat)
LAD	Left axis deviation
LAE	Left atrial enlargement
LAHB	Left anterior hemiblock
LBBB	Left bundle branch block
LVE	Left ventricular enlargement
LVH	Left ventricular hypertrophy
NPC (NPB)	Nodal premature contraction (beat)
NSR	Normal sinus rhythm
NSTEMI	Non–ST elevation myocardial infarction
NSSTTW	Nonspecific ST- and T-wave changes
NSVT	Non–sustained ventricular tachycardia
PAC (PAB)	Premature atrial contraction (beat)
PAT	Paroxysmal atrial tachycardia
PJC (PJB)	Premature junctional contraction (beat)
PNC (PNB)	Premature nodal contraction (beat)
PVC (PVB)	Premature ventricular contraction (beat)
RAE	Right atrial enlargement
RBBB	Right bundle branch block
RSR	Regular sinus rhythm
RVH	Right ventricular hypertrophy
SVT	Supraventricular tachycardia
VF	Ventricular fibrillation
VPC (VPB)	Ventricular premature contraction (beat)
VT	Ventricular tachycardia

CARDIO

Methods Used to Calculate Heart Rates

Four methods can be used to calculate from an ECG rates with regular cardiac rhythms. When conduction is normal, both atrial and ventricular rates are identical. When the rhythm is irregular, each beat in a 30- or 60-second rhythm strip should be counted to estimate the rate.

- Multiply the number of QRS complexes in a 6-second strip (most ECG paper has markers every 1, 3, or 6 sec) by 10 (chart speed = 25 mm/sec). Estimate the portion of an RR interval when only a portion of one is contained at the end of 6 seconds.
- Divide 300 by the number of whole or partial large boxes between two consecutive R waves.
- Find an R wave that falls on a large box line and count how many large boxes are in the interval before the next R wave. Memorize the values for each large box interval.

Heart Rate	Number of Large Boxes
300	1
150	2
100	3

75	4
60	5
50	6
43	7

• Divide 1,500 by the number of small boxes between consecutive R waves.

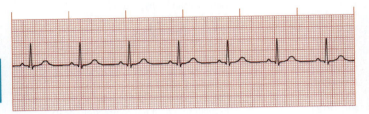

Normal sinus rhythm.

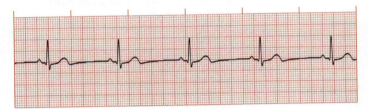

Sinus bradycardia.

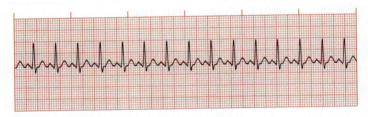

Sinus tachycardia.

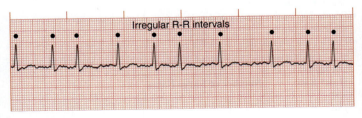

Atrial fibrillation.

CARDIO

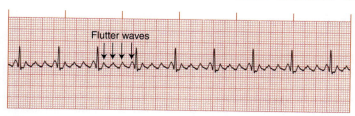

Atrial flutter.

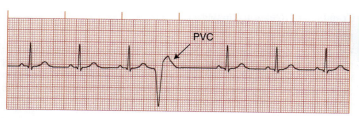

Premature ventricular contractions.

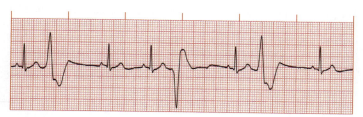

Multifocal premature ventricular contractions.

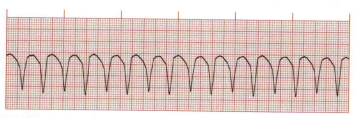

Ventricular tachycardia.

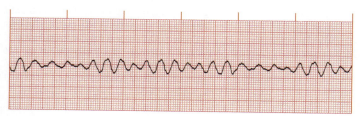

Ventricular fibrillation.

From:
Jones, SA: ECG Notes: Interpretation and Management Guide. FA Davis, Philadelphia, 2005.

Examine the Rhythm and Determine if Regular or Irregular

Assess the regularity of the RR intervals. A regular rhythm has equally sized spaces between all intervals. An intermittently irregular rhythm is generally regular with occasional disruptions (e.g., extra beats). A regularly irregular rhythm has a cyclical pattern of varying RR intervals. An irregularly irregular rhythm has no recurring pattern; RR intervals vary in an inconsistent manner.

Examples of Irregular Rhythms

Rhythm Names

Rhythms are generally named by the beat that initiates conduction to the ventricles and the rate. For example, *sinus bradycardia* is a slow rate originating in the SA node, a *junctional* (or *nodal*) *rhythm* is a normal rate originating in the AV junction, and *ventricular tachycardia* is a rapid rhythm originating in the ventricles.

Identifying P Waves

The presence of P waves indicates that myocardial conduction is initiated in the atria. A normal impulse initiated in the SA node has a P wave that is upright, rounded, and 1 to 3 mm tall. The P waves that are abnormally shaped include *flutter* (F) waves, which are also called *saw-toothed* and have a regular pattern; *fibrillation* (f), which are small, grossly irregular deflections on the baseline; and *premature* P waves, which look different and usually have a different PR interval than the regular P waves in a rhythm strip. (Premature beats are discussed in the section Identifying Extra Waves or Complexes.)

Evaluating the PR Interval for Duration and Relationship of P Wave to QRS Complex

The normal PR interval is between 0.12 and 0.20 s (3–5 small boxes). A shorter-than-normal PR interval indicates increased AV conduction or an atrial impulse that does not originate in the SA node. A longer-than-normal PR interval indicates a slowing of conduction from the SA node into the AV junction. A prolonged PR interval defines *atrioventricular heart block*. With normal conduction, a QRS complex should follow each P wave.

Type of Block	Characteristics
First degree	Prolonged PR interval; all P waves are followed by a QRS complex.
Second-degree Mobitz type I (Wenckebach)	Progressive lengthening of the PR interval until one P wave is not conducted (no QRS follows a P wave). Occurs as a regular irregularity.
Mobitz type II	Atrial rate is regular, but some impulses are not conducted from the SA node through the AV junction. Ratio of conduction (e.g., 2:1 or 3:1) is regular. Occurs as a regular irregularity.

CARDIO

Third degree (complete)	No conduction of impulse through the AV junction; no relationship between atrial and ventricular activity. Atrial and ventricular rhythms may be regular, but the ventricular rate is initiated below the AV node and is slow and independent of atrial activity.

Evaluation of QRS Complex for Shape and Duration

All QRS complexes should be identical to one another. The normal duration of a QRS complex is 0.06–0.10 seconds (1.5–2.5 small boxes). Bundle branch blocks (BBBs) signify conduction interference down either the right or left bundle. Although both demonstrate a widened QRS complex, an RBBB has a notched and widened R component, and an LBBB has only a widened R. Bundle branch blocks are best diagnosed with a 12-lead ECG. Irregularities in ventricular conduction include flutter, fibrillation, and PVCs. Flutter and fibrillation usually develop following ventricular tachycardia and show a progressive degeneration of organized myocardial electrical activity.

Identifying Extra Waves or Complexes

Extra waves or complexes signify myocardial irritability. The problem may be atrial, junctional (nodal), and/or ventricular. The severity of a dysrhythmia is related to the location, frequency, and number of sites where extra beats are initiated.

Supraventricular Dysrhythmias

Premature atrial contractions (PACs) arise from an ectopic atrial focus. Their P waves look different from normal and also usually have a different PR interval. *Premature junctional (nodal) contractions* (PJCs) originate in the AV junction; the P wave may be inverted owing to retrograde conduction and may occur before, following, and buried within the QRS complex. Both PACs and PJCs have normally shaped QRS complexes and are generally not dangerous unless frequent or associated with signs and symptoms of altered hemodynamics.

Premature ventricular contractions (PVCs) are the most dangerous and are classified by frequency and irritable foci. The PVCs are not preceded by a P wave, are conducted abnormally through the ventricles, and are characterized by wide, bizarre QRS complexes. *Unifocal PVCs* arise from a single irritable focus and are identically shaped; *multifocal PVCs* come from different sites and do not look alike. Frequency of PVCs is described by the terms *single quadrigeminy* (one PVC every fourth beat), *trigeminy* (one every third beat), and *bigeminy* (every other beat is a PVC). Paired PVCs are called *couplets* and a run of PVCs is called a *salvo*. As PVCs signify ventricular irritability, multiple sites and increasing frequency are potentially lethal because the cardiac rhythm may disintegrate into ventricular tachycardia, fibrillation, or asystole. More than six PVCs per minute is considered dangerous. Particularly lethal is a PVC that falls on a T wave (R on T phenomenon). It does not allow the ventricle to repolarize, and ventricular fibrillation is likely to ensue.

Major Risk Factors for Coronary Heart Disease

Cigarette smoking
Hypertension (blood pressure $\geq$140/90 mm Hg)
Low HDL cholesterol
Family history (Coronary heart disease in male first-degree relative at an age
    younger than 55 years or coronary heart disease in female first-degree rel-
    ative younger than 65 years)
Age (men $\geq$45 years and women $\geq$55 years)
Physical inactivity

Cholesterol

TABLE 5.29 **Normal Values for Fasting Lipoprotein Levels**

Lipid	Values (in mg/dL)	Classification
LDL cholesterol	<100	Optimal
	100–129	Near optimal/above optimal
	130–159	Borderline high
	160–189	High
	$\geq$190	Very high
Total cholesterol	<200	Desirable
	200–239	Borderline high
	$\geq$240	High
HDL cholesterol	<40	Low
	$\geq$60	High

FROM: National Heart Lung Blood Institute. *ATP III Guidelines-At-A-Glance.* http://
www.nhlbi.nih.gov/guidelines/cholesterol/atglance.pdf. Accessed January 21, 2012.
LDL = low-density lipoprotein; HDL = high-density lipoprotein.

Metabolic Syndrome

The presence of three or more of the following five modifiable cardiovascular risk factors places an individual at risk for cardiovascular disease and
type 2 diabetes.

- Waist circumference
  - >102 cm (>40 in.) for men
  - >88 cm (>35 in.) for women
- Blood pressure
  - $\geq$130 mm Hg systolic and/or
  - $\geq$85 mm Hg diastolic

- Fasting glucose
  - ≥110 mg/dL or 6.1 mmol/L
- Triglycerides
  - ≥150 mg/dL or 1.69 mmol/L
- HDL cholesterol
  - <40 mg/dL (1.04 mmol/L) in men
  - <50 mg/dL (1.29 mmol/l) in women

From:

National Heart Lung Blood Institute. ATP III Guidelines-At-A-Glance.
http://www.nhlbi.nih.gov/guidelines/cholesterol/atglance.pdf. Accessed January 21, 2012.

Cardiac Dysfunction

CARDIO

TABLE 5.30 Diagnostic Tests for Cardiac Dysfunction

Procedure	Description
Cardiac catheterization (for angiography)	The coronary arteries are injected with a contrast material, and the arterial system can be visualized with cinefluoroscopy: narrowing or occlusion of arteries can be evaluated.
Cardiac catheterization	Catheterization is used to measure intracardiac, transvalve, and pulmonary artery pressures and measure blood gas pressures to determine cardiac output and evaluate shunting.
Continuous hemodynamic monitoring	Pulmonary artery catheterization (Swan-Ganz) provides immediate cardiopulmonary pressure measurements. An invasive bedside (intensive care unit) procedure that evaluates left ventricular function. A balloon-tipped, flow-directed catheter, connected to a transducer and a monitor, is used to allow measurements of pulmonary artery pressure; pulmonary capillary wedge pressure; cardiac output; and mixed venous saturation, which evaluates pulmonary vascular resistance and tissue oxygenation.
Electron beam computed tomography (EBCT)	A noninvasive test that can be used to detect the buildup of calcium in the coronary arteries. EBCT is much faster than standard computed tomography, and therefore can obtain an accurate image while the heart is beating.

(table continues on page 462)

◗ **TABLE 5.30** **Diagnostic Tests for Cardiac Dysfunction** (continued)

Procedure	Description
Echocardiography a. Transthoracic (TTE)	The reflections of ultrasound waves from cardiac surfaces are analyzed. It is used to evaluate left ventricular systolic function and the structure and function of cardiac walls, valves, and chambers; it can identify abnormal conditions such as tumors or pericardial effusion.
b. Transesophageal (TEE)	Transesophageal echocardiography is performed through the esophagus and stomach by a modified gastroscopy probe with one or two ultrasound transducers at its tip. TEE provides better image resolution and superior images of posterior cardiac structures. Continuous imaging is possible during operations or invasive procedures.
Electrocardiogram (ECG)	Surface electrodes record the electrical activity of the heart. A 12-lead ECG provides 12 views of the heart; it is used to assess cardiac rhythm, to diagnose the location, extent, and acuteness of myocardial ischemia and infarction; and to evaluate changes with activity.
Exercise stress tests	Numerous protocols for exercise tests have been used to assess responses to increased workloads with steps, treadmills, or bicycle ergometers. In conjunction with ECG and blood pressure recordings, patients are evaluated for exercise capacity, cardiac dysrhythmias, and diagnosis, prognosis, and management of coronary artery disease.
Hemodynamic monitoring	See Continuous hemodynamic monitoring.
Holter monitoring	Continuous ambulatory ECG monitoring done by recording the cardiac rhythm for a period of time (from 24 hours up to a month). Used to evaluate cardiac rhythm, efficacy of medications, transient symptoms that may indicate cardiac disease, and pacemaker function; and to correlate symptoms with activity.
Pharmacological stress tests	A noninvasive assessment for patients with coronary disease who are unable to achieve adequate cardiac stress with exercise. An incremental infusion of dobutamine or adenosine is given causing an increase in the myocardial oxygen demand. Echocardiographic evaluation of cardiac wall motion abnormalities is performed with simultaneous evaluation of ECG and BP.

CARDIO

Procedure	Description
Phonocardiography	This test records cardiac sounds. Times the events of the cardiac cycle and confirms auscultatory findings.
Radionuclide angiography	Red blood cells tagged (marked) with a radionuclide are injected into blood. Ventricular wall motion can be evaluated and the ejection fraction determined; abnormal blood flow with valve and congenital defects can also be detected; techniques include gated-pool equilibrium studies and first-pass techniques.
Technetium-99m scanning (hot spot imaging)	Technetium-99m injected into blood is taken up by damaged myocardial tissue; this identifies and localizes acute myocardial infarctions
Thallium-201 myocardial perfusion imaging (cold spot imaging)	Thallium-201 injected into blood at peak exercise; scanning identifies ischemic and infarcted myocardium, which does not take up thallium-201. The test is used to diagnose coronary artery disease and perfusion, particularly when ECG is equivocal.

CARDIO

Ratings of Perceived Exertion

🔶 TABLE 5.31 Borg Scales for Rating of Perceived Exertion (RPE)

The original scale (6–20) is on the left and the 10-point category ratio (CR) scale is on the right.

Borg RPE Scale	CR10 Scale
6 No exertion at all	0 Nothing at all
7	0.5 Extremely weak (just noticeable)
8 Extremely light	1 Very weak
9 Very light	2 Weak (light)
10	3 Moderate
11 Light	4
12	5 Strong (heavy)
13 Somewhat hard	6
14	7 Very strong

(table continues on page 464)

TABLE 5.31 Borg Scales for Rating of Perceived Exertion (RPE) (continued)

Borg RPE Scale	CR10 Scale
15 Hard (heavy)	8
16	9
17 Very hard	10 Extremely strong ("maximal")
18	
19 Extremely hard	* Absolute maximum (Highest possible)
20 Maximal exertion	

Copyright Gunnar Borg. Reproduced with permission. From: Borg, G: *Borg's Perceived Exertion and Pain Scales.* Human Kinetics, Champaign, IL, 1998.
For more information: Borg, GA: Psychophysical bases of perceived exertion. *Med Sci Sports Exerc* 14:377, 1982.

Exercise Testing

TABLE 5.32 Commonly Used Treadmill Exercise Testing Protocols

Bruce Protocol			
Stage	mph	Grade %	Duration of Stage (min)
I	1.7	10	3
II	2.5	12	3
III	3.4	14	3
IV	4.2	16	3
V	5.0	18	3
Balke Protocol			
Begins at 3.3 mph, 0% grade. Each minute grade increases 1%.			

TABLE 5.33 **YMCA Cycle Ergometer Test**

Uses two to four consecutive 3-min workloads (multistage test). Goal is to achieve a heart rate between 110% and 85% of age-predicted maximal heart rate for at least two consecutive stages. Heart rate is monitored during each stage for the final 15 sec of each minute.

First stage	150 kg-m/min for 3 min

Second stage	If the heart rate during the third minute of the first stage is:
	    <80 beats/min, the second stage is 750 kg-m/min for 3 min
	    80–89 beats/min, the second stage is 600 kg-m/min for 3 min
	    90–100 beats/min, the second stage is 450 kg-m/min for 3 min
	    >100 beats/min, the second stage is 300 kg-m/min for 3 min

Third stage	Add 150 kg-m/min to the work rate for the second stage and perform this rate for 3 min
Fourth stage (if required)	Add 150 kg-m/min to the work rate for the second stage and perform this rate for 3 min

CARDIO

6-Minute Walk Test (6MWT)

The 6-minute walk test is a submaximal exercise test to measure endurance of patients with cardiovascular and pulmonary problems. Recommended that the test is performed indoors, in a flat, straight 30-meter corridor that is seldom traveled. The turnaround points should be marked with a cone. The distance walked in 6 minutes is required. The patient is allowed to rest as necessary, although timing continues during the rest(s).

Conditions

Dysrhythmias

Determining the Clinical Significance of a Dysrhythmia

Dysrhythmias result in varying degrees of abnormal hemodynamics. Cardiac output is decreased with very slow or very rapid rates.

Dysrhythmias Classified by Their Effect on Cardiac Output
Dysrhythmias Associated With Normal or Near Normal Hemodynamics (Generally Benign)

- Sinus rhythm with premature atrial contractions
- Sinus rhythm with premature junctional contractions
- Artificial pacemaker rhythm with 1:1 capture
- Atrial fibrillation with an average ventricular response between 60 and 100/min
- Atrial flutter with an average ventricular response between 60 and 100/min
- Sinus rhythm with first-degree AV block
- Sinus rhythm with occasional premature ventricular contractions
- Sinus bradycardia averaging 50–60/min
- AV junctional rhythm averaging 50–60/min

- Sinus rhythm with second-degree AV block Mobitz type 1
- Isorhythmic AV dissociation

Dysrhythmias With Normal or Near Normal Hemodynamics but That Are Potentially Dangerous

- Sinus rhythm with short episodes of ventricular tachycardia
- Sinus rhythm with short episodes of paroxysmal supraventricular tachycardia
- Accelerated junctional rhythms
- Artificial pacemaker rhythm with premature ventricular contractions that are new, multifocal, or couplets
- Sinus rhythm with second-degree AV block Mobitz type 2
- Atrial flutter or fibrillation with tachycardia ventricular rates
- Sinus rhythm with sinus arrest
- Sinus bradycardia with rates below 50/min

Dysrhythmias With Significantly Altered Hemodynamics

- Ventricular tachycardia (with pulses)
- Sinus rhythm or atrial fibrillation with complete heart block
- Very slow (40/min or below) sinus, junctional, or idioventricular rhythms
- Malfunctioning artificial pacemakers with idioventricular rhythms

Dysrhythmias Associated With Absent Hemodynamics—Lethal Conditions

- Ventricular fibrillation
- Asystole
- Pulseless ventricular tachycardia or flutter
- Agonal idioventricular complexes
- Electromechanical dissociation
- Third-degree AV heart block with ventricular standstill

● TABLE 5.34 Common Forms of Arrhythmias

Classification	Characteristic Rhythm
Sinus Arrhythmias	
Sinus tachycardia	>100 beats/min
Sinus bradycardia	<60 beats/min
Sick sinus syndrome	Severe bradycardia (<50 beats/min); periods of sinus arrest
Supraventricular Arrhythmias	
Atrial fibrillation and flutter	Atrial rate >300 beats/min
Atrial tachycardia	Atrial rate >140–200 beats/min
Premature atrial contractions	Variable

Classification	Characteristic Rhythm
Atrioventricular Junctional Arrhythmias	
Junctional rhythm	40–55 beats/min
Junctional tachycardia	100–200 beats/min
Conduction Disturbances	
Atrioventricular block	Variable
Bundle branch block	Variable
Fascicular block	Variable
Ventricular Arrhythmias	
Premature ventricular contractions	Variable
Ventricular tachycardia	140–200 beats/min
Ventricular fibrillation	Irregular, totally uncoordinated rhythm

From: Ciccone, CD: *Pharmacology in Rehabilitation,* ed. 4. FA Davis, Philadelphia, 2007, p 324, with permission.

Drug Treatment for Dysrhythmias

TABLE 5.35 Classification of Antiaryhthmic Drugs

Generic Names	Trade Names
Class I: Sodium Channel Blockers	
Subclass A Disopyramide	Norpace
Procainamide	Promine, Pronestyl, Procan
Quinidine	Cardioquin, Duraquin, others
Subclass B Lidocaine	Xylocaine
Mexiletine	Mexitil
Moricizine*	Ethmozine
Subclass C Flecainide	Tambocor
Propafenone	Rythmol

(table continues on page 468)

CARDIO

⬤ TABLE 5.35 Classification of Antiaryhthmic Drugs (continued)

Generic Names	Trade Names
Class II: Betablockers	
Acebutolol	Sectral
Atenolol	Tenormin
Esmolol	Brevibloc
Metoprolol	Lopressor
Nadolol	Corgard
Propranolol	Inderal
Sotalol	Betapace
Timolol	Blocadren
Class III: Drugs That Prolong Repolarization	
Amiodarone†	Cordarone
Bretylium	Bretylol
Dofetilide	Tikosyn
Ibutilide	Corvert
Class IV: Calcium Channel	
Blockers Diltiazem	Cardizem, Dilacor
Verapamil	Calan, Isoptin, Verlan

From: Ciccone, CD: *Pharmacology in Rehabilitation,* ed. 4. FA Davis, Philadelphia, 2007, p 325, with permission.
*Also has some class IC properties.
†Also has some properties from the other three drug classes.

Hypertension

Clinical Significance of Blood Pressure and Related Measures of Cardiac Function

■ TABLE 5.36 **Changes in Blood Pressure, Cardiac Output, and Peripheral Vascular Resistance With Age**

Age (yr)	Blood Pressure (mm Hg)			Blood Flow		Peripheral Vascular Resistance†	
	Systolic/Diastolic	Mean Arterial Pressure	Cardiac Index* (L/min/m²)	Cardiac Output L/min)	mm Hg / L / min	dyne · sec · cm¹
10	90/60	70	3.7	4.4	14.7	1,180
20	110/70	83	3.5	6.0	13.0	1,040
30	115/75	88	3.4	5.8	14.3	1,140
40	120/80	93	3.3	5.6	15.7	1,260
50	125/82	96	3.2	5.4	16.9	1,350
60	130/85	100	3.0	5.1	18.6	1,480
70	135/88	104	2.9	4.9	20.2	1,600
80	140/90	107	2.8	4.8	21.3	1,700

From: Wilson, RF: *Critical Care Manual: Applied Physiology and Principles of Therapy*, ed. 2. FA Davis, Philadelphia, 1992, p 24, with permission.
*Assuming a body surface area of 1.2 m² at age 10 and 1.7 m² thereafter.
†Assuming a central venous pressure (CVP) of 5 mm Hg.

CARDIO

🔴 TABLE 5.37 Classification of Blood Pressures in Adults

Category	Blood Pressure (in mm Hg)
Normal	Systolic <120; diastolic <80
Prehypertension	Systolic 120–139; diastolic 80–89
Hypertension Stage 1 Stage 2	Systolic ≥140; diastolic >90 Systolic 140–159; diastolic 90–99 Systolic ≥160; diastolic >100

From: *The Seventh Report of the Joint National Committee on Prevention, Detection, Evaluation, and Treatment of High Blood Pressure.* 2004. http://www.nhlbi.nih.gov/guidelines/hypertension/jnc7full.pdf. Accessed January 21, 2012.

🔴 TABLE 5.38 Classification of Blood Pressures in Children and Adolescents

Category	Systolic or Diastolic Blood Pressure, Percentile
Normal	<90th
Prehypertension	90th to <95th or if blood pressure exceeds 120/80 even if <90th percentile up to <95th percentile
Hypertension Stage 1 Stage 2	95th to 99th percentile plus 5 mm Hg >99th percentile plus 5 mm Hg

Screening for Hypertension

For the adult general population the *Seventh Report of the Joint National Committee on Prevention, Detection, Evaluation, and Treatment of High Blood Pressure* recommends the following:

- Screening every 2 years for persons with blood pressure less than 120/80 mm Hg
- Screening every year for persons with systolic blood pressure of 120 to 139 mm Hg or diastolic blood pressure of 80 to 89 mm Hg
- Recheck in 2 months for those with stage I hypertension (systolic blood pressure of 140 to 159 mm Hg or diastolic blood pressure of 90 to 99 mm Hg)
- Evaluate or refer to source of care in 1 month for those with stage II hypertension (systolic blood pressure of ≥140 mm Hg or diastolic blood pressure of ≥90 mm Hg)
- for those with higher pressures (e.g., 180/110 mm Hg), evaluate and treat immediately or within 1 week depending on clinical situation and complications.

TABLE 5.39 Drug Treatment for Hypertension and Cardiac Disease: Stepped-Care Approach to Hypertension

STEP 1: In patients with mild hypertension, drug therapy is usually initiated with a single agent (monotherapy) from one of the following classes: a diuretic, a beta blocker, an angiotensin converting enzyme (ACE) inhibitor, or a calcium channel blocker.

STEP 2: If a single drug is unsuccessful in reducing blood pressure, a second agent is added. The second drug can be from one of the initial classes not used in step 1, or it can be from a second group that includes the centrally acting agents (clonidine, guanabenz), presynaptic adrenergic inhibitors (reserpine, guanethidine), alpha-1 blockers (prazosin, doxazosin), and vasodilators (hydralazine, minoxidil).

STEP 3: A third agent is added, usually from one of the classes listed in step 2 that has not already been used. Three different agents from three different classes are often administered concurrently in this step.

STEP 4: A fourth drug is added from still another class.

From: Ciccone, CD: *Pharmacology in Rehabilitation,* ed. 4. FA Davis, Philadelphia, 2007, p 300, with permission.

CARDIO

TABLE 5.40 Antihypertensive Drug Categories

Category	Primary Site(s) of Action	Primary Antihypertensive Effect(s)
Diuretics	Kidneys	Decrease in plasma fluid volume
Sympatholytics	Various sites within the sympathetic division of the autonomic nervous system	Decrease sympathetic influence on the heart and/or peripheral vasculature
Vasodilators	Peripheral vasculature	Lower vascular resistance by directly vasodilating peripheral vessels
Inhibition of the renin-angiotensin system (ACE inhibitors and angiotensin II receptor blockers)	Peripheral vasculature and certain organs with a functional renin-angiotensin system (heart, kidneys)	ACE inhibitors: prevent the conversion of angiotensin I to angiotensin II. Angiotensin II receptor blockers: block the effects of angiotensin II on the vasculature and various other tissues
Calcium channel blockers	Limit calcium entry into vascular smooth muscle and cardiac muscle	Decrease vascular smooth-muscle contraction; decrease myocardial force and rate of contraction

From: Ciccone, CD: *Pharmacology in Rehabilitation,* ed. 4. FA Davis, Philadelphia, 2007, p 291, with permission.
ACE = angiotensin converting enzyme.

TABLE 5.41 Sympatholytic Drugs Used to Treat Hypertension

Beta Blockers
Acebutolol (Sectral)
Atenolol (Tenormin)
Betaxolol (Kerlone)
Bisoprolol (Zebeta)
Carteolol (Cartrol)
Labetalol (Normodyne; Trandate)
Metoprolol (Lopressor, others)
Nadolol (Corgard)
Oxprenolol (Trasicor)
Penbutolol (Levatol)
Pindolol (Visken)
Propranolol (Inderal)
Sotalol (Betapace)
Timolol (Blocadren)
Alpha-Blockers
Doxazosin (Cardura)
Phenoxybenzamine (Dibenzyline)
Prazocin (Minipress)
Terazosin (Hytrin)

Presynaptic Adrenergic Inhibitors
Guanadrel (Hylorel)
Guanethidine (Ismelin)
Reserpine (Serpalan, others)

Centrally Acting Agents
Clonidine (Catapres)
Guanabenz (Wytensin)
Guanfacine (Tenex)
Methyldopa (Aldomet)

Ganglionic Blockers
Mecamylamine (Inversine)
Trimethaphan (Arfonad)

From: Ciccone, CD: *Pharmacology in Rehabilitation,* ed. 4. FA Davis, Philadelphia, 2007, p 293, with permission.

TABLE 5.42 Antihypertensive Vasodilators, Angiotensin-Converting Enzyme (ACE) Inhibitors, and Calcium Channel Blockers

Vasodilators	
Diazoxide (Hyperstat)	Minoxidil (Loniten)
Hydralazine (Apresoline)	Nitroprusside (Nipride, Nitropress)
ACE Inhibitors	
Benazepril (Lotensin)	Moexipril (Univasc)
Captopril (Capoten)	Perindopril (Aceon)
Enalapril (Vasotec)	Quinapril (Accupril)
Fosinopril (Monopril)	Ramipril (Altace)
Lisinopril (Prinivil, Zestril)	Trandolapril (Mavik)
Angiotensin II Receptor Blockers	
Candesartan (Atacand)	Telmisartan (Micardis)
Irbesartan (Avapro)	Valsartan (Diovan)
Losartan (Cozaar)	

Calcium Channel Blockers	
Amlodipine (Norvasc)	Nicardipine (Cardene)
Bepridil (Vascor)	Nifedipine (Adalat, Procardia)
Diltiazem (Cardizem)	Nimodipine (Nimotop)
Felodipine (Plendil)	Verapamil (Calan, Isoptin)
Isradipine (DynaCirc)	

From: Ciccone, CD: *Pharmacology in Rehabilitation,* ed 4. FA Davis, Philadelphia, 2007, p 296, with permission.
ACE = angiotensin-converting enzyme.

CARDIO

● TABLE 5.43 Summary of Common Beta Blockers

Generic Name	Trade Name(s)	Selectivity	Primary Indications*
Acebutolol	Sectral	Beta-1	Hypertension, arrhythmias
Atenolol	Tenormin	Beta-1	Angina pectoris, hypertension, prevent reinfarction
Betaxolol	Kerlone	Beta-1	Hypertension
Bisoprolol	Zebeta	Beta-1	Hypertension
Carteolol	Cartrol	Nonselective	Hypertension
Labetalol	Normodyne, Trandate	Nonselective	Hypertension
Metoprolol	Lopressor, Toprol-XL	Beta-1	Angina pectoris, hypertension, prevent reinfarction
Nadolol	Corgard	Nonselective	Angina pectoris, hypertension
Penbutolol	Levatol	Nonselective	Hypertension
Pindolol	Visken	Nonselective	Hypertension
Propranolol	Inderal	Nonselective	Angina pectoris, arrhythmias, hypertension, prevent reinfarction, prevent vascular headache

(table continues on page 474)

TABLE 5.43 Summary of Common Beta Blockers (continued)

Generic Name	Trade Name(s)	Selectivity	Primary Indications*
Sotalol	Betapace	Nonselective	Arrhythmias
Timolol	Blocadren	Nonselective	Hypertension, prevent reinfarction, prevent vascular headache

From: Ciccone, CD: *Pharmacology in Rehabilitation,* ed. 4. FA Davis, Philadelphia, 2007, p 282, with permission.
*Only indications listed in the United States product labeling are included in this table. All drugs are fairly similar pharmacologically, and some may be used for appropriate cardiovascular conditions not specifically listed in product labeling.

Angina Pectoris

Angina pectoris is an oppresive pain or pressure in the chest caused by ischemia to the cardiac tissue. The pain may radiate to other parts of the body including the left > right arm, the posterior neck, lower jaw, upper back, between the shoulder blades, and the abdomen.

TABLE 5.44 Diuretic Drugs Used to Treat Hypertension

Thiazide Diuretics
Bendroflumethiazide (Naturetin)
Chlorothiazide (Diuril)
Chlorthalidone (Hygroton, others)
Hydrochlorohiazide (Esidrix, others)
Hydroflumethiazide (Diucardin, Saluron)
Methylothiazide (Enduron, others)
Metolazone (Diulo, Mykrox, Zaroxolyn)
Polythiazide (Renese)
Quinethazone (Hydromox)
Trichlormethiazide (Metahydrin, Naqua)

Loop Diuretics
Bumetanide (Bumex)
Ethacrynic acid (Edecrin)
Fusosemide (Lasix, others)

Potassium-Sparing Diuretics
Amiloride (Midamor)
Spironolactone (Aldactone)
Triamterene (Dyrenium)

From: Ciccone, CD: *Pharmacology in Rehabilitation,* ed. 4. FA Davis, Philadelphia, 2007, p 291, with permission.

Levels of Angina

1+ Light or barely noticeable
2+ Moderate, bothersome
3+ Severe and very uncomfortable
4+ Most severe pain ever experienced

TABLE 5.45 Types of Angina Pectoris

Classification	Cause	Drug Therapy
Stable angina	Myocardial oxygen demand exceeds oxygen supply; usually brought on by physical exertion	Sublingual/lingual nitroglycerin in typically used at the onset of an acute episode; a beta blocker or a long-acting nitrate is often used to prevent attacks
Variant angina	Myocardial oxygen supply decreases due to coronary vasospasm; may occur while patient is at rest	Treated primarily with a calcium channel blockers
Unstable angina	Myocardial oxygen supply decreases at the same time that oxygen demand increases; can occur at any time secondary to atherosclerotic plaque rupture within the coronary artery	May require a combination of drugs – that is, a calcium channel blocker plus a beta-blocker. Anticoagulant drugs are also helpful in preventing thrombogenesis and coronary occlusion

From: Ciccone, CD: *Pharmacology in Rehabilitation,* ed. 4. FA Davis, Philadelphia, 2007, p 313, with permission.

See Tables 5.42 and 5.43 on pages 472–473 for calcium channel blockers and beta blockers that may also be used for treatment of angina.

CARDIO

TABLE 5.46   Organic Nitrates Used for the Treatment of Angina Pectoris

Dosage Form	Onset of Action	Duration of Action
Nitroglycerin		
Oral	20–45 min	4–6 hr
Buccal (extended release)	2–3 min	3–5 hr
Sublingual/lingual	1–3 min	30–60 min
Ointment	30 min	4–8 hr
Transdermal patches	Within 30 min	8–24 hr
Isosorbide Dinitrate		
Oral	15–40 min	4–6 hr
Oral (extended release)	30 min	12 hr
Chewable	2–5 min	1–2 hr
Sublingual	2–5 min	1–2 hr
Isosorbide Mononitrate		
Oral	30–60 min	6–8 hr
Amyl Nitrite		
Inhaled	30 sec	3–5 min

From: Ciccone, CD: *Pharmacology in Rehabilitation,* ed. 4. FA Davis, Philadelphia, 2007, p 308, with permission.

Acute Myocardial Infarction

Myocardial infarction (heart attack) is the development of ischemia due to cardiac artery occlusion that results in the death of cardiac tissue. The incidence in the U.S. population is 1.5 million persons annually and is reponsible for 500,000 deaths per year.

Signs and Symptoms

Signs and symptoms of acute myocardial infarction include a pain similar to that for angina pectoris but may be more intense. There is a heaviness, squeezing, or tight feeling in the chest; nausea and vomiting; lightheadedness; dyspnea and hypotension; sweating; weakness; and apprehension. There may be fever, shock, and cardiac failure. Symptoms may not follow this classic pattern in women who may also report shortness of breath and chronic unexplained fatigue. Women may also report continuous pain in the midthoracic or interscapular regions and neck or shoulder pain. Silent attacks, without symptoms, may also occur. These are more frequent among persons with diabetes, nonwhites, adults older than 75 years, and smokers.

Myocardial Enzymes

Tissue necrosis causes enzymes to be released into the blood. Enzymes released by myocardial damage demonstrate a characteristic pattern and duration of pressure in the blood.

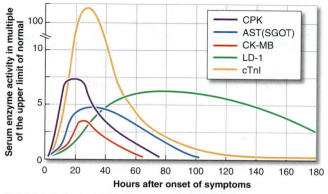

Stylized depiction (assembled from multiple sources) of the time-activity curves of CPK, CK-MB, LD-1, AST (SGOT), and cTnI following onset of acute myocardial infarction (defined on the basis of sentinel-persistent chest pain).

TABLE 5.47 Myocardial Enzymes

Abbreviation for Enzyme	Enzyme (normal value)	Description
AST (formerly called SGOT)	Aspartate aminotransferase (serum glutamic oxaloacetic transaminase) (<45 U/mL)	Enzyme appears in serum within hours, peaks at 12–24 hr, falls to normal within 2–7 days. AST is also released due to damage to muscle, brain tissue, and other internal organs.
CPK (CK)	Creatine phosphokinase (20–232 U/mL)	Enzyme appears in serum within hours, peaks within 24 hr, falls to normal within 3–5 days. CPK is also released due to damage to brain tissue and skeletal muscle.
CK-MB	Creatine kinase myocardial band isoenzyme (0–8 ng/mL)	Isoenzyme of CPK more specific for myocardial damage; appears in serum at 3–6 hr, peaks at 12–24 hr, falls to normal within 48 hr.
REL INDEX	Relative index (0–2.5%)	Relative index calculations are only of value if CK-MB is >8 ng/mL and CPK exceeds upper limit. An index >2.5% is highly suggestive of myocardial damage.

(table continues on page 478)

CARDIO

⬤ TABLE 5.47 Myocardial Enzymes (continued)

Abbreviation for Enzyme	Enzyme (normal value)	Description
LDH (LD)	Lactate dehydrogenase (<600 U/mL)	Enzyme begins to rise 12–24 hr, peaks by day three, and returns to normal within 8–12 days. LDH is also released due to damage to brain, red blood cell tissue, kidney, lung, and spleen.
cTnI	Cardiac troponin I (<0.6 ng/mL)	Sensitive and specific marker of myocardial injury. Appears in serum at 3–6 hr, peaks at 14–48 hr, returns to normal in 7–14 days.
BNP	Brain natriuretic peptide ≤100 pg/mL)	Diagnostic for congestive heart failure. Prognostic marker for acute coronary syndromes.

Electrocardiographic Changes After Myocardial Infarctions

Serial 12-lead ECG recordings are used to diagnose the presence and evolution of AMI. Injury is localized by the presence of abnormal waves on specific ECG leads. The standard 12-lead electrocardiogram includes limb leads I to III, aVR, aVL, and aVF; and chest leads V1 to V6.

⬤ TABLE 5.48 Changes in 12-Lead Electrocardiographs (ECG) Associated With Location of Infarction

Infarction site:
1. Anterior infarction   Q or QS in V1–V4
2. Lateral infarction   Q or QS in lead I, aVL
3. Inferior infarction   Q or QS in leads II, III, aVF
4. Posterior infarction   Large R waves in V1–V3
                                ST depression V1, V2, or V3

From: O'Sullivan, SB, and Schmitz, TJ: *Physical Rehabilitation,* ed. 5. FA Davis, Philadelphia, 2007, p 603.

Surgical Management of Coronary Artery Disease

Coronary Artery Bypass Grafts

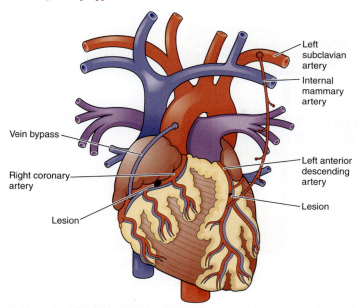

Coronary artery bypass graft procedures. (A) Saphenous vein bypass graft. Leg vein is sutured to ascending aorta and to right coronary artery beyond critical stenosis, creating vascular conduit to shunt blood around blockage to ischemic myocardium. (B) Mammary artery graft procedure. Mammary artery is anastomosed to anterior descending branch of left coronary artery distal to blockage so blood flow is reestablished.

Pacemakers

Pacemakers are implanted to help manage conduction or rhythm disturbances. The pulse generator is surgically implanted into a subcutaneous pouch in the pectoral or abdominal area. Endocardial leads are positioned in the right atrium, right ventricle, or both. The lead wire is connected to the pulse generator to complete the circuit. The pulse generator senses electrical activity in the heart and stimulates the heart according to the pacemaker type and program parameters. Many surgeons may limit use of the arm closest to the lead insertion for ~2 weeks after insertion, until the lead wires are firmly attached to the myocardial wall.

Percutaneous Transluminal Coronary Angioplasty

Percutaneous transluminal coronary angioplasty (PTCA) is a nonsurgical technique using a balloon-tipped catheter to achieve coronary reperfusion. Under fluoroscopic guidance the PTCA catheter is advanced across the middle of the coronary lesion. The balloon is inflated and reduces the constriction by physically splitting the atheromatous plaque and stretching the arterial wall. Many PTCAs involve stent placement. The rehabilitation clinician should be aware of risk for bleeding at the groin insertion site and may need to modify activities.

CARDIO

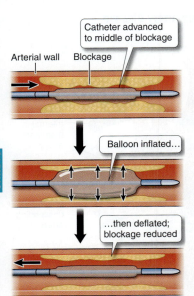

Percutaneous transluminal coronary angioplasty (PTCA) with stent placement.

Heart Failure

Heart failure results when the myocardium is unable to maintain adequate circulation of the blood for respiration and metabolism. There may be failure of the right or left ventricle or both.

TABLE 5.49 Pacemaker Classification System

Pacemakers are commonly identified using a three-letter code as per the first three columns. Pacemakers that also have the capacity to respond to physiological stimuli are identified by the code in the fourth column.

Chamber(s) Paced	Chamber(s) Sensed	Response to Sensing	Rate Responsive Pacing
O = None	O = None	O = None	R = Rate responsive
A = Atrium	A = Atrium	T = Triggered	
V = Ventricle	V = Ventricle	I = Inhibited	
D = Dual (A&V)	D = Dual (A&V)	D = Dual (T&I)	

Based on: O'Sullivan, SB, and Schmitz, T: *Physical Rehabilitation,* ed. 5. FA Davis, Philadelphia, 2007, p 634.

TABLE 5.50 New York Heart Association Classifications of Chronic Heart Failure

Functional Classification	Description
Class I	Patients with cardiac disease but without resulting limitations of physical activity. Ordinary physical activity does not cause undue fatigue, palpitation, dyspnea, or anginal pain.
Class II	Patients with cardiac disease resulting in slight limitation of physical activity. Patients are comfortable at rest. Ordinary physical activity results in fatigue, palpitation, dyspnea, or anginal pain.
Class III	Patients with cardiac disease resulting in marked limitation of physical activity. Patients are comfortable at rest. Less than ordinary physical activity causes fatigue, palpitation, dyspnea, or anginal pain.
Class IV	Patients with cardiac disease resulting in inability to carry on any physical activity without discomfort. Symptoms of cardiac insufficiency or of the anginal syndrome may be present even at rest. If any physical activity is undertaken, discomfort is increased.
Class A	Patients with cardiac disease whose physical activity need not be restricted in any way.
Class B	Patients with cardiac disease whose ordinary physical activity need not be restricted but who should be advised against severe or competitive efforts.
Class C	Patients with cardiac disease whose ordinary physical activity should be moderately restricted and whose more strenuous efforts should be discontinued.
Class D	Patients with cardiac disease whose ordinary physical activity should be markedly restricted.
Class E	Patients with cardiac disease who should be at complete rest or confined to bed or chair.

Reprinted by permission of the American Heart Association, New York.

CARDIO

TABLE 5.51 Types of Heart Failure

Type	Description
Backward	Venous return to the heart is reduced, with resulting venous stasis and congestion.
Congestive	Systemic congestion (edema, enlarged liver, elevated venous pressure) due to right heart failure and/or pulmonary congestion due to left heart failure.
Forward	Cardiac output is greatly reduced due to left ventricular failure, as after myocardial infarction when the ventricle has lost contractility.
High output	Cardiac failure that results from conditions that increase the amount of circulation, as with a large arteriovenous fistula or anemia.
Low output	Failure of the heart to maintain adequate cardiac output due to insufficient venous return, as with hemorrhage.

TABLE 5.52 Comparisons of Right- and Left-Sided Heart Failure

Right	Left
Elevated end-diastolic right ventricular pressure	Elevated end-diastolic left ventricular pressure Pulmonary congestion
Systemic congestion	Pulmonary edema
Enlarged liver	Dyspnea, orthopnea
Ascites	Paroxysmal nocturnal dyspnea
Jugular venous distention	Cough
Dependent (pitting) edema	Bronchospasm (cardiac asthma)
Fatigue	Fatigue
Anorexia and bloating	Oliguria
Oliguria, nocturia	Cyanosis (central)
Cyanosis (capillary stasis)	Tachycardia

Right	Left
Pleural effusion (R > L) Unexplained weight gain Etiology:	
	Etiology: Hypertension
Mitral stenosis	Coronary artery disease
Pulmonary parenchymal or vascular disease	Aortic valve disease Cardiomyopathies
Pulmonic or tricuspid valvular disease	Congenital heart defects Infective endocarditis
Infective endocarditis	High-output conditions Various connective tissue disorders

CARDIO

Valvular Dysfunction

🔶 TABLE 5.53 Primary Drugs Used in Congestive Heart Failure

Drug Group	Primary Effect
Agents That Increase Myocardial Contraction Force (positive inotropic agents)	
Digitalis Glycosides Digoxin (Lanoxin) Digitoxin (Digitaline)	Increase myocardial contractility by elevating intracellular calcium levels and facilitating actin-myosin interaction in cardiac cells; may also help normalize autonomic effects on the heart
Other Positive Inotropes Amrinone (generic) Milrinone (Primacor)	Enhance myocardial contractility by prolonging effects of cAMP, which increases intracellular calcium levels and promotes stronger actin-myosin interaction in cardiac cells
Dopamine (Intropin) Dobutamine (Dobutrex)	Stimulate cardiac beta-1 adrenergic receptors, which selectively increases myocardial contraction force
Agents That Decrease Cardiac Workload	
Angiotensin-Converting Enzyme (ACE) Inhibitors Benazepril (Lotensin) Captopril (Capoten) Enalapril (Vasotec) Fosinopril (Monopril) Lisinopril (Prinivil, Zestril) Quinapril (Accupril) Ramipril (Altace) Trandolapril (Mavik) For others, see Table 5.42.	Reduce peripheral vascular resistance by preventing angiotensin II–induced vasoconstriction and vascular hypertrophy/remodeling; also help prevent sodium and water retention by limiting aldosterone secretion, and promote vasodilation by prolonging the effects of bradykinin

(table continues on page 484)

CARDIO

● **TABLE 5.53** **Primary Drugs Used in Congestive Heart Failure** (continued)

Drug Group	Primary Effect
Agents That Decrease Cardiac Workload	
Angiotensnin II Receptor Blockers* Eprosartan (Teveten) Losartan (Cozaar) Valsartan (Diovan)	Reduces angiotensin ii-induced peripheral vascular resistance and cardiovascular hypertrophy/remodeling by blocking angiotensin II receptors on the heart and vasculature
Beta Adrenergic Blockers Acebutolol (Sectral) Atenolol (Tenormin) Carteolol (Cartrol) Carvedilol (Coreg) Labetalol (Normodyne, Trandate) Metoprolol (Lopressor) For others, see Table 5.43.	Prevent sympathetic-induced overload on the heart by blocking the effects of epinephrine and norepinephrine on the myocardium; some agents (e.g., carvedilol) may also promote peripheral vasodilation
Diuretics†	Decrease the volume of fluid the heart must pump by promoting the excretion of excess sodium and water; also reduce fluid accumulation (congestion) in the lungs and other tissues
Vasodilators Hydralazine (Apresoline) Nesiritide (Natrecor) Nitrates (isosorbide dinitrate, others) Prazosin (Minipress)	Promote dilation in the peripheral vasculature, which decreases the amount of blood returning to the heart (cardiac preload) and decreases the pressure against which the heart must pump (cardiac afterload)

From: Ciccone, CD: *Pharmacology in Rehabilitation,* ed. 4. FA Davis, Philadelphia, 2007, pp 335–356, with permission.
*Angiotensin ii-receptor blockers are not currently approved for treating heart failure; they are used primarily as an alternative if patients cannot tolerate ACE inhibitors.
†Various thiazide, loop, or potassium-sparing diuretics can be used, depending on the needs of each patient. See Table 5.44 for specific diuretic agents.

Congenital Heart Defects

The incidence of congenital cardiac anomalies is 8 per 1,000 live births. Rubella is the most common infection related to congenital cardiovascular defects. Other possible causes include exposure to x-rays, alcohol, infections or drugs, maternal diabetes, family history, and some hereditary dysplasias such as Down syndrome. Cardiac defects can be classified as cyanotic or acyanotic and then further categorized by whether pulmonary circulation is normal or increased.

Cyanotic lesions are present when the abnormality causes deoxygenated blood to enter the systemic circulation without passing through the lungs. This can result from admixture, as occurs with right-to-left shunts; pulmonary hypoperfusion; or transposition of the great vessels, which results in poor communication between the systemic and pulmonary circulations.

Common Congenital Heart Defects

Heart defects are second to prematurity as the most common cause of death in the first year of life. Medical and surgical advances have resulted in many children surving to adulthood with corrected and uncorrected defects.

Acyanotic Defects

atrial septal defect (ASD): A communication between the atria, most commonly in the foramen ovale region. Accounts for a third of all persons with congenital heart defects who survive to adulthood. Good prognosis if corrected. If not corrected, older children may have growth failure and symptoms of congestive heart failure. Adults may demonstrate fatigue or dyspnea on exertion.

ventricular septal defect (VSD): A communication between the ventricles. Allows for shunting of oxygenated blood from the left ventricle to mix with unoxygenated blood from the right ventricle. Most common congenital heart defect. Many close spontaneously. May demonstrate symptoms of pulmonary artery hypertension, congestive heart failure, dyspnea, fatigue, and intolerance of exercise. May present with frequent respiratory infections and poor growth and development.

coarction of the aorta: A constriction of the aorta near the site of the ligamentum arteriosum and can be preductal (proximal to the ductus arteriosus) or postductal (distal to the ductus arteriosus). May manifest as higher blood pressure in the upper extremities compared to the lower extremities. Infants may demonstrate congestive heart failure. Children may report headaches, fainting, hypertension, fatigue, or cold feet. Adults may be asymptomatic or report dyspnea, headaches, hypertension, dizziness, or syncope. Exercise testing recommended before participation in athletics. Increased risk of aortic dissection with pregnancy.

patent ductus arteriosus (PDA): Persistance of a communication between the main pulmonary artery and the aorta. Usually spontaneous closure by day four in normal term infants. Common in children born to mothers affected by rubella, infants born at altitudes over 10,000 feet, and premature infants weighing less than 1,500 g. In premature infants most common sympton is congestive heart failure. If does not close spontaneously may require catheterization or ductal ligation. Large defects may require a transplant.

Cyanotic Defects

transposition of the great vessels: Reversal of the great arteries. The pulmonary artery arises from the left ventricle and the aorta and coronary arteries arise from the right ventricle. Cyanosis frequent due to poorly oxygenated blood. Surgery usually recommended in first year of life with excellent long-term outcome.

tetraology of Fallot: Combination of ventricular septal defect, right ventricular outflow obstruction, overriding aorta, and right ventricular hypertrophy. Cyanosis results due to shunting of blood right to left and increases risk for arrhythmias and death. Excitement and other events that cause tachypnea can increase cyanosis and should be avoided. Squatting or knee-chest position, as well as administration of oxygen, may help cyanotic episodes. Palliative and corrective surgery may improve oxygenated blood flow.

CARDIO

⬤ TABLE 5.54   Valvular Dysfunction

Type	Description
Atresia	Congenital absence or closure.
Prolapse	Typically of the mitral valve; valve cusp falls back into atrium during systole.
Regurgitation	Incompetent valve closure allows blood to flow backwards; this is also called *insufficiency*.
Stenosis	Valve becomes stiff and fibrotic, obstructing the passage of blood through the valve.

Interventions

Exercise Prescription

Energy Consumption
Metabolic Equivalents

Metabolic equivalents (METs) are used to compare the energy cost of various activities to the resting state. Oxygen consumption in a resting state is estimated to be approximately 3.5 mL O_2/kg per minute, which is 1 MET. The oxygen consumption of an individual for a given activity is usually expressed in liters per minute or milliliters per kilogram per minute. Energy expenditure in calories depends on the weight of the individual. When the individual's weight and oxygen consumption are known, the energy expenditure in calories can be estimated.

Conversions
1 MET = 3.5 mL O_2/kg/min
1 MET = 1 kcal/kg/min
1 L O_2/min = 5 kcal

   Example: A 110-pound (50-kg) person performs a 5-MET activity for 20 minutes.

Oxygen consumption = 5 × 3.5 mL O_2/kg/min = 17.5 mL O_2/kg/min
Expressed in liters per minute = 5 × 3.5 mL O_2/kg/min × 50 kg = 875 mL O_2/min divided by 1,000 (to convert milliliters to liters) = 0.875 L O_2/min
Calories consumed = 0.875 × 5 kcal/min = 4.375 kcal/min
Total caloric consumption = 4.375 kcal/min × 20 min = 87.5 kcal

● TABLE 5.55 Normal Values for Maximal Oxygen Uptake at Different Ages

Age (yr)		Men	Women
20–29			
	mL O$_2$/kg/min	43 ± 7.2	36 ± 6.9
	METs	12	10
30–39			
	mL O$_2$/kg/min	42 ± 7.0	34 ± 6.2
	METs	12	10
40–49			
	mL O$_2$/kg/min	40 ± 7.2	32 ± 6.2
	METs	11	9
50–59			
	mL O$_2$/kg/min	36 ± 7.1	29 ± 5.4
	METs	10	8
60–69			
	mL O$_2$/kg/min	33 ± 7.3	27 ± 4.7
	METs	9	8
70–79			
	mL O$_2$/kg/min	29 ± 7.3	27 ± 5.8
	METs	8	8

From: Fletcher, GF, et al: Exercise standards for testing and training: a statement for healthcare professionals from the American Heart Association. *Circulation* 104(14):1694–1740, 2001.

Values are expressed as mean ± standard deviation. MET indicates metabolic equivalent; 1 MET = 3.5 mL O$_2$/kg/min.

Approximate Metabolic Equivalent Values for Various Activities

These values should be used as guidelines only. There is much individual variation in energy expenditure depending on how an activity is performed (e.g., speed, technique). One MET equals 3.5 mL O$_2$/kg per minute.

CARDIO

Activity	METs
Auto repair	3–4
Backpacking	7
Badminton	4.5–7
Basketball	4.5–8
Bedside commode	3
Bicycling, 10–11.9 mph	6
Bicycling, 12–13.9 mph	8
Bicycling, leisure <10 mph	4
Biycling, stationary 100 watts	5.5
Bowling	3
Canoeing, rowing, kayaking	3–12
Carpentry, general	3.5
Carrying small children	3
Chopping wood	6
Cleaning gutters	5
Cleaning house, vigorous effort (e.g. washing windows)	3
Climbing hills with 0- to 9-pound load	7
Cooking, standing or sitting	2
Dancing (aerobic)	6.5–13
Dancing (ballroom fast, e.g., disco, folk, square)	3.7–7.4
Desk work	1.5–2.5
Dressing, undressing	2
Driving car	2
Field hockey	8
Fishing (from bank)	3.5–4
Fishing (stream wading)	6
Gardening; digging, spading, composting	5
Gardening (raking)	4–4.3
Gardening (weeding)	4.5
Golf (power cart)	3.5
Golf (walk, carry bag)	4.5
Grooming (washing, shaving, brushing teeth, etc.)	2
Handball	8–12
Hiking (cross-country)	6
Horseback riding, general	4
Housework, multiple tasks light effort	2.5
Housework, multiple tasks vigorous effort	4
Hunting, general	5
Ironing, standing	2.3
Judo	10
Mopping	3.5
Mountain climbing	8
Mowing lawn, hand mower	6
Mowing lawn, power mower	5.5
Mowing lawn, riding mower	2.5
Music playing, piano or organ	2.5
Paddleball, racquetball	6–10
Painting, inside house	3
Painting, outside house	5

Activity	METs
Putting away groceries	2.5
Rope jumping, fast	12
Rope jumping, slow	8
Running, 10 mph (6 min/mi)	16
Running, 5 mph (12 min/mi)	8
Running, 6 mph (10 min/mi)	10
Running, 7.5 mph (8 min/mi)	12.5
Sailing	3–5
Scuba diving	7
Sexual activity, vigorous effort	1.5
Showering	2
Shuffleboard	3
Skating, ice or roller	7
Skiing, cross-country	7–14
Skiing, downhill	5–8
Sledding, tobogganing	7
Snow removal, operating snowblower	4.5
Snow shoveling	6
Snowshoeing	8
Soccer	7–10
Squash	12
Stair climbing, down	3
Stair climbing, up	8
Swimming	4–10
Table tennis	4
Tennis	5–7
Touch football	8
Using bedpan	4
Vacuuming	3.5
Volleyball	3–8
Walking with crutches	5
Walking, 2 mph	2.5
Walking, 2.5 mph	3
Walking, 3 mph	3.3
Walking, 3.5 mph	3.8
Walking, 4 mph	5
Walking, 4.5 mph	6.3
Walking, 5 mph	8
Walking, less than 2 mph	2
Washing dishes	2.3
Wheelchair propulsion	2

CARDIO

Examples of Methods of Exercise Prescription

Exercise Prescription by Heart Rate

The age-adjusted maximum heart rate (AAMHR) for an individual can be estimated by subtracting age from 220. The training heart rate (THR) can then be calculated by multiplying by the percentage of the desired intensity.

THR range in beats/min = 0.65 (220 − age) to 0.90 (220 − age)

The Karvonen equation uses the individual's resting heart rate to establish a THR range:

THR range in beats/min = 0.65 to 0.9 (AAMHR – resting HR) + resting HR

Exercise Prescription by Metabolic Equivalents

Activities of appropriate intensity can be selected if an individual's functional capacity in METs is known. An intensity of 60%–70% of the functional capacity is considered an appropriate training range. If 60% of maximum MET is used, add the maximum MET level to 60, divide this by 100, and multiply this value by maximum METs.

Example for an individual with a 5-MET maximum: (60 + 5)/100 = 0.65

0.65 × 5 METs = 3.25 METs (average training intensity)

Physical Activity Guidelines

Key Guidelines for Children and Adolescents

- Children and adolescents should do 60 minutes (1 hr) or more of physical activity daily.
  - Aerobic: Most of the 60 or more minutes a day should be either moderate- or vigorous-intensity aerobic physical activity, and should include vigorous-intensity physical activity at least 3 days a week.
  - Muscle-strengthening: As part of their 60 or more minutes of daily physical activity, children and adolescents should include muscle-strengthening physical activity on at least 3 days of the week.
  - Bone-strengthening: As part of their 60 or more minutes of daily physical activity, children and adolescents should include bone-strengthening physical activity on at least 3 days of the week.
- It is important to encourage young people to participate in physical activities that are appropriate for their age, that are enjoyable, and that offer variety.

Key Guidelines for Adults

- All adults should avoid inactivity. Some physical activity is better than none, and adults who participate in any amount of physical activity gain some health benefits.
- For substantial health benefits, adults should do at least 150 minutes (2 hr and 30 min) a week of moderate-intensity, or 75 minutes (1 hr and 15 min) a week of vigorous-intensity aerobic physical activity, or an equivalent combination of moderate- and vigorous intensity aerobic activity. Aerobic activity should be performed in episodes of at least 10 minutes, and preferably, it should be spread throughout the week.
- For additional and more extensive health benefits, adults should increase their aerobic physical activity to 300 minutes (5 hr) a week of moderate intensity, or 150 minutes a week of vigorous intensity aerobic physical activity, or an equivalent combination of moderate- and vigorous-intensity activity. Additional health benefits are gained by engaging in physical activity beyond this amount.
- Adults should also do muscle-strengthening activities that are moderate or high intensity and involve all major muscle groups on 2 or more days a week, as these activities provide additional health benefits.

Key Guidelines for Older Adults

The Key Guidelines for Adults also apply to older adults. In addition, the following guidelines apply only to older adults:

- When older adults cannot do 150 minutes of moderate-intensity aerobic activity a week because of chronic conditions, they should be as physically active as their abilities and conditions allow.
- Older adults should do exercises that maintain or improve balance if they are at risk of falling.
- Older adults should determine their level of effort for physical activity relative to their level of fitness.
- Older adults with chronic conditions should understand whether and how their conditions affect their ability to do regular physical activity safely.

Key Guidelines for Safe Physical Activity

To participate in physical activity safely and reduce the risk of injuries and other adverse events, people should do the following:

- Understand the risks and yet be confident that physical activity is safe for almost everyone.
- Choose to participate in types of physical activity that are appropriate for their current fitness level and health goals, because some activities are safer than others.
- Increase physical activity gradually over time whenever more activity is necessary to meet guidelines or health goals. Inactive people should "start low and go slow" by gradually increasing how often and how long activities are done.
- Protect themselves by using appropriate gear and sports equipment; looking for safe environments; following rules and policies; and making sensible choices about when, where, and how to be active.
- Be under the care of a health-care provider if they have chronic conditions or symptoms. People with chronic conditions and symptoms should consult their health-care provider about the types and amounts of activity appropriate for them.

Key Guidelines for Women During Pregnancy and the Postpartum Period

- Healthy women who are not already highly active or doing vigorous-intensity activity should get at least 150 minutes of moderate-intensity aerobic activity a week during pregnancy and the postpartum period. Preferably, this activity should be spread throughout the week.
- Pregnant women who habitually engage in vigorous-intensity aerobic activity or who are highly active can continue physical activity during pregnancy and the postpartum period, provided that they remain healthy and discuss with their health-care provider how and when activity should be adjusted over time.

Key Guidelines for Adults With Disabilities

- Adults with disabilities, who are able to, should get at least 150 minutes a week of moderate-intensity or 75 minutes a week of vigorous-intensity aerobic activity, or an equivalent combination of moderate- and vigorous-intensity aerobic activity. Aerobic activity should be performed in episodes of at least 10 minutes, and preferably, it should be spread throughout the week.

- Adults with disabilities, who are able to, should also do muscle-strengthening activities of moderate or high intensity that involve all major muscle groups on 2 or more days a week, as these activities provide additional health benefits.
- When adults with disabilities are not able to meet the guidelines, they should engage in regular physical activity according to their abilities and should avoid inactivity.
- Adults with disabilities should consult their health-care provider about the amounts and types of physical activity that are appropriate for their abilities.

Key Messages for People With Chronic Medical Conditions

- Adults with chronic conditions obtain important health benefits from regular physical activity.
- When adults with chronic conditions do activity according to their abilities, physical activity is safe.
- Adults with chronic conditions should be under the care of a health-care provider. People with chronic conditions and symptoms should consult their health-care provider about the types and amounts of activity appropriate for them.

> *From:*
> *Physical Activity Guidelines for Americans. http://www.health.gov/paguidelines/guidelines/summary.aspx. Accessed January 21, 2012.*

Cardiac Rehabilitation

Cardiac rehabilitation is a multidisciplinary and comprehensive long-term program that includes exercise; education; and counseling to modify the risk of heart disease, foster healthy behaviors, and improve the functional status of the person with heart disease. Cardiac rehabilitation includes three phases:

- Phase I: includes exercise and education begun during inpatient hospitalization following a coronary event. The role of the rehabilitation specialist includes monitoring of activity tolerance, educating the patient regarding adverse symptoms to activity, and preparing the patient for discharge to home.
- Phase II: includes supervised exercise, education, and counseling as an outpatient following exercise tolerance testing. The duration of this phase may be from 3 to 6 months.
- Phase III: a life-long maintenance phase.
- Some programs will consider a fourth phase as the period between hospital discharge and the exercise tolerance test that precedes phase II. This phase allows for monitoring by the team as the patient transitions to home and prepares for more intense activities.

Components of Phase I Cardiac Rehabilitation

- Vital sign monitoring before and after activity, including heart rate, blood pressure, respiratory rate, perceived exertion, signs and symptoms of intolerance, and ECG monitoring.
- Progression of activity from approximately 1 to 5 METs.
- Assessment of function for discharge to home.

- Education concerning the purpose of cardiac rehabilitation, identification of cardiovascular risk factors, signs of activity intolerance, and instruction in home exercise program.

Cardiac Rehabilitation/Secondary Prevention Programs (Phase II)
Core Components
- Patient assessment
- Nutritional counseling
- Weight management
- Blood pressure management
- Lipid management
- Diabetes management
- Tobacco cessation
- Psychosocial management
- Physical activity counseling
- Exercise training

CARDIO

TABLE 5.56 Summary of Metabolic Calculations to Estimate Energy Expenditure (in mL/kg/min) During Common Physical Activities

Activity	Sum these components			Limitations
	Resting component	Horizontal component	Vertical component/ resistance component	
Walking	3.5	0.1 × speed (in m/min)	1.8 × speed (in m/min) × grade	Most accurate for speeds of 1.9–3.7 mph (50–100 m/min)
Running	3.5	0.2 × speed (in m/min)	0.9 × speed (in m/min) × grade	Most accurate for speeds >5 mph (134 m/min)
Stepping	3.5	0.2 × steps per min	1.33 × (1.8 × step height [in m] × steps per min)	Most accurate for stepping rates of 12–30 steps per min
Leg cycling	3.5	3.5	(1.8 × work rate [in kg-m/min]/ body mass (in kg)	Most accurate for work rates of 300–1,200 kg-m/min (50–200 W)
Arm cycling	3.5		(3 × work rate [in kg· m/min])/ body mass (in kg)	Most accurate for work rates between 150–750 kg-m/min (25125 W)

Modified from: *ACSM's Guidelines for Exercise Testing and Prescription*, ed. 8. Lippincott Williams & Wilkins, Philadelphia, 2009, p 158.

Clinical Indications and Contraindications for Inpatient and Outpatient Cardiac Rehabilitation

Indications

- Medically stable post-myocardial infarction (MI)
- Stable angina
- Coronary artery bypass graft surgery (CABG)
- Percutaneous transluminal coronary angioplasty (PTCA) or other transcatheter procedure
- Compensated congestive heart failure (CHF)
- Cardiomyopathy
- Heart or other organ transplantation
- Other cardiac surgery, including valvular and pacemaker insertion (including implantable cardioverter defibrillator [ICD])
- Peripheral arterial disease (PAD)
- High-risk cardiovascular disease (CVD) ineligible for surgical intervention
- Sudden cardiac death syndrome
- End-stage renal disease
- At risk for coronary artery disease (CAD) with diagnoses of diabetes mellitus, dyslipidemia, hypertension, obesity, or other diseases and conditions
- Other patients who may benefit from structured exercise and/or patient education based on physician referral and consensus of the rehabilitation team

Contraindications

- Unstable angina
- Resting systolic BP (SBP) >200 mm Hg or resting diastolic BP (DBP) >100 mm Hg that should be evaluated on a case-by-case basis
- Orthostatic BP drop of >20 mm Hg with symptoms
- Critical aortic stenosis (i.e., peak SBP gradient of >50 mm Hg with an aortic valve orifice area of <0.75 cm^2 in an average-size adult)
- Acute systemic illness or fever
- Uncontrolled atrial or ventricular dysrhythmias
- Uncontrolled sinus tachycardia (>120 beats/min)
- Uncompensated CHF
- Third-degree atrioventricular (AV) block without pacemaker
- Active pericarditis or myocarditis
- Recent embolism
- Thrombophlebitis
- Resting ST-segment depression or elevation (>2 mm)
- Uncontrolled diabetes mellitus
- Severe orthopedic conditions that would prohibit exercise
- Other metabolic conditions, such as acute thyroiditis, hypokalemia, hyperkalemia, or hypovolemia

From:

ACSM's Guidelines for Exercise Testing and Prescription, ed. 8. Lippincott Williams & Wilkins, Philadelphia, 2009, p 209, with permission.

CARDIO

⬤ TABLE 5.57 Core Components of Exercise Training in Cardiac Rehabilitation/Secondary Prevention Programs

Evaluation	Symptom-limited exercise testing, including ECG monitoring, is strongly recommended. Stratification of patient risk to determine the level of supervision and monitoring. Use risk stratification as recommended by the American Heart Association (AHA) and the American Association of Cardiovascular and Pulmonary Rehabilitation (AACVPR).
Interventions	Individualized exercise prescription for aerobic and resistance training based on evaluation findings, risk stratification, comorbidities and goals. Aerobic exercise: 3–5 days/wk; 50%–80% of exercise capacity; 20–60 min/session. May include walking, treadmill, cycling, rowing, stair climbing, ergometers, and other forms of continuous or interval training as appropriate. Resistance exercise: 2–3 days/wk; 10–15 repetitions/set to moderate fatigue; 1–3 sets of 8–10 different upper and lower body exercises. May include calisthenics, elastic bands, cuff/hand weights, dumbbells, free weights, pulleys, or weight training machines. Include warm-up, cool-down, and flexibility exercises in each exercise session. Provide progressive updates to the exercise regimen and modify if clinical status changes. Supplement the formal exercise regimen with physical activity at home most days of the week (≥ 5).
Expected outcomes	Understanding of safety issues during exercise, including warning signs/symptoms. Increased cardiorespiratory fitness and enhanced flexibility muscular endurance and strength. Reduced symptoms, attenuated physiological responses to physical activities, and improved psychosocial well-being. Reduced cardiovascular risk and mortality.

Modified from: Balady, GJ, et al: Core components of cardiac rehabilitation/secondary prevention programs: 2007 update; a scientific statement from the American Heart Association Exercise, Cardiac Rehabilitation, and Prevention Committee; the Council on Clinical Cardiology; the Councils on Cardiovascular Nursing, Epidemiology and Prevention, and Nutrition, Physical Activity, and Metabolism; and the American Association of Cardiovascular and Pulmonary Rehabilitation. *Circulation* 115(20):2675–2682, 2007.

TABLE 5.58 Effects of Medications on Heart Rate, Blood Pressure, Electrocardiographic Findings (ECG), and Exercise Capacity

Medication	Heart Rate	Blood Pressure	ECG	Exercise Capacity
Beta blockers (including carvedilol and labetalol)	↓* rest and exercise	↓ rest and exercise	↓ HR* rest ↓ ischemia† exercise	↑ in patients with angina; ↓ or ↔ in patients without angina
Nitrates	↑ rest ↓ or ↔ exercise	↓ rest ↓ or ↔ exercise	↑ HR rest ↑ or ↔ HR exercise ↓ ischemia† exercise	↑ in patients with angina; ↔ in patients without angina; ↑ or ↔ in patients with chronic heart failure (CHF)
Calcium channel blockers Amlodipine Felodipine Isradipine Nicardipine Nifedipine Nimodipine Nisoldipine	↓ or ↔ rest and exercise	↓ rest and exercise	↑ or ↔ HR rest and exercise ↓ ischemia† exercise	↑ in patients with angina; ↓ or ↔ in patients without angina
Diltiazem Verapamil	↓ rest and exercise	↓ rest and exercise	↓ HR rest and exercise ↓ ischemia† exercise	

(table continues on page 498)

CARDIO

TABLE 5.58 Effects of Medications on Heart Rate, Blood Pressure, Electrocardiographic Findings (ECG), and Exercise Capacity (continued)

Medication	Heart Rate	Blood Pressure	ECG	Exercise Capacity
Digitalis	↓ in patients with atrial fibrillation and possibly CHF; not significantly altered in patients with sinus rhythm	↔ rest and exercise	May produce non-specific ST-T wave changes rest; may produce ST segment depression exercise	Improved only in patients with atrial fibrillation or in patients with CHF
Diuretics	↔ rest and exercise	↔ or ↓ rest and exercise	↔ or PVCs rest May cause PVCs and false-positive test results if hypokalemia occurs; may cause PVCs if hypomagne-semia occurs exercie	↔, except possibly in patients with CHF
Vasodilators, nonadrenergic	↑ or ↔ rest and exercise	↓ rest and exercise	↑ or ↔ HR rest and exercise	↔, except ↑ or ↔ in patients with CHF
ACE inhibitors and angiotensin II receptor blockers	↔ rest and exercise	↓ rest and exercise	↔ rest and exercise	↔, except ↑ or ↔ in patients with CHF
α-Adrenergic blockers	↔ rest and exercise	↓ rest and exercise	↔ rest and exercise	↔

Medication	Heart Rate	Blood Pressure	ECG	Exercise Capacity
Antiadrenergic agents without selective blockade	↓ or ↔ rest and exercise	↓ rest and exercise	↓ or ↔ HR rest and exercise	↔
Antiarrhythmic agents	All antiarrhythmic agents may cause new or worsened arrythmias (proarrhythmic effect)			
Class I Quinidine Disopyramide	↑ or ↔ rest and exercise	↓ or ↔ rest ↔ exercise	↑ or ↔ HR rest; May prolong QRS and QT intervals rest Quinidine may cause false-negative test results exercise	↔
Procainamide	↔ rest and exercise	↔ rest and exercise	May prolong QRS and QT intervals Procainamide may cause "false-positive" test results ↔ rest and exercise	↔
Phenytoin Tocainide Mexiletine	↔ rest and exercise ↔ rest and exercise	↔ rest and exercise ↔ rest and exercise	May prolong QRS and QT intervals rest ↔exercise ↓ HR rest	↔ ↔

(table continues on page 500)

CARDIO

TABLE 5.58 Effects of Medications on Heart Rate, Blood Pressure, Electrocardiographic Findings (ECG), and Exercise Capacity (continued)

Medication	Heart Rate	Blood Pressure	ECG	Exercise Capacity
Moricizine Propafenone	↓ rest ↓ or ↔ exercise	↔ rest and exercise	↓ or ↔ HR exercise	↔
Class II Beta-blockers (see previous entry)				
Class III Amiodarone Sotalol	↓ rest and exercise	↔ rest and exercise	↓ HR rest ↔ HR exercise	↔
Class IV Calcium channel blockers (see previous entry)				
Bronchodilators	↔ rest and exercise	↔ rest and exercise	↔ rest and exercise	Bronchodilators ↔ exercise capacity in patients limited by bronchospasm
Anticholinergic agents	↑ or ↔ rest and exercise	↔	↑ or ↔ HR; may produce PVCs rest and exercise	
Xanthine derivities				
Sympathomimetic agents	↑ or ↔ rest and exercise	↑, ↔, or ↓ rest and exercise	↑ or ↔ HR rest and exercise	↔

CARDIO

Medication	Heart Rate	Blood Pressure	ECG	Exercise Capacity
Cromolyn sodium	↔ rest and exercise	↔ rest and exercise	↔ rest and exercise	↔
Steroidal anti-inflammatory agents	↔ rest and exercise	↔ rest and exercise	↔ rest and exercise	↔
Antilipidemic agents	Clofibrate may provoke arrhythmias, angina in patients with prior myocardial infarction Nicotinic acid may ↓ BP All other hyperlipidemic agents have no effect on HR, BP, and ECG			↔
Psychotropic medications: Minor tranquilizers	May ↓ HR and BP by controlling anxiety; no other effects			
Antidepressants	↑ or ↔ rest and exercise	↓ or ↔ rest and exercise	Variable rest	
Major tranquilizers	↑ or ↔ rest and exercise	↓ or ↔ rest and exercise	Variable rest	
Lithium	↔ rest and exercise	↔ rest and exercise	May result in T-wave changes and arrhythmias rest and exercise	

(table continues on page 502)

CARDIO

TABLE 5.58 Effects of Medications on Heart Rate, Blood Pressure, Electrocardiographic Findings (ECG), and Exercise Capacity (continued)

Medication	Heart Rate	Blood Pressure	ECG	Exercise Capacity
Nicotine	↑ or ↔ rest and exercise	↑ rest and exercise	↑ or ↔ HR; may provoke ischemia, arrhythmias rest and exercise	↔, except ↓ or ↔ in patients with angina
Antihistamines	↔ rest and exercise	↔ rest and exercise	↔ rest and exercise	↔
Cold medications with sympatho-mimetic agents	Effects similar to those described in *Sympathomimetic agents*, although magnitude of effects is usually diminished			↔
Thyroid medications: only levothyroxine	↑ rest and exercise	↑ rest and exercise	↑ HR; may provoke arrhythmias; ↑ ischemia rest and exercise	↔, unless angina worsened
Alcohol	↔ rest and exercise	Chronic use may have role in ↑ BP rest and exercise	May provoke arrhythmias rest and exercise	↔
Hypoglycemic agents: insulin and oral agents	↔ rest and exercise	↔ rest and exercise	↔ rest and exercise	↔

CARDIO

Medication	Heart Rate	Blood Pressure	ECG	Exercise Capacity
Blood modifiers (anticoagulants and antiplatelets)	↔ rest and exercise	↔ rest and exercise	↔ rest and exercise	↔, ↑ or ↔ in patients limited by intermittent claudication (for cilostazol only)
Pentoxifylline	↔ rest and exercise	↔ rest and exercise	↔ rest and exercise	↔ in patients limited by intermittent claudication
Antigout medications	↔ rest and exercise	↔ rest and exercise	↔ rest and exercise	↔
Caffeine	Variable effects depending on previous use Variable effects on exercise capacity May provoke arrythmias			
Anorexiants/diet pills	↑ or ↔ rest and exercise	↑ or ↔ rest and exercise	↑ or ↔ rest and exercise	Increased HR and BP common with norepinephrine reuptake inhibitors (e.g., sibutramine)

Modified from: *ACSM's Guidelines for Exercise Testing and Prescription*, ed 8. Lippincott Williams & Wilkins, Philadelphia, 2009, pp 286–291.

PVCs = premature ventricular contraction; ↑, increase; ↔, no effect; ↓, decrease.

*Beta blockers with intrinsic sympathomimetic activity (ISA) lower resting heart rate only slightly.

†May prevent or delay myocardial ischemia.

TABLE 5.59 Guidelines for Electrocardiographic (ECG) Monitoring in Exercise Training

Activity Classification	ECG Monitoring
A: apparently healthy	Not required
B: known stable coronary artery disease, low risk for cardiac complications during vigorous exercise	Monitored and supervised for activity instruction (usually 6–12 sessions)
C: moderate to high risk for cardiac complications during exercise and/or unable to self-regulate or to understand recommended activity levels	Monitored and supervised (usually 12 sessions or more)

Based on: Fletcher, GF, et al: Exercise standards for testing and training: A statement for healthcare professionals from the American Heart Association. *Circulation* 104(14):1694–1740, 2001.

CARDIO

PULMONARY

Anatomy

Upper Respiratory Tract

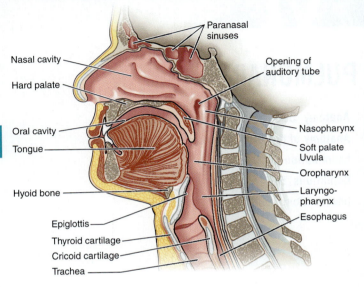

- Paranasal sinuses
- Nasal cavity
- Hard palate
- Opening of auditory tube
- Oral cavity
- Tongue
- Nasopharynx
- Soft palate
- Uvula
- Oropharynx
- Hyoid bone
- Laryngo-pharynx
- Epiglottis
- Esophagus
- Thyroid cartilage
- Cricoid cartilage
- Trachea

PULM

Trachea and Bronchial Tree

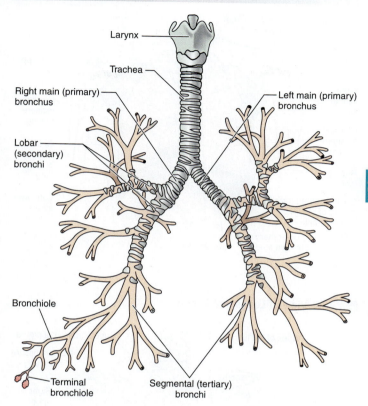

Larynx

Trachea

Right main (primary) bronchus

Left main (primary) bronchus

Lobar (secondary) bronchi

Bronchiole

Terminal bronchiole

Segmental (tertiary) bronchi

Anterior View of Lungs and Thorax

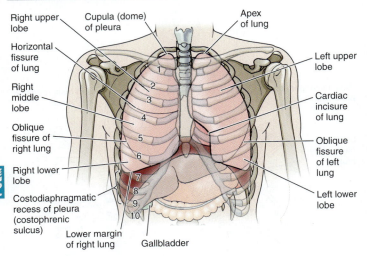

Right upper lobe
Cupula (dome) of pleura
Apex of lung
Horizontal fissure of lung
Left upper lobe
Right middle lobe
Cardiac incisure of lung
Oblique fissure of right lung
Oblique fissure of left lung
Right lower lobe
Costodiaphragmatic recess of pleura (costophrenic sulcus)
Left lower lobe
Lower margin of right lung
Gallbladder

Posterior View of Lungs and Thorax

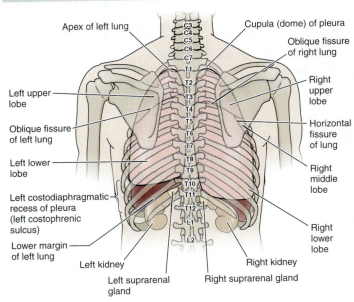

Apex of left lung
Cupula (dome) of pleura
Oblique fissure of right lung
Left upper lobe
Right upper lobe
Oblique fissure of left lung
Horizontal fissure of lung
Left lower lobe
Right middle lobe
Left costodiaphragmatic recess of pleura (left costophrenic sulcus)
Right lower lobe
Lower margin of left lung
Left kidney
Right kidney
Left suprarenal gland
Right suprarenal gland

PULM

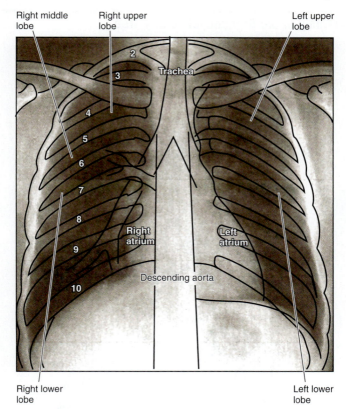

Normal posteroanterior (PA) chest radiograph.

Anatomy of the Bronchopulmonary Tree

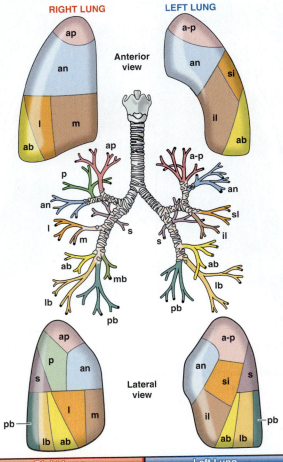

RIGHT LUNG   **LEFT LUNG**

Anterior view

Lateral view

PULM

Right Lung			Left Lung	
Right upper lobe	**Right middle lobe**	**Right lower lobe**	**Left upper lobe**	**Left lower lobe**
ap - apical	**l** - lateral	**s** - superior	**a-p** - apical-posterior	**s** - superior
an - anterior	**m** - medial	**ab** - anterior basal	**an** - anterior	**ab** - anterior medial basal
P - posterior		**lb** - lateral basal	**sl** - superior lingula	**lb** - lateral basal
		pb - posterior basal	**il** - inferior lingula	**pb** - posterior basal
		mb - medial basal		

Examination

Terms Associated With the Examination of the Pulmonary System

barrel chest: An increased anterior-posterior diameter of the thorax, barrel chest is sometimes associated with pulmonary emphysema.

cyanosis: A bluish tinge to the skin, cyanosis is caused by low oxygen saturation of hemoglobin.

digital clubbing: An abnormal finding, digital clubbing is flattening of the normal angle between the base of the nail and its cuticle as well as enlargement of the terminal phalanx.

flail chest: When ribs are broken in two or more places, this segment of the chest wall moves paradoxically during ventilation.

fremitus: Palpable vibrations felt through the chest wall (see *tactile fremitus* and *vocal fremitus*).

palpation: The chest is palpated for areas of tenderness, symmetry, amount, and synchrony of thoracic excursion during ventilation, integrity of the rib cage, and position of the mediastinum and vibrations.

pectus carinatum: The sternum protrudes forward and is abnormally prominent; also called *pigeon* or *chicken breast*.

pectus excavatum: The sternum is abnormally depressed; it is also called *funnel chest*.

percussion: See separate listing on page 514.

tactile fremitus: Palpable vibrations are felt during ventilation. (See *fremitus* and *vocal fremitus*.)

vocal fremitus: Palpable felt vibrations when the patient is speaking. (See *fremitus* and *tactile fremitus*.)

PULM

TABLE 6.1 Terms Used to Describe Breathing

Term	Explanation
Apnea	Absence of breathing
Apneusis	Cessation of respiration in the inspiratory position
Biot's breathing	Several short breaths or gasps followed by irregular periods of apnea
Bradypnea	Abnormally slow rate of breathing
Cheyne-Stokes respiration	Cycles of gradual increase in rate and depth of respiration with apneic pauses between cycles
Dyspnea	Complaint of shortness of breath

(table continues on page 512)

TABLE 6.1 Terms Used to Describe Breathing (continued)

Term	Explanation
Eupnea	Normal rate and rhythm of breathing
Hyperpnea	Increased breathing; increased depth with or without increased rate
Hyperventilation	Increased ventilation; technically a decrease in $PaCO_2$
Hypoventilation	Decreased ventilation; technically an increase in $PaCO_2$
Kussmaul's breathing	Deep gasping respirations associated with diabetic acidosis and coma ("air hunger")
Orthopnea	Dyspnea that occurs when patient assumes recumbent position
Paroxysmal nocturnal dyspnea	Dyspnea that comes on at night and suddenly awakens the patient
Tachypnea	Abnormally rapid rate of breathing

Respiratory Rate

TABLE 6.2 Normative Values by Age

Age	Respiratory Rate (breaths/min)
Newborn	25–50
3 years	20–30
10 years	16–22
16 years	15–20
Adult	12–20
Older adult	15–22

Data from: O'Sullivan, SB, and Schmitz, TJ: *Physical Rehabilitation,* ed. 5. FA Davis, Philadelphia, 2007, p 82.

Pulmonary Auscultation

Breath sounds are classified as normal or abnormal and with or without accompaniments (adventitious breath sounds). Normal breath sounds vary, depending on what area is being auscultated.

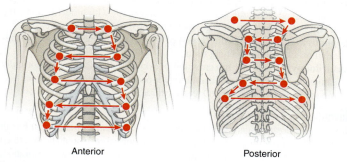

Anterior   Posterior

Auscultation of lungs.

🟠 TABLE 6.3 Normal Breath Sounds

Type	Location Auscultated	Description of Sound
Tracheal	Trachea	Inspiration and expiration are equal in duration; loud, high pitched, and hollow; short pause between inspiration and expiration
Bronchial	Over manubrium, between clavicles, or between scapulae	Inspiration shorter than expiration; loud, high pitched, short pause inspiration and expiration
Bronchovesicular	Over large airways near sternum and between scapulae	Inspiration should equal expiration in duration, lower intensity than bronchial; medium pitched, no pause between inspiration and expiration
Vesicular	Over peripheral lung tissue	Long inspiration with short expiration; relatively faint and low pitched; no pause between inspiration and expiration

Abnormal Breath Sounds

When tracheal, bronchial, or bronchovesicular breath sounds are auscultated over a lung that should sound vesicular, the breath sound is abnormal. Sound is transmitted better through solid or consolidated lung tissue, and increased transmission is indicative of pathology. Sometimes these abnormal breath sounds are termed *tubular*. An abnormal intensity of a breath sound is also noted when present.

bronchophony: Abnormal transmission of spoken words. Typically, the patient is asked to say the letter *E* or the number *99*; with bronchophony, the *E* will sound like an *A* and is sometimes noted as "E to A change."

egophony: The nasal, bleating sound of spoken or whispered words auscultated over consolidated lung tissue.

pectoriloquy: Abnormal transmission of whispered syllables that normally cannot be heard distinctly. Examining for pectoriloquy usually involves asking the patient to whisper, "One, two, three."

Adventitious Breath Sounds

Adventitious breath sounds are accompaniments to normal or abnormal breath sounds. Adventitious breath sounds are always abnormal and should be described by name and by when they are heard during respiration (inspiration, expiration, early, late, etc.). They are further classified into three major categories: continuous breath sounds, noncontinuous breath sounds, and rubs.

continuous breath sounds: Most prominent during expiration, they are thought to be caused by the vibrations of air passing through airways narrowed by inflammation, bronchospasm, or secretions. Frequently they are present in asthma and chronic bronchitis. The noises of wheezes are described as squeaky, snoring, or groaning.

friction rub: Caused by the rubbing of pleural surfaces against one another, usually as a result of inflammation or neoplastic processes. A friction rub sounds similar to footsteps on packed snow or creaking old leather and is more commonly heard during inspiration, but this can be highly variable. A friction rub may be accompanied by pain during inspiration.

noncontinuous breath sounds: Most common during inspiration, they are thought to be caused by the sound of gas bubbling through secretions or by the opening of alveoli and small airways that have collapsed because of fluid, poor aeration, or inflammation. These sounds are frequently associated with congestive heart failure, atelectasis, and pulmonary fibrosis. Noncontinuous breath sounds are described as sounding like soda pop fizzing or hair rubbed through the fingers next to the ear. They should be called *crackles*; other terms used are *rales* and *crepitations*. Descriptive terms used with crackles are *fine* or *coarse*.

rhonchi: Low-pitched and sonorous.

wheezes: High-pitched, sibilant, and musical.

Percussion of the Pulmonary System

percussion: An evaluation technique in which the examiner strikes the distal end of the middle finger of one hand over the middle finger of the other hand, which is placed firmly over the chest wall. The resonance created by this maneuver has a variable pitch and feel, depending on the density of the underlying tissue. Four different percussion notes are described.

🟧 TABLE 6.4 Percussion Sounds

Note (sound)	Characteristics of Normal Location	Underlying Tissue
Flat	Muscle on extremity	No underlying air
Dull	Liver, heart, viscera	Primarily soft tissue, some air
Normal resonance	Lung	Air and soft tissue
Hyper-resonant (tympanic)	Stomach	Primarily air

Pulmonary Function Tests

Terms Used In Pulmonary Function Testing

🟧 TABLE 6.5 Pulmonary Function Abbreviations

Abbreviation	Term
A-aDo$_2$	Alevolar-arterial O_2 difference (gradient)
CSTAT	Static lung compliance
DLCO	Diffusing capacity for CO (mL/min/mm Hg)
ERV	Expiratory reserve volume
FEF$_{25\% - 75\%}$	Mean forced expiratory flow during the middle of FVC
FEV$_1$(L)	Forced expiratory volume in 1 sec, in liters
FEV$_1$ %FVC	Forced expiratory volume in 1 sec as percentage of FVC
FiO$_2$	Percentage of inspired O_2
FRC	Functional residual capacity
FVC	Forced vital capacity
[H$^+$]	Hydrogen ion concentration (nanomole/L)
MEP	Maximal expiratory pressure (cm H_2O)
MIP	Maximal inspiratory pressure (cm H_2O)
MVV	Maximal voluntary ventilation

(table continues on page 516)

PULM

⬤ **TABLE 6.5 Pulmonary Function Abbreviations** (continued)

Abbreviation	Term
PAO_2	Partial pressure of alveolar O_2
$PACO_2$	Partial pressure of alveolar CO_2
PaO_2	Partial pressure of arterial O_2
$PaCO_2$	Partial pressure of arterial CO_2
P_B	Barometric pressure
PCO_2	Partial pressure of CO_2
$PETCO_2$	Partial pressure of end tidal CO_2
PEF	Peak expiratory flow (L/min)
PIO_2	Partial pressure of inspired O_2
PO_2	Partial pressure of O_2
Pv	Partial pressure of mixed venous (pulmonary arterial) blood
PvO_2	Partial pressure of mixed venous O_2
$PvCO_2$	Partial pressure of mixed venous CO_2
Q	Perfusion; volume of blood that circulates through the heart and lungs in 1 min
Raw	Airway resistance
RV	Residual volume
TLC	Total lung capacity
TV	Tidal volume
VC	Vital capacity
V	Ventilation; volume of air exchanged in 1 min
V_A	Alveolar ventilation (L/min)
VCO_2	CO_2 production (L/min)
VO_2	O_2 consumption (L/min)

For more information: Mason, RJ, et al: *Murray and Nadel's: Textbook of Respiratory Medicine,* ed. 4. WB Saunders, Philadelphia, 2005.
The Merck Manual, ed 18. Merck & Co, Rahway, NJ, 2006.

Common Pulmonary Function Tests

body plethysmography: Measures total lung capacity and airway resistance. It allows the RV to be accurately determined and is most useful for diagnosing obstructive disorders.

diffusing capacity (DLCO): The patient inspires a small amount of CO; the CO in the end-expired gas is analyzed and the amount of CO that diffused into the blood is calculated. Low DLCO may indicate thickening of alveolar-capillary membranes and/or abnormal ventilation-perfusion relationships.

flow-volume loops: Graphically plot maximal inspiratory and expiratory volumes and flows; visual examination of the shape of the loop used for detecting intrathoracic and extrathoracic obstruction and restriction.

nitrogen washout test: Measures the distribution of ventilation and closing volume (the volume during expiration when small airways collapse). Concentration of N_2 is measured over complete expiration after breathing 100% O_2. An abnormal curve of N_2 concentration reflects asynchronous alveolar emptying and small airway closure, characteristic of obstructive disorders.

spirometry: Measures lung volumes and capacities (with the exception of residual volume [RV] and total lung capacity [TLC]), flow rates, and the maximal voluntary ventilation [MVV]; used as a general screening test for detection of abnormal breathing patterns, lung obstruction and/or restriction, efficacy of medication (bronchodilation), estimate ventilatory reserve, and patient compliance.

ventilation-perfusion (V/Q) scan: A radioactive tracer is injected into the circulation and/or the patient inhales a radioactive gas or aerosol. Distribution and matching of ventilation to perfusion can then be examined. Disorders that might be detected by a V/Q scan include vascular occlusion (pulmonary embolism), lung consolidation, and obstructive and restrictive diseases.

PULM

Lung Volumes and Capacities

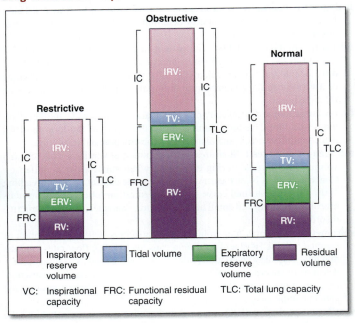

PULM

Obstructive

Restrictive

Normal

Legend:
- Inspiratory reserve volume
- Tidal volume
- Expiratory reserve volume
- Residual volume

VC: Inspirational capacity   FRC: Functional residual capacity   TLC: Total lung capacity

TABLE 6.6 Normative Values for Resting Lung Volumes and Capacities*

Tidal volume	500 mL
Inspiratory reserve volume	3,000 mL
Expiratory reserve volume	1,100 mL
Residual volume	1,200 mL
Inspiratory capacity	3,500 mL
Functional residual capacity	2,300 mL
Vital capacity	4,600 mL
Total lung capacity	5,800 mL

For more information: Brannon, FJ, et al: *Cardiopulmonary Rehabilitation: Basic Theory and Application*, ed. 2. FA Davis, Philadelphia, 1998, pp 48–52.
Jones, SA: *Pocket Anatomy & Physiology*. FA Davis, Philadelphia, 2009, pp 211–214.
*Approximate values for healthy young men. Normative volumes and capacities will vary according to the age, height, race, gender, and body position of the person.

TABLE 6.7 Severity of Pulmonary Impairments (% of predicted normal)

Severity	VC	FEV₁	FEV₁/FVC	MEF	TLC	DLCO
Normal	>80	>80	>70	>65	>80	>80
Mild	66–80	66–80	60–70	50–65	66–80	61–80
Moderate	50–65	50–65	45–59	35–49	50–65	40–60
Severe	<50	<50	<45	<35	<50	<40

Classification of Pulmonary Impairments

obstructive: Characterized by reductions in expiratory air flows with or without reductions in the vital capacity. Total lung capacity may be increased with severe hyperinflation.

restrictive: Characterized by a decreased vital capacity with normal expiratory air flows.

Arterial Blood Gases and Oxygenation

arterial blood gas (ABG) studies: Provide information about how well the lungs are functioning to provide oxygen, eliminate carbon dioxide, and, with the kidneys, regulate the blood's acid-base balance. Serious consequences can result from abnormal ABGs.

TABLE 6.8 Normal Arterial Blood Gas Values

Arterial	Premature	Term Infant	Child	Adult
pH	7.35–7.39	7.26–7.41	7.35–7.45	7.35–7.45
PaCO₂	38–44 mm Hg	34–54 mm Hg	35–45 mm Hg	35–45 mm Hg
PaO₂	65–80 mm Hg	60 mm Hg	75–100 mm Hg	75–100 mm Hg
O₂ sat	40%–90%	40%–95%	95%–98%	95%–98%
CO₂ content	19–27 mEq/L	20–28 mEq/L	18–27 mEq/L	23–29 mEq/L
Base excess	−1 to −2 mEq/L	−7 to −1 mEq/L	−4 to +2 mEq/L	−2 to +2 mEq/L

⬤ TABLE 6.9 Gas Pressure (mm Hg)

Gas	Dry Air	Moist Tracheal Air	Alveolar Gas	Arterial Blood	Mixed Venous Blood
P_{O_2}	159.1	149.2	104	100	40
P_{CO_2}	0.3	0.3	40	40	46
P_{H_2O}	0.0	47.0	47	47	47
P_{N_2}	600.6	563.5	569	573	573
P_{TOTAL}	760	760	760	760	706

⬤ TABLE 6.10 Interpretation of Abnormal Acid-Base Balance

Type	pH	$PaCO_2$	CO_2	Causes	Signs and Symptoms
Respiratory alkalosis	↑	↓	WNL	Alveolar hyperventilation	Dizziness, syncope, tingling, numbness, early tetany
Respiratory acidosis	↓	↑	WNL	Alveolar hypoventilation	Early: anxiety, restlessness, dyspnea, headache; late: confusion, somnolence, coma
Metabolic alkalosis	↑	WNL	↑	Bicarbonate ingestion, vomiting, diuretics, steroids, adrenal disease	Vague symptoms: weakness, mental dullness, possibly early tetany
Metabolic acidosis	↓	WNL	↓	Diabetic, lactic, or uremic acidosis, prolonged diarrhea	Secondary hyperventilation (Kussmaul's breathing), nausea and vomiting, cardiac dysrhythmias, lethargy, and coma

↑ = increase; ↓ = decrease; WNL = within normal limits.

Oxygenation

The PaO_2 and the hemoglobin oxygen saturation (O_2 sat) provide information about how well the lungs are functioning as an oxygenator.

hypoxemia: An abnormally low amount of oxygen in the blood.

hypoxia: Refers to a low amount of oxygen, usually at the tissue level.

Noninvasive Oxygen Monitoring

Ear oximetry is useful for monitoring oxygen saturation during exercise. Capillary oxygen saturation is measured by spectrophotometry using a device that attaches to the ear. Transcutaneous skin electrodes are also used to assess oxygen saturation in pediatric patients; transcutaneous oxygen pressure (TCO_2) correlates well with the PaO_2, although the TCO_2 value tends to be lower.

TABLE 6.11 Causes of Hypoxemia

Type	Description	Causes
Hypoventilation	Low level of ventilation causes increase in $PaCO_2$ with concomitant decrease in PaO_2.	Drug overdose, anesthesia, pathology of medulla, abnormalities of spinal pathways, poliomyelitis, diseases and pathology of respiratory muscles, chest wall trauma, kyphoscoliosis, upper airway obstruction
Diffusion impairment	Blood-gas barrier is thickened.	Asbestosis, sarcoidosis, interstitial fibrosis, collagen diseases, alveolar cell carcinoma
Shunt	Blood reaches arterial system without passing through ventilated regions of the lungs; can be anatomic or physiological.	Congenital cardiac defects, infectious and inflammatory processes
V/Q inequality	Mismatching of ventilation to blood flow	Chronic obstructive lung disease, interstitial lung disease, vascular disorders
Decreased inspired oxygen	Partial pressure of oxygen lowers as barometric pressure decreases.	High altitudes

PULM

Oxygen Therapy

high-flow: All of the gas the patient breathes is delivered by a mask or tube, which allows for precise control of FiO_2. Venturi or "Venti" masks are high-flow systems that mix room air with oxygen to provide a precise FiO_2.

low-flow: This system provides only part of the patient's minute volume and uses masks, nasal cannula, or prongs. The tidal volume should be between 300 and 700 mL and the ventilatory rate below 25 per minute to use a low-flow system. Due to variability in ventilation, the FiO_2 can only be estimated.

TABLE 6.12 Estimated Fraction of Inspired Oxygen With Low-Flow Devices

Low-Flow Device	Estimated FiO$_2$ (%)
Room air	21
Nasal prongs	
1 L/min	24
2 L/min	28
3 L/min	32
4 L/min	36
5 L/min	40
6 L/min	44
Oxygen mask	
5–6 L/min	40
6–7 L/min	50
7–8 L/min	60
Mask with reservoir bag	
6 L/min	60
7 L/min	70
8 L/min	80
9 L/min	90
10 L/min	99+

Sputum Analysis

Sputum is described in terms of quantity, viscosity, color, and odor. The frequency, time of day, and ease of expectoration is also noted. Laboratory analysis is necessary to establish a definitive diagnosis. These tests include Gram stain for bacteria, culture and sensitivity for infectious agent, and appropriate antibiotic, acid-fast bacillus stain to detect the tuberculosis bacillus, and cytology to examine for cellular constituents and malignancy.

TABLE 6.13 Sputum

Term	Description
Fetid	Foul-smelling, typical of anaerobic infection; typically occurs with bronchiectasis, lung abscess, or cystic fibrosis
Frothy	White or pink-tinged, foamy, thin sputum associated with pulmonary edema
Hemoptysis	Expectoration of blood or bloody sputum; amount may range from blood-streaked to massive hemorrhage and is present in a variety of pathologies
Mucoid	White or clear, not generally associated with bronchopulmonary infection but is present with chronic cough (acute or chronic bronchitis, cystic fibrosis)
Mucopurulent	Mixture of mucoid sputum and pus, yellow to pale green, associated with infection
Purulent	Pus, yellow or greenish sputum, often copious and thick, common with acute and chronic infection
Rusty	Descriptive of the color of sputum; classic for pneumococcal pneumonia (also called *prune juice*)
Tenacious	Thick, sticky sputum

PULM

Exercise Testing the Patient With Pulmonary Disease

TABLE 6.14 Protocols Used for Exercise Testing the Patient With Pulmonary Disease

Mode	Protocol	For More Information
Walk tests	Walk as far as possible in 6 min.*	*Guyatt, G, Berman, L, and Townsend, M: Long-term outcome after respiratory rehabilitation. CMAJ 137:1089–1095, 1987.*
	Walk as far as possible in 12 min.	*Cooper, KH: A means of assessing maximal oxygen intake: Correlation between field and treadmill walking. JAMA 203:201–204, 1968.*
Cycle tests	Begin at 100 kpm, increase 100 kpm every min.	*Jones, NL: Exercise testing in pulmonary evaluation: Rationale, methods and the normal respiratory response to exercise. N Eng J Med 293:541–544, 1975.*
	Begin at 100 kpm, increase 100 kpm every minute or 50 kpm every min when FEV_1 <1 L/s.	*Berman, LB, and Sutton, JR: Exercise for the pulmonary patient. J Cardiopulm Rehabil Prev 6:52–61, 1986.*
Treadmill tests	2 mph constant 0 grade; 3.5% grade every 3 min.	*Naughton, JP, Balke, B, and Poarch, R: Modified work capacity studies in individuals with and without coronary artery disease. J Sports Med 4:208–212, 1964.*
	3.3 mph constant 0 grade; 3.5% grade every 2 min.	*Balke, B, and Ware, R: An experimental study of physical fitness of Air Force personnel. US Armed Forces Med J 10:675–688, 1959.*
Shuttle walk test	Walk back and forth at a steady pace around 2 cones that are placed 9 m apart; pace is increased each min; 12 levels of speed beginning at 0.50 m/s and ending at 2.37 m/s.	*Singh, SJ, et al: Development of a shuttle walking test of disability in patients with chronic airways obstruction. Thorax 47:1019–1024, 1992.*
Step test	Step up and down a 15-cm-high single-step at a rate of 30 steps per min for 3 min.	*Balfour-Lynn, IM, et al: A step in the right direction: Assessing exercise tolerance in cystic fibrosis. Pediatr Pulmonol 25:278–284, 1998.*

*See description of 6-minute walk test in Section V, Cardiovascular, p 465.

PULM

TABLE 6.15 Rating of Perceived Shortness of Breath

Score	Description
0	Nothing at all
0.5	Very, very slight (Just noticeable)
1	Rest; very slight
2	Slight (Light)
3	Moderate
4	Somewhat severe
5	Severe (Heavy)
6	
7	Very severe
8	
9	
10	Very, very severe (Almost maximum)
*	Maximal

From: Mahler, DA, et al: Continuous measurement of breathlessness during exercise: Validity, reliability, and responsiveness. *J Appl Physiol* 90:2188–2196, 2001.

Exercise Termination Criteria for the Patient With Pulmonary Disease

The symptom-limited endpoint of an exercise test for pulmonary patients may be quite different from that for cardiac patients. Criteria for stopping a pulmonary exercise test may include but not be limited to the following:

- Maximal shortness of breath
- A fall in PaO_2 of >20 mm Hg or a PaO_2 <55 mm Hg
- A rise in $PaCO_2$ of >10 mm Hg or a $PaCO_2$ >65 mm Hg
- Cardiac ischemia or dysrhythmias
- Symptoms of fatigue
- Increase in diastolic blood pressure readings of 20 mm Hg, systolic hypertension >250 mm Hg, decrease in blood pressure with increasing workloads
- Leg pain
- Total fatigue
- Signs of insufficient cardiac output
- Reaching a ventilatory maximum

From:

Brannon, FJ, et al: Cardiopulmonary Rehabilitation: Basic Theory and Application, ed. 2. FA Davis, Philadelphia, 1998, p 300, with permission.

PULM

Conditions

TABLE 6.16　Typical Signs and Symptoms of Pulmonary Diseases

Pathological Process	Chest Wall Movement	Mediastinal Position	Percussion Note	Breath Sounds	Vocal Sounds	Adventotopis	Cough–Sputum	Miscellaneous
Asthma	Normal or symmetrically decreased	Midline	Normal or hyperresonant	Vesicular with prolonged expiration	Normal or diminished	Wheezing cough	Dry or productive of tenacious mucoid sputum with plugs	Anxiety, severe bronchospasm may restrict air flow to the extent that no wheezing is heard
Atelectasis	Reduced on affected side	Shifted toward affected side	Dull or flat	Decreased or absent	Reduced or absent with large area collapsed; egophony and whispering pectoriloquy with smaller collapse	None or coarse rales	None, hacking or productive, particularly if atelectasis is due to mucous plugging	May have fever; may have pain

PULM

Pathological Process	Chest Wall Movement	Mediastinal Position	Percussion Note	Breath Sounds	Vocal Sounds	Adventotopis	Cough–Sputum	Miscellaneous
Chronic or acute bronchitis	Normal or symmetrically decreased	Midline	Normal	Vesicular with prolonged expiration	Normal	Wheezing and rhonchi	Productive of mucoid or purulent sputum with infection	May have fever
Bronchiectasis	May be reduced over affected area	Midline or toward affected area	Abnormal, may be dull or hyperresonant	Bronchial or broncho-vesicular	Increased	Coarse rales, rhonchi	Usually copious amounts of purulent sputum; possibly foul smelling; hemoptysis may occur	Physical exam depends on amount of fluid ectatic areas
Pulmonary effusion or empyema	Reduced or absent on affected side	Away from affected side	Dull or flat	Decreased or absent; high pitched bronchial may be present	Reduced or absent	May have pleural rub	Absent or nonproductive	

(table continues on page 528)

PULM

TABLE 6.16 Typical Signs and Symptoms of Pulmonary Diseases (continued)

Pathological Process	Chest Wall Movement	Mediastinal Position	Percussion Note	Breath Sounds	Vocal Sounds	Adventitous	Cough–Sputum	Miscellaneous
Pneumonia (lung consolidation)	Reduced on affected side	Midline	Dull	Broncho-vesicular, bronchial	Egophony, whispering pectoriloquy	Fine rales early; coarse later	Dry, hacking, or productive; sputum may be purulent, bloody	Fever; may have pleuritic pain
Lung abcess, cavitation	Normal or reduced on affected side	Midline or toward affected side	Abnormal (dull or hyperreso-nant)	Bronchial, amorphic	Increased, egophony, whispering pectoriloquy	Coarse rales	Productive of purulent foul-smelling sputum	Physical exam depends on amount of fluid in affected area; abscess may develop distal to bronchial obstruction; lung cancer should be ruled out; may have fever

PULM

Pathological Process	Chest Wall Movement	Mediastinal Position	Percussion Note	Breath Sounds	Vocal Sounds	Advemtotopis	Cough–Sputum	Miscellaneous
Emphysema	Normal or symmetrically decreased	Midline	Normal or hyperresonant	Harsh vesicular with prolonged expiration; may be decreased or distant	Normal or reduced	None, rhonchi, rales	Variable	
Pulmonary edema	Normal or symmetrically reduced	Midline	Normal, may be dull at lung bases	Vesicular	Normal	Rales, generally symmetric	Irritating, frothy white or pink sputum	
Pulmonary embolism	Reduced on affected side	Midline	Normal or dull	May be reduced	Normal	Rales, wheezing, pleural friction rub	Dry, hacking, or productive; may have hemoptysis	May have pleuritic pain, apprehension

(table continues on page 530)

TABLE 6.16 Typical Signs and Symptoms of Pulmonary Diseases (continued)

Pathological Process	Chest Wall Movement	Mediastinal Position	Percussion Note	Breath Sounds	Vocal Sounds	Adventotopis	Cough–Sputum	Miscellaneous
Cystic fibrosis	Normal or reduced	Midline	Normal, dull or hyperresonant	Vesicular, bronchovesicular, bronchial	May have egophony	Rales, wheezing	Productive of large amounts of tenacious mucoid, mucopurulent, or purulent sputum; may have hemoptysis	Physical exam depends on extent of disease and amount of retained secretions
Pneumothorax	Reduced on affected side (but hemithorax may be enlarged)	Away from affected side	Hyperresonant, tympanic	Decreased, distant, or absent	Decreased	None	Dry	May have local or referred pain
Laryngotracheobronchitis (croup)	Retractions	Midline	Normal	Vesicular, prolonged inspiration	Normal	Stridor, wheezing, rales	Barking, productive of viscous sputum	Low-grade fever
Bronchiolitis	Retractions	Midline	Hyperresonant	Vesicular, prolonged expiration	Normal	Wheezing, rales	Hacking, productive of mucoid to purulent sputum	Typically follows an upper respiratory tract infection

PULM

Chronic Obstructive Pulmonary Disease (COPD)

TABLE 6.17 Differential Features of Chronic Pulmonary Conditions

Feature	Emphysema	Chronic Bronchitis
Family history	Occasional (α_1 antitrypsin deficiency)	Occasional (cystic fibrosis)
Atopy	Absent	Absent
Smoking history	Usual	Usual
Sputum character	Absent or mucoid	Predominantly neutrophilic
Chest x-ray	Useful if bullae, hyper-inflation, or loss of peripheral vascular markings are present	Often normal; occasional hyperinflation
Spirometry	Obstructive pattern unimproved with bronchodilator	Obstructive pattern improved with bronchodilator

TABLE 6.18 Stages of Chronic Obstructive Pulmonary Disease

Stage	Signs
Early	Examination may be negative or show only slight prolongation of forced expiration (which can be timed while auscultating over the trachea—normally 3 sec or less); slight diminution of breath sounds at the apices or bases; scattered rhonchi or wheezes, especially on expiration, often best heard over the hila anteriorly. The rhonchi often clear after cough.
Moderate	Above signs are usually present and more pronounced, often with decreased rib expansion; in addition there is: Use of the accessory muscles of respiration. Retraction of the supraclavicular fossae in inspiration. Generalized hyper-resonance. Decreased area of cardiac dullness. Diminished heart sounds at base. Increased anteroposterior distance of the chest.*
Advanced	Examination usually shows the above findings to a greater degree and often shows: Evidence of weight loss. Depression of the liver. Hyperpnea and tachycardia with mild exertion. Low and relatively immobile diaphragm.

(table continues on page 532)

⬤ TABLE 6.18 Stages of Chronic Obstructive Pulmonary Disease (continued)

Stage	Signs
	Contraction of abdominal muscles on inspiration. Inaudible heart sounds, except in the xiphoid area cyanosis.
Cor pulmonale	Increased pulmonic second sound and close splitting. Right-sided diastolic gallop. Left parasternal heave (right ventricular overactivity). Early systolic pulmonary ejection click, with or without systolic ejection murmur. With failure, there is: Distended neck veins, functional tricuspid insufficiency. V waves, and hepatojugular reflux. Hepatomegaly. Peripheral edema.

*Misplaced confidence may be placed in relating the shape of the thorax to the presence or absence of obstructive lung disease. It has been shown that the classic "barrel chest" with poor rib separation may be due solely or largely to dorsal kyphosis. In such patients, ventilatory function may nonetheless be normal because of good diaphragmatic motion.

⬤ TABLE 6.19A GOLD Classification System for Severity of Chronic Obstructive Pulmonary Disease

Stage	Characteristics
I: mild COPD	$FEV_1/FVC < 70\%$ $FEV_1 \geq 80\%$ predicted With or without chronic symptoms (cough, sputum production)
II: moderate COPD	$FEV_1/FVC < 70\%$ $50\% \leq FEV_1 < 80\%$ predicted With or without chronic symptoms (cough, sputum production)
III: severe COPD	$FEV_1/FVC < 70\%$ $30\% \leq FEV_1 < 50\%$ predicted With or without chronic symptoms (cough, sputum production)
IV: very severe COPD	$FEV_1/FVC < 70\%$ $FEV_1 < 30\%$ predicted or $FEV_1 < 30\%$ predicted plus chronic respiratory failure

From: Fabbri, L, Pauwels, RA, and Hurd, SS; GOLD Scientific Committee. Global Strategy for the Diagnosis, Management, and Prevention of Chronic Obstructive Pulmonary Disease: GOLD Executive Summary updated 2003. *COPD* 1:105–141, 2004.
Classification based on postbronchodilator FEV_1.
FEV_1 = forced expiratory volume in 1 second; FVC = forced vital capacity; respiratory failure = arterial partial pressure of oxygen (PaO_2) < 8.0 kPa (60 mm Hg) with or without arterial partial pressure of CO_2 ($PaCO_2$) > 6.7 kPa (50 mm Hg) while breathing air at sea level.

PULM

Drugs Used to Treat COPD

TABLE 6.19B Suggested Pharmacological Management Based on the GOLD Classification of Severity of Lung Disease

Stage	Suggested Management
I: mild COPD	Avoidance of risk factors; Influenza vaccination; Add short-acting bronchodilator when needed.
II: moderate COPD	Add regular treatment with one or more long-acting bronchodilators; Add rehabilitation.
III: severe COPD	Add inhaled glucocorticoids if repeated exacerbations.
IV: very severe COPD	Add long-term oxygen if chronic respiratory failure; Consider surgical treatments.

From: Fabbri, L, Pauwels, RA, and Hurd, SS; GOLD Scientific Committee. Global Strategy for the Diagnosis, Management, and Prevention of Chronic Obstructive Pulmonary Disease: GOLD Executive Summary updated 2003. *COPD* 1:105–141, 2004.

PULM

■ TABLE 6.20 Beta-Adrenergic Bronchodilators

Drug	Primary Receptor	Route of Administration	Onset of Action (min)	Time to Peak Effect (hr)	Duration of Action (hr)
Albuterol	Beta-2	Inhalation Oral	5–15 15–30	1–1.5 2–3	3–6 8 or more
Epinephrine	Alpha, beta-1,2	Inhalation Intramuscular Subcutaneous	3–5 Variable 6–15	— — 0.3	1–3 <1–4 <1–4
Formoterol	Beta-2	Inhalation	1–3	—	12
Isoetharine	Beta-2	Inhalation	1–6	0.25–1	1–4
Isoproterenol	Beta-2	Inhalation Intravenous Sublingual	2–5 Immediate 15–30	— — —	0.5–2 <1 1–2
Metaproterenol	Beta-2	Inhalation (aerosol) Oral	Within 1 Within 15–30	1 Within 1	1–5 Up to 4
Pirbuterol	Beta-2	Inhalation	Within 5	0.5–1	5
Salmeterol	Beta-2	Inhalation	10–20	3–4	12
Terbutaline	Beta-2	Inhalation Oral Parenteral	15–30 Within 60–120 Within 15	1–2 Within 2–3 Within 0.5–1	3–6 4–8 1.5–4

From: Ciccone, CD: *Pharmacology in Rehabilitation*, ed. 4. FA Davis, Philadelphia, 2007, p 375, with permission.

⬤ TABLE 6.21 Xanthine Derivative Bronchodilators

Generic Name	Trade Name(s)	Dosage Forms
Aminophylline	Phyllocontin	Oral; extended-release oral; rectal; injection
Dyphylline	Dilor, Lufyllin	Oral; injection
Oxtriphylline	Choledyl	Oral; extended-release oral
Theophylline	Aerolate, Lanophyllin, Theo-Dur, many others	Oral; extended-release oral; injection

From: Ciccone, CD: *Pharmacology in Rehabilitation,* ed 4. FA Davis, Philadelphia, 2007, p 377, with permission.

PULM

⬤ TABLE 6.22 Corticosteroids Used in Obstructive Pulmonary Disease

Generic Name	Trade Name(s)	Dosage Forms*
Beclomethasone	Beclovent, Vanceril	Inhalation
Betamethasone	Celestone	Oral; IV or IM injection
Budesonide	Pulmicort	Inhalation
Cortisone	Cortone	Oral; IM injection
Dexamethasone	Decadron, others	Oral; IV or IM injection
Flunisolide	AeroBid	Inhalation
Hydrocortisone	Cortef	Oral; IV or IM injection
Methylprednisolone	Medrol	Oral; IV injection
Prednisolone	Prelone, others	Oral
Prednisone	Deltasone, others	Oral
Triamcinolone	Azmacort, others	Inhalation; oral; IM injection

From: Ciccone, CD: *Pharmacology in Rehabilitation,* ed 4. FA Davis, Philadelphia, 2007, p 379, with permission.
IM = intramuscular; IV = intravenous.
*Dosage forms that use the inhalation route are often preferred in asthma and other obstructive pulmonary diseases. Systemic administration by the oral route or by injection is typically reserved for acute or severe bronchoconstrictive disease.

Asthma

TABLE 6.23 Differential Features of Reactive Airway Disease

Feature	Asthma
Family history	Frequent
Atopy	Frequent
Smoking history	Infrequent
Sputum character	Predominantly eosinophilic
Chest x-ray	Often normal; hyperinflation during acute attack
Spirometry	Obstructive pattern usually shows good response to bronchodilator

Seasonal Allergies
Antihistamine Drugs Used in Symptomatic Treatment of Seasonal Allergies

TABLE 6.24 Antihistamines Drugs Used in Symptomatic Treatment of Seasonal Allergies

Generic Name	Trade Name(s)*	Dosage†	Sedation Potential‡
Azatadine	Optimine	1–2 mg every 8–12 hr	Low
Brompheniramine	Bromphen, Dimetapp, others	4 mg every 4–6 hr	Low
Carbinoxamine	Rondec, others	4–8 mg every 6–8 hr	Low to moderate
Cetirizine	Zyrtec	5–10 mg once a day	Very low
Chlorpheniramine	Chlor-Trimeton, Telachlor, others	4 mg every 4–6 hr	Low
Clemastine	Tavist	1.34 mg twice daily or 2.68 mg 1–3 times daily	Low

Generic Name	Trade Name(s)*	Dosage†	Sedation Potential‡
Cyproheptadine	Periactin	4 mg every 6–8 hr	Moderate
Desloratadine	Clarinex, Aerius	5 mg once a day	Very low
Dexchlorpheniramine	Polaramine, Dexchlor	2 mg every 4–6 hr	Low
Dimenhydrinate	Dramamine, others	50–100 mg every 4 hr	High
Diphenhydramine	Benadryl, others	25–50 mg every 4–6 hr	High
Doxylamine	Unisom Nighttime Sleep-Aid	12.5–25 mg every 4–6 hr	High
Fexofenadine	Allegra	60 mg twice daily or 180 mg/d	Very low
Hydroxyzine	Atarax, Vistaril	25–100 mg 3–4 times a day	Moderate
Loratadine	Claritin	10 mg once a day	Very low
Phenindamine	Nolahist	25 mg every 4–6 hr	Low
Pyrilamine	Codimal, others	25–50 mg every 8 hr	Moderate
Tripelennamine	PBZ	25–50 mg every 4–6 hr	Moderate
Triprolidine	Actifed, others	2.5 mg every 6–8 hr	Low

From: Ciccone, CD: *Pharmacology in Rehabilitation,* ed 4. FA Davis, Philadelphia, 2007, p 372, with permission.
*Some trade names reflect the combination of the antihistamine with other agents (decongestants, antitussives, and so forth).
†Normal adult dosage when taken orally for antihistamine effects.
‡Sedation potential is based on comparison with other antihistamines and may vary considerably from person to person.

Interventions

Postural Drainage

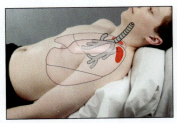

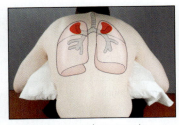

Upper lobes apical segments

Bed or drainage table flat.

Patient leans back on pillow at 30° angle against therapist.

Therapist claps with markedly cupped hand over area between clavicle and top of scapula on each side.

Upper lobes posterior segments

Bed or drainage table flat.

Patient leans over pillow at 30° angle.

Therapist stands behind and claps over upper back on both sides.

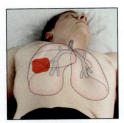

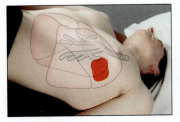

Right middle lobe

Foot of table or bed elevated 16 inches.

Patient lies head down on left side and rotates 1/4 turn backward. Pillow may be placed behind from shoulder to hip. Knees should be flexed.

Therapist claps over right nipple area. In females with breast development or tenderness, use cupped hand with heel of hand under armpit and fingers extending forward beneath the breast.

Left upper lobe lingular segments

Foot of table or bed elevated 16 inches.

Patient lies head down on right side and rotates 1/4 turn backward. Pillow may be placed behind from shoulder to hip. Knees should be flexed.

Therapist claps with moderately cupped hand over left nipple area. In females with breast development or tenderness, use cupped hand with heel of hand under armpit and fingers extending forward beneath the breast.

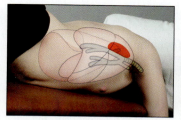

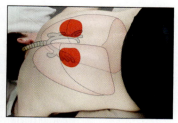

Lower lobes lateral basal segments

Foot of table or bed elevated 20 inches.

Patient lies on abdomen, head down, then rotates 1/4 turn upward. Upper leg is flexed over a pillow for support.

Therapist claps over uppermost portion of lower ribs. (Position shown is for drainage of right lateral basal segment. To drain the left lateral basal segment, patient should lie on his right side in the same posture.)

Lower lobes posterior basal segments

Foot of table or bed elevated 20 inches.

Patient lies on abdomen, head down, with pillow under hips. Therapist claps over lower ribs close to spine on each side.

PULM

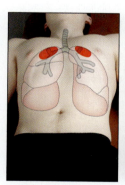

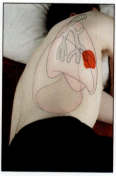

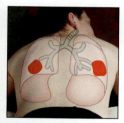

Lower lobes superior segments

Bed or table flat.

Patient lies on abdomen with two pillows under hips.

Therapist claps over middle of back at tip of scapula on either side of spine.

Upper lobes anterior segments

Bed or drainage table flat.

Patient lies on back with pillow under knees.

Therapist claps between clavicle and nipple on each side.

Lower lobes anterior basal segments

Foot of table or bed elevated 20 inches.

Patient lies on side, head down, pillow under knees.

Therapist claps with slightly cupped hand over lower ribs. (Position shown is for drainage of <u>right</u> anterior basal segment. To drain the left anterior basal segment, patient should lie on his right side in the same posture.)

Airway Clearance Techniques

● TABLE 6.25 Airway Clearance Techniques

Technique	Description	Precautions
Postural drainage	A technique in which the patient is positioned to facilitate gravity drainage of secretions from the airways. Positions should be maintained for 5–10 min. See figure on pages 538–539.	Avoid significant changes in patient's vital signs, increase in intracranial pressure with head down positions, and stress to intravascular lines and indwelling tubes. Avoid Trendelenburg positions for patients with gastroesophageal reflux disease or at high risk for gastroesophageal reflux disease.
Percussion	A technique of clapping the chest wall. Percussion can be applied using either manual or mechanical techniques. Often combined with postural drainage.	Avoid redness or petechiae of skin (indicates improper hand positioning by therapist, or patient coagulopathy). May be performed in the presence of rib fractures, chest tubes and subcutaneous emphysema; should produce a hollow sound; should not cause undue pain; does not need to be forceful to be effective if performed properly.
Vibration	The application of fine shaking of the chest wall during the expiratory phase.	Avoid pinching or shearing of soft tissue and digging of fingers into soft tissue. Should not be performed over rib fractures or unstable thoracic spine injuries; be sure to vibrate chest wall, not just shake soft tissue; forcefulness should vary according to patient's needs and tolerance.
Autogenic drainage	This is a 3-level breathing sequence beginning at low lung volumes, followed by breathing at mid-lung volumes, followed by deep breathing and huff coughing. Performed independently by the patient in upright sitting.	Patient needs to be motivated and needs to learn the proper performance of the techniques.

PULM

Technique	Description	Precautions
Directed coughing	A technique that mimics the attributes of an effective spontaneous cough; the cough can be manually assisted by application of external pressure to the epigastric region or thoracic cage during the expiratory phase (as in the patient with neuromuscular disease); sometimes called *quad coughing.*	Coughing ability may be improved by manual support of the postoperative patient's incision; stomas following tracheal tube removal should be covered with an airtight dressing to improve cough efficiency; an effective cough must be preceded by a large inspiration; methods of cough stimulation, including "huffing," vibration, summed breathing, external tracheal compression and oral pharyngeal stimulation, may be used.
Suctioning	To clear secretions from the trachea of patients who have an artificial airway in place.	In intubated patients, suctioning is performed routinely and is an integral part of chest therapy; frequency of suctioning is determined by the quantity of secretions; the suctioning procedure should be limited to a total of 15 sec; the suction catheter can reach only to the level of the main-stem bronchus; it is more difficult to cannulate the left main-stem bronchus than the right; nasotracheal suctioning should be avoided.
Manual hyperinflation	This is a technique to improve secretion clearance by use of a manual ventilation device, an end-inspiratory pause, and a fast, unobstructed exhalation.	Avoid barotrauma; hyperinflation can produce alterations in cardiac output.
Forced expiratory technique (FET)	Sometimes called *huff coughing,* this technique consists of one or 2 huffs from mid-to-low lung volumes with the glottis open, followed by relaxed diaphragmatic breathing.	Requires patient cooperation; avoid excessive fatigue.

PULM

(table continues on page 542)

■ TABLE 6.25 **Airway Clearance Techniques** (continued)

Technique	Description	Precautions
Active cycle breathing	This technique includes breathing control, forced expiratory technique, thoracic expansion techniques, and may include postural drainage and percussion.	Avoid Trendelenburg positions for patients with gastroesophageal reflux disease or at high risk for gastroesophageal reflux disease. Requires patient cooperation.
Positive expiratory pressure (PEP)	With this technique the patient exhales against a pressure of 10–20 cm H_2O.	Risk of pneumothorax; sinusitis; epistaxis; ear infection.
Oscillatory positive expiratory pressure (PEP)	This technique uses a device that produces PEP with oscillations in the airway during the expiratory phase.	Risk of pneumothorax; sinusitis; epistaxis; ear infection.
High frequency chest wall oscillation	This technique uses an inflatable vest that attaches by hoses to an air pulse generator producing pressures to about 50 cm H^2O at frequencies of 5–25 Hz.	Do not use for persons with chest tubes, indwelling catheter or other devices in chest area.
Exercise	Exercise, including ambulation, can mobilize secretions, in addition to improve pulmonary function and activity limitations of the patient.	Avoid stress to intravascular lines and indwelling tubes, orthostatic hypotension, significant changes in vital signs, and dyspnea.

For more information: Hess, DR: Evidence for secretion clearance techniques. *Cardiopulmonary Phys Ther J* 13:7–22, 2002;
Frownfelter, D, and Dean, E: *Cardiovascular and Pulmonary Physical Therapy: Evidence and Practice,* ed. 4. Mosby, St. Louis, 2006;
Mackenzie, CF, Imle, PC, and Ciesla, NL: *Chest Physiotherapy in the Intensive Care Unit,* ed. 2. Williams & Wilkins, Baltimore, 1989, pp 358–359.

VII

INTEGUMENTARY

Anatomy

Skin

The most superficial, and thinnest, layer of skin is the epidermis, which lies on top of the dermis. The dermis is thicker than the epidermis and contains many glands and nerve endings. Below the dermis is subcutaneous tissue, which is the thickest layer and is composed primarily of fat. Collectively, the skin functions to provide protection from the outside world, regulate temperature, provide tactile input, absorb ultraviolet radiation, and metabolize vitamin D. Skin is also a major component of appearance.

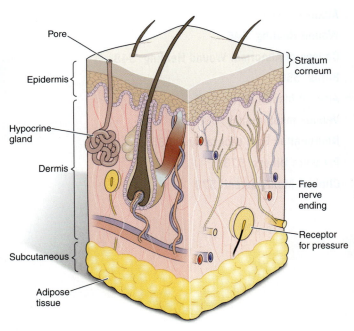

Complete skin section.

🔴 TABLE 7.1 **Types of Cells and Location in Skin**

Layer of Skin	Cell Type	Function
Epidermis	Keratinocytes (squamous cells)	Synthesis of keratin
	Melanocytes	Synthesis of melanin
	Langerhan's cells	Immune response
	Basal cells	Epidermal production
	Eccrine unit	Thermoregulation by perspiration
	Apocrine unit	Sweat production
	Hair follicle	Protection
	Nails	Protection
	Sebaceous glands	Produces sebum (oil for lubrication of skin)
Dermis	Fibroblasts	Collagen synthesis
	Collagen	Insoluble connective tissue protein
	Elastin	Primary protein in elastic tissue
	Macrophages	Phagocytosis; initiate growth and repair through growth factor production
	Mast cells	Provide histamine for vasodilation
	Lymphatic glands	Removal of microbes and interstitial waste
	Blood vessels	Thermoregulation; provides metabolic skin requirements
	Nerve fibers	Sensory perception
Subcutaneous tissue	Adipose	Protection from trauma, energy storage, thermoregulation

INTEG

Wound Healing

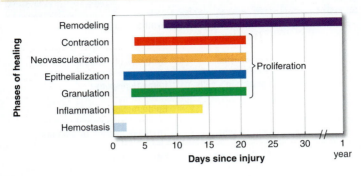

Normal wound healing.

TABLE 7.2 Stages of Wound Healing

Stage of Healing (time after injury)	Major Cellular Component	Description
Hemostasis (0–2 days)	Platelets	Platelets are the first cells to arrive at the site of injury. They attach to exposed collagen at the area of injury and release chemicals that attract more platelets, ultimately forming a platelet plug to temporarily stop bleeding. Platelets are also vital to the healing process because of the growth factors they release.
Inflammation (4–6 days)	Leukocytes	White blood cells arrive at the wound site in response to the coagulation cascade. Leukocytes are divided into granulocytes and monocytes. Granulocytes are more abundant, and include neutrophils, basophils, and eosinophils, with neutrophils being the most common of the three. Neutrophils arrive first and are phagocytic, as are eosinophils. They are only necessary for wound healing in the presence of infection. Basophils release histamine, which increases the vascular permeability at the wound site. The most

Stage of Healing (time after injury)	Major Cellular Component	Description
		important inflammatory cells are the macrophages, which are monocytes. Macrophages are also phagocytic, but unlike neutrophils their presence is crucial to wound healing in all wounds. In addition to phagocytosis, the macrophages play a critical role in stimulating the proliferative phase of healing.
Proliferation (4–14 days)		
Granulation	Fibroblasts	The attraction of fibroblasts to the wound is initiated by macrophages that are present from the inflammatory phase. Fibroblasts produce a wound matrix that consists of collagen, elastin, and proteoglycans. The stimulus for fibroblast activity is low oxygen conditions, as are typical in a wound.
Epithelialization	Keratinocytes	In superficial wounds, keratinocytes begin migrating across the wound from the edges, as well as from any hair follicles in the wound bed. This is best accomplished in a moist environment and will continue until the skin edges meet the leading skin edge from the other side of the wound. A healthy matrix laid down by the fibroblasts is crucial for the keratinocytes to migrate over the top.
Neovascularization	Endothelial cells	New blood vessel formation occurs in conjunction with the fibroblast activity to create a well-vascularized layer of granulation tissue. The endothelial cells stimulate the production of new blood vessels and also transport oxygen and nutrients into the wound environment. Other factors that contribute to new blood vessel formation are

INTEG

(table continues on page 548)

TABLE 7.2 Stages of Wound Healing (continued)

Stage of Healing (time after injury)	Major Cellular Component	Description
		low oxygen tension, lactic acid, biogenic amines, and several growth factors including those released by fibroblasts and macrophages.
Contraction	Myofibroblasts	Myofibroblasts are specialized fibroblasts that have characteristics of smooth muscle cells, and thus are capable of contracting. In full-thickness wounds, contraction peaks at 2 wk and accounts for up to a 40% reduction in wound size. Contraction is regulated by cellular actin and enhanced by fibronectin. Wound contraction is not a factor in superficial wounds where re-epithelialization can occur from within the wound.
Remodeling (7 days to > 1 yr)	Collagen and collagenase	After the proliferative phase is complete, a haphazard arrangement of matrix materials (primarily collagen) is present. Over a period of time lasting up to 1 year after injury, the collagen is remodeled. Type III collagen is converted to the more stable type I collagen and fibers are aligned parallel to the lines of tension on the scar. This is accomplished by a delicate balance of collagen production and collagen breakdown by collagenase.

Causes of Abnormal Wound Healing

Infection

Whether a wound becomes infected or not depends on the interplay between the host response and the characteristics of the invading pathogen. Host defenses depend primarily on an intact immune system consisting of granulocytes (neutrophils, eosinophils, basophils), which are the first responders, as well as macrophages and lymphocytes (T cells and B cells). An adequate response is also dependent on sufficient blood flow to the area of interest and proper nutrition. Two characteristics of the invading organism that have the greatest influence on whether an infection will develop are dose and virulence. *Dose* refers to the quantity of the bacteria that is present, and *virulence* refers to potency, or the ability to produce a severe disease. If the host defenses are strong enough, a wound can be colonized with bacteria and not exhibit any signs of infection, and will heal without complications. With a healthy host response, the quantitative definition of infection is 10^5 organisms/gram of tissue for most forms of bacteria.

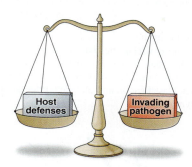

TABLE 7.3 The Infection Continuum

Sterile	Contaminated	Colonized	Critically Colonized	Systemic Infection
Only occurs in the operating room	All open wounds are contaminated. Bacteria are present, but not adhering to the wound.	All chronic wounds are colonized. Bacteria adhering to the wound, but not impairing wound healing.	Bacteria are adhered to the wound and replicating. Leads to activation of the local immune response, but no signs of systemic infection.	Bacteria present in amounts that are overwhelming the host response. Will have signs and symptoms of systemic infections, including worsening of the wound.

Refer to Section XII, General Medicine, pages 790–801, for further information on types and treatment of bacterial infections.

Burns

Burn Classifications

The Nature of the Burn Wound

Based on cellular events, a typical burn wound that is more severe than a superficial burn can be said to have three zones. In the zone of coagulation, there is cell death. In the zone of stasis, cells are injured and will usually die within 24–48 hours unless there is adequate treatment. In the zone of hyperemia, there is minimal cell damage. The extent of each wound is dependent on the intensity and duration of the heat source, skin thickness, vascularity, age, and pigmentation.

Classification of Burn Injury

Most medical literature now classifies burn injuries by the depth of the skin tissue destroyed rather than by the previously used classification of first-, second-, and third-degree burns. The following figures identify the extent of the burn wound for each classification and include a brief description of general clinical signs and symptoms.

INTEG

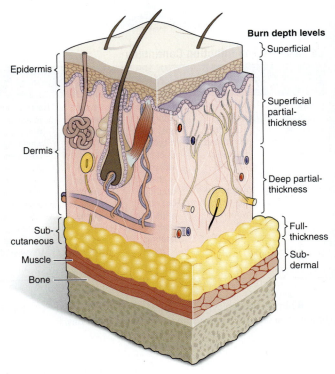

Skin section showing burn depth levels of different types of burns.

Estimating Burn Areas

Rule of Nines

The rule of nines is used to estimate the percentage of body area burned. Body areas are said to constitute either 9% of the area or some number divisible by 9. The head and each upper extremity are 9% (4.5% on each surface). The posterior surface of the trunk (the back) is 18%, as is the anterior surface of the trunk. The genital area is 1%, and each lower extremity is 18% (9% on each surface). Although the rule of nines is very practical, it provides only gross estimates of the areas and has been supplanted for exact estimates by use of Lund-Browder charts.

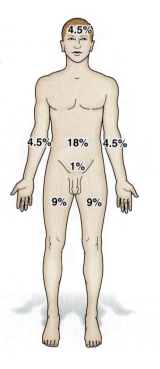
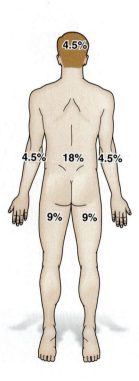

INTEG

Lund-Browder Charts

The rule of nines is widely used to estimate body surface area, but more accurate estimates of areas are thought to be obtainable by use of Lund-Browder charts. These take into account changes that occur during normal growth. The total estimate for a child or an adult is obtained by adding the relative percentages for each body area according to the appropriate age group. This accounts for changes in the proportion of the head and lower extremities to body surface area during growth.

Young Children

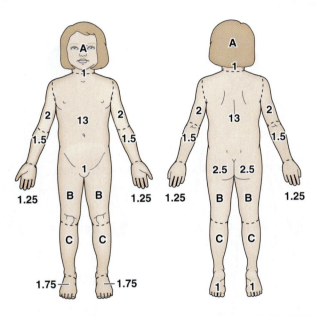

TABLE 7.4 Estimation of Body Surface Areas in Young Children

	Age in Years		
Area	0	1–4	5–9
A. Each surface of the head	9.5	8.5	6.5
B. Each surface of the thigh	2.75	3.25	4.0
C. Each surface of the leg	2.5	2.5	2.75

Children and Adults

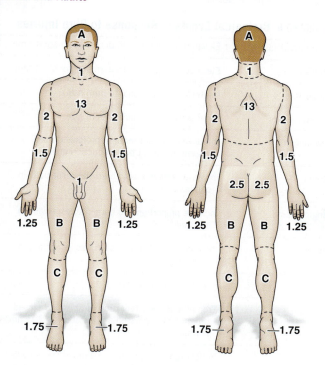

TABLE 7.5 Estimation of Body Surface Areas in Children and Adults

Area	Age in Years		
	10–14	15	Adult
A. Each surface of the head	5.5	4.5	3.5
B. Each surface of the thigh	4.25	4.5	4.75
C. Each surface of the leg	3.0	3.25	3.5

Based on: Lund, CC, and Browder, NC: The estimation of area of burns. *Surg Gynecol Obstet* 79:352–358, 1944.

Biological Events in Burns

⬤ **TABLE 7.6** **Biological Events in Response to Burn Injuries**

Free fatty acids	Elevated proportional to burn size for short time.
Triglycerides	Elevated proportional to burn size for short time.
Cholesterol	Depressed proportional to burn size.
Phospholipids	Depressed proportional to burn size.
Fibrinogen	Initial fall with subsequent prolonged rise. Consumption great but production greater.
Renin	Increase proportional to burn size, especially in children.
Angiotensin	Increase proportional to burn size, especially in children.
ACTH	Increase proportional to burn size, especially in children.
Protein	Rapid and persistent drop.
Albumin	Prompt and persistent drop until wound closed; production depressed and catabolism 2–3 times normal.
Globulin	Initial drop with rise to supranormal levels by 5–7 days; catabolism 2–3 times normal, but production vastly increased.
IgG	Immediate depression followed by slow rise.
IgM	Altered little by burn in adults but in children follows pattern of IgG.
IgA	Altered little by burn in adults but in children follows pattern of IgG.
Red blood cells	Immediate loss proportional to burn size and depth. Life span 30% of normal owing to plasma factor.
White blood cells	Initial and prolonged rise. May drop with sepsis.
Cardiac output	Precipitous drop to 20%–40% of normal with slow spontaneous recovery in 24–36 hr. Myocardial depressant factor demonstrated.
Blood viscosity	Sharp rise proportional to hematocrit.

INTEG

Carboxyhemoglobin	Not significant after 72 hr (<2%). Most prominent with inhalation injury (80%). Exists with or without surface burns.
BSP	Retention proportional to burn size with rapid rise and persistence for several weeks.
Cortisol	Prompt rise to 2–4 times normal.
Aldosterone	Usually returns to normal by end of first week but may remain elevated for long periods. Varied response to ACTH often nil in early period.
Peripheral resistance	Rises sharply—slow fall.
Pulmonary vascular resistance	Rises sharply—slow fall.
Pulmonary artery pressure	Prompt rise and slow return.
Left atrial pressure	Normal or low. High with failure.
PO_2	Low with delay or inadequate therapy.
pH	Prompt response to therapy.
PCO_2	Initial alkalosis or hyperventilation promptly resolves.
Blood lactate	May rise to high levels with hyperventilation or poor perfusion.
Excess lactate	Mild elevations characteristic but may rise to high levels with inadequate or delayed resuscitation.
ALT AST Alk phos	Prompt rise with peak at 2–3 days and persistence for several weeks owing to liver damage, not release of skin enzymes.
Renal function	Renal plasma flow depressed more than glomerular filtration rates. Free water clearances down. All values promptly return to normal with adequate resuscitation.
Evaporative water loss	Donor sites and partial-thickness burns have intermediate loss rates. Full-thickness burns lose at same rate as open pan of water. Estimate (25 + % burn) × M^2 body surface. Fifteen to 20 times normal skin rates.

(table continues on page 556)

INTEG

TABLE 7.6 Biological Events in Response to Burn Injuries (continued)

Pulmonary function (in absence of pneumonia)	Proportional to magnitude of burn; independent of inhalation injury. Minute ventilation (V_e) increased up to 500%; peak at 5 days. Static compliance (CSTAT) usually normal but may change with onset pneumonia. Lung clearance index (LCI) normal until terminal. Oxygen consumption greatly increased. Forced vital capacity (FVC) normal even with V_e increase; may drop with pneumonia.

From: O'Sullivan, SB, and Schmitz, TJ: *Physical Rehabilitation: Assessment and Treatment,* ed. 3. FA Davis, Philadelphia, 1994, p 518, with permission.
ACTH = adrenocorticotropic hormone; alk phos = alkaline phosphatase; ALT = alanine transaminase; AST = aspartate transaminase; BSP = bromsulphalein.

Arterial Insufficiency

Risk Factors for Peripheral Arterial Disease

Modifiable
- Smoking
- Diabetes
- Hypertension
- Hypercholesterolemia
- Obesity

Nonmodifiable
- Age >70 years
- Male gender
- Diabetes
- Hypercoagulable states
- Hyperhomocysteinemia

TABLE 7.7 Arterial Wound Characteristics

Location	Dorsum of foot, lateral leg, toes
Pain	May be severe
Edema	Initially not present. May occur if limb remains in dependent position.
Size	Variable; dependent on site of vascular compromise
Depth	Typically deep; may involve tendon, capsule, bone

Shape	Punched out appearance
Exudate	Minimal
Color	Pale red if circulation diminished; yellow or black if circulation diminished further
Skin temperature	Cool to touch
Pulses	Diminished or absent

Peripheral Arterial Assessment

Pulse Palpation and Grading

For the lower extremity, a thorough vascular examination should include assessment of the iliac, femoral, popliteal, dorsalis pedis, and posterior tibial arteries. Palpation is complicated by edema, scar tissue, and induration. Pulses are graded as absent or present, but several scales exist to classify the strength of the pulse further. Because several scales exist, it is recommended that the description be included with the score, that is, 3+ (normal pulse). The agreement between clinicians in determining whether lower extremity pulses are present or absent has been reported as fair to nearly perfect agreement, but the ability to distinguish between normal and reduced pulses is very poor. Training has been shown to improve agreement between investigators in the assessment of the posterial tibial and dorsalis pedis arteries.

Grading Pulses

0 = No palpable pulse
1+ = Barely perceptible pulse
2+ = Diminished pulse
3+ = Normal pulse
4+ = Bounding pulse; possible aneurysm.

Ankle-Brachial Index (ABI) Testing

The ankle-brachial index is a ratio of the systolic blood pressure in the ankle (dorsalis pedis or posterior tibial artery) to the systolic blood pressure in the brachial artery of the arm. The test is performed with the patient in supine position, and requires only a blood pressure cuff and a handheld Doppler probe. A normal value is 1.0 and values less than 0.97 have been shown to be 96% to 97% sensitive and 94% to 100% selective for patients with occlusions or stenoses identified angiographically.

INTEG

TABLE 7.8 Ankle-Brachial Index (ABI) Interpretation

ABI	Clinical Significance
1.2	Individuals with long-standing diabetes mellitus may have an ABI of this magnitude, indicating noncompressible, calcified large lower extremity arteries (i.e., posterior tibial and/or popliteal arteries). In this case, an ABI provides useful information for several decades. The ABI is not useful in this instance.
1.0	Normal arterial blood flow. Compression therapy not indicated.
0.8–1.0	Mild arterial occlusive disease. May have no symptoms. Compression therapy with monitoring and caution.
0.5–0.8	Moderate arterial occlusive disease. Vascular specialist referral needed.
< 0.5	Severe arterial occlusive disease. Vascular specialist referral needed. Compression therapy absolutely contraindicated. No débridement because of high risk for necrosis and infection.

From: McCulloch, JM, and Kloth, LC: *Wound Healing: Evidence-Based Management,* ed. 4. FA Davis, Philadelphia, 2010, p 96, with permission.

Skin Temperature Assessment

Large changes in skin temperature can be assessed by palpation. At temperatures around 30°C changes as small as 1°C may be noticeable. There may be a large amount of variability and the assessment is fairly subjective. For a quantifiable, objective temperature assessment, infrared thermometers can be used and will give a reading to within one tenth of a degree. A unilateral cold foot usually indicates arterial disease. Stoffers et al calculated a sensitivity of 0.10 and specificity of 0.98 in a trial involving 2,455 patients.

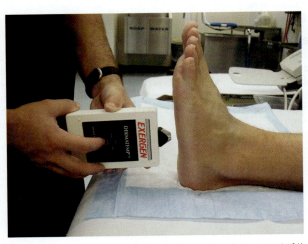

Infrared thermometer used to assess the temperature on the plantar aspect of the foot.

Capillary Refill

The examiner applies pressure to the pulp of any toe for several seconds until blanching is present. When the pressure is removed, the normal color should return within 3 seconds. If it takes longer than this, it is indicative of poor perfusion to the capillary beds in small vessel disease. Capillary refill has been found to be of limited diagnostic value, in part due to the fact that the capillaries may be refilling from veins in the area, and not due to an intact capillary network.

Rubor of Dependency and Venous Filling Time

The rubor of dependency and venous filling time tests are noninvasive tests of the arterial system, and can be performed together. In both tests, the patient is positioned supine. The color on the plantar aspect of the foot should be noted. The leg is passively elevated to 45° for 1 minute by the examiner. In the presence of arterial disease, drastic blanching will be noted on the plantar aspect of the foot while it is elevated. The leg is then placed in a dependent position. The rubor of dependency test will result in the return of the normal color within 15 seconds if the arterial system is intact. If the test is positive for arterial insufficiency, the plantar aspect of the foot will turn dark red and take at least 30 seconds for color to return. The venous filling time is measured by monitoring the veins in the dorsum of the foot. If the veins refill within 15 seconds of being put in a dependent position there is normal perfusion. If venous distention takes longer than 30 seconds, it is positive for arterial compromise.

In several studies, color change was identified as a weak predictor of arterial disease, with a positive likelihood ratio ranging from 1.6 to 2.8. It did not improve the clinical prediction after multivariate analysis. Venous filling time greater than 20 seconds has a low sensitivity (0.22–0.25), but was helpful in the prediction of arterial disease, with a positive likelihood ratio of 3.6 to 4.6.

Claudication Testing

Claudication pain, which results from the increased oxygen demands of the exercising muscle, can be used to assess the extent of vascular involvement. The amount of time it takes for calf pain to result from walking at a standardized pace on level ground can be recorded. Alternatively, there are subjective grades that can be applied to claudication symptoms, such as the one below.

TABLE 7.9 Grades of Claudication Symptoms

Grade	Description
I	Definite discomfort or pain, but only of initial or modest levels
II	Moderate discomfort or pain from which the patient's attention can be diverted
III	Intense pain from which the patient's attention cannot be diverted
IV	Excruciating and unbearable pain

Based on: *ACSM's Guidelines for Exercise Testing and Prescription,* ed. 8. Lippincott Williams & Wilkins, Philadelphia, 2009, p 120.

Venous Insufficiency

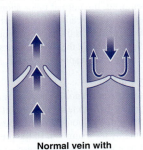 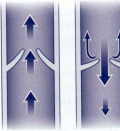

Normal vein with competent valves

Abnormal vein with incompetent valves allowing blood to backflow

Competent and incompetent vessels.

Risk Factors for Venous Insufficiency

- History of varicose veins
- Deep venous thrombophlebitis
- Previous vein surgery
- Obesity
- Age (in males)
- Clotting disorders
- Venous hypertension
- Pregnancy
- Lower extremity trauma
- Lower extremity dependency
- Family history of venous problems

TABLE 7.10 Typical Venous Wound Presentation

Location	Proximal to medial malleolus
Shape	Irregular shape
Size	May be very large
Depth	Superficial
Color	Typically red, often with layer of yellow fibrin on wound surface
Drainage	Moderate to heavy

Periwound	Hemosiderin staining and lipodermatosclerosis
Edema	Moderate to severe
Pulses	Present
Pain	Aching; worse with prolonged dependent positions and improved with elevation

Peripheral Venous System Assessment

Percussion Test

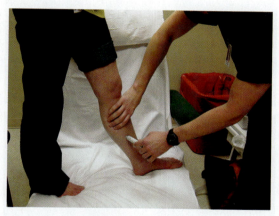

The percussion test is a noninvasive assessment of the valves of the venous system. With the patient standing, the examiner places the Doppler along the vein at a distal location while percussing the vein proximally. An increase in blood flow noted with the Doppler indicates incompetent venous valves between the area of palpation and percussion.

INTEG

Trendelenburg Test

The Trendelenburg test is a noninvasive assessment of the peripheral venous system that can be used to differentiate between superficial or perforating incompetent veins as the causative factor in venous insufficiency.

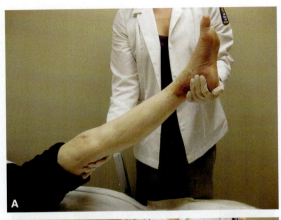

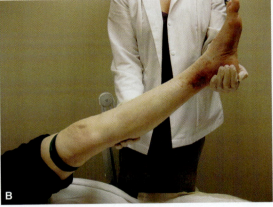

Trendelenburg. (A) Patient lying supine with leg passively elevated 45° for 1 min to drain venous system. (B) A tourniquet is loosely applied to occlude the superficial venous system without compromising arterial flow.

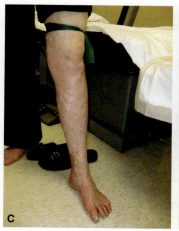 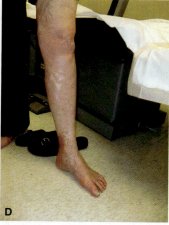

(C) The patient is assisted to a standing position rapidly with the tourniquet in place. Filling of the superficial veins within 5 sec indicates incompetence of the valves in the perforating veins below the tourniquet. (D) The tourniquet is then removed and the superficial veins are monitored for additional, immediate filling. If this occurs within the first 5 sec, it is indicative of valvular incompetence of the superficial veins.

Deep Venous Thrombosis Assessment

A deep venous thrombosis (DVT), or blood clot in a vein, has the potential to cause serious injury or even death, and thus must be evaluated carefully. Suspect a DVT if a patient presents with resting calf pain and edema distal to the calf. Other signs associated with a DVT include warmth, tenderness, and redness distal to the obstruction. Previous tests such as Homan's sign and the cuff test are potentially dangerous as they could dislodge a clot, and frequently result in false positive tests. The following clinical prediction model has been used to determine which patients are at a low probability for having a DVT. A low probability score on the Wells Clinical Prediction model indicates a 95% probability that a DVT is not present. When combined with a negative D-dimer, this probability increases to 99%.

Well's Clinical Decision Rules for Deep Venous Thrombosis

One point assigned for the presence of each of the following:

- Active cancer (within 6 mo of diagnosis or receiving palliative care)
- Paralysis, paresis, or recent immobilization of lower extremity
- Bedridden for more than 3 days or major surgery in the last 4 weeks
- Localized tenderness in the center of the posterior calf, the popliteal space, or along the femoral vein in the anterior thigh/groin
- Entire lower extremity swelling
- Unilateral calf swelling (more than 3 mm larger than uninvolved side)

- Unilateral pitting edema
- Collateral superficial veins (nonvaricose)

Subtract two points if:

- An alternative diagnosis is as likely (or more likely) than DVT (e.g., cellulitis, postoperative swelling, calf strain)

Total Score:

- −2 to 0   Low probability of DVT (3%)
- 1 to 2   Moderate probability of DVT (17%)
- 3 or more   High probability of DVT (75%)

Medical consultation is advised in the presence of low probability; medical referral is required with moderate or high score.

CEAP Classification of Venous Disease

Chronic venous disorders can be classified using the CEAP classification system. The CEAP classification is divided into a Clinical classification, Etiological classification, Anatomic classification, and a Pathophysiological classification.

TABLE 7.11 Clinical Classification from CEAP Classification

C_0	No visible or palpable signs of venous disease
C_1	Telangiectasies or reticular veins
C_2	Varicose veins
C_3	Edema
C_{4a}	Pigmentation or eczema
C_{4b}	Lipodermatosclerosis or atrophie blanche
C_5	Healed venous ulcer
C_6	Active venous ulcer
S	Symptomatic, including ache, pain, tightness, skin irritation, heaviness, and muscle cramps, and other complaints attributable to venous dysfunction
A	Asymptomatic

Neuropathic Foot Ulcerations

🔴 TABLE 7.12 Risk Factors for Diabetic Foot Ulcers

Foot Issues	Diabetic Issues	Neuropathic Issues	Skin Issues	Miscellaneous Issues
Higher plantar temperature	Duration of diabetes	Absent Achilles tendon reflex	No extremity hair	Male
Elevated foot pressures	Poor glucose control	Insensate to 5.07 (10-g) monofilament	Dryness	Taller height
Footwear rubbing	Needs insulin	Subjective neuropathic symptoms	Redness	History of amputation
More callosities	Higher fasting glucose	Elevated vibration threshold	Previous ulcers	Alcohol/tobacco abuse
Rigid foot deformities	Poor diabetes knowledge		Ulcer resulting from surgery	Divorce/living alone
Trauma			Occupational hazards	Immobile
			Trauma	TcPO$_2$ < 30 mm Hg
				Poor vision
				Vascular disease
				Age
				Immunopathy
				Nephropathy

From: McCulloch, JM, and Kloth, LC: *Wound Healing: Evidence-Based Management,* ed. 4. FA Davis, Philadelphia, 2010, pp 71, with permission.
TcPO$_2$ = transcutaneous partial pressure of oxygen.

Neuropathic Foot Examination

History

Assess for history of diseases/conditions that predispose patient to neuropathy, including:

- Diabetes
  - Assess both blood sugar levels and hemoglobin A_1C levels. Hemoglobin A_1C levels relate to the average blood sugar over the past 3 months, and will not be affected by eating or fasting prior to testing to the same degree that blood glucose levels will.
  - According to the American Diabetes Association the goal hemoglobin A_1C = 7% or less
- Hansen's disease
- Spina bifida
- Chronic alcoholism
- Peripheral nerve injury
- Charcot-Marie-Tooth disease
- Lumbosacral spine injury
- Neuro-syphilis

Sensory Testing

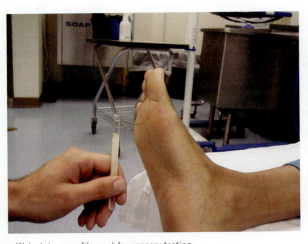

Semmes-Weinstein monofilament for sensory testing.

Sensory testing is performed with a 5.07 (10-g) Semmes-Weinstein monofilament to assess for loss of protective sensation. Touch each spot shown in the figure below with enough force to bend the monofilament 1 inch. Instruct the patient to close his or her eyes and respond yes when the monofilament is felt. Inability to perceive the monofilament in any one spot is considered positive for a loss of protective sensation.

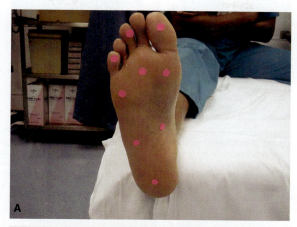

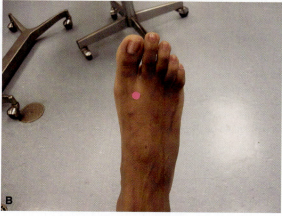

The locations for monofilament testing using the 10-site method. (A) Plantar. (B) Dorsal.

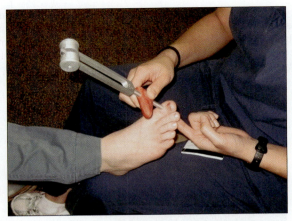

Vibratory threshold testing using a 128-Hz tuning fork. Multiple studies have found the assessment of peripheral neuropathy with a tuning fork to be reproducible and accurate, and more sensitive to change than monofilament testing. The vibrating tuning fork is placed on the dorsal aspect of the great toe interphalangeal joint. Several methods to interpret the results exist. The time the vibration is felt by the patient can be recorded and compared to established norms, or to other areas of the body with intact sensation.

Motor Testing

Strength Testing

Manual muscle testing is used for extrinsic and intrinsic foot musculature. (See pp. 126, 130–131 in Section III, Musculoskeletal, for further information on muscle testing.)

Limitations of Motion

Normal gait requires a minimum of 10° of ankle dorsiflexion and 55° of metatarsophalangeal extension. Limitations to either of these ranges will lead to increased forefoot pressures in the late stance phases of gait, or will result in shortened step length on the affected side to avoid excessive forefoot weight-bearing.

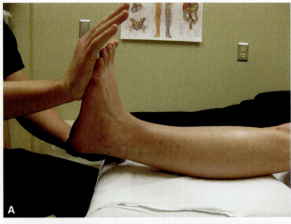

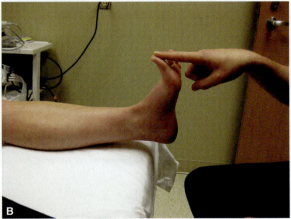

Passive range of motion assessment of (A) dorsiflexion and (B) great toe extension.

Identification of Deformities

Deformities predispose the foot to ulceration by creating high-pressure areas. These areas are even more susceptible to breakdown when combined with sensory impairment.

TABLE 7.13 The Impact of Selected Deformities on Ulceration

Deformity	Areas at Risk for Ulceration
Bunion	Medial first metatarsophalangeal joint
Claw toes	Plantar aspect of metatarsal heads, dorsal aspect of interphalangeal joints, most distal aspect of distal phalanx
Hammer toes	Plantar aspect of metatarsal heads, dorsal aspect of interphalangeal joints
Charcot fractures	Plantar midfoot; varying other areas dependent upon degree of deformity
Plantarflexed first ray	Plantar aspect of first metatarsal head and great toe
Hallux limitus	Plantar aspect of great toe
Hallux valgus	Dorsal and medial first metatarsal head
Pes cavus	Heel and metatarsal heads
Pes planus	Medial aspect of foot
Equinovarus	Lateral aspect of foot
Previous amputations	Adjacant weight-bearing areas

Adapted from: Mahoney E: Diabetic foot ulcerations. In McCulloch, JM, and Kloth, LC: *Wound Healing: Evidence-Based Management,* ed. 4. FA Davis, Philadelphia, 2010, p 215, with permission.

Skin Inspection

A thorough skin assessment should be performed to identify areas of high stress. Potential problem areas can be detected by looking for redness, increased local temperature, swelling, maceration (see Fig. 7.16), callus, preulceration, or ulceration. The presence of any of these factors may indicate infection or inflammation due to stress on the tissue and warrants further investigation. Calluses are indicative of high-pressure areas, and frequently may be covering an underlying ulceration. Heavy callus should be removed by a trained professional to reduce pressure on the tissue underneath. Skin temperature can be assessed to within one-tenth of a degree using an infrared thermometer (see Fig. 7.8 in arterial assessment section of this chapter).

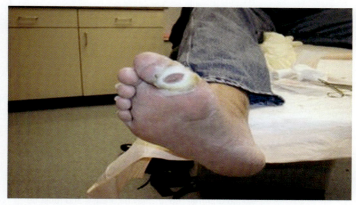

Diabetic foot ulcer with periwound maceration.

Vascular Testing

Signs of poor perfusion to the foot include:

- Absent or diminished pulses in the foot
- Capillary refill greater than three seconds
- Hairless, shiny, atrophic skin
- Claudication or rest pain
- Rubor of dependency

For further information on vascular testing, refer to the vascular assessment section of this chapter.

Footwear Assessment

- The shape of the shoe conforms to the shape of the foot.
- There is a ⅜- to ½-inch space between the end of the shoe and the longest toe.
- The first metatarsophalangeal joint is at the widest part of the shoe.
- The toe box is deep and wide enough for toe spread and toe clearance.
- Laces or straps adjust for a snug fit over the instep.
- There is a snug fit around the heel.

From:

Mahoney, E: Diabetic foot ulcerations. In McCulloch, JM, and Kloth, LC: Wound Healing: Evidence-Based Management, ed. 4. FA Davis, Philadelphia, 2010, p 216, with permission.

INTEG

🟠 **TABLE 7.14** **Characteristics of the Typical Neuropathic Foot Ulcer**

Location	Forefoot, specifically metatarsal heads and toes. Also any area bearing weight as a result of a deformity, typically over a bony process
Size	Variable; dependent upon duration of ulceration, degree of deformity, and precise location on the foot, among other factors
Shape	Typically round
Depth	Often deep. May include exposed bone
Periwound	Hyperkeratotic margins. Maceration often present from wound drainage. Callus may be present and must be removed to assess for underlying wound.
Wound bed	Typically red, unless vascular compromise is present.
Drainage	Drainage tends to be high if not off-loaded properly, and decreases when pressure is relieved. Drainage is reduced in the presence of arterial compromise, and increased with venous pathology.

Wagner Ulcer Classification

Grade	Description
0	Intact skin
1	Superficial ulcer
2	Deep ulcer
3	Deep, infected ulcer
4	Partial-foot gangrene
5	Full-foot gangrene

🟠 **TABLE 7.15** **The University of Texas Classification System for Diabetic Foot Wounds**

Stage	0	1	2	3
A	Preulcerative or postulcerative lesion completely epithelialized	Superficial wound not involving tendon, capsule, or bone	Wound penetrating to tendon or capsule	Wound penetrating to bone or joint
B	Infection	Infection	Infection	Infection

Stage	0	1	2	3
C	Ischemia	Ischemia	Ischemia	Ischemia
D	Infection and ischemia	Infection and ischemia	Infection and ischemia	Infection and ischemia

From: McCulloch, JM, and Kloth, LC: *Wound Healing: Evidence-Based Management,* ed. 4. FA Davis, Philadelphia, 2010, p 79, with permission.

Pressure Ulcers

Risk Factors for Pressure Ulcer Development

- Immobility (number one risk factor)
- Incontinence/excess moisture
- Increased age
- Respiratory disease
- Protein calorie malnutrition
- Patients undergoing surgery
- Low body mass index
- Patients in critical care facilities
- Diabetes
- Neurological impairment
- Vascular disease
- Diminished mentation
- Prolonged surgical procedures under general anesthesia
- Previous ulceration site

Pressure Ulcer Staging

According to the National Pressure Ulcer Advisory Panel (NPUAP), the definition of a pressure ulcer is "localized injury to the skin and/or underlying tissue usually over a bony prominence, as a result of pressure, or pressure in combination with shear and/or friction."[1] An individual's susceptibility to a pressure ulcer is determined by an interaction of many factors, primarily those listed in the table above. The NPUAP classifies pressure ulcers based on the depth of injury, with stage I being the most superficial, and stage IV the deepest. In addition, two new stages, suspected deep tissue injury and unstageable, were added in 2007. The following is a definition of each stage as defined by the NPUAP:

---

[1]See NUPAP website, http://www.npuap.org

TABLE 7.16 Staging Pressure Ulcers

Stage I	Intact skin with non-blanchable redness of a localized area usually over a bony prominence. Darkly pigmented skin may not have visible blanching; its color may differ from the surrounding area. It may also be painful, firm, soft, warmer, or cooler than adjacent skin. It is a warning sign for at-risk patients.
Stage II	Partial thickness loss of dermis presenting as a shallow open ulcer with a red-pink wound bed, without slough. May also present as an intact or open/ruptured serum-filled blister.
Stage III	Full thickness tissue loss. Subcutaneous fat may be visible but the fascia and structures beneath the fascia (bone, tendon, ligaments, muscle, joint capsule) are not exposed. Slough may be present but does not obscure the depth of tissue loss. May include undermining and tunneling.
Stage IV	Full thickness tissue loss with exposed bone, tendon, or muscle. Slough or eschar may be present on some parts of the wound bed. Often includes undermining and tunneling.
Suspected deep tissue injury	Purple or maroon localized area of discolored intact skin or blood-filled blister due to damage of underlying soft tissue from pressure and/or shear. The area may be preceded by tissue that is painful, firm, mushy, boggy, warmer, or cooler as compared to adjacent tissue.
Unstageable	Full thickness tissue loss in which the base of the ulcer is covered by slough (yellow, tan, gray, green, or brown) and/or eschar (tan, brown, or black) in the wound bed.

From: National Pressure Ulcer Advisory Panel. http://www.npuap.org. Accessed January 21, 2012. With permission.

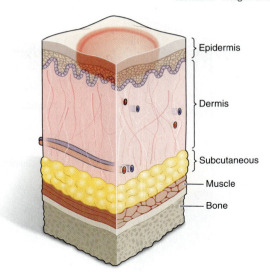

Stage I pressure ulcer.

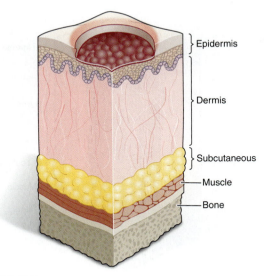

Stage II pressure ulcer.

INTEG

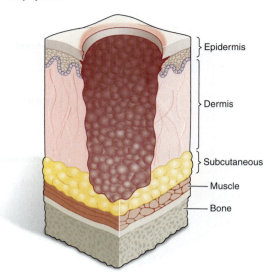

Stage III pressure ulcer.

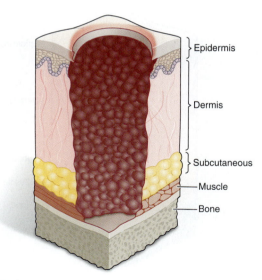

Stage IV pressure ulcer.

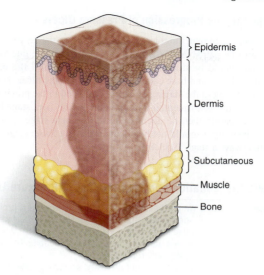

Suspected deep tissue injury.

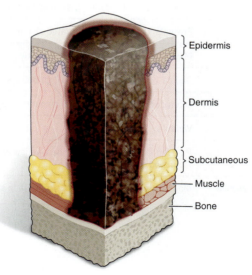

Unstageable pressure ulcer.

Documenting the Progression of Pressure Ulcers

To accurately document the stage of a pressure ulcer, the deepest portion of the wound must be palpable or visible. It this is not possible due to eschar, then the wound should be documented as unstageable until the eschar can be débrided. If the wound base can be examined, then the ulcer should be documented according to the staging guidelines outlined in the previous chart. Following the initial assessment, if a wound deteriorates (i.e., stage II regresses to stage III) it should then be documented as the new stage. Conversely, as a wound is healing, it should not be documented as a lesser stage (once a stage IV ulcer, always a stage IV ulcer).

TABLE 7.17 Location and Presentation of Pressure Ulcers

Location	Weight-bearing areas, typically over bony prominences, dependent upon position. Majority of ulcers in one of five locations.
	Supine: sacrum, heel, lateral malleolus (if leg remains externally rotated)
	Seated: ischial tuberosity, sacrum, greater trochanter
	Side lying: greater trochanter, lateral malleolus
Pain	Loss of sensation is often a predisposing factor. In patients with sensation, pain may be severe.
Edema	Presents as taut, shiny, indurated skin in periwound area
Size	May be very large if not addressed early
Depth	Should be staged using NPUAP guidelines
Shape	Often circular, may have large amounts of undermining
Exudate	Variable
Color	Pale red if circulation diminished, yellow or black if circulation diminished further
Skin temperature	May be warmer or cooler than surrounding skin

INTEG

Clinical Management

Date: _____ Time: _____ **Treatment duration:** _____

Diagnosis: _____

Subjective: Pain: **Last dressing change:**

Comments:

Objective examination: Size: cm^2

    Mode of arrival: L: W: D:

    Assistive device: Drainage amount:

    Wearing prescribed   Drainage type:
    dressings/ footwear?   Periwound:

    Wound Location: Nails:

    If other, enter location: Edema:

    Wound stage: Sensation:

    Wound color: Pulses:

Color	Pre-debridement	Post-debridement
	%	%
	%	%
	%	%

	(L)	(R)
DP		
PT		
Popliteal		
ABI		

Odor: Special Tests: Results:

Treatment: Comments:

Wound cleansed with

Debridement performed today?   Debriment type:

Modalities:

Dressings: Offloading:

Patient education:

Comments:

Assessment:

Tolerance to treatment:

Comments:

Plan:

Comments:

Follow-up:

INTEG

INTEG

● TABLE 7.18 Dressings and Topical Agents (arranged from least occlusive to most occlusive)

Common Dressing Classes	Purpose	Indications	Contraindications
Gauze	Absorptive dressing that is permeable to water. May be soaked with saline or impregnated with other agents.	1. Secondary dressing for all wound types 2. Used as wound packing for deep wounds with low exudates 3. Saline soaked dressings will débride wound if allowed to dry out	1. Dry gauze on healthy granulation tissue
Calcium alginate	Forms a gel and creates a moist wound healing environment to assist with granulation and autolysis.	1. Moderate to heavy exudates 2. Active bleeding 3. Loose packing of tunnels and tracts	1. Allergy to seaweed 2. Deep fistulas or cavities in which complete removal of dressing cannot be assured 3. Full thickness burns
Impregnated gauze	Helps prevent gauze from sticking to wound base. Absorptive capacity is typically low, but varies depending on what the gauze is impregnated with. Can increase occlusiveness of primary dressing.	1. Minimal exudating wounds 2. As a secondary dressing to promote moist environment 3. Over skin grafts and graft donor sites	1. Moderate to heavily exudating wounds

Common Dressing Classes	Purpose	Indications	Contraindications
Hydrofibers	Highly absorbent and moisture retentive dressing, turns to gel when wet, which provides occlusive environment. Protects periwound skin from maceration by locking fluid in the dressing.	1. Moderate to heavily draining wounds 2. Forms intimate contact with wound bed 3. Maintain moist wound environment if pre-moistened	1. Not intended for lightly draining wounds unless premoistened
Semipermeable films	Transparent membrane is permeable to oxygen and moisture vapor, but not bacteria. Provides moist environment, promotes autolysis, protects from trauma, and bacteria. No absorptive capability.	1. Superficial wounds with minimal exudate 2. Allows for visualization of the wound without dressing removal 3. Secondary dressing with absorptive dressing to increase occlusion	1. Not intended for infected wounds 2. Moderate to heavily draining wounds 3. Caution on fragile skin due to adhesives
Semipermeable foams	Maintain moist environment by absorbing excess exudate and protects the wound from bacteria and moisture. Varying degrees of absorption and occlusion. May be adhesive or nonadhesive.	1. Moderate to heavy drainage, depending on individual dressing type 2. Moderate degree of padding	1. Non-draining wounds 2. Full-thickness burns 3. Avoid adhesives will fragile periwound skin

(table continues on page 582)

🔵 **TABLE 7.18 Dressings and Topical Agents (arranged from least occlusive to most occlusive)** (continued)

Common Dressing Classes	Purpose	Indications	Contraindications
Hydrocolloids	Considered most occlusive of moisture retentive dressings. Some are semipermeable and some are completely occlusive. Provide absorption for minimal to moderate drainage, promotes autolysis by maintaining moist environment. Protects against trauma and bacteria.	1. Autolytic débridement 2. Stimulates granulation 3. Stage I–III pressure ulcers, depending on absorptive capacity of specific dressing 4. Wounds with minimal to moderate drainage 5. Protects from friction	1. Infected wounds 2. Fragile peri-wound tissue 3. Heavy drainage
Hydrogels	Can be in sheet or amorphous gel form. Adds moisture to dry wounds, can absorb small amounts of wound exudate, and promotes autolysis. Gel form requires a secondary dressing.	1. Dry to minimally draining wounds of various etiologies 2. May be used on infected wounds if patient on antibiotics 3. Necrotic wounds to promote débridement	4. Heavily draining wounds

Specialty Dressing Classes	Purpose	Indications	Contraindications
Collagen	Functions as wound scaffolding and is hydrophilic so is capable of absorbing large amounts of drainage. Promotes hemostasis and granulation.	1. Partial or full thickness pressure ulcers and burns free of necrotic tissue 2. Often used over meshed skin grafts or donor sites	1. Dry wounds 2. Allergy or sensitivity to any of the animal sources of collagen

INTEG

Specialty Dressing Classes	Purpose	Indications	Contraindications
	Require secondary dressing. Often animal derived.	3. Promotes autolytic débridement by maintaining wound moisture	
Antimicrobials	Includes silver, iodine, methylene blue and gentian violet. Available in powders, gels, ointments, sheets of varying sizes. Allow for topical delivery of antimicrobial agent. Varying ability to absorb drainage. Often impregnated into other classifications of dressings and will share the characteristics of that class.	1. Suspected or confirmed local infection 2. Prophylaxis to prevent infection	1. Not intended for long-term use without improvement 2. Not to be used as a replacement for systemic antibiotics 3. Concern that misuse could lead to resistant organisms
Skin protectants	Protects peri-wound skin from breakdown caused by moisture and caustic agents, typically due to incontinence and/or wound exudate.	1. Indicated for at risks areas of skin, including skin folds, perineum, under adhesive dressings, and around wound and stoma sites	1. Not intended for use on the wound bed

(table continues on page 584)

INTEG

TABLE 7.18 **Dressings and Topical Agents (arranged from least occlusive to most occlusive)** (continued)

Specialty Dressing Classes	Purpose	Indications	Contraindications
Enzymes	Removal of non-viable, collagenous material from the wound. Adjunct to, or used in place of, sharps débridement.	1. Presence of nonviable tissue 2. Effective on wounds that cannot be débrided with sharps	1. Sensitivity to components of the enzyme
Biological dressings (Refer to package insert for specific dressing instructions. Most require application by a physician.)	Grafts or dressings that are developed from human or animal sources. Some have growth factors or active viable tissue to stimulate healing, and others are acellular.	1. Burns and non-healing ulcerations 2. Often used when autografts are not optimal	1. Allergy to the donor source

Compression Therapy

Compression therapy can be divided into two major groups, the first being wraps and bandages, and the second being compression pumps. They are used in combination for the treatment of venous insufficiency, promotion of venous ulceration healing, prevention of deep vein thrombosis, and, in the cases of specialized pumps, treatment of lymphedema.

TABLE 7.19 **Compression Bandages and Wraps**

Bandage Type	Resting Pressure	Working Pressure	Example
Non-stretch	Low	High	Unna boot, Circaid
Short-stretch	Low	High	Crepe-type dressing
Long-stretch	High	Variable	Elastic bandage

A high working pressure will help to assist with venous blood flow by providing a rigid dressing that the calf muscle can pump against. Care must be taken with long-stretch bandages because the resting pressure may be higher than the diastolic blood pressure when the patient is lying down, which can lead to ischemic changes.

General considerations for compression wraps include the following:

- The smaller the radius of curvature of the limb, the greater the sub-bandage pressure will be.
  - This leads to breakdown at bony prominences.
- As the number of layers of compression increases, the sub-bandage pressure increases.
  - Figure-eight wrap has more layers than spiral wrapping, so it exerts more pressure.
- A wider bandage will exert less sub-bandage pressure.
  - A 6-inch wrap will provide less pressure than a 4-inch wrap applied in the same manner.
- As the tension applied to the bandage increases, the sub-bandage pressure will increase.
  - It is important to maintain a constant tension while applying a bandage.

Intermittent Compression Pump Guidelines

1. Gently cleanse the wound.
2. Cover the extremity with a plastic bag and place in the compression sleeve.
3. Elevate the extremity slightly.
4. Pump for 30 to 60 minutes at a pressure less than diastolic.
5. Use a compression/relaxation ratio of 90:30 seconds to allow for reperfusion of the tissues.
6. Apply compression bandaging to limb once pumping is complete.
7. Treat a minimum of one to two times per week.

Adapted from:

McCulloch, JM: Compression therapy. In McCulloch, JM, and Kloth, LC: Wound Healing: Evidence-Based Management, ed. 4. FA Davis, Philadelphia, 2010, p 597.

TABLE 7.20 Contraindications to Pneumatic Compression Therapy

Absolute Contraindications	Relative Contraindications
Arterial insufficiency	Congestive heart failure
Active cellulitis	Kidney disease
DVT	Lymphedema (unless specialty pump available)

● **TABLE 7.21 Compression Garment Classes**

Over the Counter	Prescription	Class	Uses
10–15 mm Hg	20–30 mm Hg	Class 1: Light compression	Light circulatory disorders, varicose vein prevention, pregnancy, edema prevention in lymphedema
15–20 mm Hg	30–40 mm Hg	Class 2: Medium compression	Venous insufficiency, varicose veins, pregnancy, mild lymphedema
	40–50 mm Hg	Class 3: High compression	Advanced venous disease, varicosities, and severe lymphedema

Note: These values are approximate, and may vary by manufacturer.

● **TABLE 7.22 Off-Loading Devices for the Foot**

Device	Fluctuating Edema Present	Balance Issues Present	Infection Present	Comments
Total contact cast	✗	✗	✗	Considered the gold standard for plantar forefoot ulcers. Requires training to apply safely.
Posterior walking splint	✓	✗	✓	Allows for dressing changes. Requires training to apply safely.
Prefabricated cast walkers	✓	✗	✓	Easy application. Can off-load any portion of the foot. Shown to be as effective as casting if it is not removed.

Device	Fluctuating Edema Present	Balance Issues Present	Infection Present	Comments
Wedge shoes	✓	✗	✓	Intended for off-loading the forefoot only and requires adequate dorsiflexion range of motion to accommodate the elevated forefoot. Should never be used bilaterally. Off-loading can be improved with the addition of a soft insert or an adhesive felt foam dressing.
DH shoe	✓	✓	✓	Extra depth of shoe allows for bulky dressings to be worn. Pegs can be removed to off-load any aspect of the foot. The flexible sole allows for a more normal gait pattern, but transfers weight to the forefoot.
Heel wedge	✓	✗	✓	Only intended to off-load plantar heel ulcers. Need to encourage short step length with foot contact at the midfoot rather than the heel.

All devices should be used with an appropriate assistive device.

INTEG

Electrotherapy

🟠 **TABLE 7.23** **Electrical Stimulation Parameters for Wound Healing**

Stimulation Parameters	LVPC Devices	HVPC Devices	DC Devices (continuous)
Voltage (V)	25–50	50–150	0.001–10
Current (mA)	30–35	0.3–0.6	0.2–0.8
Pulse frequency (pps)	50–130	50–100	NA
Pulse duration (μsec)	130	20–60	NA

Modified from: Kloth, LC, and Zhao, M: Endogenous and exogenous electrical fields for wound healing. In McCulloch, JM, and Kloth, LC: *Wound Healing: Evidence-Based Management,* ed. 4. FA Davis, Philadelphia, 2010, p 476, with permission.
DC = direct current; HVPC = high-voltage pulsed current; LVPC = low-voltage pulsed current; NA = not available.

INTEG

Polarity Suggestions for Use of Electrotherapy With Noninfected Wounds

Negative polarity: Begin with cathode on the wound and continue as long as regular wound measurements indicate that wound healing is steadily progressing, as evidenced by increased granulation and decreased exudation.

Positive polarity: When wound measurements indicate that healing is not progressing or is regressing, change to positive polarity and continue as long as healing progress continues.

Negative polarity: Change polarity again if there is no healing progress and maintain for 7 to 14 treatments, as long as healing progress is being made.

Precautions and Contraindications for Use of Electrotherapy With Wound Healing

Precautions

- Skin irritation under the nontreatment electrode in contact with the skin (occurrence is more common with direct current or monophasic pulsed current than with high-voltage pulsed current)

Contraindications

- Basal or squamous cell carcinoma in the wound or periwound tissues or melanoma
- Untreated osteomyelitis present in bone in the base of the wound
- Placement of electrodes so current flows through the pericardial area, carotid sinus, phrenic nerve, parasympathetic nerves or ganglia, muscles of the larynx, or any type of external or implanted electronic pacemaker device

Débridement

Definitions

autolysis: Removal of nonviable material from the wound through the use of the body's own phagocytic cells. This is the most selective form of débridement, and can be promoted with the addition of moisture-retentive dressings.

débridement: The removal of necrotic and/or infected tissue from the wound.

enzymatic débridement: A selective form of débridement that uses topical enzymes to break down devitalized tissue. Requires a physician order and prescription.

mechanical débridement: Encompasses a variety of débridement methods including wet-to-dry dressings, cleansing with gauze, pulsatile lavage, and whirlpool. Depending on the method, it may range from nonselective to semiselective débridement.

sharp débridement: The removal of nonviable tissue with sterile instruments, including curettes, scissors, tweezers, and scalpels. All state practice acts allow physical therapists to perform sharp débridement, but states vary on the decision to allow physical therapy assistants to débride. Further information can be obtained by accessing the state practice acts for each state at http://www.apta.org.

surgical débridement: The removal of viable and nonviable tissue with sterile, sharp instruments. This is not a part of the physical therapist's practice act because it involves viable tissue. It may only be performed by a physician, podiatrist, or certified physician assistant.

ultrasonic débridement: The use of sound wave energy to selectively débride nonviable tissue.

INTEG

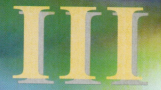

PART III

Specialty Areas of Practice

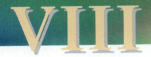

SECTION

VIII

PEDIATRICS

Conditions

Classification of Birth Injuries

Cerebral Birth Injury

Cerebral birth injury is damage to the nervous system by complications during pregnancy, labor, delivery, or the immediate neonatal period. It is associated with a number of predisposing factors related to maternal health, maternal age, social status, labor and delivery, birth weight, gestation, and parity. The most common mechanisms are asphyxia (which may be chronic or acute) and trauma.

intraventricular hemorrhage—not related to trauma: More common in premature infants and with respiratory distress syndrome.

compression head injury—compression of the head: Most likely in full-term or postmature infants, many of whom are large for their gestational age. May present as subarachnoid, subdural, or (infrequently) cerebellar hemorrhage.

Fractures

Most of these lesions heal without treatment; however, the infant may be more comfortable when the fracture is immobilized.

skull fractures: Fissure fractures are not uncommon but are usually of little significance. Depressed fractures (a "pond" fracture) may result from pressure on the sacral promontory. The majority resolve spontaneously.

clavicle fractures: This fracture may occur during breech delivery if the baby's arms become displaced or may be the result of a difficult vertex delivery. Recovery is likely without treatment; however, the upper arm may be immobilized against the chest. The baby should always be examined for a concurrent brachial plexus injury.

humeral fractures: This fracture may occur when a displaced arm is pulled down during a breech delivery. The baby should always be examined for nerve damage.

femoral fractures: This fracture may occur when a leg is pulled down during delivery of a breech presentation with extended legs. The fracture may be immobilized by bandaging the affected limb to the abdomen.

Nerve Lesions

abducens palsy: Transient abducens palsy occurs in a significant proportion of children born after prolonged labor and those who are delivered by forceps. Usually there is full recovery after a few days or weeks.

facial palsy: Pressure from a forceps blade may injure the extracranial part of the facial nerve. Facial palsy occasionally occurs following a spontaneous vaginal delivery. Recovery may be expected within 2–3 weeks.

Erb's palsy: Trauma to the C5 and C6 spinal roots due to excessive traction on the neck during a delivery, such as a difficult breech extraction or vertex delivery, where there has been difficulty with delivery of the shoulders. The affected arm lies limply at the infant's side, with the hand pronated and wrist slightly flexed. Recovery is usually complete within 2 weeks.

other brachial plexus injuries: The C4 root may be implicated in addition to Erb's palsy, thereby affecting function of the diaphragm with possible resultant acute respiratory distress. Much less common is damage to the lower roots (C7–T1).

radial palsy: Involvement of the radial nerve usually by subcutaneous fat necrosis or spontaneously due to pressure as a result of malposition in utero. Complete recovery is expected.

spinal cord injuries: These lesions are rare; however, they may occur following a breech delivery or with spinal fractures or subluxations. They occur most commonly in the cervical and thoracic region and are produced by traction on the vertebral column during delivery. There may also be an additional lesion to the brachial plexus due to tearing of the cervical roots from the spinal cord.

> **For more information:**
> McIntosh, N, Helms, P, and Smyth, RL (eds): Forfar and Arneil's Textbook of Pediatrics, ed. 7. Churchill Livingstone, New York, 2003.

Cerebral Palsy

The definition of cerebral palsy and classifications of the types of cerebral palsy have changed over time. In 2006, an executive committee recommended the following definition and classification following the International Workshop on Definition and Classification of Cerebral Palsy and input from others in the field.

I. Definition of Cerebral Palsy

Cerebral palsy (CP) describes a group of permanent disorders of the development of movement and posture, causing activity limitation, that are attributed to nonprogressive disturbances that occurred in the developing fetal or infant brain. The motor disorders of cerebral palsy are often accompanied by disturbances of sensation, perception, cognition, communication, and behavior, by epilepsy, and by secondary musculoskeletal problems.

II. Classification of Cerebral Palsy

The definition of cerebral palsy covers a wide range of clinical presentations and activity limitations, therefore classification according to the following components is useful.

1. Motor abnormalities
   a. Nature and typology of the motor disorder:
   b. Functional motor abilities
2. Associated impairments
3. Anatomic and radiologic findings
   a. Anatomic distribution
   b. Radiologic findings
4. Causation and timing

Types of Movement Disorders

spasticity: Characterized by increased muscle tone (hyperreflexia), stereotyped and limited movements, pathological stretch reflexes with clonus, persistence of primitive and tonic reflexes, and poor development of postural reflex mechanisms.

athetosis (dyskinetic syndrome): Characterized by an abnormal amount and type of involuntary motion with varying amounts of tension, normal reflexes, and asymmetric involvement. Abnormal movements are exaggerated by voluntary movement, postural adjustments, and changes in emotion or speech. Often associated with impaired speech and poor respiratory and oral-motor control; related to erythroblastosis and birth asphyxia.

   rotary athetosis: Common type that involves muscles that function as rotators; rotary motion usually slow. Feet describe circular motion, hands pronate and supinate, and shoulders internally and externally rotate. There are varying degrees of muscle tension.

   tremor (tremor-like) athetosis: Common type that involves irregular and uneven involuntary contraction and relaxation involving flexors and extensors, abductors, and adductors. Rotary motion is not seen.

   dystonic athetosis: Extremities, head, neck, and trunk assume distorted positions. There is increased muscle tone. Different abnormal positions may be assumed over time.

   choreoathetosis: Involuntary, unpredictable, small movements of the distal parts of the extremities.

   tension athetosis: A state of increased muscle tension blocking involuntary athetoid movements. Tension is not constant. Tension must be the dominant characteristic for this classification to be applicable; normally a temporary classification.

   nontension athetosis: Involuntary movements without increased muscle tone; a temporary classification identifying a treatment phenomena and is frequently seen as an initial symptom of cerebral palsy in small babies.

   flailing athetoid: A rare type of athetosis. Arms and legs are thrown violently from shoulder and hip, but there is little involvement of hands, wrists, fingers, or knees.

ataxia: Ataxia is associated with developmental deficits of the cerebellum and characterized by disturbance in the sense of balance and equilibrium, dyssynergias, and low postural tone. Distribution is bilateral, affecting trunk and legs more than arms and hands, as well as a widespread stance and gait. Ataxia often follows initial stage of hypotonia. Associated problems include nystagmus, poor eye tracking, delayed and poorly articulated speech, astereognosis, and poor depth perception.

hypotonia: Often a transient stage in the evolution of athetosis or spasticity, and characterized by decreased muscle tone, real or apparent weakness, and increased range of movement. A child typically assumes "froglike" position when placed supine and uses hands to support trunk during sitting.

PEDS

Predicted Gross Motor Development in Children With Cerebral Palsy

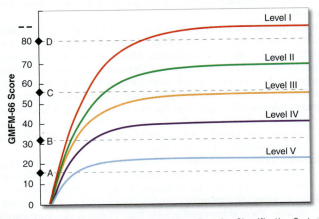

Predicted Average Development by the Gross Motor Function Classification System Levels. The diamonds on the vertical axis identify 4 Gross Motor Function Measure-66 (GMFM-66) items that predict when children are expected to have a 50% chance of completing that item successfully. The GMFM-66 item 21 (diamond A) assesses whether a child can lift and maintain his/her head in a vertical position with trunk support by a therapist while sitting; item 24 (diamond B) assesses whether when in a sitting position on a mat, a child can maintain sitting unsupported by his/her arms for 3 sec; item 69 (diamond C) measures a child's ability to walk forward 10 steps unsupported; and item 87 (diamond D) assesses the task of walking down 4 steps alternating feet with arms free.

From:

Rosenbaum, PL, et al: *Prognosis for gross motor function in cerebral palsy: Creation of motor development curves. JAMA* 288:1357–1363, 2002.

PEDS

Prediction of Ambulation in Children With Spastic Cerebral Palsy

TABLE 8.1 Prognosis of Children With Spastic Cerebral Palsy (Based on Gross Motor Skills)

Gross Motor Skill	Age (mo)	Prognosis
Head control	<9 9–19 >20	Good Guarded Poor
Sitting	<24 24–35 >36	Good Guarded Poor
Crawling	<30 30–61 >61	Good Guarded Poor

Adapted from: Campos du Paz, A, Burnett, S, and Braga, L: Walking prognosis in cerebral palsy. *Dev Med Child Neurol* 130–134, 1994.

PEDS

Prognosis Based on Postural Reactions and Primitive Reflexes

When the child is at least 12 months old, score one point for each of the following primitive reflexes if obligatory:

- Asymmetrical tonic neck reflex
- Symmetrical tonic neck reflex
- Moro
- Neck righting
- Extensor thrust

Score one point for each of the following postural reactions if absent:

- Foot placement
- Parachute

Prognosis for ambulation:

0 points = good
1 point = guarded
2+ points = poor

Adapted from:

Bleck, EE: Locomotor prognosis in cerebral palsy. Dev Med Child Neurol 17:18–25, 1975.

Gross Motor Function Classification System for Cerebral Palsy

Classification according to the highest level of mobility a child aged 6 to 12 years is expected to achieve.

Level I: Walks without restriction; limitations in more advanced gross motor skills.

Level II: Walks without assistive devices; limitations walking outdoors and in the community.

Level III: Walks with assistive mobility devices; limitations walking outdoors and in the community.

Level IV: Self-mobiltiy with limitations; children are transported or use power mobility outdoors and in the community.

Level V: Self-mobility is severely limited even with the use of assistive technology.

Muscular Dystrophy

Classification of Muscular Dystrophies

The following classification of muscular dystrophies is based on genetic criteria and distribution of muscle degeneration. Each category is followed by a list of characteristic features.

Duchenne Muscular Dystrophy (DMD)

- DMD is a degenerative muscle disease that affects primarily males, either by X-linked recessive inheritance through a maternal carrier or by spontaneous mutation of genes coding for dystrophin protein.
- Diagnosis is typically made by age 5 years, when physical abilities fall noticeably below those of peers.
- Signs include progressive symmetrical weakness first affecting proximal muscles of the hips, pelvis, and shoulder girdle.
- Calf muscle pseudohypertrophy, trouble climbing stairs, difficulty jumping and running, and Gowers' sign when arising from the floor are typical presenting factors.
- Waddling, wide-based lordotic gait, toe walking, and frequent falls are characteristic with disease progression, alongside contractures and scoliosis.
- DMD is associated with non-progressive learning difficulties; IQ is normally distributed but shifted down by two standard deviations. Autism spectrum disorders are also more prevalent than in the general population.
- Many boys with DMD lose the ability to walk between ages 8 and 13; full-time power wheelchair use is common by age 12.
- Cardiac and respiratory functions are affected in later disease stages.
- Improved medical and rehabilitative management, including corticosteriod therapy, has led to improvements in function, health, and longevity; children diagnosed today have the possibility of living into their fourth decade.

Becker Muscular Dystrophy (BMD)

- An X-linked recessive dystrophy resembling DMD, but less severe.
- Often with onset in adolescence or adulthood, although may also present in childhood.
- As in DMD, characterized by progressive weakness of trunk, pelvis, and proximal upper and lower extremities, alongside muscle pseudohypertrophy.
- Initially, difficulty in gait, climbing stairs, and rising from the floor.
- Contractures and skeletal deformities occur eventually, but these are less severe than in DMD.
- Early myocardial disease may develop.

ment is less common than in DMD.

- Cogniti~~v~~ ~~ses~~ slowly and with much variability; most survive well into ~~ul~~thood.
- Disea~~~~
  ~~humeral~~ **Dystrophy (FSH or FSHD)**
  ~~~~le disease that affects both sexes equally, with variable age of onset, in childhood or early adolescence.

  ~~er~~ized by slowly progressive weakness of the face and proximal upper ~~it~~y muscles, including scapular stabilizers.

  ~~al~~ signs, such as sleeping with eyes slightly open and facial weakness with blowing or drinking from a straw, may be evident in early childhood.
- Significant impairment and functional limitation delayed until later in the first decade.
- If walking becomes difficult, power mobility will be needed, as arm weakness will not allow independent manual chair use.
- Severe scapular winging is a hallmark of the adult stage.
- Highly resistive upper extremity exercise and muscle fatigue should be avoided, as they can contribute to progression of muscle weakness.
- Wide range of clinical severity, with near-normal life expectancy.

Limb-Girdle Muscular Dystrophy (LGMD)

- A heterogeneous group of disorders characterized by progressive weakness of the hip and shoulder muscles.
- Variability in heritability, age of onset, progression, and the distribution and severity of weakness.
- Onset can occur in childhood with presentation mimicking DMD, but more often in late adolescence or early adulthood.
- Patients may eventually require wheelchair use, but skeletal deformities are not frequent.
- Mortality in late stages relates to cardiopulmonary complications, including pneumonia.

Emery Dreifuss Muscular Dystrophy (EDMD)

- Two different genetic forms: X-linked (EMD1) and autosomal (EMD2).
- Generally presents by 10 years of age, although contractures and weakness can begin from the neonatal period through early adulthood.
- Clinical features of EMD1 include contractures of the ankle, elbow and posterior neck muscles, slowly progressive scapulohumeroperoneal weakness, and muscle wasting.
- Onset of contractures often occurs before weakness develops.
- Toe walking is common on initial presentation.
- Cardiac impairments, including conduction abnormalities that cause syncope and require a pacemaker, are consistently present in adulthood and related to sudden death.

Other types of childhood muscular dystrophy include congenital muscular dystrophies (CMD) and myotonic muscular dystrophy (MMD), also known as Steinert disease.

PEDS

Vignos Functional Rating Scale for Duchenne Muscular~~~ ~~~phy

1. Walks and climbs stairs without assistance.
2. Walks and climbs stairs with aid of railing.
3. Walks and climbs stairs slowly with aid of railing (over 25 sec for standard steps).
4. Walks, but cannot climb stairs.
5. Walks assisted, but cannot climb stairs or get out of chair.
6. Walks only with assistance or with braces.
7. In wheelchair: sits erect and can roll chair and perform bed and wheelchair ADL.
8. In wheelchair: sits erect and is unable to perform bed and wheelchair ADL without assistance.
9. In wheelchair: sits erect only with support and is able to do only minimal ADL.
10. In bed: can do no ADL without assistance.

ADL = activities of daily living.

From:

Stuberg, WA: Muscular dystrophy and spinal muscular atrophy. In Campbell, SK, Vander Linden, DW, and Palisano, R: Physical Therapy for Children, ed. 2. WB Saunders, Philadelphia, 2000, p 345, with permission.

TABLE 8.2 Classification of Spinal Muscular Atrophy

Type	Onset	Inheritance	Course
Acute child-onset, type I, Werdnig-Hoffmann (acute)	0–3 mo	Recessive	Rapidly progressive; severe hypotonia; death within first year
Chronic childhood-onset, type II, Werdnig-Hoffmann (chronic)	3 mo–4 yr	Recessive	Rapid progress that stabilizes; moderate to severe hypotonia; shortened life span
Juvenile-onset, type III, Kugelberg-Welander	5–10 yr	Recessive	Slowly progressive; mild impairment

Reprinted from: Stuberg, WA: Muscular dystrophy and spinal muscular atrophy. In Campbell, SK, Vander Linden, DW, and Palisano, R: *Physical Therapy for Children,* ed. 2. WB Saunders, Philadelphia, 2000, p 357, with permission from Elsevier.

Types of Spina Bifida

A normal spine with an intact spinal cord is seen on the left. Illustrations of types of spina bifida (midline closure defects) are to the right. Although defects may occur anywhere along the vertebral column, they are most common in the lumbar and lumbosacral regions.

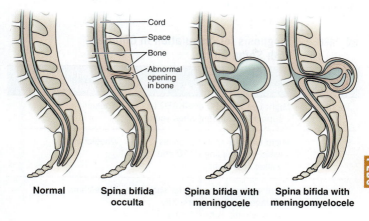

Cord
Space
Bone
Abnormal opening in bone

Normal   Spina bifida   Spina bifida with   Spina bifida with
                 occulta   meningocele   meningomyelocele

Spina bifida occulta is a failure of the vertebral lamina to develop and is usually asymptomatic; however, it may be associated with other birth defects. Spina bifida with meningocele is a midline defect with herniation of the meninges. Depending on the severity of the herniation and associated problems, there may or may not be any neural defect. Spina bifida with meningomyelocele is a midline defect with herniation of neural tissue. In addition to neural deficits, this condition may be life threatening due to complications such as infection (meningitis) and hydrocephalus.

TABLE 8.3 Prognosis for Ambulation in Children With Spina Bifida

Level	Orthoses/Assistive Device	Long-Term Prognosis/ Community Mobility
Thoracic	Might use THKAFO or HKAFO for supported standing when young	Wheelchair
L1–2	Might walk for short distances when young using KAFO and walker or crutches	Wheelchair
L3	Might walk at home and for short distances in the community when young using KAFO and crutches or walker	Wheelchair
L4	Community ambulation with AFO and crutches, especially when young	Ambulation; wheelchair for long distances
L5	Community ambulation without orthoses or with foot orthoses; may use crutches for long distances because of fatigue	Ambulation; may use wheelchair for sports
Sacral	Community ambulation without orthoses or with foot orthoses	Ambulation; may use wheelchair for sports

Based on Ratliffe, KT: *Clinical Pediatric Physical Therapy: A Guide for the Physical Therapy Team.* Mosby, St. Louis, MO, 1998.
AFO = ankle-foot orthosis; HKAFO = hip-knee-ankle-foot orthosis; KAFO = knee-ankle-foot orthosis; THKAFO = trunk-hip-knee-ankle-foot orthosis

🔵 TABLE 8.4 Signs and Symptoms of Shunt Malfunction

Any Age	Infants	Toddlers	School-Aged Children
Vomiting Irritability	Bulging fontanelle	New nystagmus	Handwriting changes
Lethargy Seizures	High-pitched cry	New strabismus	Decreased school performance
Edema, redness along shunt tract	Increased rate of growth in head circumference Thinning of skin over scalp	Personality changes	Memory changes

From: Tappit-Emas, E: Spina bifida. In Tecklin, JS (ed): *Pediatric Physical Therapy,* ed. 3. Lippincott, Philadelphia, 1999, pp 163–222.

Down Syndrome

🔵 TABLE 8.5 Development of Skills in Children With Down Syndrome

Skill	Children With Down Syndrome		Typical Children	
	Average Age (mo)	Range (mo)	Average Age	Range (mo)
Smiling	2	1 1/2> –3	1	1/2–3
Rolling	6	2–12	5	2–10
Sitting	9	6–18	7	5–9
Crawling	11	7–21	8	6–11
Creeping	13	8–25	10	7–13
Standing	10	10–32	11	8–16
Walking	20	12–45	13	8–18
Talking, words	14	9–30	10	6–14
Talking, sentences	24	18–46	21	14–32
Eating finger food	12	8–28	8	6–16

(table continues on page 604)

PEDS

TABLE 8.5 Development of Skills in Children With Down Syndrome (continued)

Skill	Children With Down Syndrome		Typical Children	
	Average Age (mo)	Range (mo)	Average Age (mo)	Range (mo)
Using spoon/ fork	20	12–40	13	8–2
Toilet training – bladder	48	20–95	32	18–60
Toilet training – bowel	42	28–90	29	16–48
Undressing	40	29–72	32	22–42
Putting clothes on	58	38–98	47	34–58

From Pueschel, SM: *A Parent's Guide to Down Syndrome: Toward a Brighter Future.* Paul H. Brooks, Baltimore, 1990.

Autism

Common Characteristics of Children With Autism

The following characteristics are common, but not universal:

Motor Development

- Impaired skilled motor tasks and gestures (most common motor finding).
- Delayed gross and fine motor development; rate of development often slows at age 2 to 3 years.
- Muscle tone and reflex abnormalities (especially hypotonia when young).
- Impaired motor imitation.
- Generalized deficit in praxis (in addition to imitation).
- Poor balance and coordination.
- Unusual gait patterns, such as toe walking.
- Repetitive and stereotypic movements of body, limbs, and fingers.
- Delayed learning of complex motor skills, such as tricycle riding.
- Lack of anticipation during movement preparation phases.

Communication and Social Development

- Deficits in joint attention (coordinating attention between people and objects).
- Orienting and attending to a communication partner.
- Shifting gaze between people and objects.
- Sharing affect or emotional states with another person.

- Following the gaze and point of another person.
- Sharing experiences by drawing another persons' attention to objects or events.
- Difficulty learning conventional or shared meaning for symbols, such as conventional gestures, conventional meanings for a word, and pretend play.
- Some have limited ability to use speech for communication; most who can speak go through a period of echolalia.
- Some have idiosyncratic or unconventional means of communication, including behaviors that others perceive as problems.
- Low rates of initiation of interaction with others and response to them.
- Less attention to others' emotions than other children.

From:

National Research Council Committee on Educational Interventions for Children With Autism. Division of Behavioral and Social Sciences and Education. Educating Children With Autism. National Academy Press, Washington, DC, 2001.

Other

- Unusual responses to sensory input.
- Cerebellar abnormalities.
- Attention deficits and hyperactivity.
- Visual spatial skills often more advanced than other areas.
- Oral-motor problems, feeding problems, and limited food preferences.
- Sleep disturbances, particularly of sleep-wake cycles.

Intervention for Children With Autism Spectrum Disorders to Improve Motor Function

Although children with autism spectrum disorders commonly have motor delays or deficits, no consistent research exists to support the effectiveness of interventions designed to improve motor function. General recommendations include the following:

- Be aware of the difficulty many children have with imitation.
- Individualize interventions to accomplish functional goals.
- Integrate interventions into functional activities within daily routines in natural environments.
- Focus on activities that are meaningful to the child and overall goals for the child.
- Provide short duration interventions with frequent and systematic documentation of progress.
- Measure outcomes in sensory and motor function, specific activities, and participation.
- Modify interventions if the child is not making progress toward functional goals.
- Assess and structure the physical and sensory environments to accommodate a child's sensory and motor function.

From:

McEwen, IR, Meiser, MJ, and Hansen, LH: Children with motor and intellectual disabilities. In Campbell, SK, Palisano, RJ, and Orlin, M: Physical Therapy for Children, ed. 4. Saunders, Philadelphia, 2011.

PEDS

Juvenile Rheumatoid Arthritis

Criteria for The Diagnosis of Juvenile Rheumatoid Arthritis

I. General

Juvenile rheumatoid arthritis (JRA) is a common autoimmune or autoinflammatory disease of childhood characterized by peripheral joint synovitis with soft tissue inflammation and effusion. A new nomenclature, juvenile idiopathic arthritis (JIA), is also used for JRA, and may eventually replace the original term. Many distinct subtypes of JRA have been identified and several classification schemas exist, including those of the American College of Rheumatology (ACR), the European League Against Rheumatism (EULAR), and the International League of Associations for Rheumatology (ILAR). The ACR criteria, first developed in 1977, have been well validated and continue to be the most widely known; they are included in this section.

The ACR identifies JRA as a category of diseases with three principal types: (1) systemic, (2) pauciarticular or oligoarthritis, and (3) polyarticular or polyarthritis. The onset subtypes may be further classified into the subsets below. This classification describes the criteria for JRA diagnosis.

Age at onset: <16 yr
Arthritis: swelling or effusion or the presence of two or more of the following
- Limitation of range of motion
- Tenderness or pain with motion
- Increased heat in ≥1 joint

Duration of disease: ≥6 wk
Onset type defined by articular involvement in the first 6 months after onset:
- Polyarthritis: ≥5 inflamed joints
- Oligoarthritis: ≤4 inflamed joints
- Systemic disease: arthritis with intermittent fever and skin rash

Exclusion of other forms of juvenile arthritis such as psoriatic juvenile idiopathic arthritis, enthesitis-related arthritis, and undifferentiated arthritis, which are included in the 1997 International League of Associations for Rheumatology (ILAR) classification criteria.

Adapted from: Cassidy, JT, et al (eds): *Textbook of Pediatric Rheumatology,*
ed. 5. Elsevier Saunders, Philadelphia, 2005.

II. Presentation and Prognosis of JRA by Type

- Pauciarticular JRA
  - Characterized by periods of remission and flare, although different in each child; some may have just one or two flares and never have symptoms again, while others may flare frequently.
  - Leg length discrepancy from asymmetric knee synovitis and bone growth may contribute to flexion contractures and gait abnormalities.

- Uveitis (eye inflammation) may lead to scarring or blindness in 15% to 20% of children.
- Active arthritis extends into adulthood in 40% to 50% of patients.
- Radiographic joint damage is seen within 5 years of onset.
- Polyarticular JRA and Systemic JRA
  - Active arthritis extends into adulthood in 50% to 70% of patients.
  - Long-term disabilities arise in 30% to 40%.
  - Radiographic joint damage is seen within 5 years of onset.
  - Mortality rate is 0.4% to 2% (greater with systemic JRA than with polyarticular JRA).

III. Disease Management

- Treatment goals are to control inflammation, relieve pain, prevent or control joint damage and maximize joint and body function and participation.
- The trend in JRA management has shifted in the last 10 to 15 years and now tends to be more aggressive earlier in the disease course, with the aim of preventing and slowing the progression of joint damage.

Medical Management

- Generally includes NSAIDs, corticosteroids, disease-modifying antirheumatic drugs such as methotrexate and sulfasalazine, or biological response modifiers.
- Growth horomone may be used to address growth dysfunction.
- Joint replacement or soft tissue releases may be used later in the disease process.
- Nutrition and weight management are important to help maintain healthy weight and minimize excessive joint forces.

Rehabilitation Management

- Strengthening and range of motion exercises are important adjuncts to maximize functional abilities.
- Joint splinting, particularly for knee and wrist extension, can help maintain range of motion and relieve pain.
- Moist heat, gentle range of motion exercises, and, ocassionally, cryotherapy can help relieve characteristic morning stiffness.
- Most children can take part fully in physical activities and non-contact sports when symptoms are under control. During a disease flare, limiting certain activities may be necessary, depending on the joints involved.

PEDS

Examination

Classification of Infants by Birth Weight

● TABLE 8.6 Classification of Infants by Birth Weight

Classification	Birth Weight
Normal	2,500 g–4,500 g
Low birth weight (LBW)	1,500 g–2,499 g
Very low birth weight (VLBW)	1,000 g–1,499 g
Extremely low birth weight	800–999 g
Micropremie	<800 g

Apgar Scores

● TABLE 8.7 Apgar Scores

Sign	Score (for each item)		
	0	1	2
Heart rate	Absent	Slow (<100)	>100
Respiratory effort	Absent	Slow, irregular	Good; crying
Muscle tone	Limp	Some flexion of extremities	Active motion
Reflex irritability	No response	Grimace	Cough or sneeze
Color	Blue, pale	Body pink; extremities blue	Completely pink

Physical Development

CDC Growth Charts: United States

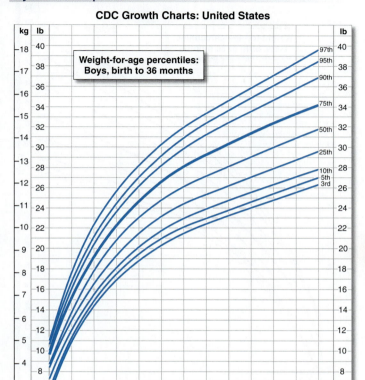

Weight-for-age percentiles:
Boys, birth to 36 months

CDC Growth Charts: United States.

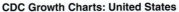

CDC Growth Charts: United States

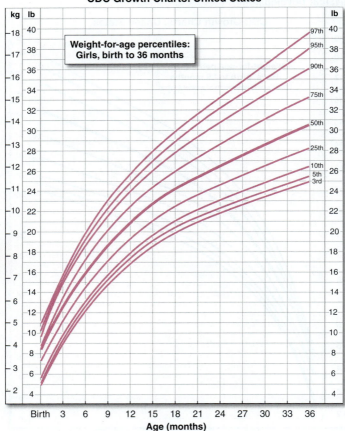

Weight-for-age percentiles: Girls, birth to 36 months

PEDS

Fontanels

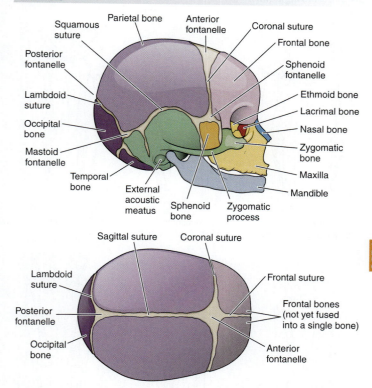

The fontanels of the infant are shown in the figure. The posterior fontanel closes between 2 and 3 months of age; the anterior fontanel closes between 16 and 18 months of age.

Lower Limb Alignment

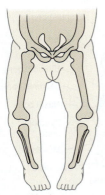

Newborn—
moderate genu varum

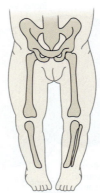

6 months—
minimal genu varum

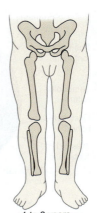

1 to 2 years—
legs straight

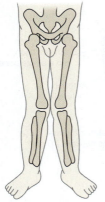

2 to 4 years—
physiologic genu valgum

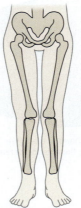

16-year-old females—
slight genu valgum

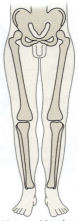

16-year-old males—
slight genu varum

PEDS

Reflexes and Postural Reactions

TABLE 8.8 Reflex Testing

Reflex	Stimulus	Response
Primitive/Spinal		
Flexor withdrawal	Noxious stimulus (pinprick) to sole of foot; tested in supine or sitting position	Toes extend, foot dorsi-flexes, entire leg flexes uncontrollably. Onset: 28 wk Integrated: 1–2 mo
Crossed extension	Noxious stimulus to ball of foot of extremity fixed in extension; tested in supine position	Opposite lower extremity flexes, then adducts and extends. Onset: 28 wk gestation Integrated: 1–2 mo
Traction	Grasp forearm and pull up from supine into sitting position	Grasp and total flexion of the upper extremity occur. Onset: 28 wk gestation Integrated: 2–5 mo
Moro	Sudden change in position of head in relation to trunk: drop infant backward from sitting position	Extension, abduction of upper extremities, hand opening, and crying followed by flexion, adduction of arms across chest occur. Onset: 28 wk gestation Integrated: 5–6 mo
Startle	Sudden loud or harsh noise	Sudden extension or abduction of arms; crying occurs. Onset: birth Integrated: persists
Grasp	Maintained pressure to palm of hand (palmar grasp) or to ball of foot under toes (plantar grasp)	Flexion of fingers or toes is maintained. Onset: palmar: birth; plantar: 28 wk Integrated: palmar: 4–6 mo; plantar: 9 mo
Tonic/Brain Stem		
Asymmetrical tonic neck (ATNR)	Rotation of the head to one side	Flexion of skull limbs, extension of the jaw limbs, "bow and arrow" or "fencing" posture occur. Onset: birth Integrated: 4–6 mo

(table continues on page 614)

PEDS

● **TABLE 8.8 Reflex Testing** (continued)

Reflex	Stimulus	Response
Symmetrical tonic neck (STNR)	Flexion or extension of the head	With head flexion: flexion of arms, extension of legs occur; with head extension: extension of arms, flexion of legs occur. Onset: 4–6 mo Integrated: 8–12 mo
Symmetrical tonic labyrinthine (TLR or STLR)	Prone or supine position	With prone position: increased flexor tone/flexion of all limbs occurs; with supine: increased extensor tone/extension of all limbs occur. Onset: birth Integrated: 6 mo
Positive supporting	Contact to the ball of the foot in upright standing position	Rigid extension (cocontraction) of the lower extremities occurs. Onset: birth Integrated: 6 mo
Associated reactions	Resisted voluntary movement in any part of the body	Involuntary movement in a resting extremity occurs. Onset: birth–3 mo Integrated: 8–9 yr
Neck righting action on the body (NOB)	Passively turn head to one side; tested in supine	Body rotates as a whole (log rolls) to align the body with the head. Onset: 4–6 mo Integrated: 5 yr
Body righting action on the body (BOB)	Passively rotate upper or lower trunk segment: tested in supine	Body segment not rotated follows to align the body segments. Onset: 4–6 mo Integrated: 5 yr
Labyrinthine head righting (LR)	Occlude vision; alter body position by tipping body in all directions	Head orients to vertical position with mouth horizontal. Onset: birth–2 mo Integrated: persists
Optical righting (OR)	Alter body position by tipping body in all directions	Head orients to vertical position with mouth horizontal. Onset: birth–2 mo Integrated: persists

Reflex	Stimulus	Response
Body righting action on head (BOH)	Place in prone or supine position	Head orients to vertical position with mouth horizontal. Onset: birth–2 mo Integrated: 5 yr
Protective extension (PE)	Displace center of gravity outside the base of support	Arms or legs extend and abduct to support and to protect the body against falling. Onset: arms: 4–6 mo; legs: 6–9 mo Integrated: persists
Equilibrium reactions—tilting (ER)	Displace the center of gravity by tilting or moving the support surface (e.g., with a movable object such as an equilibrium board or ball)	Curvature of the trunk toward the upward side along with extension and abduction of the extremities on that side occurs; protective extension on the opposite (downward) side occurs. Onset: prone 6 mo; supine 7–8 mo; sitting 7–8 mo; quadruped 9–12 mo; standing 12–21 mo. Integrated: persists
Equilibrium reactions—postural fixation	Apply a displacing force to the body, altering the center of gravity in its relation to the base of support; can also be observed during voluntary activity	Curvature of the trunk toward the external force with extension and abduction of the extremities on the side to which the force was applied occurs. Onset: prone 6 mo; supine 7–8 mo: sitting 7–8 mo; quadruped 9–12 mo; standing 12–21 mo Integrated: persists

Typical Movement Development

Every child develops at their own pace. The following are from the Centers of Disease Control (CDC) as a general guide to development:

BY THE END OF 3 MONTHS

- Raises head and chest when lying on stomach
- Supports upper body with arms when lying on stomach
- Stretches legs out and kicks when lying on stomach or back
- Opens and shuts hands
- Pushes down on legs when feet are placed on a firm surface

PEDS

- Brings hand to mouth
- Takes swipes at dangling objects with hands
- Grasps and shakes hand toys

BY THE END OF 7 MONTHS

- Rolls both ways (front to back, back to front)
- Sits with, and then without, support on hands
- Supports whole weight on legs
- Reaches with one hand
- Transfers object from hand to hand
- Uses hand to rake objects

BY 1 YEAR

- Reaches sitting position without assistance
- Crawls forward on belly
- Assumes hands-and-knees position
- Creeps on hands and knees
- Gets from sitting to crawling or prone (lying on stomach) position
- Pulls self up to stand
- Walks holding on to furniture
- Stands momentarily without support
- May walk two or three steps without support

BY 2 YEARS

- Walks alone
- Pulls toys behind her while walking
- Carries large toy or several toys while walking
- Begins to run
- Stands on tiptoe
- Kicks a ball
- Climbs onto and down from furniture unassisted
- Walks up and down stairs holding on to support

BY 3 YEARS

- Climbs well
- Walks up and down stairs, alternating feet (one foot per stair step)
- Kicks ball
- Runs easily
- Pedals tricycle
- Bends over easily without falling

BY 4 YEARS

- Hops and stands on one foot up to five seconds
- Goes upstairs and downstairs without support
- Kicks ball forward
- Throws ball overhand
- Catches bounced ball most of the time
- Moves forward and backward with agility

BY 5 YEARS

- Stands on one foot for 10 seconds or longer
- Hops, somersaults
- Swings, climbs
- May be able to skip

From:

Centers for Disease Control and Prevention. http://www.cdc.gov/ncbddd/actearly/milestones/index.html. Accessed January 21, 2012.

PEDS

PEDS

TABLE 8.9 Typical Development in Other Domains

Age*	Developmental Domain		
	Social and Emotional	Vision	Hearing and Language
3 mo	• Begins to develop a social smile • Enjoys playing with other people and may cry when playing stops • Becomes more expressive and communicates more with face and body • Imitates some movements and facial expressions	• Watches faces intently • Follows moving objects • Recognizes familiar objects and people at a distance • Starts using hands and eyes in coordination	• Smiles at the sound of a voice • Begins to babble • Begins to imitate some sounds • Turns head toward direction of sound
7 mo	Social and Emotional • Enjoys social play • Interested in mirror images • Responds to other people's expressions of emotion and appears joyful often	Vision • Develops full color vision • Distance vision matures • Ability to track moving objects improves Cognitive • Finds partially hidden object • Explores with hands and mouth • Struggles to get objects that are out of reach	Language • Responds to own name • Begins to respond to "no" • Can tell emotions by tone of voice • Responds to sound by making sounds • Uses voice to express joy and displeasure

	Developmental Domain		
Age*	Social and Emotional	Vision	Hearing and Language
1 yr	• Shy or anxious with strangers • Cries when mother or father leaves • Enjoys imitating people in his play • Shows specific preferences for certain people and toys • Tests parental responses to his actions during feedings • Tests parental responses to his behavior • May be fearful in some situations • Prefers mother and/or regular caregiver over all others • Repeats sounds or gestures for attention • Finger-feeds self • Extends arm or leg to help when being dressed	• Explores objects in many different ways (shaking, banging, throwing, dropping) • Finds hidden objects easily • Looks at correct picture when the image is named • Imitates gestures • Begins to use objects correctly (drinking from cup, brushing hair, dialing phone, listening to receiver)	• Babbles chains of sounds • Pays increasing attention to speech • Responds to simple verbal requests • Responds to "no" • Uses simple gestures, such as shaking head for "no" • Babbles with inflection (changes in tone) • Says "dada" and "mama" • Uses exclamations, such as "Oh-oh!" • Tries to imitate words

(table continues on page 620)

PEDS

PEDS

TABLE 8.9 Typical Development in Other Domains (continued)

	Developmental Domain		
	Social and Emotional	**Vision**	**Hearing and Language**
Age*	Social and Emotional	Emotional	Cognitive	Language

Age*	Social and Emotional	Emotional	Cognitive	Language
2 yr	• Imitates behavior of others, especially adults and older children • More aware of herself as separate from others • More excited about company of other children	• Demonstrates increasing independence • Begins to show defiant behavior • Separation anxiety increases toward midyear then fades	• Finds objects even when hidden under two or three covers • Begins to sort by shapes and colors • Begins make-believe play	• Points to object or picture when it's named • Recognizes names of familiar people, objects, and body parts • Says several single words (by 15 to 18 months) • Uses simple phrases (by 18 to 24 months) • Uses 2- to 4-word sentences • Follows simple instructions • Repeats words overheard in conversation
3 yr	• Imitates adults and playmates • Spontaneously shows affection for familiar playmates • Can take turns in games • Understands concept of "mine" and "his/hers"	• Expresses affection openly • Expresses a wide range of emotions • By 3, separates easily from parents • Objects to major changes in routine	• Makes mechanical toys work • Matches an object in hand or room to a picture in a book • Plays make-believe with dolls, animals, and people • Sorts objects by shape and color • Completes puzzles with three or four pieces • Understands concept of "two"	• Follows a two- or three-part command • Recognizes and identifies almost all common objects and pictures • Understands most sentences • Understands placement in space ("on," "in," "under")

	Developmental Domain		
Age*	Social and Emotional	Vision	Hearing and Language
			• Uses 4- to 5-word sentences • Can say name, age, and sex • Uses pronouns (I, you, me, we, they) and some plurals (cars, dogs, cats) • Strangers can understand most words
4 yr	• Interested in new experiences • Cooperates with other children • Plays "Mom" or "Dad" • Increasingly inventive in fantasy play • Dresses and undresses • Negotiates solutions to conflicts • More independent	• Correctly names some colors • Understands the concept of counting and may know a few numbers • Tries to solve problems from a single point of view • Begins to have a clearer sense of time • Follows three-part commands • Recalls parts of a story • Understands the concepts of "same" and "different" • Engages in fantasy play	• Imagines that many unfamiliar images may be "monsters" • Views self as a whole person involving body, mind, and feelings • Often cannot tell the difference between fantasy and reality	• Has mastered some basic rules of grammar • Speaks in sentences of five to six words • Speaks clearly enough for strangers to understand • Tells stories

(table continues on page 622)

PEDS

PEDS

■ **TABLE 8.9 Typical Development in Other Domains** (continued)

Age*	Developmental Domain			
	Social and Emotional	Vision		Hearing and Language
5 yr	• Wants to please friends • Wants to be like friends • More likely to agree to rules • Likes to sing, dance, and act • Shows more independence and may even visit a next-door neighbor by self	• Can count 10 or more objects • Correctly names at least four colors • Better understands the concept of time • Knows about things used every day in the home (money, food, appliances)	• Aware of gender • Able to distinguish fantasy from reality • Sometimes demanding, sometimes eagerly cooperative	• Recalls part of a story • Speaks sentences of more than five words • Uses future tense • Tells longer stories • Says name and address

From: Centers for Disease Control and Prevention. http://www.cdc.gov/ncbddd/actearly/milestones/index.html
For more information about speech and language development, visit the American-Speech-Language-Hearing Association at http://www.asha.org/public/speech/development/chart.htm and the National Institute on Deafness and Other Communication Disorders at http://www.nidcd.nih.gov/health/voice/thebasics_speechandlanguage.asp. Websites accessed March 20, 2010.

Vital Signs

🔴 TABLE 8.10 Vital Signs and Blood Gas Values for Children

	Newborn	Older Infant and Child
Respiratory rate (breaths/min)	40–60	20–30 (≤6 yr) 15–20 (>6 yr)
Heart rate (beats/min)	120–200	100–180 (≤3 yr) 70–150 (≥3 yr)
PO_2 (mm Hg)	60–90	80–100
PCO_2 (mm Hg)	30–35	30–35 (≤2 yr) 20–24 (>2 yr)
Blood pressure (mm Hg) Systolic	60–90	75–130 (≤3 yr) 90–140 (>3 yr)
Diastolic	30–60	45–90 (≤3 yr) 50–80 (>3 yr)
Arterial oxygen saturation (%)	87–89 (low)	95–100
	94–95 (high) 90–95 (preterm infant)	

Data from: Comer, DM: Pulse oximetry: Implications for practice. *J Obstet Gynecol Neonatal Nurs* 21:35, 1992; and Pagtakhan, RD, and Chernick, V: Intensive care for respiratory disorders. In Kendig, EL, and Chernick, V (eds): *Disorders of the Respiratory Tract in Children,* ed. 4. WB Saunders, Philadelphia, 1983, pp 145–168, with permission from Elsevier
Adapted from: Kelly, MK: Children requiring long-term ventilator assistance. In Campbell, SK, Vander Linden, DW, and Palisano, RJ: *Physical Therapy for Children,* ed. 3. WB Saunders, Philadelphia, 2006, pp 793–817, with permission from Elsevier.

Pain

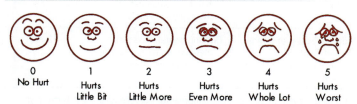

| 0
No Hurt | 1
Hurts Little Bit | 2
Hurts Little More | 3
Hurts Even More | 4
Hurts Whole Lot | 5
Hurts Worst |

FACES Pain Scale. The child is asked to choose the face that best describes his/her pain and the appropriate number is recorded. The rating scale is recommended for children age 3 years and older. *From: Hockenberry, MJ, and Wilson, D: Wong's Essentials of Pediatric Nursing, ed. 8. Mosby, St. Louis, MO, 2009. Used with permission.*

Functional Reach

TABLE 8.11 Functional Reach Scores in Typical Children Age 5 to 15 Years

Age	Mean Reach (cm)	95% CI (cm)	Critical Reach* (cm)
5–6	21.17	16.79–24.91	16.79
7–8	24.21	20.56–27.96	20.56
9–10	27.21	25.56–31.64	25.56
11–12	32.79	29.68–36.18	29.68
13–15	32.30	29.58–36.08	29.58

From: Donahoe, B, Turner, D, and Worrell, T: The use of functional reach as a measurement of balance in boys and girls without disabilities ages 5 to 15 years. *Pediatr Phys Ther* 6:189–193, 1994.
*Reach scores below critical values (2 SD) may indicate a delay in reach skills.

PEDS

Measurement Instruments

TABLE 8.12 Measurement Instruments Used in Pediatrics

Name	Type of Test	Age
Alberta Infant Motor Scale (AIMS)	Motor performance: assesses postural control in supine, prone, sitting, and standing	Birth–18 mo
Assessment, Evaluation, and Programming System for Infants and Children	Behavioral, motor performance; social skills: assesses fine motor, gross motor, adaptive, cognitive, social-communication, social	1 mo–3 yr
Battelle Developmental Inventory (2nd ed) (BDI-2)	Developmental: assesses personal-social, adaptive, motor, communication, and cognitive ability	Birth–7 yr 11 mo
Bayley Scales of Infant and Toddler Development (3rd ed) (Bayley-III)	Developmental: assesses cognitive, language, social-emotional, motor, and adaptive behavior	1–42 mo
Brigance Inventory of Early Development	Developmental: represents a comprehensive profile of developmental status examining gross motor, fine motor, self-help, prespeech, speech	Birth–7 yr

Name	Type of Test	Age
	and language, general knowledge and comprehension, early academic skills	
Bruininks-Oseretsky Test of Motor Proficiency (2nd ed) (BOT-2)	Developmental: assesses fine manual control, manual coordination, body coordination, strength, and agility	4–21 yr
The Carolina Curriculum for Infants and Toddlers With Special Needs (2nd ed)	Behavioral: assesses cognition, communication, gross motor, fine motor, self-help	Birth–24 mo
Choosing Options and Accommodations for Children (COACH)	Educational program planning based on family priorities and team decision making	3–21 yr
DeGangi-Berk Test of Sensory Integration (TSI)	Sensory: assesses underlying sensory motor mechanisms; postural control, bilateral motor integration, reflex integration	3–5 yr
Denver Development Screening Test II (DDST-II), (Denver II)	Developmental: detects potential developmental problems in the areas of gross motor, fine motor, language, personal-social	1 wk–6.5 yr
Early Learning Accomplishment Profile (ELAP)	Developmental: determines skill levels through task analyses; gross motor, fine motor, cognitive, language, self-help, social-emotional	Birth–36 mo
Functional Independence Measure for Children (Wee-FIM)	Functional: measures severity of disability; self-care, sphincter control, mobility, locomotion, communication, social, cognition, gross motor, fine motor, language, personal-social, adaptive	6 mo–7 yr
Gross Motor Function Measure (GMFM)	Developmental: measures gross motor function of children with cerebral palsy; lying and rolling, sitting, crawling, and kneeling, standing, walking, and running and jumping	Best suited for children 2–5 yr with cerebral palsy or Down syndrome

(table continues on page 626)

PEDS

⬤ **TABLE 8.12 Measurement Instruments Used in Pediatrics** (continued)

Name	Type of Test	Age
Hawaii Early Learning Profile (HELP)	Behavioral: determines developmental level; cognition, language, gross motor, fine motor, social, self-help	Birth–36 mo
Home Observation for Measurement of the Environment (HOME)	Determines the impact of home environment on the child; emotional and verbal responsiveness of parents, acceptance of child, organization of environment, provision of appropriate play materials, parental involvement, opportunities for stimulation	Birth–36 mo
Infant Monitoring Questionnaires (IMQ)	Developmental: determines developmental level through parent report; communication, gross motor, fine motor, adaptive, personal-social	4–36 mo
The Infant Motor Screen (IMS)	Neurological: tone, primitive reflexes, automatic, responses	Preterm infants at corrected ages 4–16 mo
Infant Neurological International Battery (INFANIB)	Neurological: tone, reflexes, automatic responses, head and trunk control	Birth–9 mo
Infant Toddler Scale for Every Baby (ITSE)	Developmental: cognitive, communication, physical, social-emotional, adaptive	3–42 mo
Miller Assessment of Preschoolers (MAP)	Developmental: identifies children with mild to moderate delays; sensorimotor, cognitive	33–68 mo
Movement Assessment Battery for Children (2nd ed) (Movement ABC-2)	Developmental: identifies and describes motor impairments	3–16 yr 11 mo
Movement Assessment of Infants (MAI)	Neurological: tone, reflexes, automatic reactions, volitional movement	Birth–12 mo

PEDS

Name	Type of Test	Age
Naturalistic Observation of Newborn Behavior (NONB)	Behavioral: used to develop a profile of infants' physiological and behavioral responses to environmental demands and care giving; behavioral state, autonomic responses, motor	Birth–4 wk post-term
Neonatal Behavioral Assessment Scale (NBAS)	Determines interactive behavior and neuromotor status; state, tone, reflexes, interactive behavior	Birth–1 mo
Neonatal Oral-Motor Assessment Scale (NOMAS)	Identifies oral motor dysfunction; jaw and tongue patterns during nutritive and non-nutritive sucking	Neonate
Neurobehavioral Assessment of Preterm Infant (NAPI)	Adaptive-transactive, neurological: determines neurobehavioral status and effects of intervention; state, behavior, reflexes, motor patterns, tone	32–42 wk gestation
The Neurological Assessment of the Preterm and Full-Term Newborn Infant	Neurological: Evaluates functional neurological status; tone, posture, spontaneous movement, primitive reflexes, tendon reflexes	Infants 38–42 wk gestation
Nursing Child Assessment Satellite Training Teaching and Feeding Scales (NCAST)	Adaptive-transactive: assesses parental responsiveness to infant and infant-caregiver interaction; sensitivity to cues, response to distress, social-emotional growth, cognitive growth, clarity of cues, responsiveness to parent	Teaching birth–3 yr, feeding birth–1 yr
Peabody Developmental Motor Scales (2nd ed)	Developmental: gross motor, fine motor	Birth–71 mo
Pediatric Evaluation of Disability Inventory (PEDI)	Functional: self-care, mobility, and social function	6 mo–7.5 yr
Quick Neurological Screening Test (QNST)	Neuromotor: determines risk for learning disabilities; motor maturity, fine and gross motor control, motor planning, spatial organization, visual and auditory perception, balance	6–17 yr

PEDS

(table continues on page 628)

TABLE 8.12 Measurement Instruments Used in Pediatrics (continued)

Name	Type of Test	Age
Scales of Independent Behavior (SIB)	Developmental, functional: motor, social and communication, personal and community living, behavior problems	Birth to adulthood
Screening Test for Evaluating Preschoolers (First Step)	Developmental: identifies children in need of comprehensive evaluation; cognition, communication, motor, social-emotional, adaptive	33–74 mo
Sensory Integration and Praxis Test (SIPT)	Sensory: assesses vestibular, proprioception, kinesthesia, tactile, visual	4–8 yr 11 mo
Test of Infant Motor Performance (TIMP)	Motor performance: identifies deficits in postural control; ability to orient and stabilize head in space and in response to stimulation, selective control of distal movements, antigravity control of trunk and extremities	32 wk gestation to 4 mo post-term
Test of Sensory Functions in Infants (TSFI)	Sensory: assesses tactile, deep pressure, visual-tactile integration, adaptive motor, ocular-motor, reactivity to vestibular stimulation	4–18 mo
Test of Visual-Motor Integration (TVMI)	Developmental: assesses visual-motor skills	4–17 yr
Toddler and Infant Motor Evaluation (TIME)	Motor performance: assesses repertoires of movements through observations; neurological foundations, stability, mobility, motor organization	Birth–42 mo
Transdisciplinary Play Based Assessment	Adaptive-transactive, developmental: determines developmental skill levels, learning style, and interaction through structured play; cognition, communication and language; sensorimotor, social-emotional	6 mo–6 yr

Based on: Long, TM, and Toscano, K: *Handbook of Pediatric Physical Therapy*, ed. 2. Lippincott Williams & Wilkins, Philadelphia, 2002, pp 96–162.

Normal Distribution

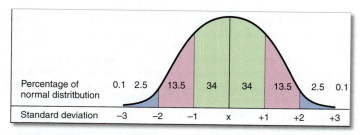

Percentage of normal distribution		0.1	2.5	13.5	34	34	13.5	2.5	0.1
Standard deviation		−3	−2	−1	x	+1	+2	+3	

The normal distribution is used to interpret children's scores on norm-referenced tests. For example, the mean Intelligence Quotient (IQ) is equal to 100 with a standard deviation of 15. An IQ of 115 is interpreted as one standard deviation above the mean. Approximately 68% of the area under the normal curve is ±1 standard deviation from the mean; approximately 95% of the area under the normal curve is ±2 standard deviations from the mean; and approximately 99.75% of the area under the normal curve is ±3 standard deviations from the mean. A z-score may also be used to standardize a score. A z-score is calculated by subtracting the obtained score on a test from the mean score and dividing by the standard deviation. For example a z-score of −1 represents a score that is one standard deviation below the mean, a z-score of −2 represents a score two standard deviations below the mean. Positive z-scores represent scores above the mean.

PEDS

Public Laws

Individuals With Disabilities Education Act (IDEA) of 2004

General Description: IDEA (Pub L. No. 108–4467, Sec. 601[d]) (1) ensures that all children with disabilities have available to them a free appropriate public education that emphasizes special education and related services designed to meet their unique needs and prepare them for further education, employment, and independent living; (2) provides for early intervention services for infants and toddlers with disabilities and their families; and (3) ensures that the rights of children with disabilities and their parents are protected. Part B of IDEA covers programs for children and youth age 3 years and above. Part C covers early intervention service for infants and toddlers birth through age 3.

Part B Eligibility

Under IDEA, students are eligible for special education and related services (such as physical therapy and occupational therapy) if they are within the age range specified by the state's plan for special education (usually age 3 through 21 years), meet the eligibility criteria for one of the 13 categories of disabilities specified in IDEA, and require special education and related services because of the disability. The 13 categories are autism, deaf-blindness, deafness, hearing impairment, mental retardation, multiple disabilities, orthopedic impairments, other health impairment, serious emotional disturbance, specific learning disability, speech or language impairment, traumatic brain injury, and visual impairment including blindness (CFR Sec. 300.8 [c]).

For children ages 3 through 9, or a subset of that age range, states and local education agencies (LEA) may choose to use the category of developmental delay, rather than label a child with a particular disability. Children must have delay in one or more of the following areas: physical development, cognitive development, communication development, social or emotional development, or adaptive development, and because of the delay need special education and related services (CFR Sec. 300.8 [b]).

Part C Eligibility

Infants and toddlers (and their families) are eligible for early intervention services if they meet the definition of "infants and toddlers with disabilities." To be eligible for services, children must be age birth through 3 years who need early intervention services because of delays in cognitive, physical, communication, social or emotional, and/or adaptive development, or have a diagnosed condition with a high probability of resulting in developmental delay, such as Down syndrome. At the discretion of the state, children without a diagnosed condition who are at risk for developmental delay may be eligible. The amount of developmental delay, the specific conditions, and the type of risk required for a child to be eligible for early intervention services are left to the states' discretion, within federal guidelines.

Physical Therapy and Occupational Therapy Services

Under Part B, physical therapy and occupational therapy are related services, which IDEA defines as supportive services "required to assist a child with a disability to benefit from special education" (CFR Sec. 300.34 [a]). Under Part C, physical therapy and occupational therapy are early intervention services. CFR Sec. 303.13 defines early intervention services as services that "are designed to meet the developmental needs of an infant or toddler with a disability as requested by the family, the needs of the family to assist appropriately in the infant's or toddler's development, as identified by the individualized family service plan team" in physical, cognitive, communication, social or emotional, or adaptive development.

The specific early intervention, special education, and related services that a child needs are decided by each child's team, which includes the child's parents and the professionals involved with the child. For children and families in early intervention, the team identifies the unique needs of the child (and family, if the family wishes) and writes the service plan, including outcomes, on an individualized family service plan (IFSP). For children receiving special education and related services, the team identifies the child's unique needs and writes the service plan, including goals and objectives/benchmarks on an individualized education program (IEP).

IFSP and IEP goals are not discipline-specific (such as physical therapy goals, occupational therapy goals, and speech goals); goals relate to activities the child needs and wants to do. Only after the team identifies the goals does it decide which services are needed. If the team decides the child needs physical therapy or occupational therapy, then the child receives it. Children who meet eligibility criteria for Part B or Part C services can receive therapy without meeting additional criteria, such as obtaining certain scores on tests of motor development. Therapy services should be provided in the most appropriate environment, as defined by IDEA. This usually means services are provided in the home and other natural environments for children in early intervention programs, and in least restrictive environments, such as school, community settings, and work sites for students receiving Part B services.

Section 504

General Description: Children with disabilities who are not eligible for services under IDEA may qualify for services under Section 504 of the Rehabilitation Act of 1973. Children with disabilities are entitled to services under Section 504 if they are of an age during which (1) all children without disabilities would receive such services, (2) the state provides a free and appropriate public education, and (3) it is mandatory to provide such services to individuals with disabilities. Although the first criterion usually is not applicable to physical therapy or occupational therapy, the second and third criteria apply if a student needs therapy at school to accommodate for a disability.

Definition of Disability Under Section 504

Under Section 504, a person has a disability who (1) has a physical or mental impairment that substantially limits one or more major life activities, (2) has a record of having a physical or mental impairment that limits one or more life activities, or (3) does not have an impairment, but is regarded as having an impairment. Students who need physical therapy in school usually meet the first criterion. Major life activities are defined as "functions such as caring for one's self, performing manual tasks, walking, seeing, hearing, speaking, breathing, learning and working."

Physical Therapy and Occupational Therapy Services

Some students' limitations in major life activities require physical therapy or occupational therapy to accommodate the limitations or to participate in school activities. A student with mobility limitations, for example, might need to learn how to move from place to place on a new school campus or a student might need to learn to use the bathroom at school. Services that a student needs are written into a 504 plan.

Based on:

McEwen, IR (ed): IDEA: Providing Physical Therapy Services Under Parts B & C of the Individuals With Disabilities Education Act, ed. 2. Section on Pediatrics, American Physical Therapy Association, Alexandria, VA, 2009.

Team Models

Three common models of team functioning for services with children and families are multidisciplinary, interdisciplinary, and transdisciplinary. The following classic characteristics of each type of team suggest that the models are distinct, but many teams have characteristics of more than one model.

● TABLE 8.13 Team Models

	Multidisciplinary	Interdisciplinary	Transdisciplinary
Assessment	Separate assessments by team members	Separate assessments by team members	Team members and family conduct a comprehensive assessment together
Parent Participation	Parents meet with individual team members	Parents meet with team or team representative	Parents are full, active, and participating members of the team
Service Plan Development	Team members develop separate plans for their disciplines	Team members share their separate plans with one another	Team members and the parents develop a service plan based on family priorities, needs, and resources
Service Plan Responsibility	Team members are responsible for implementing their section of the plan	Team members are responsible for sharing information with one another as well as for implementing their sections of the plan	Team members are responsible and accountable for how the primary service provider implements the plan
Lines of Communication	Informal lines	Periodic case-specific team meetings	Regular team meetings where continuous transfer of information, knowledge, and skills are shared among team members

	Multidisciplinary	Interdisciplinary	Transdisciplinary
Guiding Philosophy	Team members recognize the importance of contributions from other disciplines	Team members are willing and able to develop, share, and be responsible for providing services that are a part of the total service plan	Team members make a commitment to teach, learn, and work across discipline boundaries to implement unified service plan
Staff Development	Independent and within own discipline	Independent within as well as outside of discipline	An integral component of team meetings for learning across disciplines and team building

PEDS

From: Wordruff, G, and McGonigel, MJ: Early intervention team approaches: The transdisciplinary model. In Jordan, J, et al (eds). *Early Childhood Special Education: Birth to Three.* The Council for Exceptional Children and its Division for Early Childhood, Reston, VA, 1988, pp 163–181.

Seven Principles of Family-Centered Services

1. The overriding purpose of providing family-centered help is family "empowerment," which in turn benefits the well-being and development of the child.
2. Mutual trust, respect, honesty, and open communication characterize the family-provider relationship.
3. Families are active participants in all aspects of services. They are the ultimate decision makers in amount, type of assistance, and the support they seek to use.
4. The ongoing "work" between families and providers is about identifying family concerns (priorities, hopes, needs, goals, or wishes) and finding family strengths and the services and supports that will provide the necessary resources to meet those needs.
5. Efforts are made to build on and use families' informal community support systems before relying solely on professional, formal services.
6. Providers across all disciplines collaborate with families to provide resources that best match what the family needs.
7. Support and resources need to be flexible, individualized, and responsive to the changing needs of families.

From:

Family Centered Services: Guiding Principles for Delivery of Family Centered Services. http://www.extension.iastate.edu/culture/files/FamlCntrdSrvc.pdf. *Accessed March 20, 2010. This resource also includes examples of behaviors and practices under each principle.*

Cultural Competence

Cultural competence refers to a program's ability to honor and respect those beliefs, interpersonal styles, attitudes, and behaviors both of families who are clients and the multicultural staff who are providing services. In doing so, it incorporates these values at the levels of policy, administration, and practice. Achieving cultural competence is a process, not an endpoint.

Major Values and Principles

- The family as defined by each culture is the primary system of support and preferred intervention
- The system must recognize that racial and ethnic populations have to be at least bicultural and that this status may create a unique set of issues to which the system must be equipped to respond
- Individuals and families make different choices based on cultural forces; these choices must be considered if education/service delivery are to be helpful and appropriate
- Practice is driven in the service delivery system by culturally preferred choices, not by culturally blind or culturally free interventions
- Inherent in cross-cultural interactions are dynamics that must be acknowledged, adjusted to, and accepted. The system must sanction and in some cases mandate the incorporation of cultural knowledge into policy making, education, and practice
- Cultural competence involves determining an individual or family's cultural identity and levels of acculturation and assimilation to more effectively apply the helping principle of "starting where the individual or family is"
- Cultural competence involves working in conjunction with natural, informal support and helping networks within culturally diverse communities (e.g., neighborhood, civic, and advocacy associations; ethnic, social, and religions organizations; and, where appropriate, spiritual healers)
- Cultural competence extends the concept of self-determination
- Cultural competence seeks to identify and understand the needs and help-seeking behaviors of individuals and families. Cultural competence seeks to design and implement services that are tailored or matched to the unique needs of individuals, children, and families
- An agency or education program staffing pattern that reflects the makeup of the population within the geographic locale helps ensure the delivery of effective services
- Cultural competence embraces the principles of equal access and non-discriminatory practices in service delivery and education

Guidelines for Using Interpreters

1. Always use an interpreter unless you are fluent in the language.
2. Avoid asking family members, particularly children, to interpret.
3. Try to use an interpreter of the same sex as the patient/client.
4. Talk to the patient/client; do not direct questions or comments to the interpreter.
5. Plan what to say ahead of time. Do not confuse the interpreter by restating or hesitating.
6. Use simple language, with short questions and comments; carefully avoid jargon and slang.
7. If you get a response you do not expect, restate the question or comment. The interpreter may have misunderstood you or the patient/client.
8. Wait patiently for the interpretation, which can seem to take a long time.
9. Ask patients/clients to repeat instructions and other information you want to be sure they understand.
10. If you think the patient/client understands some English, speak slowly, not loudly.
11. Learn basic words and sentences in the language.

PEDS

Based on:

Putsch, RW III. Cross-cultural communication: The special case of interpreters in health care. JAMA 254:3344–3348, 1985.

Child Abuse and Neglect

The federal Child Abuse Prevention and Treatment Act (CAPTA) (42 U.S.C.A. §5106g), amended by the Keeping Children and Families Safe Act of 2003, describes the minimum acts or behaviors that define child abuse and neglect. States have developed their own laws based on the federal definitions, which include reporting requirements for professionals and others. Complete definitions and state-specific information are available from the Child Welfare Information Gateway at http://www.childwelfare.gov. For information about filing a report, call Childhelp USA at 1–800–4-A-CHILD (1-800-422-4453) or local child protective service agencies.

Federal Definition of Abuse and Neglect

- Any recent act or failure to act on the part of a parent or caretaker which results in death, serious physical or emotional harm, sexual abuse or exploitation; or
- An act or failure to act which presents an imminent risk of serious harm

General Signs of Abuse and Neglect

The child:

- Shows sudden changes in behavior or school performance.
- Has not received help for physical or medical problems brought to the parents' attention.
- Has learning problems (or difficulty concentrating) that cannot be attributed to specific physical or psychological causes.
- Is always watchful, as though preparing for something bad to happen.
- Lacks adult supervision.
- Is overly compliant, passive, or withdrawn.
- Comes to school or other activities early, stays late, and does not want to go home.

The parent:

- Shows little concern for the child.
- Denies the existence of—or blames the child for—the child's problems in school or at home.
- Asks teachers or other caretakers to use harsh physical discipline if the child misbehaves.
- Sees the child as entirely bad, worthless, or burdensome.
- Demands a level of physical or academic performance the child cannot achieve.
- Looks primarily to the child for care, attention, and satisfaction of emotional needs.

The parent and child:

- Rarely touch or look at each other.
- Consider their relationship entirely negative.
- State that they do not like each other.

Signs of Physical Abuse

Consider the possibility of physical abuse when the **child:**

- Has unexplained burns, bites, bruises, broken bones, or black eyes.
- Has fading bruises or other marks noticeable after an absence from school.
- Seems frightened of the parents and protests or cries when it is time to go home.
- Shrinks at the approach of adults.
- Reports injury by a parent or another adult caregiver.

Consider the possibility of physical abuse when the **parent or other adult caregiver:**

- Offers conflicting, unconvincing, or no explanation for the child's injury.
- Describes the child as "evil," or in some other very negative way.
- Uses harsh physical discipline with the child.
- Has a history of abuse as a child.

Signs of Neglect

Consider the possibility of neglect when the **child:**

- Is frequently absent from school.
- Begs or steals food or money.
- Lacks needed medical or dental care, immunizations, or glasses.
- Is consistently dirty and has severe body odor.
- Lacks sufficient clothing for the weather.
- Abuses alcohol or other drugs.
- States that there is no one at home to provide care.

Consider the possibiltiy of neglect when the **parent or other adult caregiver:**

- Appears to be indifferent to the child.
- Seems apathetic or depressed.
- Behaves irrationally or in a bizarre manner.
- Is abusing alcohol or other drugs.

Signs of Sexual Abuse

Consider the possibility of sexual abuse when the **child:**

- Has difficulty walking or sitting.
- Suddenly refuses to change for gym or to participate in physical activities.
- Reports nightmares or bedwetting.
- Experiences a sudden change in appetite.
- Demonstrates bizarre, sophisticated, or unusual sexual knowledge or behavior.
- Becomes pregnant or contracts a venereal disease, particularly if under age 14.
- Runs away.
- Reports sexual abuse by a parent or another adult caregiver.

Consider the possibility of sexual abuse when the **parent or other adult caregiver:**

- Is unduly protective of the child or severely limits the child's contact with other children, especially of the opposite sex.
- Is secretive and isolated.
- Is jealous or controlling with family members.

Signs of Emotional Maltreatment

Consider the possibility of emotional maltreatment when the **child:**

- Shows extremes in behavior, such as overly compliant or demanding behavior, extreme passivity, or aggression.
- Is either inappropriately adult (e.g., parenting other children) or inappropriately infantile (e.g., frequently rocking or head banging).
- Is delayed in physical or emotional development.
- Has attempted suicide.
- Reports a lack of attachment to the parent.

PEDS

Consider the possibility of emotional maltreatment when the **parent or other adult caregiver:**

- Constantly blames, belittles, or berates the child.
- Is unconcerned about the child and refuses to consider offers of help for the child's problems.
- Overtly rejects the child.

From:

Child Welfare Information Gateway, a service of the Children's Bureau, Administration for Children and Families, U.S. Department of Health and Human Services. http://www.child welfare.gov/. Accessed March 20, 2010.

Sports Participation

Physical activity is encouraged for many chronic health conditions (see Physical Activity Guidelines, Section V, Cardiovascular, pp 490–492). Certain conditions may limit participation or pose an increased risk of injury. In addition to the information on sports participation for children and adolescents with medical conditions provided in the accompanying table, other variables to consider include the following:

- The amount of contact
- Cardiovascular demands
- Current health status of the athlete
- The sport played, including position and level of competition
- The maturity of the competitor
- The relative size of the athlete participating in collision or contact sports
- The availability of protective equipment
- The availability and efficacy of treatment
- Has rehabilitation or other treatments have been completed
- Whether the sport can be modified to allow for safer participation
- The ability of the athlete's parents and coach to understand and to accept risks involved with participation

TABLE 8.14 Medical Conditions of Children and Adolescents and Sports Participation

Condition	May Participate and Explanation
Atlantoaxial instability	Qualified yes. Athlete (particularly if he or she has Down syndrome or juvenile rheumatoid arthritis with cervical involvement) needs evaluation to assess risk of spinal cord injury during sports participation, especially when using a trampoline
Bleeding disorder	Qualified yes. Athlete needs evaluation

Condition	May Participate and Explanation
Cardiovascular disease	
Carditis	No. May result in sudden death with exertion
Hypertension	Qualified yes. Those with hypertension >5 mm Hg above the 99th percentile for age, gender, and height should avoid heavy weightlifting and power lifting, bodybuilding, and high-static component sports. Those with sustained hypertension (>95th percentile for age, gender, and height) need evaluation. The National High Blood Pressure Education Program Working Group report defined prehypertension and stage 1 and stage 2 hypertension in children and adolescents younger than 18 years of age.
Congenital heart disease	Qualified yes. Consultation with a cardiologist is recommended. Those who have mild forms may participate fully in most cases; those who have moderate or severe forms or who have undergone surgery need evaluation.
Dysrhythmia Long-QT syndrome Malignant ventricular arrhythmias Symptomatic Wolff-Parkinson-White syndrome Advanced heart block Family history of sudden death or previous sudden' cardiac event Implantation of a cardi overter-defibrillator	Qualified yes. Consultation with a cardiologist is advised. Those with symptoms (chest pain, syncope, near-syncope, dizziness, shortness of breath, or other symptoms of possible dysrhythmia) or evidence of mitral regurgitation on physical examination need evaluation. All others may participate fully.
Heart murmur	Qualified yes. If the murmur is innocent (does not indicate heart disease), full participation is permitted. Otherwise, athlete needs evaluation (see Structural/acquired heart disease, especially Hypertrophic cardiomyopathy and Mitral valve prolapse).
Structural/acquired heart disease Hypertrophic cardiomyopathy Coronary artery anomalies Arrhythmogenic right ventricular cardiomyopathy Acute rheumatic fever with carditis	Qualified yes. Consultation with a cardiologist is recommended. The 36th Bethesda Conference provided detailed recommendations. Most of these conditions carry a significant risk of sudden cardiac death associated with intense physical exercise. Hypertrophic cardiomyopathy requires thorough and repeated evaluations, because disease may change manifestations during later adolescence. Marfan syndrome with an aortic aneurysm also can cause sudden death during intense physical exercise. Athlete who has ever received chemotherapy with

(table continues on page 640)

⬤ TABLE 8.14 Medical Conditions of Children and Adolescents and Sports Participation (continued)

Condition	May Participate and Explanation
Ehlers-Danlos syndrome, vascular form Marfan syndrome Mitral valve prolapse Anthracycline use Vaculitis/vascular disease Kawasaki disease (coronary artery vasculitis) Pulmonary hypertension	anthracyclines may be at increased risk of cardiac problems because of the cardiotoxic effects of the medications, and resistance training in this population should be approached with caution; strength training that avoids isometric contractions may be permitted. Athlete needs evaluation. Qualified yes. Consultation with a cardiologist is recommended. Athlete needs individual evaluation to assess risk on the basis of disease activity, pathological changes, and medical regimen.
Cerebral palsy	Qualified yes. Athlete needs evaluation to assess functional capacity to perform sports-specific activity.
Diabetes mellitus	Yes. All sports can be played with proper attention and appropriate adjustments to diet (particularly carbohydrate intake), blood glucose concentrations, hydration, and insulin therapy. Blood glucose concentrations should be monitored before exercise, every 30 min during continuous exercise, 15 min after completion of exercise, and at bedtime.
Diarrhea, infectious	Qualified no. Unless symptoms are mild and athlete is fully hydrated, no participation is permitted, because diarrhea may increase risk of dehydration and heat illness (see Fever).
Eating disorders	Qualified yes. Athlete with an eating disorder needs medical and psychiatric assessment before participation.
Eyes Functionally 1-eyed athlete Loss of an eye Detached retina or family history of retinal detachment at young age High myopia Connective tissue disorder, such as Marfan or Stickler syndrome	Qualified yes. A functionally 1-eyed athlete is defined as having best-corrected visual acuity worse than 20/40 in the poorer-seeing eye. Such an athlete would suffer significant disability if the better eye were seriously injured, as would an athlete with loss of an eye. Specifically, boxing and full-contact martial arts are not recommended for functionally 1-eyed athletes, because eye protection is impractical and/or not permitted. Some athletes who previously underwent intraocular eye surgery or had a serious eye injury may have increased risk of injury because of weakened eye

Condition	May Participate and Explanation
Previous intraocular eye surgery or serious eye injury	tissue. Availability of eye guards approved by the American Society for Testing and Materials and other protective equipment may allow participation in most sports, but this must be judged on an individual basis.
Eyes Conjunctivitis, infectious	Qualified no. Athlete with active infectious conjunctivitis should be excluded from swimming.
Fever	No. Elevated core temperature may be indicative of a pathological medical condition (infection or disease) that is often manifest by increased resting metabolism and heart rate. Accordingly, during athlete's usual exercise regimen, the presence of fever can result in greater heat storage, decreased heat tolerance, increased risk of heat illness, increased cardiopulmonary effort, reduced maximal exercise capacity, and increased risk of hypotension because of altered vascular tone and dehydration. On rare occasions, fever may accompany myocarditis or other conditions that may make usual exercise dangerous.
Gastrointestinal Malabsorption syndromes (celiac disease or cystic fibrosis)	Qualified yes. Athlete needs individual assessment for general malnutrition or specific deficits resulting in coagulation or other defects; with appropriate treatment, these deficits can be treated adequately to permit normal activities.
Gastrointestinal Short-bowel syndrome or other disorders requiring specialized nutritional support, including parenteral or enteral nutrition	Qualified yes. Athlete needs individual assessment for collision, contact, or limited-contact sports. Presence of central or peripheral. indwelling, venous catheter may require special considerations for activities and emergency preparedness for unexpected trauma to the device(s).
Heat illness, history of	Qualified yes. Because of the likelihood of recurrence, athlete needs individual assessment to determine the presence of predisposing conditions and behaviors and to develop a prevention strategy that includes sufficient acclimatization (to the environment and to exercise intensity and duration), conditioning, hydration, and salt intake, as well as other effective measures to improve heat tolerance and to reduce heat injury risk (such as protective equipment and uniform configurations).

PEDS

(table continues on page 642)

🔲 TABLE 8.14 Medical Conditions of Children and Adolescents and Sports Participation (continued)

Condition	May Participate and Explanation
Hepatitis, infectious (primarily hepatitis C)	Yes. All athletes should receive hepatitis B vaccination before participation. Because of the apparent minimal risk to others, all sports may be played as athlete's state of health allows. For all athletes, skin lesions should be covered properly, and athletic personnel should use universal precautions when handling blood or body fluids with visible blood.
HIV infection	Yes. Because of the apparent minimal risk to others, all sports may be played as athlete's state of health allows (especially if viral load is undetectable or very low). For all athletes, skin lesions should be covered properly, and athletic personnel should use universal precautions when handling blood or body fluids with visible blood. However, certain sports (such as wrestling and boxing) may create a situation that favors viral transmission (likely bleeding plus skin breaks). If viral load is detectable, then athletes should be advised to avoid such high-contact sports.
Kidney, absence of one	Qualified yes. Athlete needs individual assessment for contact, collision, and limited-contact sports. Protective equipment may reduce risk of injury to the remaining kidney sufficiently to allow participation in most sports, providing such equipment remains in place during activity.
Liver, enlarged	Qualified yes. If the liver is acutely enlarged, then participation should be avoided because of risk of rupture. If the liver is chronically enlarged, then individual assessment is needed before collision, contact, or limited-contact sports are played. Patients with chronic liver disease may have changes in liver function that affect stamina, mental status, coagulation, or nutritional status.
Malignant neoplasm	Qualified yes. Athlete needs individual assessment.
Musculoskeletal disorders	Qualified yes. Athlete needs individual assessment.
Neurological disorders History of serious head or spine trauma or abnormality,	Qualified yes. Athlete needs individual assessment for collision, contact, or limited-contact sports.

Condition	May Participate and Explanation
including craniotomy, epidural bleeding, subdural hematoma, intracerebral hemorrhage, second-impact syndrome, vascular malformation, and neck fracture	
History of simple concussion (mild traumatic brain injury), multiple simple concussions, and/or complex concussion	Qualified yes. Athlete needs individual assessment. Research supports a conservative approach to concussion management, including no athletic participation while symptomatic or when deficits in judgment or cognition are detected, followed by graduated return to full activity.
Myopathies	Qualified yes. Athlete needs individual assessment.
Recurrent headaches	Yes. Athlete needs individual assessment.
Recurrent plexopathy (burner or stinger) and cervical cord neuropraxia with persistent defects	Qualified yes. Athlete needs individual assessment for collision, contact, or limited-contact sports; regaining normal strength is important benchmark for return to play.
Seizure disorder, well controlled	Yes. Risk of seizure during participation is minimal.
Seizure disorder, poorly controlled	Qualified yes. Athlete needs individual assessment for collision, contact, or limited-contact sports. The following noncontact sports should be avoided: archery, riflery, swimming, weightlifting, power lifting, strength training, and sports involving heights. In these sports, occurrence of a seizure during activity may pose a risk to self or others.
Obesity	Yes. Because of the increased risk of heat illness and cardiovascular strain, obese athlete particularly needs careful acclimatization (to the environment and to exercise intensity and duration), sufficient hydration, and potential activity and recovery modifications during competition and training.
Organ transplant recipient (and those taking immunosuppressive medications)	Qualified yes. Athlete needs individual assessment for contact, collision, and limited-contact sports. In addition to potential risk of infections, some medications (e.g., prednisone) may increase tendency for bruising.
Ovary, absence of one	Yes. Risk of severe injury to remaining ovary is minimal.

(table continues on page 644)

PEDS

⬤ **TABLE 8.14 Medical Conditions of Children and Adolescents and Sports Participation** (continued)

Condition	May Participate and Explanation
Pregnancy, postpartum	Qualified yes. Athlete needs individual assessment. As pregnancy progresses, modifications to usual exercise routines will become necessary. Activities with high risk of falling or abdominal trauma should be avoided. Scuba diving and activities posing risk of altitude sickness should also be avoided during pregnancy. After the birth, physiological and morphological changes of pregnancy take 4 to 6 weeks to return to baseline.
Respiratory conditions Pulmonary compromise, including cystic fibrosis	Qualified yes. Athlete needs individual assessment but, generally, all sports may be played if oxygenation remains satisfactory during graded exercise test. Athletes with cystic fibrosis need acclimatization and good hydration to reduce risk of heat illness.
Asthma	Yes. With proper medication and education, only athletes with severe asthma need to modify their participation. For those using inhalers, recommend having a written action plan and using a peak flowmeter daily. Athletes with asthma may encounter risks when scuba diving.
Acute upper respiratory infection	Qualified yes. Upper respiratory obstruction may affect pulmonary function. Athlete needs individual assessment for all except mild disease (see Fever).
Rheumatologic diseases Juvenile rheumatoid arthritis Juvenile dermatomyositis, idiopathic myositis Systemic lupus erythematosis Raynaud phenomenon	Qualified yes. Athletes with systemic or polyarticular juvenile rheumatoid arthritis and history of cervical spine involvement need radiographs of vertebrae C1 and C2 to assess risk of spinal cord injury. Athletes with systemic or HLA-B27-associated arthritis require cardiovascular assessment for possible cardiac complications during exercise. For those with micrognathia (open bite and exposed teeth), mouth guards are helpful. If uveitis is present, risk of eye damage from trauma is increased; ophthalmologic assessment is recommended. If visually impaired, guidelines for functionally 1-eyed athletes should be followed. Athlete with juvenile dermatomyositis or systemic lupus erythematosis with cardiac involvement requires cardiology assessment before participation. Athletes receiving systemic corticosteroid therapy are at higher risk of osteoporotic fractures and avascular necrosis, which should be

PEDS

Condition	May Participate and Explanation
	assessed before clearance; those receiving immunosuppressive medications are at higher risk of serious infection. Sports activities should be avoided when myositis is active. Rhabdomyolysis during intensive exercise may cause renal injury in athletes with idiopathic myositis and other myopathies. Because of photosensitivity with juvenile dermatomyositis and systemic lupus erythematosis, sun protection is necessary during outdoor activities. With Raynaud phenomenon, exposure to the cold presents risk to hands and feet.
Sickle cell disease	Qualified yes. Athlete needs individual assessment. In general, if illness status permits, all sports may be played; however, any sport or activity that entails overexertion, overheating, dehydration, or chilling should be avoided. Participation at high altitude, especially when not acclimatized, also poses risk of sickle cell crisis.
Sickle cell trait	Yes. Athletes with sickle cell trait generally do not have increased risk of sudden death or other medical problems during athletic participation under normal environmental conditions. However, when high exertional activity is performed under extreme conditions of heat and humidity or increased altitude, such catastrophic complications have occurred rarely. Athletes with sickle cell trait, like all athletes, should be progressively acclimatized to the environment and to the intensity and duration of activities and should be sufficiently hydrated to reduce the risk of exertional heat illness and/or rhabdomyolysis. According to National Institutes of Health management guidelines, sickle cell trait is not a contraindication to participation in competitive athletics, and there is no requirement for screening before participation. More research is needed to assess fully potential risks and benefits of screening athletes for sickle cell trait.
Skin infections, including herpes simplex, molluscum contagiosum, verrucae (warts), staphylococcal and streptococcal	Qualified yes. During contagious periods, participation in gymnastics or cheerleading with mats, martial arts, wrestling, or other collision, contact, or limited-contact sports is not allowed.

(table continues on page 646)

PEDS

⬤ TABLE 8.14 Medical Conditions of Children and Adolescents and Sports Participation (continued)

Condition	May Participate and Explanation
infections (furuncles [boils], carbuncles, impetigo, methicillin-resistant Staphylococcus aureus [cellulitis and/or abscesses]), scabies, and tinea	
Spleen, enlarged	Qualified yes. If the spleen is acutely enlarged, then participation should be avoided because of risk of rupture. If the spleen is chronically enlarged, then individual assessment is needed before collision, contact, or limited-contact sports are played.
Testicle, undescended or absence of one	Yes. Certain sports may require a protective cup.

Based on: Rice, SG; American Academy of Pediatrics Council on Sports Medicine and Fitness: Medical conditions affecting sports participation. *Pediatrics* 121(4):841–848, 2008.

"Needs evaluation" means that a physician with appropriate knowledge and experience should assess the safety of a given sport for an athlete with the listed medical condition. Unless otherwise noted, this need for special consideration is because of variability in the severity of the disease, the risk of injury for the specific sport, or both.

GERIATRICS

Demographics

The Graying of America

- The growth rate of the population 65 years and older exceeded the growth rate of the total population when baby boomers began reaching age 65 in 2011.
- Starting in 2012, nearly 10,000 Americans will turn 65 every day and by 2030 20% of the population will be 65 and older.
- The "oldest old"—those aged 85 and over—are one of the fastest growing age groups: currently, the oldest old are 10% of the elderly population and 1% of the total U.S. population. By 2050, the oldest old are projected to be 24% of elderly population and 5% of the total U.S. population.
- In the United States, the elderly population is more racially diverse than in the past. In 2000, 16.5% of the elderly population was nonwhite or Hispanic; this percentage is expected to increase to about 31% by 2040.
- The average 75-year-old has three chronic conditions and takes five different prescription drugs.
- In the United States, the growing percentage of elderly people will have enormous effects on the distribution and cost of health care. Two-thirds of current health-care costs in older adults are for treating chronic illnesses.
- In 2001, chronic diseases were the leading causes of death among older adults.

Based on:

Beers, MH, and Berkow, R (eds): Merck Manual of Geriatrics, ed. 3. Merck Research Laboratories, Whitehouse Station, NJ, 2000, section 1, chapter 2, Demographics (updated September 2005). website: http://www.merck.com/mkgr/mmg/sec1/ch2/ch2a.jsp. Accessed July 20, 2009.
Merck Institute of Aging and Health. The State of Aging and Health in America 2004. http://www.cdc.gov/aging/pdf/State_of_Aging_and_Health_in_America_2004.pdf. Accessed July 20, 2009.

TABLE 9.1 **Proportion of Persons ≥ 65 Years and ≥ 85 Years in the Population Including Projections Through 2040 (number in thousands)**

Year	Total Population (all ages)	≥ 65 years		≥ 85 years	
		Number	Percentage of Total Population	Number	Percentage of Total Population ≥ 65
1940	132,122	9,031	6.8	370	4.1
1960	179,323	16,560	9.2	929	5.6
1980	226,546	25,550	11.3	2,240	8.8
2000	281,422	34,992	12.4	4,240	12.1

	≥ 65 years		≥ 85 years	
Year	Total Population (all ages)	Number	Percentage of Total Population	Number	Percentage of Total Population ≥ 65
2020	335,805	54,632	16.3	7,269	13.3
2040	391,946	80,049	20.4	15,409	19.2

From: Beers, MH, and Berkow, R (eds): *Merck Manual of Geriatrics,* ed. 3. Merck Research Laboratories, Whitehouse Station, NJ, 2000, section 1, chapter 2, Demographics (updated September 2005). http://www.merck.com/mkgr/mmg/sec1/ch2/ch2a.jsp. Accessed July 20, 2009.
Source: U.S. Census Bureau: U.S. interim projections by age, sex, race and Hispanic origin. 2004. http://www.censuc.gov/ipc/www/usinterimproj/.

TABLE 9.2 Leading Causes of Death Among Persons 65 and Older in 2002

Cause of Death	Number of Deaths	Death Rate (per 100,000 population)	Percentage of All Deaths in Those ≥65 Years Old
Heart disease	576,301	1,618.7	31.8
Malignant neoplasms	391,001	1,098.3	21.6
Cerebrovascular disease	143,293	402.5	7.9
Chronic lower respiratory disease	108,313	304.2	6.0
Influenza and pneumonia	58,826	165.2	3.2
Alzheimer's disease	58,289	163.7	3.2
Diabetes mellitus	54,715	153.7	3.0
Nephritis, nephrotic syndrome, and nephrosis	34,316	96.4	1.9
Accidents	33,641	94.5	1.9
Septicemia	26,670	74.9	1.5

(table continues on page 650)

GERI

● **TABLE 9.2 Leading Causes of Death Among Persons 65 and Older in 2002** (continued)

Cause of Death	Number of Deaths	Death Rate (per 100,000 population)	Percentage of All Deaths in Those ≥65 Years Old
All other causes, residual	326,355	916.7	18.0
All causes	1,811,720	5,088.8	100.0

Based on: Beers, MH, and Berkow, R (eds): *Merck Manual of Geriatrics,* ed. 3. Merck Research Laboratories, Whitehouse Station, NJ, 2000, section 1, chapter 2, Demographics (updated September 2005). http://www.merck.com/mkgr/mmg/tables/2t3.jsp. Accessed July 20, 2009.

Source: Anderson, RN, and Smith, BL: Deaths: Leading causes for 2002. *National Vital Statistics Report* 53(17), 2005, table 1. National Center for Health Statistics, Hyattsville, MD.

Falls Among Older Adults

How Big Is the Problem?

- More than one-third of adults 65 and older fall each year in the United States.
- Falls result in disability, functional decline, and reduced quality of life.
- Falls are the leading cause of injury-related deaths: every hour an older adult dies as a result of a fall.
- Approximately 1.8 million adults 65 and older were treated in emergency departments for nonfatal fall-related injuries, and more than 433,000 of these patients were hospitalized.
- The rates of fall-related deaths among older adults rose significantly over the past decade.

Outcomes Linked to Falls

- Many older adults who fall, even those who are not injured, develop a fear of falling. This fear may cause them to limit their activities, leading to reduced mobility and physical fitness, and increasing their actual risk of falling.
- People age 75 and older who fall are four to five times more likely to be admitted to a long-term care facility for a year or longer.
- Twenty to 30% of people who fall suffer moderate to severe injuries such as bruises, hip fractures, or head traumas.
- More than 90% of hip fractures among adults age 65 and older are caused by falls, most often by falling sideways onto the hip.
- About one out of five hip fracture patients dies within a year of their injury.
- Osteoporosis increases the likelihood of a hip fracture.
- Rates of fall-related fractures among older adults are more than twice as high for women as for men.

- Falls are the most common cause of traumatic brain injuries (TBI). In 2000, TBI accounted for 46% of fatal falls among older adults.
- Men are more likely to die from a fall. After adjusting for age, the fall fatality rate in 2004 was 49% higher for men than for women.
- There is little difference in fatal fall rates between whites and blacks from ages 65 to 74.
- After age 75, white men have the highest fatality rates, followed by white women, black men, and black women.
- White women have significantly higher rates of fall-related hip fractures than black women.

Cost of Falls Among Older Adults

- By 2020, the annual direct and indirect cost of fall injuries is expected to reach $54.9 billion (in 2007 U.S. dollars).
- Hip fractures are the most frequent type of fall-related fractures. The cost of hospitalization for hip fracture averaged about $18,000.
- In a study of people age 72 and older, the average health-care cost of a fall-related injury totaled $19,440, not including doctors' services.

Falls in Nursing Homes

- By 2030 the number of adults 65 and older who live in nursing homes is expected to rise to about 3 million.
- Each year, a typical nursing home with 100 beds reports 100 to 200 falls.
- As many as 75% of nursing home residents fall each year: twice the rate of falls for older adults living in the community.
- About 1,800 older adults living in nursing homes die each year from fall-related injuries.

Most falls in older adults occur indoors. No specific time of day or time of year is associated with falling. Among the elderly, most falls occur during usual activities such as walking. Indoor falls occur most often in the bathroom, bedroom, and kitchen. About 10% of falls occur on stairs (the first and last steps are the most dangerous), with descent being more hazardous than ascent. Common sites of outdoor falls are curbs and steps. In institutions, the most common sites of falls are the bedside (during transfers into or out of bed) and the bathroom.

Based on:

Fact Sheets. http://www.cdc.gov/HomeandRecreationalSafety/Falls/index.html. Accessed July 18, 2009.

Fall Risk Factors

The cause of most falls is multifactorial, involving the interaction of risk factors. There are four categories of risk factors: biological, behavioral, environmental, and socioeconomic. Socioeconomic factors indirectly increase the risk for falling. The risk of falling increases dramatically as the number of risk factors increases. Likewise, a reduction in the number of risk factors decreases the risk of falling.

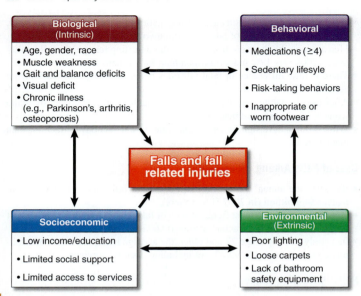

Biological (Intrinsic)
- Age, gender, race
- Muscle weakness
- Gait and balance deficits
- Visual deficit
- Chronic illness (e.g., Parkinson's, arthritis, osteoporosis)

Behavioral
- Medications (≥4)
- Sedentary lifestyle
- Risk-taking behaviors
- Inappropriate or worn footwear

Falls and fall related injuries

Socioeconomic
- Low income/education
- Limited social support
- Limited access to services

Environmental (Extrinsic)
- Poor lighting
- Loose carpets
- Lack of bathroom safety equipment

GERI

Risk factor model for falls and fall-related injuries in older adults. Adapted from: World Health Organization. WHO Global report on falls prevention in older adults. 2007.

TABLE 9.3 Most Common Risk Factors for Falls

Risk Factor	Significant/Total*	Mean RR-OR†	Range
Muscle weakness	10/11	4.4	1.5–10.3
History of falls	12/13	3.0	1.7–7.0
Gait deficit	10/12	2.9	1.3–5.6
Balance deficit	8/11	2.9	1.6–5.4
Use assistive device	8/8	2.6	1.2–4.6
Visual deficit	6/12	2.5	1.6–3.5
Arthritis	3/7	2.4	1.9–2.9
Impaired ADL	8/9	2.3	1.5–3.1
Depression	3/6	2.2	1.7–2.5
Cognitive impairment	4/11	1.8	1.0–2.3
Age >80 yr	5/8	1.7	1.1–2.5

Based on: Guideline for the prevention of falls in older persons. American Geriatrics Society, British Geriatrics Society, and American Academy of Orthopaedic Surgeons Panel on Falls Prevention. *J Am Geriatr Soc* 49(5):664–672, 2001. ADL = activities of daily living.
*Number of studies with significant relative risk ratio or odds ratio in univariate analyses/Total number of studies that included factor.
†Relative risk ratio (RR) calculated for prospective studies. Odds ratio (OR) calculated for retrospective studies.

Biological Factors

Changes in Postural Control
Decreased proprioception
Slower righting reflexes
Decreased muscle strength and range of motion, especially of the lower extremity
Increased postural sway
Orthostatic hypotension

Changes in Gait
Lower foot swing height
Slower gait
Increased variability

Declining Visual Abilities
Depth perception
Dark adaptation
Contrast sensitivity
Declining visual fields
Visuospatial function
Increased sensitivity to glare

Chronic Illnesses
Parkinson's disease
Stroke
Arthritis
Dementia

Based on:

Instability and falls. In Kane, RL, et al: Essentials of Clinical Geriatrics, ed. 6. McGraw-Hill, New York, 2009.

GERI

● TABLE 9.4 Medical Conditions That Predispose Older Adults to Falls

Function Impairment	Disorder
BP regulation	Anemia
	Arrhythmias
	Cardioinhibitory carotid sinus hypersensitivity
	COPD
	Dehydration
	Infections (e.g., pneumonia, sepsis)
	Metabolic disorders (e.g., thyroid disorders, hypo-glycemia, hyperglycemia with hyperosmolar dehydration)
	Neurocardiogenic inhibition after micturition
	Postural hypotension
	Postprandial hypotension
	Valvular heart disorders

(table continues on page 654)

● **TABLE 9.4** **Medical Conditions That Predispose Older Adults to Falls** (continued)

Function Impairment	Disorder
Central processing	Delirium Dementia
Gait	Arthritis Bunions Corns and calluses Foot deformities Muscle weakness
Neuromotor function	Cerebellar degeneration Myelopathy (e.g., due to cervical or lumbar spondylosis) Parkinson's disease Peripheral neuropathy Stroke Vertebrobasilar insufficiency
Postural control	Same as for BP regulation and gait
Proprioception	Peripheral neuropathy (such as that due to diabetes mellitus) Vitamin B_{12} deficiency
Vestibular function	Acute labyrinthitis Benign paroxysmal positional vertigo Hearing loss Meniere's disease
Vision	Cataract Glaucoma Macular degeneration (age-related)

Based on: Beers, MH, and Berkow, R (eds): *Merck Manual of Geriatrics,* ed. 3. Merck Research Laboratories, Whitehouse Station, NJ, 2000, section 2, chapter 20, Falls (updated May 2005). http://www.merck.com/mkgr/mmg/tables/20t1.jsp. Accessed July 20, 2009.
BP = blood pressure; COPD = chronic obstructive pulmonary disease.

Behavioral Factors

Polypharmacy/use of certain medications
Excess alcohol use
Physical inactivity
Inappropriate or worn footwear

TABLE 9.5 Major Classes of Medications and Mechanisms That Are Associated With Increased Fall Risk in Older Adults

Medication Class	Medications Included in Class	Mechanism
Benzodiazepines (long and short acting)	Flurazepam, diazepam, alprazolam, lorazepam	Sedation, dizziness, decrease neuromuscular function, cognitive impairment
Antidepressants	Tricyclic antidepressants (TCA), selective serotonin reuptake inhibitors (SSRI)	Postural hypotension, sedation, blurred vision, confusion, ataxia
Antipsychotics	Chlorpromazine, haloperidol, risperidone, olanzapine	Postural hypotension, dizziness, blurred vision, sedation
Antiepileptics	Barbiturates, phenytoin, valproic acid, carbamazepine	Ataxia, cognitive impairment, sedation
Antihypertensives Centrally acting antihypertensives	Clonidine, methyldopa, reserpine, minoxidil	Postural hypotension, sedation
Beta blockers	Propranolol, atenolol, metoprolol	Postural hypotension, sedation
Thiazide diuretics	Hydrochlorothiazide (HCTZ), metolazone, chlorthalidone	Postural hypotension, lethargy
ACE inhibitors	Captopril, enalapril, lisinopril	Postural hypotension
Cardiac Medications Nitrates	Nitroglycerin, isosorbide dinitrate	Postural hypotension, syncope

(table continues on page 656)

GERI

⬤ **TABLE 9.5** **Major Classes of Medications and Mechanisms That Are Associated With Increased Fall Risk in Older Adults** (continued)

Medication Class	Medications Included in Class	Mechanism
Antiarrhythmics	Procainamide, quinidine, tocainide, flecainide	Hypotension, arrhythmias
Cardiac glycosides	Digoxin	Lethargy, confusion

Based on: Cameron, KA: The role of medication modification in fall prevention. In National Council on Aging: *Falls Free: Promoting a National Falls Prevention Action Plan*. Research Review Papers, 2004, pp 29–39; table 1, p 33.
For more information: Leipzig, RM, Cumming, RG, and Tinetti, ME: Drugs and falls in older people: A systematic review and meta-analysis: I. Psychotropic drugs. *J Am Geriatr Soc* 47(1):30–39, 1999.
Leipzig, RM, Cumming, RG, and Tinetti, ME: Drugs and falls in older people: A systematic review and meta-analysis: II. Cardiac and analgesic drugs. *J Am Geriatr Soc* 47(1):40–50, 1999.
Hartikainen, S, Lönnroos, E, and Louhivuori, K: Medication as a risk factor for falls: Critical systematic review. *J Gerontol A Biol Sci Med Sci* 62(10):1172–1181, 2007.

Environmental Factors

Poor lighting
Slick or irregular floor surfaces
Cluttered environments
Furniture that is too low or too high
Unsafe stairways
Bathroom fixtures that are too low or too high or that do not have arm support
Incorrect size, type, or use of assistive devices
Poorly designed public spaces

Environmental Modifications to Reduce the Likelihood of Falls Among Older Persons

Bathroom

Bathtub: eliminate slippery surfaces by installing materials with a high coefficient of friction, install grab bars, eliminate unstable towel racks near the tub and shower
Toilet seat: raise seat if too low
Cabinets: check for adequate room lighting and safe distances required to reach objects
Medications: assure that there is correct and legible labeling of adequate size to be read

Stairs

Step heights: reduce to 6 in. or less if possible
Handrails: install rails if they are not present, and extend the rail beyond the top and bottom steps

Inclines: assure that all inclined surfaces are not too long to be managed by the person using them, and make certain there are places where someone can rest

Surfaces: install nonskid material on all steps

Lighting: assure proper lighting, including night lights and the use of color contrast materials at step edges

Kitchen

Cabinets: make cabinets at heights where persons do not have to reach excessively to access them

Floor: eliminate slippery surfaces including waxed surfaces that are slippery

Appliances: assure that there is correct and legible labeling of adequate size to be read for all controls

Tables: check the stability of table legs; assure that curved legs do not impede walking paths

Chairs: check for sturdiness and eliminate friction-free legs (rollers, etc.)

General Considerations

Rugs: eliminate frayed edges, curves, or materials that do not contrast with undersurface

Appliances: arrange electrical cords that could impede walkways

Chairs: provide chairs with arms for body support or assistance from sit-to-stand position; eliminate unstable furniture (tables and chairs)

Positioning: arrange furniture to minimize obstacles in major thoroughfares

Temperature: check temperature controls to assure a comfortable environment

GERI

Based on:

Tideiksaar, R: *Preventing falls: Home hazard checklist to help older patients protect themselves.* Geriatrics 41:26, 1986.

Beers, MH, and Berkow, R (eds): *Merck Manual of Geriatrics, ed. 3.* Merck Research Laboratories, Whitehouse Station, NJ, 2000, section 2, chapter 20, Falls (updated May 2005). Available from http://www.merck.com/mkgr/mmg/sec1/ch2/ch2a.jsp. Accessed July 20, 2009.

Tinetti, M: *Preventing falls in elderly persons.* N Engl J Med 348;1, 2003.

Instability and falls. In Kane, RL, Ouslander, JG, and Abrass, IB (eds): *Essentials of Clinical Geriatrics, ed. 6.* McGraw-Hill, New York, 2009.

Assessment and Management of Falls

Based on Fall Prevention Guidelines, the intensity of assessment should vary according to the target population (2001; Fig. 10.2). Low-risk seniors should be asked annually about falls as part of routine primary care health visits. All seniors who report a single fall should be observed performing the Get-Up-and-Go test. High-risk seniors—such as those with recurrent falls, living in a nursing home, prone to injurious falls or presenting after a fall—require a more comprehensive and detailed fall assessment, including fall circumstances.

Guidelines for the Prevention of Falls

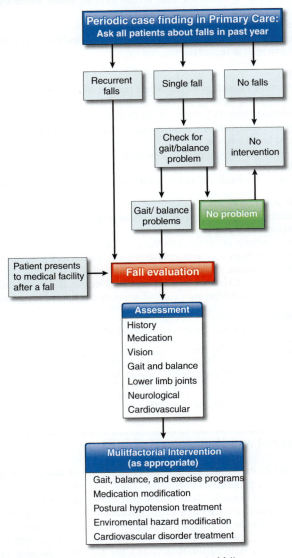

Algorithm summarizing the assessment and management of falls.

● TABLE 9.6 Recommended Clinical Assessment and Management of Fall Risk for Older Persons Living in the Community

Assessment and Risk Factor	Management
Circumstances of previous falls*	Changes in environment and activity to reduce the likelihood of recurrent falls
Medication use • High-risk medications (e.g., benzodiazepines, sleeping medications, neuroleptics, antidepressants, anticonvulsants, or class IA antiarrhythmics)*†‡ • Four or more medications‡	Review and reduction of medications
Vision* • Acuity <20/60 • Decreased depth perception • Decreased contrast sensitivity • Cataracts	Ample lighting without glare; avoidance of multifocal glasses while walking; referral to an ophthalmologist
Postural blood pressure (after ≥5 min in a supine position, immediately after standing, and 2 min after standing)‡ • ≥20 mm Hg (or ≥20%) drop in systolic pressure, with or without symptoms, either immediately or after 2 min of standing	Diagnosis and treatment of underlying cause, if possible; review and reduction of medications; modification of salt restriction; adequate hydration; compensatory strategies (e.g., elevation of head of bed, rising slowly, or dorsiflexion exercises); pressure stockings; pharmacologic therapy if the above strategies fail
Balance and gait†‡ • Patient's report or observation of unsteadiness • Impairment on brief assessment (e.g., the Get Up and Go test or performance-oriented assessment of mobility)	Diagnosis and treatment of underlying cause, if possible; reduction of medications that impair balance; environmental interventions; referral to physical therapist for assistive devices and for gait and progressive balance training
Targeted neurological examination • Impaired proprioception* • Impaired cognition* • Decreased muscle strength†‡	Diagnosis and treatment of underlying cause, if possible; increase in proprioceptive input (with an assistive device or appropriate footwear that encases the foot and has a low heel and thin sole); reduction of medications that impede cognition; awareness on the part of caregivers of cognitive deficits; reduction of environmental risk factors; referral to physical therapist for gait, balance, and strength training

GERI

(table continues on page 660)

TABLE 9.6 Recommended Clinical Assessment and Management of Fall Risk for Older Persons Living in the Community (continued)

Assessment and Risk Factor	Management
Targeted musculoskeletal examination • Examination of legs (joints and range of motion) and examination of feet*	Diagnosis and treatment of the underlying cause, if possible; referral to physical therapist for strength, range-of-motion, and gait and balance training and for assistive devices; use of appropriate footwear; referral to podiatrist
Targeted cardiovascular examination† • Syncope • Arrhythmia (if there is known cardiac disease, an abnormal electrocardiogram, and syncope)	Referral to cardiologist; carotid-sinus massage (in the case of syncope)
Home-hazard evaluation after hospital discharge†‡	Removal of loose rugs and use of night-lights, nonslip bathmats, and stair rails; other interventions as necessary

Based on: Tinetti, ME: From clinical practice. Preventing falls in elderly persons. *N Engl J Med* 348(1):42–49, 2003.
*Recommendation of this assessment is based on observational data that the finding is associated with an increased risk of falling.
†Recommendation of this assessment is based on one or more randomized controlled trials of a single intervention.
‡Recommendation of this assessment is based on one or more randomized controlled trials of a multifactorial intervention strategy that included this component.

Components of a Successful Fall Prevention Program

• *Education* about falls and fall risk factors
• *Exercises* that improve mobility, strength, and balance that are taught by trained personnel
• *Medication review* conducted by pharmacist or health-care providers to identify side effects or interactions that may contribute to falls
• *Vision exams* by optometrist or ophthalmologist
• *Home safety assessment* and home modification by occupational therapists or trained personnel

TABLE 9.7 Characteristics of Successful Fall Prevention Intervention Studies

Study	Focus	Providers	Structure	Total Contact Time
Barnet 2003	Balance, coordination, strength, reaction time, aerobic capacity	Certified exercise instructors	Group exercise classes	37 hr
Campbell 1997	Strength, balance, home exercises	Physical therapist or nurse	1:1 at home	4 hr
Clemson 2004	Fall prevention strategies, self-efficacy, behavior	Occupational therapist and trained experts	Small group classes + home visit	17 hr
Close 1999	Identify risk factors, referrals, recommendations	Physician and occupational therapist	1:1	1.75 hr
Cumming 1999	Home hazards	Occupational therapist	1:1	2 hr
Day 2002	Strength, balance, vision, home hazards	Certified exercise instructors	Group exercise classes	15 hr
Hornbrook 1994	Risky behaviors, physical fitness, home hazards	Trained personnel, physical therapist	Group exercise classes + home visit	7.5 hr
Li 2001,2002	Balance, physical performance	Experienced tai chi instructor	Group classes	78 hr
Lord 2003	Strength, coordination, balance, gait, ADL	Trained exercise instructors	Group exercise classes	96 hr

(table continues on page 662)

GERI

TABLE 9.7   Characteristics of Successful Fall Prevention Intervention Studies (continued)

Study	Focus	Providers	Structure	Total Contact Time
Nikolaus 2003	Home hazards	Team of nurses, physical therapists, occupational therapists, social worker, secretary	1:1	8 hr
Rubenstein 2000	Strength, endurance, mobility, balance	Trained exercise instructor or physical therapist	Group exercise classes	54 hr
Tinetti 1994	Fall risk factors	Primary care physician, physical therapist	Varied	Varied
Wagner 1994	Fall risk factors	Trained nurse-educator	1:1 home visit + behavioral intervention	Varied
Wolf 1996	Strength, balance, walking speed, physical functioning	Tai chi master	Group classes + home practice	12 hr

Based on: Stevens, JA, and Sogolow, ED: Preventing falls: What works. A CDC compendium of effective community-based interventions from around the world. National Center for Injury Prevention and Control. Atlanta, GA. 2008, pp 67–69. ADL = activities of daily living.

GERI

Geriatric Assessment

🔶 TABLE 9.8 Ten-Minute Screen for Geriatric Conditions

Problem	Screening Measure	Positive Screen
Vision	Ask this question: "Because of your eyesight, do you have trouble driving a car, watching television, reading or doing any of your daily activities?" If the patient answers "yes," test each eye with the Snellen eye chart while the patient wears corrective lenses (if applicable).	"Yes" to question and inability to read at greater than 20/40 on the Snellen eye chart
Hearing	Use an audioscope set at 40 dB. Test the patient's hearing using 1,000 and 2,000 Hz.	Inability to hear 1,000 or 2,000 Hz in both ears or inability to hear frequencies in either ear
Leg mobility	Time the patient after giving these directions: "Rise from the chair. Then walk 20 feet briskly, turn, walk back to the chair and sit down."	Unable to complete task in 15 sec
Urinary incontinence	Ask this question: "In the past year, have you ever lost your urine and gotten wet?" If the patient answers "yes," ask this question: "Have you lost urine on at least 6 separate days?"	"Yes" to both questions
Nutrition and weight loss	Ask this question: "Have you lost 10 pounds over the past 6 months without trying to do so?" If the patient answers "yes," weigh the patient.	"Yes" to the question or a weight of less than 45.5 kg (100 lb)
Memory	Three-item recall	Unable to remember all three items after 1 min
Depression	Ask this question: "Do you often feel sad or depressed?"	"Yes" to the question

(table continues on page 664)

GERI

🔵 TABLE 9.8 Ten-Minute Screen for Geriatric Conditions (continued)

Problem	Screening Measure	Positive Screen
Physical disability	Ask the patient these six questions: • "Are you able to do strenuous activities, like fast walking or bicycling?" • "Are you able to do heavy work around the house, like washing windows, walls, or floors?" • "Are you able to go shopping for groceries or clothes?" • "Are you able to get to places that are out of walking distance?" • "Are you able to bathe—sponge bath, tub bath, or shower?" • "Are you able to dress: put on a shirt, button and zip your clothes, or put on your shoes?"	"No" to any of the questions

Based on: Miller, KE, Zylstra, RG, and Standridge, JB: The geriatric patient: A systematic approach to maintaining health. *Am Fam Physician* 61(4):1089–1094, 2000.

GERI

Assessment of Mental Functions in Older Persons

Clinical Assessment

1. Appearance—poor grooming habits, inappropriate or unkempt clothing indicating neglect or difficulty with activities of daily living (ADL)
2. Cognition—mini-mental status exam (see below)
3. Mood—observation of posture, facial expressions, and speed of movements or expression of thoughts; noting any comments of helplessness, worthlessness, hopelessness, guilt, or shame; directly asking questions regarding mood, feelings, appetite, and/or sleep changes (see below for depression scales and clinical manifestations of depression.)
4. Anxiety disorders—inquire about any specific fears (phobias) that appear irrational with regard to places, people, or things; obsessive thoughts (recurrent thoughts, ideas) or compulsions (unwanted behaviors that are repeated). Ask, "Do you have thoughts that keep coming to your mind that are difficult to get rid of?" or "Do you feel you have to do certain tasks repeatedly, more than you might really need to?" Obsessions in the elderly may indicate depression.
5. Delusions/hallucinations—see Acute Confusional (delirium) States in Older Persons, below.

TABLE 9.9 Clinical Manifestations of Depression in Older Adults

Item	Symptoms
Mood	Depressed attitude, irritability, or anxiety (however, the patient may smile or deny subjective mood change and instead complain of pain or other somatic distress) Crying spells (however, the patient may complain of inability to cry or to experience emotions)
Associated psychological manifestations	Lack of self-confidence; low self-esteem; self-reproach Poor concentration and memory Reduction in gratification; loss of interest in usual activities; loss of attachments; social withdrawal Negative expectations; hopelessness; helplessness; increased dependency Recurrent thoughts of death Suicidal thoughts (rare, but serious when present)
Somatic manifestations	Psychomotor retardation; fatigue Agitation Anorexia and weight loss Insomnia
Psychotic manifestations	Delusions of worthlessness and sinfulness Delusions of ill health (nihilistic, somatic, or hypochondriacal) Delusions of poverty Depressive auditory, visual, and (rarely) olfactory hallucinations

Based on: Beers, MH, and Berkow, R (eds): *Merck Manual of Geriatrics,* ed. 3. Merck & Co, Whitehouse Station, NJ, 2000, section 4, chapter 33, Depression, table 33-3. http://www.merck.com/mkgr/mmg/tables/33t3.jsp. Accessed July 30, 2009.

Depression Scales Used for Geriatric Patients

Beck Depression Inventory: This test addresses 21 characteristics associated with depression, and each item is scored from 0 to 3. A score greater than 21 suggests depression.

Center of Epidemiologic Studies Depression Scale (CES-D): This test contains 20 items. For each item, respondents are asked to report the number of days that they have experienced symptoms during the previous week. Scores above 19 indicate the likelihood of depression.

General Health Questionnaire: This 60-item test is self-administered and is designed to detect mental distress. The scaled version contains 28 items that test four categories: somatic symptoms, anxiety and insomnia, social dysfunction, and depression. Scores of 4 or 5 are often seen as a cutoff, with higher scores indicating depression.

Geriatric Depression Scale: This questionnaire consists of 30 "yes" or "no" items. The test is scored by assigning a point for each answer matching the "yes" or "no" response assigned to it. Scores above 10 or 11 indicate depression.

Zung Self-Rating Depression Scale: This scale contains 20 statements rated by four possible levels of applicability to self, and each is scored on a 1 to 4 basis. The scale uses a Likert scale, with a total raw score of 80 possible. An index is generated by dividing the raw score by 80; therefore, a score of 1 is the maximum score. Eighty-eight percent of patients diagnosed as depressed from a psychiatric examination had a score of 0.50 or higher, and the same percentage of patients who were not depressed had scores of less than 0.50.

TABLE 9.10 Geriatric Depression Scale (short form)

1. Are you basically satisfied with your life?	Yes	No
2. Have you dropped many of your activities and interests?	Yes	No
3. Do you feel that your life is empty?	Yes	No
4. Do you often get bored?	Yes	No
5. Are you in good spirits most of the time?	Yes	No
6. Are you afraid that something bad is going to happen to you?	Yes	No
7. Do you feel happy most of the time?	Yes	No
8. Do you often feel helpless?	Yes	No
9. Do you prefer to stay at home rather than go out and do new things?	Yes	No
10. Do you feel you have more problems with memory than most?	Yes	No
11. Do you think it is wonderful to be alive now?	Yes	No
12. Do you feel pretty worthless the way you are now?	Yes	No
13. Do you feel full of energy?	Yes	No
14. Do you feel that your situation is hopeless?	Yes	No
15. Do you think that most people are better off than you are?	Yes	No

*Score:*____/15	One point for "No" to questions 1, 5, 7, 11, 13 One point for "Yes" to other questions	Normal 3±2 Mildly depressed 7±3 Very depressed 12±2

Based on: Beers, MH, and Berkow, R (eds): *Merck Manual of Geriatrics,* ed. 3. Merck & Co, Whitehouse Station, NJ, 2000, section 4, chapter 33, Depression, table 33-4. http://www.merck.com/mkgr/mmg/tables/33t3.jsp. Accessed July 30, 2009.
Adapted from: Sheikh, JI, and Yesavage, JA: Geriatric depression scale (GDS): Recent evidence and development of a shorter version. In Brink, TL (ed): *Clinical Gerontology: A Guide to Assessment and Intervention.* Haworth Press, 1986, Binghamton, NY, pp 165–173. By The Haworth Press, Inc.

GERI

Acute Confusional (delirium) States in Older Persons

- Delirium is very common among the elderly.
- Of general medical patients age 70 years or older admitted to the hospital, 10% to 20% are delirious at admission, and 10% to 20% become delirious during hospitalization.
- The incidence of postoperative delirium among patients age 70 and older is 15% to 25% after elective procedures and 35% to 65% after emergency procedures (e.g., hip fracture surgery).
- The hallmark of delirium is acute cognitive dysfunction with impaired attentiveness, which develops acutely.
- A patient with delirium has acute fluctuations in mental status, with varying levels of inattention and altered levels of consciousness.
- Risk factors include advanced old age, underlying dementia, functional impairment, and medical comorbidity and its treatments.
- Hospitalized patients with delirium are at 10 times greater risk for medical complications (including death), longer hospital stay, and increased need for discharge placement.
- Management of delirium includes treating underlying disorders, removing contributing factors, behavioral control, avoiding iatrogenic complications, and supporting patient and family.

Factors that can precipitate delirium (using the mnemonic DELIRIUM) are the following:

*D*rug use (especially when the drug is introduced or the dosage is adjusted)
*E*lectrolyte and physiological abnormalities (e.g., hyponatremia, hypoxemia)
*L*ack of drugs (withdrawal)
*I*nfection (especially urinary tract or respiratory infection)
*R*educed sensory input (e.g., blindness, deafness, darkness, change in surroundings)
*I*ntracranial problems (e.g., stroke, bleeding, meningitis, postictal state)
*U*rinary retention and fecal impaction
*M*yocardial problems (e.g., myocardial infarction, arrhythmia, heart failure)

🔶 TABLE 9.11 Selected Drugs That May Induce Delirium

Medication Class	Medications Included in Class
Sedative-Hypnotics*	
Benzodiazepines (especially long-acting)	Diazepam, flurazepam, chlordiazepoxide
Barbiturates (severe withdrawal syndrome)	
Chloral hydrate	
Alcohol	

(table continues on page 668)

● **TABLE 9.11 Selected Drugs That May Induce Delirium** (continued)

Medication Class	Medications Included in Class
Antidepressants (especially highly anticholinergic tertiary amines)	Amitriptyline, imipramine, doxepin
Anticholinergics	Diphenhydramine, oxybutynin, benztropine, atropine, scopolamine
Opioids	Meperidine
Antipsychotics (most likely with low-potency, highly anticholinergic drugs)	Clozapine
Anticonvulsants	Phenytoin
Antiparkinsonian drugs	Levodopa/carbidopa, bromocriptine, trihexyphenidyl, amantadine
H₂ blockers	Famotidine, cimetidine, ranitidine, nizatidine

Based on: Beers, MH, and Berkow, R (eds): *Merck Manual of Geriatrics*, ed. 3. Merck & Co, Whitehouse Station, NJ, 2000, section 5, chapter 39, Delirium, table 39-1. http://www.merck.com/mkgr/mmg/tables/39t1.jsp. Accessed August 7, 2009.
*Delirium may result from initiation or withdrawal.

● **TABLE 9.12 Comparison of Delirium and Dementia**

Delirium	Dementia
Sudden onset	Insidious onset
Precise time of onset	Uncertain time of onset
Usually reversible	Slowly progressive
Short duration (usually days to weeks)	Long duration (years)
Fluctuations (usually over minutes to hours)	Good days and bad days
Abnormal levels of consciousness	Normal level of consciousness
Typically, an association with drug use or withdrawal or with acute illness	Typically, no association with drug use or acute illness
Almost always worse at night (sundowning)	Often worse at night
Inattention	Attention not sustained
Variable disorientation	Disorientation to time and place

GERI

Delirium	Dementia
Typically slow, incoherent, and inappropriate language	Possible difficulty finding the right word
Impaired but variable recall	Memory loss, especially for recent events

Based on: Beers, MH, and Berkow, R (eds): *Merck Manual of Geriatrics,* ed. 3. Merck & Co, Whitehouse Station, NJ, 2000, section 5, chapter 39, Delirium, Table 39-2. http://www.merck.com/mkgr/mmg/tables/39t2.jsp. Accessed August 7, 2009.

Based on:

Beers, MH, and Berkow, R (eds): Merck Manual of Geriatrics, ed, 3. Merck Research Laboratories, Whitehouse Station, NJ, 2000, section 5, chapter 39, Delirium. http://www.merck.com/mkgr/mmg/ tables/39t2.jsp. Accessed August 7, 2009.

TABLE 9.13 Confusion Assessment Method*

Criteria	Evidence
Acute change in mental status	Observation by a family member, caregiver, or primary care physician
Symptoms that fluctuate over minutes or hours	Observation by nursing staff or other caregiver
Inattention	Patient history Poor digit recall, inability to recite the months backwards
Altered level of consciousness	Hyperalertness, drowsiness, stupor, or coma
Disorganized thinking	Rambling or incoherent speech

Based on: Beers, MH, and Berkow, R (eds): *Merck Manual of Geriatrics,* ed. 3. Merck & Co, Whitehouse Station, NJ, 2000, section 5, chapter 39, Delirium, table 39-4. http://www.merck.com/mkgr/mmg/tables/39t4.jsp. Accessed July 30, 2009.
*The first three criteria plus the fourth or fifth criterion must be present to confirm a diagnosis of delirium.

TABLE 9.14 Cognition

Elements Tested	Types of Items	Tested Instruments Used
Attention span/ concentration	Block designs	Evaluation Scale
Intelligence	Correct observed behaviors	Extended Dementia Scale
Learning ability	Math problems	Face-Hand Test

(table continues on page 670)

TABLE 9.14 Cognition (continued)

Elements Tested	Types of Items	Tested Instruments Used
Memory: distant	Puzzles or word problems	Geriatric Interpersonal Dementia Rating Scale
Memory: recent	Recall of distant news events	Memory and Information Test
Orientation	Recall of birth date	Mental Status Questionnaire
Perceptual ability	Recall of old personal events	Mini-Mental State Exam
Problem solving/ judgment	Recall of messages	Misplaced Objects Test
Psychomotor ability	Recall of time	PGC Mental Status
Social intactness	Recall of place Recall of recent events Recall of own name Simulated situations Vocabulary tests	Quick Test Set Test Short Portable MSQ VIRO Orientation Scale Visual Counting Test WAIS (complete or abridged) Wechsler Memory Scale

Based on: Kane, RA, and Kane, RL: *Assessing the Elderly: A Practical Guide to Measurement.* Lexington Books, Lexington, MA, 1981, pp 81–94.

TABLE 9.15 Affective Functioning

Elements Tested	Types of Items Tested	Instruments Used
Demoralization	Appetite disturbances	Affect Balance Scale
Depression, endogenous	Psychophysiological apathy	Beck Depression Inventory
Depression, reactive	Sadness	Hopkins Symptom Checklist
Suicidal risk	Sense of failure Sleep disturbances Suicidal thoughts Symptoms Tearfulness Withdrawal	Zung Self-Rating Depression Scale

GERI

Elements Tested	Types of Items Tested	Instruments Used
Affective impairment	Numerous items gathered through clinical observation, questionnaire, or projective testing	Emotional Problems Questionnaire
Cognitive mental health		Gerontological Apperception Test
Paranoia		London Psychogeriatric Rating Scale
Presence of psychopathology		Nurses Observation for Inpatient Evaluation
Substance abuse		OARS Mental Health Section Psychological Well-Being Interview Savage-Britton Index Screening Score of Psychiatric Symptoms Senior Apperception Test

Based on: Kane, RA, and Kane, RL: *Assessing the Elderly: A Practical Guide to Measurement.* Lexington Books, Lexington, MA, 1981, pp 81–94.

TABLE 9.16 Tests of Higher Cognitive Functions (by region of brain affected)

Lobe	Test (patient-required tasks)
Frontal	Points finger each time examiner makes fist and makes fist each time examiner points
Temporal	Dominant hemisphere: standard aphasia testing (spontaneous speech, repetition, comprehension, writing, and naming)
	Nondominant hemisphere: interprets effect of others (identifies behavior represented in photos of faces or interprets affect based on examiner's voice)
Parietal	Dominant hemisphere: names fingers, knows left from right, performs calculations using paper, reads Nondominant hemisphere: reproduces matchstick figure made by examiner
Occipital	Matches color and objects if unable to name them

Based on: Gallo, JJ, et al: *Handbook of Geriatric Assessment,* ed. 4. Jones and Bartlett, Sudbury, MA, 2006.

Mental Status Assessment Instruments Used for Geriatric Patients

Category Fluency: This test requires respondents to identify as many items as possible in each of four categories. The test is not timed, and there is a maximum of 10 items in each category for a total score of 40. Scores of less than 15 are abnormal, with 80% of demented elderly people scoring at this level.

Cognitive Capacity Screen: This test is designed to detect cognitive impairments in patients with medical illness. There are 30 questions with 1 point given per correct answer. A score less than 20 is usually associated with dementia or may be due to a low level of education. The test contains some unique questions designed to test abstraction.

Folstein Mini-Mental State Examination: This test of cognitive function has two parts. The first part assesses orientation, memory, and attention. The second part evaluates the patient's ability to name objects, follow verbal or written commands, and write a sentence. Maximum score is 30 points. Normal scores approximate 28. Individuals who score 9.7, 19, and 25 are patients with dementia, patients with depression with cognitive impairment, and patients with affective disorders, respectively.

Kokmen Short Test of Mental Status: This test examines intellectual tasks including abstract thinking. There are eight categories and a maximum score of 38 points. A score of 29 or less indicates that a patient is demented with a sensitivity of 95.5% and a specificity of 91.4% (Kokmen, E, Naessens, JM, and Offest, KA: A short test of mental status: Description and preliminary results. *Mayo Clin Proc* 62:281, 1987).

Mattis Dementia Rating Scale: This test has 144 tasks and is based on the presumption that if a respondent can answer the first question in a given section correctly, then subsequent questions in that section will also be answered correctly. Scores range from 0 to 144. Most individuals who do not have dementia will score greater than 85. Patients with dementia take 30 to 45 minutes to complete the test while older individuals who are not demented can complete it in 10 to 15 minutes.

Orientation-Memory-Concentration Test: Individuals are asked six questions. Each question is given a score based on the number of errors and a weighted factor. When the weighted score is 10 or more, the patient is mentally impaired. Normally older persons score 6 or less. The memory phase and counting backward questions are answered incorrectly by respondents who are developing dementia (Katzman, R, Braun, T, and Fuld, P: Validation of a short orientation-memory-concentration test of cognitive impairment. *Am J Psychiat* 140:734, 1983).

Short Portable Mental Status Questionnaire: This test has 10 questions addressing personal history, calculation, remote memory, and orientation. More than three errors suggest mental impairment. Accuracy of answers and education of the respondent must be considered. For example, verification of mother's maiden name must be ascertained.

GERI

Mini-Mental State Exam

	Score	Points		Score	Points

Orientation

What is the

Year?	_____	1
Season?	_____	1
Date?	_____	1
Day?	_____	1
Month?	_____	1

Where are we

Country/ Neighborhood?	_____	1
State?	_____	1
Town/city?	_____	1
Name/address of building?	_____	1
Floor?	_____	1

Registration

Name three objects, with 1-sec and pause between each. Give 1 point for each object the patient can name. Repeat the objects until the patient learns all three. Score for the first trial. _____ 3

Attention and Calculation

Ask the patient to subtract 7 from 100 and continue to subtract 7 from the remainder (i.e., serial 7's). Give 1 point for each correct answer. Stop after 5 answers. _____ 5

Recall

Ask the patient to name the three objects learned during registration. Give 1 point for each object the patient can name. _____ 3

Naming

Point to a pencil and a watch. Give 1 point for each object the patient can name. _____ 2

Repitition

Have the patient repeat, "No ifs, ands, or buts." _____ 1

Comprehension

Have the patient follow a three-stage command: "Take the paper in your right hand. Fold the paper in half. Put the paper on the floor." Give 1 point for each stage the patient can perform. _____ 1

Reading

Have the patient read and obey the following written command: "Close your eyes." _____ 1

Writing

Have the patient write a sentence of his or her choice. Give 1 point if the sentence contains a subject and an object and makes sense. Ignore spelling errors. _____ 1

Drawing

Enlarge the design printed below to 1 to 5 cm per side and have the patient copy it. Give 1 point if all the sides and angles are preserved and if the intersecting sides form a quadrangle. _____ 1

Total score _____ 30

Mini-Mental State Examination.

Sleep Patterns in Older Persons

Screening Questions

A long-standing National Institutes of Health Consensus Statement on sleep disorders in the elderly recommends that health-care practitioners ask the following questions during screening:

Is the person satisfied with his or her sleep?

Does sleep or fatigue intrude on activities?

Does the bed partner or other persons notice unusual behavior (e.g., snoring, interrupted breathing, leg movements) by the patient during sleep?

Definitions of Sleep Patterns in Older Persons

transient insomnia: Poor sleep over a few nights; may be caused by stress, work, or time zone changes.

short-term insomnia: Poor sleep over less than 1 month; may be related to acute medical or psychological conditions.

long-term insomnia:

problems falling asleep of over 1-month duration that may be related to anxiety, poor sleep habits, medical problems, medication-related sleep disorders, or changes in activity levels, or

frequent awakening that may be related to depression, medication-related sleep disorders, sleep apnea, medical problems, or changes in activity levels

GERI

Based on:

Beers, MH, and Berkow, R (eds): Merck Manual of Geriatrics, ed. 3. Merck Research Laboratories, Whitehouse Station, NJ, 2000, section 6, chapter 47 (updated March 2006). http://www.merck.com/mkgr/mmg/sec6/ch47/ch47a.jsp. Accessed July 30, 2009.

TABLE 9.17 Drugs That Disturb Sleep

Drug Class or Drug	Effect on Sleep
Alcohol	Evening or nighttime use may hasten initiation of sleep, but tends to disrupt sleep structure, reducing the time spent in REM sleep.
Anticholinesterase inhibitors	With evening or nighttime use, insomnia, disturbing dreams, or both may occur. In some patients, daytime use causes somnolence.
Antipsychotics	Akathisia may occur, sometimes disturbing sleep. Symptoms usually resolve when the drug is stopped.
Beta blockers	Use of beta blockers that cross the blood-brain barrier may cause nightmares. Sleep physiology is altered through CNS effects. Nocturnal dyspnea and wheezing may occur in patients with asthma or COPD.

Drug Class or Drug	Effect on Sleep
Caffeine	Use can delay initiation of sleep and cause nocturnal awakenings. This drug effect may last from about 4 hr to, in some people, much longer.
Carbidopa-levodopa	Nightmares may occur. However, inadequate treatment of Parkinson's disease may be more disruptive to sleep than carbidopa-levodopa.
Centrally acting alpha-agonist antihypertensives (e.g., clonidine, methyldopa)	Sleep physiology is altered through CNS effects.
Decongestants that contain stimulants (e.g., ephedrine, beta agonists, methylxanthines)	Nighttime use can delay initiation of sleep.
Diuretics	Nighttime use can produce nocturia, awakening patients.
H$_2$ blockers	Nocturnal delirium may occur in the elderly.
Reserpine	Insomnia and depression may occur. Sleep physiology is altered through CNS effects.
Sedative-hypnotics (e.g., benzodiazepines)	Stopping the drug may lead to rebound insomnia; tolerance (i.e., lack of effectiveness) occurs with prolonged use.
Sympathomimetic bronchodilators	CNS stimulation occurs, delaying initiation of sleep and causing nocturnal awakenings.

Based on: Beers, MH, and Berkow, R (eds): *Merck Manual of Geriatrics,* ed. 3. Merck & Co, Whitehouse Station, NJ, 2000, section 6, chapter 47 (updated March 2006). http://www.merck.com/mkgr/mmg/tables/47t1.jsp. Accessed July 30, 2009.
CNS = central nervous system; COPD = chronic obstructive pulmonary disease; H$_2$ = histamine-2; REM = rapid eye movement.

Malnutrition (protein-energy undernutrition) in Older Persons

Systemic Changes Contributing to Malnutrition (protein deficiency) in Older Persons

Circulatory: pedal edema, orthostatic hypotension, pressure sores
Musculoskeletal: fatigue, reduced muscle strength, hip fracture, lack of energy
Immunologic: reduced natural killer cell activity, decreased serum antibody response to antigens, infections, increased interactions between drugs
Other: altered thyroid function, weight changes

TABLE 9.18 Factors Contributing to Malnutrition (protein deficiency) in Older Adults

Addison's disease	Hyperthyroidism
Alcoholism	Late-life paranoia
Anorexia nervosa, anorexia tardive	Loneliness
Cancer	Malabsorption syndrome (e.g., late-onset celiac disease, pancreatic insufficiency)
Cholelithiasis	Mania
Chronic infection (e.g., tuberculosis, *Clostridium difficile* diarrhea, *Helicobacter pylori* infection)	Pheochromocytoma
Chronic obstructive pulmonary disease	Physical disability (e.g., tremors)
Dementia	Poverty
Dental problems	Stroke
Depression	Therapeutic diets
Difficulty shopping for or preparing food	Use of drugs (e.g., digoxin, theophylline)
Diminished sense of smell and taste	Withdrawal from drugs (e.g., anxiolytics and other psychoactive drugs)
Dysphagia	Xerostomia
Hypercalcemia	

Based on: Beers, MH, and Berkow, R (eds): *Merck Manual of Geriatrics,* ed. 3. Merck & Co, Whitehouse Station, NJ, 2000, section 8, chapter 61, Protein-energy undernutrition, table 61-2. http://www.merck.com/mkgr/mmg/tables/61t2.jsp. Accessed August 6, 2009.

TABLE 9.19 "Scales" Protocol For Evaluating Risk of Malnutrition in Older Adults*

Item Evaluated	Assign One Point	Assign Two Points
Sadness (as measured on the Geriatric Depression Scale—see p 666)	10–14	≥15
Cholesterol level	<160 mg/dL (<4.15 mmol/L)	—
Albumin level	3.5–4 g/dL	<3.5 g/dL
Loss of weight	1 kg (or 0.25 in., midarm circumference) in 1 mo	3 kg (or 0.5 in., midarm circumference) in 6 mo
Eating problems	Patient needs assistance	—
Shopping and food preparation problems	Patient needs assistance	—

Adapted from: Morley JE, and Miller DK: Malnutrition in the elderly. *Hosp Pract* 27(7):95–116, 1992.
Based on: Beers, MH, and Berkow, R (eds): *Merck Manual of Geriatrics,* ed. 3. Merck & Co, Whitehouse Station, NJ, 2000, section 8, chapter 61, Protein-energy undernutrition, table 61-3. http://www.merck.com/mkgr/mmg/tables/61t3.jsp. Accessed July 30, 2009.
*A total score ≥ 3 indicates that the patient is at risk of malnutrition.

Thermal Regulation in Older Persons

- The elderly are susceptible to hyperthermia and hypothermia even when they stay indoors.
- Many commonly used drugs predispose older adults to hyperthermia or hypothermia.
- Diabetes increases risk of hypothermia 6-fold in the elderly.
- Hyperthermia and hypothermia increase risk of death from serious comorbidities.

TABLE 9.20 Drugs That Increase Risk for Hyperthermia

Drug Effect	Drugs
Impaired sweating	Anticholinergic drugs Antidepressants Antihistamines Antiparkinsonian drugs Antipsychotics
Hypovolemia	Diuretics

(table continues on page 678)

● TABLE 9.20 Drugs That Increase Risk for Hyperthermia (continued)

Drug Effect	Drugs
Impaired cardiovascular responsiveness Increased metabolic rate	Beta blockers Amphetamines Sympathomimetic drugs
Impaired consciousness	Ethanol Opioids Sedative-hypnotics

Based on: Beers, MH, and Berkow, R (eds): *Merck Manual of Geriatrics,* ed. 3.
  Merck & Co, Whitehouse Station, NJ, 2000, section 8, chapter 67 (updated
  February 2006). http://www.merck.com/mkgr/mmg/tables/67t1.jsp. Accessed
  July 30, 2009.

● TABLE 9.21 Factors That Increase Risk for Hypothermia

Mechanism of Action	Disorder
Decreased heat production	Diabetic ketoacidosis Hypoglycemia Hypopituitarism Hypothyroidism Myxedema Undernutrition or starvation
Reduced activity	Arthritis Dementia Falls or other injuries Paralysis Parkinson's disease or parkinsonism Stroke Weakness, generalized (polyneuropathy)
Impaired thermoregulation	Carbon monoxide poisoning* Head trauma Neuropathy (e.g., due to alcoholism or diabetes) Polio Subarachnoid hemorrhage Subdural hematoma Stroke Tumor Uremia* Wernicke's encephalopathy

GERI

Mechanism of Action	Disorder
Increased heat loss	Arteriovenous shunt Dermatitis, inflammatory (e.g., exfoliation, ichthyosis, psoriasis) Paget's disease Reduction in subcutaneous fat Undernutrition Vasodilation due to alcohol or drug use

Based on: Beers, MH, and Berkow, R (eds): *Merck Manual of Geriatrics,* ed. 3.
Merck & Co, Whitehouse Station, NJ, 2000, section 8, chapter 67 (updated February 2006). http://www.merck.com/mkgr/mmg/tables/67t2.jsp. Accessed July 30, 2009.
*Affects the hypothalamus.

💧 **TABLE 9.22 Drugs That Can Predispose Patients to Hypothermia**

Alcohol
Antidepressants
Barbiturates
Benzodiazepines
Opioids
Phenothiazines
Reserpine

Based on: Beers, MH, and Berkow, R (eds): *Merck Manual of Geriatrics,* ed. 3.
Merck & Co, Whitehouse Station, NJ, 2000 (updated February 2006), section 8, chapter 67, Hyperthermia and hypothermia.

💧 **TABLE 9.23 Effect of Aging on Laboratory Values**

Increased	Decreased
Alkaline phosphatase	Calcium, serum
Cholesterol, serum	Creatinine kinase, serum
Clotting factors VII and VIII	Creatinine clearance*
Copper, serum	Dehydroepiandrosterone (DHEA)
Ferritin, serum	1,25-dihydroxycholecalciferol, serum
Fibrinogen, serum	Estrogen, serum
Glucose, serum (postprandial)	Growth hormone
Immunoreactive parathormone, serum	Insulin-like growth factor I (IGF-I)
Interleukin-6 (IL-6)	Interleukin-1 (IL-1)
Norepinephrine, serum	Iron, serum (minimally)
Parathyroid hormone	Phosphorus, serum
Prostate-specific antigen (PSA)	Selenium, serum
	Testosterone, serum

(table continues on page 680)

⬤ **TABLE 9.23** **Effect of Aging on Laboratory Values** (continued)

Increased	Decreased
Triglycerides, serum	Thiamine, serum
Uric acid, serum	γ-tocopherol (vitamin E), plasma
	Triiodothyronine (T_3)
	Vitamin B_6, serum
	Vitamin B_{12}, serum
	Vitamin C, plasma
	Zinc, serum

Based on: Beers, MH, and Berkow, R (eds): *Merck Manual of Geriatrics,* ed. 3. Merck & Co, Whitehouse Station, NJ, 2000, appendix 1, Laboratory values. http://www.merck.com/mkgr/mmg/appndxs/app1.jsp. Accessed July 30, 2009.
*Serum creatinine may be normal, even though creatinine clearance is decreased with age, because creatinine production decreases with age.

Measures of Physical Function for Use With Community-Dwelling Adults Over Age 65

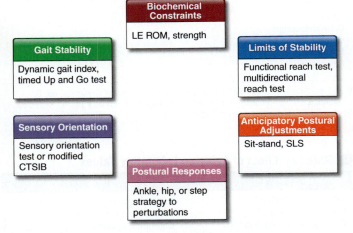

Model of systems underlying postural control and example of assessments.

A. Comprehensive physical performance
  1. Physical performance test
B. Self-report questionnaire
  1. Functional status questionnaire
  2. SF-36
  3. Sickness Impact Profile (SIP)
C. Mobility and balance—performance-based measures
  1. Berg balance scale
  2. Functional reach test

3. Gait speed
4. Dynamic gait index
5. Static balance measures (parallel, semi-tandem, tandem-stand)
6. Sensory organization test
7. Thirty-second chair stand test
8. Timed up and go—modified (TUG)
9. Walk while talk

D. Fitness for activity—performance-based measures
   1. Seated step test
   2. Six-minute walk test
E. Fitness for —self-report measures
   1. Physical Activity Scale for the Elderly (PASE)

Based on:

Hozak, FB, Wrisley, DM, and Frank, J: The Balance Evaluation Systems Test (BESTest) to differentiate balance deficits. Phys Ther 89(5):484–498, 2009.

Rikli, RE, and Jones, CJ. : Senior Fitness Test Manual. Human Kinetics, Champaign, IL, 2001.

Shumway-Cook, A, and Wollacott, M: Clinical management of the patient with a mobility disorder. In Shumway-Cook, A, and Wollacott, M: Motor Control. Theory and Practical Applications, ed. 2. Williams & Wilkins, Baltimore, 2001, pp 397–420.

VanSwearingen, JM, and Brach, JS: Making geriatric assessment work: Selecting useful measures. Phys Ther 81:1233–1252, 2001.

Physical Performance Test (PPT)

Description

Used to examine usual daily activities, including both basic activities of daily living (BADL) and instrumental activities of daily living (IADL). PPT is a performance-based global measure of physical performance. Developed and tested in the following populations: frail and well community-dwelling and institutionalized older adults. Used to describe and monitor physical performance, to screen for falls, and to predict the need for institutionalization and the likelihood of death. There are two versions of the PPT. The seven-item version consists of the following: writing a sentence, simulated eating, donning and doffing a jacket, turning 360 degrees while standing, lifting a book, picking up a penny from the floor, and walking 15.2 m (50 ft). The nine-item version includes two additional tasks of time: climbing a flight of stairs and number of flights climbed (four maximum). Time to administer the test is approximately 10 minutes.

EXAMINES

Physical performance of usual daily activities

Functional Status Questionnaire (FSQ)

Description

Used to examine physical, psychological, and social role functions in patients who are ambulatory. Self-report measure composed of six subscales that can be used individually or as a composite. Each subscale has score ranges indicating functional disabilities ("warning zones") to identify individuals with potential problems. Time to administer the test is approximately 15 minutes.

EXAMINES

Functional status

Gait Speed
Description
Examines the time required to walk a set distance. Often patient is instructed to walk at a self-selected speed that is calculated by dividing the distance traversed by the time from initiation to termination of the distance. An alternative measure is to instruct the patient to ambulate as fast as possible across a set distance. Walking speed is highly reliable so a single trial can be used. Distances range from 8 to 50 feet; moreover, walking speed has been found to be consistent for 8 versus 20 feet. Gait speed is a common measure to monitor mobility and screen for falls; therefore, extensive comparative data exist to determine clinical meaningfulness of specific findings. One method for identifying abnormal findings is to subtract two times the standard deviation (SD) from the mean.

EXAMINES
Mobility and balance

TABLE 9.24 Gait Speed Reference Values

	Men		Women	
Age	Mean (SD)	Mean −2 SD	Mean (SD)	Mean −2 SD
	Preferred Speed (ft/sec)			
60s	4.46 (.67)	3.11	4.25 (.70)	2.85
70s	4.36 (.64)	3.08	4.17 (.69)	2.79
	Maximum Speed (ft/sec)			
60s	6.34 (1.19)	3.95	5.82 (.83)	4.15
70s	6.82 (1.19)	4.44	5.74 (.92)	3.89

Based on: Bohannon, RW: Comfortable and maximum walking speed of adults aged 20–79 years: Reference values and determinants. *Age Ageing* 26(1):15–19, 1997.

Dynamic Gait Index (DGI)
Description
Used to examine ability to modify gait in response to changing task demands in community-dwelling older adults and identifying individuals who are at risk for falling. The eight items of the DGI include walking while changing speed and turning the head, walking over and around obstacles, and stair climbing. Scoring of the DGI is based on a 4-point scale from 0 to 3 with 0 indicating severe impairment and 3 indicating normal ability. A maximum total score of 24 is possible and scores of more than 19 indicate low risk for falling.

EXAMINES
Mobility and balance

Balance Measures (parallel, semi-tandem, tandem-stand)
Description
Examines the ability to stand with feet parallel, semi-tandem, and tandem. Common measure and various versions/combinations of the test exist. The length of time a patient is able to maintain balance is measured during different foot positions. FICSIT-3 static balance measure refers to a measure used in the Frailty and Injuries Cooperative Studies of Intervention Techniques trials and documents a patient's ability to maintain balance during parallel, semi-tandem, and tandem stances.

EXAMINES
Static standing balance

Sensory Organization Test
Description
Examines the way that vision, vestibular, and somatosensory systems interact to allow us to maintain our balance against the forces of gravity. This test identifies increases in postural sway associated with reducing visual or somatosensory cues for the control of standing balance.

EXAMINES
Sensory integration for static balance

GERI

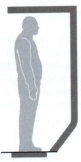
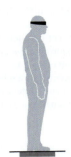
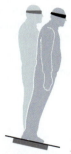
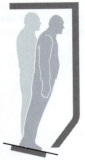
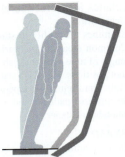
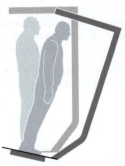

1. **Normal vision, fixed support**

2. **Absent vision, fixed support**

3. **Sway referenced vision, fixed support**

4. **Normal vision, sway referenced support**

6. **Absent vision, sway referenced support**

6. **Sway referenced vision and support**

Sensory Organization Test on Equitest device. Upper row—fixed surface support—and lower row—sway-referenced support—under conditions of normal vision (left column), no vision (center column), and sway-referenced vision (right column). These six tests provide information for assessing visual, somatosensory, and vestibular contributions to postural stability.

Thirty-Second Chair Stand Test
Description

Examines functional status, lower-extremity muscle force, and balance in older adults during the task of rising from a chair. The number of chair rises from a standard chair without upper extremity support during 30 seconds is counted. Published norms are available and are based on a nationwide sample of more than 7,000 older adults.

EXAMINES
Functional mobility

Modified Timed Up and Go
Description
Recent evidence suggests that an impaired ability to allocate attention to balance during dual-task situations may contribute significantly to falls in older adults. The TUG has been modified to assess the ability to divide attention while walking by including a cognitive condition (counting backwards by 3's) and a manual condition (carrying a cup of water) while walking as quickly as possible.

EXAMINES
Ability to divide attention while walking

Walk While Talk (WWT)
Description
The WWT consists of three conditions. The baseline condition involves walking at preferred speed without a cognitive task; the simple condition involves walking while reciting the alphabet and the complex condition involves walking while saying every other letter of the alphabet. The complex condition has been found to be highly predictive of future falls in community-dwelling older adults.

EXAMINES
Ability to divide attention while walking

Physical Activity Scale for the Elderly (PASE)
Description
Examines the physical activity level of older adults. The PASE is a self-report measure with three components measuring leisure and occupational and household activity. Can be self-administered, or an interview can be conducted (over the phone or in person).

EXAMINES
Fitness for activity

Formulation of Exercise Prescription for the Older Adult

Vital Signs by Age

TABLE 9.25 Variations in Normal Vital Signs by Age

Age	Average Value			
	Oral Temperature	Pulse	Respirations	Blood Pressure
Newborn	36.8°C (98.2°F) (axillary)	130	35	73/55
1 yr	36.8°C (98.2°F) (axillary)	120	30	90/55
5–8 yr	37.0°C (98.6°F)	100	20	95/57

(table continues on page 686)

GERI

⬤ TABLE 9.25 Variations in Normal Vital Signs by Age (continued)

Age	Oral Temperature	Pulse	Respirations	Blood Pressure
	Average Value			
10 yr	37.0°C (98.6°F)	70	20	102/62
Teen	37.0°C (98.6°F)	75	18	120/80
Adult	37.0°C (98.6°F)	80	16	120/80
Older adult (>70 yr)	36.0°C (96.8°F)	70	16	Increased diastolic

Based on: Kozer, B, et al: *Kozier & Erb's Techniques of Clinical Nursing: Basic to Intermediate Skills,* ed. 5. Pearson, Upper Saddle River, NJ, 2004, p 16.

⬤ TABLE 9.26 Target Heart Rate During Endurance Exercises by Age

Age	Target Heart Rate (beats/min)
40	126–153
50	119–145
60	112–136
70	105–128
80	98–119
90	91–111

Based on: Beers, MH, and Berkow, R (eds): *Merck Manual of Geriatrics,* ed. 3. Merck & Co, Whitehouse Station, NJ, 2000, section 3, chapter 31, Exercise, Table 31-5. http://www.merck.com/mkgr/mmg/tables/31t5.jsp. Accessed August 5, 2009.
*The target heart rate (60% to 79% of the maximal heart rate) is most useful when the maximal heart rate has been determined by an exercise stress test. The maximal heart rate, when predicted according to the patient's age alone, is not very accurate. Heart rate has a normal distribution; 95% of values occur within ±2 SD of the mean. In the elderly, 1 SD is about 17 beats/min. Thus, among 80-year-old patients with an average maximal heart rate of 150 beats/min, the maximal heart rate varies from 116 to 184 beats/min.

ACSM defines aerobic intensity differently for older and younger adults. Recommendations for younger adults are based on absolute terms (e.g., moderate intensity equals 3.0 to 6.0 MET activities). Recommendations for older adults are based on aerobic intensity relative to fitness level (e.g., walking may be moderate intensity for some and vigorous for others). A different definition of aerobic intensity is appropriate for older adults, because fitness levels can be low.

For resistance exercise for older adults, ACSM recommends performing 10 to 15 repetitions per set (as opposed to 8 to 12) to train the major muscle groups, and recommends exercise for each muscle group to occur on two or three nonconsecutive days each week.

Modified Perceived Rate of Exertion Scale

0	none	sitting
5–6	moderate	noticeable increase in heart rate and breathing; can talk, slightly breathless
7–8	vigorous	large increase in heart rate and breathing; cannot say more than a few words
10	all-out	

Recommended Physical Activity Guidelines for Older Adults

Aerobic
≥ 30 min or three bouts of ≥ 10 min
≥ 5 days/wk   **OR**
Moderate intensity
In addition to routine activities

* ≥ 20 min
* ≥ 3 days/wk
* Vigorous intensity

Strength
* 8–10 exercises of major muscle groups (legs, hips, back, abdomen, chest, shoulders, and arms).
* 10–15 repetitions
* ≥ 2 days/wk (nonconsecutive)
* Moderate to high intensity

Flexibility
* ≥ 10 min
* ≥ 2 days/wk
* Stretching to maintain or improve range of motion of major muscle groups or yoga

Balance (for those at risk for falls)
* Exercises to maintain balance (such as tai chi or individualized balance exercises)

Based on:

Nelson, ME, et al: Physical activity and public health in older adults: Recommendation from the American College of Sports Medicine and the American Heart Association. Med Sci Sports Exerc 39(8):1435–1445, 2007.

Exercise and the Immune System

The Aging Immune System
* Changes occur in both innate and adaptive immune systems.
* Older age is associated with thymic involution, decreased number of naïve T cells, and increased number of memory and effector T cells, with a reduction in T-cell repertoire.
* B-cell numbers decrease with aging. Immunoglobulin levels typically do not decline, but response to vaccine decreases with aging.
* In the innate immune system, overall numbers of natural killer (NK) cells increases; however, the function of these cells declines with aging. Aging is

GERI

often associated with chronic inflammatory state characterized by elevated levels of proinflammatory cytokines such as IL-6 and TNF-α.

- The clinical effects of immunosenescence are reflected in higher rates of malignancies, infections, and autoimmune diseases.
- Chronic inflammation itself is known to be a risk factor for vascular disease and malignancy.

Effect of Exercise on Immune Response in Older Adults

- Little evidence for acute or chronic changes in lymphocyte subsets, with the exception of CD8-positive T cells, that may be transiently elevated by acute exercise.
- No evidence that regular exercise alters phenotypic aspects of lymphocytes such as activation and/or costimulatory marker expression.
- Regular aerobic exercise may enhance cellular and humoral aspects of immunologic memory, at least in the context of influenza vaccination.
- Aerobic training, but not strength training, is associated with down-regulation of chronic inflammation and helps explain associations between exercise and reduced vascular disease.
- Aerobic training may also help prevent other diseases known to be triggered by chronic inflammation and associated with aging, such as autoimmune diseases and cancer.

Implications for Rehab Specialists

- Intense exercise (>80% of VO_2 max) is known to suppress immune function.
- It takes 6 to 24 hr for the immune system to recover from acute effects of intense exercise.
- Intense exercise during an infectious episode should be avoided by both young and elderly.
- If symptoms are located above the neck (e.g., stuffy nose or scratchy throat) exercise should be performed cautiously through the scheduled workout at half speed. If, after 10 min, the symptoms are alleviated, the workout can be finished with usual frequency, intensity, and duration. If symptoms are worse, exercise should be stopped and the person should rest.
- If there is fever or symptoms below the neck (e.g., aching muscles, cough or vomiting) exercise should not be initiated.

Based on:

Haaland, DA, et al: Is regular exercise a friend or foe of the aging immune system? A systematic review. Clin J Sport Med 18:539–548, 2008.
Kapasi, ZF, and Goodman, CC: The immune system. In, Goodman, CC, and Fuller, KS (eds): Pathology—Implications for the Physical Therapist. Saunders, Philadelphia, 2009, chapter 7, pp 241–297.

SECTION

WOMEN'S HEALTH

Clinical Anatomy of the Pelvis and Perineum

Pelvic Types

There are four basic pelvic types (see figure below), identified originally by Caldwell and Malloy in 1933, that have distinct shapes and therefore different effects on their suitability for childbirth. The average woman has a gynecoid pelvis; others may have a variation or mixture of types rather than pure android, anthropoid, or platypelloid types.

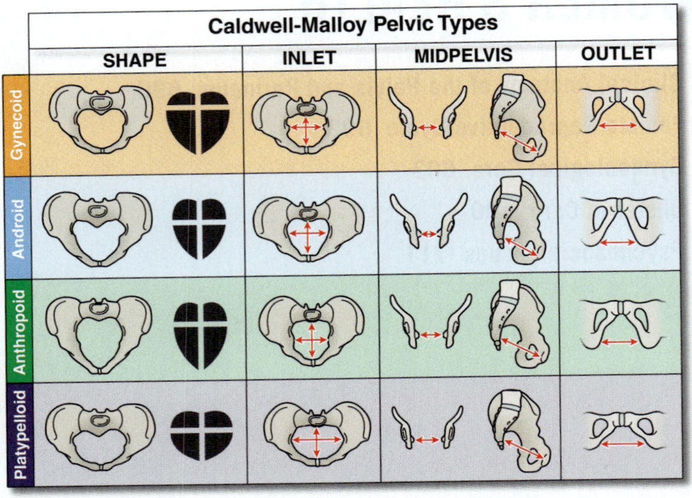

The four Caldwell-Malloy pelvic types. Differences in shape, inlet, midpelvis, and outlet dimensions are shown. *Adapted from: Ward, SL, and Hisley, SM: Maternal-Child Nursing Care. FA Davis, Philadelphia, 2009, p 123.*

For detailed anatomy of the pelvic girdle, refer to figures on pp. 691 and 692.

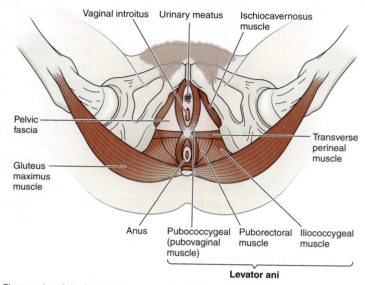

The muscles of the female pelvic floor. *Adapted from: Ward, SL, and Hisley, SM: Maternal-Child Nursing Care. FA Davis, Philadelphia, 2009, p 116.*

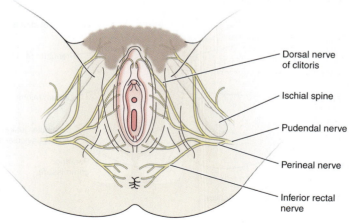

Innervation and arterial blood supply of perineum.

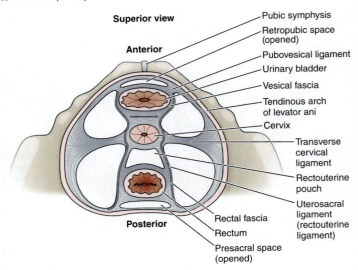

Ligaments and fascia of the perineum.

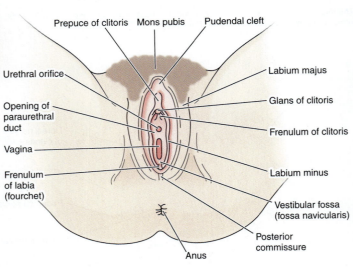

External female genetalia (vulva).

WOMEN

Female Reproductive Cycle

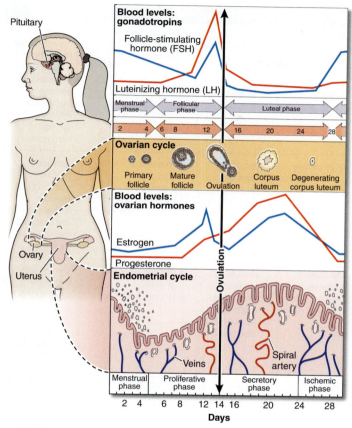

Levels of the hormones secreted from the anterior pituitary are shown relative to one another and throughout the cycle. Changes in the ovarian follicle are depicted. The relative thickness of the endometrium is also shown. *Adapted from: Ward, SL, and Hisley, SM: Maternal-Child Nursing Care. FA Davis, Philadelphia, 2009 p 126.*

Gynecological Care

Pelvic Floor Dysfunction (PFD)

The American Physical Therapy Association's (APTA's) Section on Women's Health (SOW) has defined pelvic floor dysfunction (PFD) based on common symptoms and functional presentation, as shown in Table 10.1.

WOMEN

⬤ **TABLE 10.1** **Types of Urinary Incontinence and Their Relation to Pelvic Floor Dysfunction**

Type	Description	Symptoms	Causes
Stress urinary incontinence (SUI)	Involuntary loss of urine with an increase in intra-abdominal pressure	• Loss of urine with cough, sneeze, or laughter	• Urethral hypermobility • Pelvic floor muscle weakness or damage • Decreased estrogen during menopause
Urge urinary incontinence (UUI)	Involuntary loss of urine in conjunc-tion with a strong de-sire to void	• Frequent urination • Nocturia • Urgency • Leaking when hearing water run • Changing body position (lying to sitting)	• Detrusor muscle instability • Bladder irritation from cystitis • Pelvic nerve damage
Overflow urinary incontinence (OUI)	Involuntary urine loss associated with overdis-tension of the bladder	• Chronic dribbling of urine • Urinary frequency	• Decreased detrusor contractility (e.g., from medication, diabetic neu-ropathy, other neurological disorders) • Overstretched detrusor muscle • Urethral obstruction
Mixed urinary incontinence (MUI)	Presence of both stress and urge incontinence	• Combined cues of stress and urge incontinence	• Combined mechanisms of stress and urge incontinence

Source: Irion, JM, and Irion. GL (eds): *Women's Health in Physical Therapy.* Lippincott Williams & Wilkins, Philadelphia, 2010.

Refer to pages 404–406 in Section IV, Neurology, for general information on urinary incontinence.

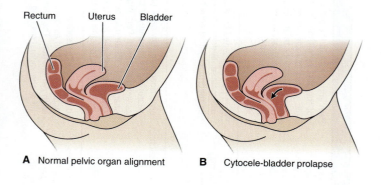

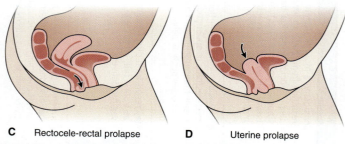

A Normal pelvic organ alignment

B Cytocele-bladder prolapse

C Rectocele-rectal prolapse

D Uterine prolapse

Normal (A) and three common types of pelvic organ proplapse (B–D). *Adapted from: Irion, JM, and Irion, GL (eds): Women's Health in Physical Therapy. Lippincott Williams & Wilkins, Philadelphia, 2010, p 119.*

WOMEN

TABLE 10.2 Pelvic Floor Pain Disorders

Disorder	Description	Causes	Symptoms
Pelvic floor muscle spasm (from levator ani syndrome, levator spasm syndrome, or pelvic floor tension myalgia)	Acute or chronic pain resulting from abnormally increased activity of the levator ani muscle complex.	Considered a musculoskeletal dysfunction resulting from spasm in levator ani muscles. Associated with low back pain, pelvic trauma, lumbar laminectomy, irritable bowel syndrome, hysterectomy, and poor posture.	Pain and spasm in the areas of the coccyx, piriformis muscle, gluteal muscle, lower back, and/or posterior thigh. May also result in constipation and painful elimination.
Incisional pain	Pelvic pain related to scar tissue and adhesions in and around the pelvic area.	Previous surgical interventions such as hysterectomy or appendectomy. Also may result from subclinical inflammatory processes such as pelvic inflammatory disease.	Pelvic pain worsened by sexual intercourse, sudden movement, or specific physical activities.
Coccydynia (coccygodynia)	Pain in and around the coccyx.	May result from direct trauma to coccyx, such as from a fall, arthritis, or as a result of vaginal delivery.	Pelvic floor pain, low back pain, sacroiliac or hip pain, or painful bowel movement. Pain may be sharp and radiate into buttocks. Often exacerbated by sitting for long periods, or stair climbing.
Dyspareunia	Recurrent or persistent pain during intercourse. Different sub-classifications depending on the occurrence of the symptoms	Numerous possible causes from dermatological disorders (e.g., vovaginitis or urethritis), insufficient vaginal lubrication, hypersensitivity from an episiotomy scar, atrophic	Burning, ripping, tearing, or aching sensation associated with penetration. The pain can be at the vaginal opening, deep

Disorder	Description	Causes	Symptoms
	(i.e., with or without a specific partner (situational vs. generalized), depth of penetration (entry vs. deep), or the episode (primary vs. secondary dyspareunia).	vaginitis, endometriosis, or psychological trauma (e.g., from past sexual abuse).	in the pelvis, or anywhere between. It may also be felt throughout the entire pelvic area and the sexual organs and may occur only with deep thrusting.
Vaginismus	Involuntary contraction or spasm of the perineal muscles resulting in painful, incomplete, or unachievable vaginal penetration.	Cause is rarely medical and often associated with a negative sexual experience or painful first pelvic examination.	May share some of the same symptoms as dyspareunia and pelvic floor muscle spasm.
Piriformis syndrome	Pain syndrome associated with the piriformis muscle, an external rotator of the hip.	Pain caused by a shortened, compressed, or spasmodic piriformis muscle. The bulk and close proximity of this muscle to the sciatic nerve are contributing factors to the presence of this syndrome.	Pain, numbness, and tingling in the low back, groin, perineum, buttock, hip, posterior thigh, or leg and foot. Symptoms typically aggravated by prolonged position of hip abduction and external rotation, such as during long periods of sitting or driving a car, or sexual intercourse.

Adapted from: Irion, JM, and Irion, GL (eds): *Women's Health in Physical Therapy.* Lippincott Williams & Wilkins, Philadelphia, 2010, pp 147–149.

WOMEN

WOMEN

TABLE 10.3 Pelvic Floor Assessment Methods

Type	Description	Use	Advantages Disadvantages
Digital palpation	The gloved and lubricated index finger of the examiner is introduced into the vagina (women) or the anus (women/men). Performed with the patient in the supine and standing position and at rest, and during contraction and relaxation.	Used to determine the muscle contraction capabilities of the pelvic floor musculature.	Simple, with minimal cost. Problem with quantification as there is no validated scale for the pelvic floor muscles. Therefore quantification of more than "absent," "weak," "normal," or "strong" is not recommended.
EMG Internal electrode	EMG sensor probe.	Able to detect muscle activity and therefore facilitates biofeedback traning with variety of visual and auditory output.	Direct contact with PFM.
Skin electrode	EMG sensors are placed on either side of the anal meatus and a second channel on hip adductor muscles.	As above.	Can be used in multiple body positions and is portable. More versatile and provides lower cost options than vaginal devices. Does not make direct contact with PFM muscles and is therefore a more indirect measure. Not a direct measure of muscle force.

Type	Description	Use	Advantages Disadvantages
Ultrasound	Probe is placed externally suprapubically, at the perineum or inserted into the vagina or rectum.	Evaluate musculature during contraction.	Noninvasive method.
Dynamometers	Probe is inserted in the vagina.	Evaluate musculature during contraction.	Only measures squeeze and not lift. Measurement may be affected by intra-abdominal pressure rises or contractions of other muscle groups such as the adductor or gluteal muscles.
Manometers	Pressure sensitive device placed in vagina.		Difficulty in locating device in same anatomical position. Only contractions with visible movement of device can be considered valid measurements of musculature.

EMG = electromyogram; PFM = pelvic floor muscle
Adapted from: Irion, JM, and Irion, GL (eds): *Women's Health in Physical Therapy.* Lippincott Williams & Wilkins, Philadelphia, 2010, pp 120–130; Bo, K, and Sherburn, M: Evaluation of female pelvic-floor muscle function and strength. *Phys Ther* 85:269–282, 2005; and Messelink B, et al: Standardisation of terminology of pelvic floor muscle function and dysfunction: Report from the Pelvic Floor Clinical Assessment Group of the International Continence Society. *Neurourol Neurodynamics* 23:374–380, 2005.

Obstetric Care

Pregnancy

Adaptations to Pregnancy

TABLE 10.4 Common Laboratory Values in Pregnancy

Laboratory Values	Usual Normal Female Value	Normal Value in Pregnancy
Serum Values Hemoglobin	11.7–15.5 g/dL (mean Hgb is 0.5–1.0 g lower in African Americans. Mexican and Asian Americans have a higher hemo-globin & hematocrit than do Cauasians)	Decreased by 1.5–2 g/dL Lowest point occurs at 30–34 wk
Hematocrit	38%–44%	Decreased by 4%–7%, lowest point at 30–34 wk
Leukocytes	$4.5–11.0 \times 10^3/mm^3$	Gradual increase of $3.5 \times 10^3/mm^3$
Platelets	$150–400 \times 10^3/mm^3$	Slight decrease
Amylase	30–110 U/L	Increased by 50%–100%
Chemistries Albumin	3.4–4.8 g/dL	Early decrease by 1 g/dL
Calcium (total)	8.2–10.2 mg/dL	Gradual decrease of 10%
Chloride	97–107 mEq/L	No significant change
Creatinine	0.5–1.1 mg/dL	Early decrease by 0.3 mg/dL
Fibrinogen	200–400 mg/dL	Progressive increase of 1–2 g/L
Glucose (fasting)	65–99 mg/dL	Gradual decrease of 10%
Potassium	3.5–5.0 mEq/L	Gradual decrease of 0.2–0.3 mEq/L

WOMEN

Laboratory Values	Usual Normal Female Value	Normal Value in Pregnancy
Protein (total)	6.0–8.0 g/dL	Early decrease of 1 g/dL then stable
Sodium	135–145 mEq/L	Early decrease of 2–4 mEq/L then stable
Urea nitrogen	8–20 mg/dL	Decrease in 1st trimester by 50%
Uric acid	2.3–6.6 mg/dL	First trimester decrease of 33%, rise at term
Urine Chemistries Creatinine	11–20 mg/kg per 24 hr	No significant change
Protein	10–140 mg per 24 hr	Up by 250–300 mg/day by the 20th week
Creatinine clearance	75–115 mL/min/ 1.73 m^2	Increased by 40%–50% by the 16th week
Serum Hormones Cortisol	8–21 g/dL	Increased by 20 g/dL
Prolactin	3.3–26.7 ng/mL	Gradual increase, 5.3–215.3 ng/mL, peaks at term
Thyroxine (T_4) total	5.5–11.0 mcg/dL	5.5–16.0 mcg/dL
Triiodothyronine (T_3) total	70–204 ng/dL	Early sustained increase of up to 50%, 116–247 ng/dL (last 4 mo of gestation)

From: Ward, SL, and Hisley, SM: *Maternal–Child Nursing Care.* FA Davis, Philadelphia, 2009, p 199, with permission.

Postural Changes in Sitting and Standing With Pregnancy

As pregnancy progresses, there is no consistent direction of postural change and postural responses are likely to be individual in nature. In sitting, some women show a progressive flattening of the lordosis, with a reversal postpartum, whereas others show no pattern or increase in the lordosis. In standing, some flatten the lumbar, thoracic, and cervical curvatures and others increase them. Anterior posture stability in standing decreases as pregnancy progresses. Altered standing posture may continue in early post-birth period.

References:
Gilleard, W, Crosbie, J, and Smith, R: *Static trunk posture in sitting and standing during pregnancy and early postbirth.* Arch Phys Med Rehabil 83:1739–1744, 2002.
Jang, J, Hsiao, KT, and Hsiao-Wecksler, ET: *Balance (perceived and actual) and preferred stance width during pregnancy.* Clin Biomechanics 23(4):468–476, 2008.

Separation of the Rectus Abdominus Pair in Pregnancy and Post-Birth

Separation of the rectus abdominus muscle into left and right halves, referred to as diastasis recti or abdominal separation, is common as pregnancy progresses. There is no consistent criterion for defining diastasis recti on the basis of the degree of separation, with values ranging from >1.5 cm to >2 finger widths used.

Post-birth, a significant reduction in the inter recti distance is seen by 4 weeks, although thickness of rectus abdominus is decreased. At 12 months, inter recti distance and muscle thickness are not fully resolved. The combination of reduced thickness and increased inter recti distance has implications for postnatal exercise and abdominal muscle function.

Biomechanics of Walking and Rising From a Chair in Pregnancy

Walking during pregnancy is generally similar to that in the nonpregnant female. As pregnancy progresses, differences include an increase in the width of the base of support, decreased pelvic and trunk rotations in the transverse plane, and a more anteriorly tilted pelvis, although the range of motion is unchanged.

Rising from a chair is altered as pregnancy progresses, with women using temporal-spatial, kinematic, and kinetic strategies to widen the base of support, minimize the propulsion, increase motion of the thoracic segment, and minimize anterior trunk-thigh apposition.

Physiological Adaptations to Pregnancy

Metabolic Adaptations of Pregnancy

↑ Resting metabolic rate
↑ Molecular fat storage
↑ Insulin sensitivity
↑ Carbohydrate utilization
↑ Requirement for calories to meet prenatal demand

Cardiovascular Adaptations of Pregnancy

↑ Blood volume
↑ Heart rate, stroke volume, and cardiac output
↓ Systemic vascular resistance
↓ Mean arterial pressure by 5 to 10 mm Hg by middle of second trimester, then returns to baseline

Respiratory Adaptations of Pregnancy

↑ Minute ventilation by almost 50%
↑ Oxygen uptake
↑ Baseline oxygen consumption by 10% to 20%

Thermoregulatory Adaptations of Pregnancy

↑ Heat produced by body, resulting from increased body weight and metabolic rate

↑ Body heat from added heat of fetoplacental unit
↓ Set point for normal body temperature
↓ Set point for sweating
↑ Dissipation of heat by:
  ↑ Blood vessel dilation
  ↑ Blood volume
  ↑ Respiration
  ↑ Blood flow to skin

Source:

Artal, R, and O'Toole, M: Guidelines of the American College of Obstetricians and Gynecologists for exercise during pregnancy and the post-partum period. Br J Sports Med 37:6–12, 2003.

Exercise and Pregnancy

ACOG Guidelines for Exercise During Uncomplicated Pregnancy and Postpartum

In January 2002, the American College of Obstetricians and Gynecologists (ACOG) published new recommendations and guidelines for exercise during pregnancy and the postpartum period,* which were reaffirmed in 2009. Uncomplicated pregnancy was no longer considered a condition for confinement, and regular exercise was promoted for its health benefits. The ACOG also published contraindications and warning signs that appear in this section.

The following general recommendations were made regarding exercise prescription, recreational activities, and competitive athletics.

Exercise Prescription

Type of Exercise
- No data to support the restriction of pregnant women from participating in aerobic activities, although some activities carry more risk than others.
- Exertion in supine activities has associated risks and should be avoided.
- Relatively low weights with multiple nonisometric repetitions are advised for resistive exercises.
- Water immersion exercise at an intensity of 60% max O_2 consumption was found to be a safe activity among pregnant women and advantageous.

Intensity of Exercise
- Pregnant women with no medical or obstetric complications can follow the same recommendations for exercise intensity as applied to nonpregnant women.
- Target heart rates should not be used to monitor exercise intensity due to the variability in maternal heart rate responses to exercise.

Duration of Exercise
- For prolonged exercises in excess of 45 minutes, attention must be paid to thermoregulation and energy balance.
- Accumulating the activity in shorter exercise periods (15-min periods) may obviate concerns related to thermoregulation and energy balance.

---

*ACOG Committee. Opinion no. 267: Exercise during pregnancy and the postpartum period. *Obstet Gynecol* 99:171–173, 2002.

WOMEN

Frequency of Exercise
- In the absence of medical or obstetric complications, pregnant women may follow the general guidelines of the CDC-ACSM to accumulate 30 minutes of exercise per day, in most, if not all, days of the week for health and general well-being.

Progression of Exercise
- Pregnant women with no medical or obstetric complications who have been sedentary before pregnancy should follow a gradual progression to achieve the recommended 30 minutes per day of exercise for general health and well-being.

Recreational Activities
- Scuba diving has associated risks and should be avoided.
- Activities that increase the risk of falls (skiing, gymnastics, horseback riding, vigorous racquet sports) or that increase stress to joints (tennis, jogging) should include cautionary advice and be evaluated on an individual basis.
- Activities with a high risk of abdominal injury or contact (ice hockey, soccer, basketball, rugby, etc.) should be avoided.

Competitive Athletics
- Same restrictions apply as faced by recreational athletes, described above.
- The relatively high-intensity, long-duration, and frequent workout schedules of most competitive athletes may place them at greater risk of thermoregulatory complications during pregnancy.

Exercise in the Postpartum Period
- Because many of the physiological and morphological changes of pregnancy persist for 4 to 6 weeks postpartum, prepregnancy exercise routines should be resumed gradually and should be individualized.
- No known maternal complications are associated with resumption of training.
- Nursing women should exercise after breastfeeding to avoid the discomfort of engorged breasts and to limit increased acidity of milk due to lactic acid buildup.

WOMEN

TABLE 10.5 ACOG Contraindications to Aerobic Exercise During Pregnancy and Postpartum

Absolute Contraindications	Relative Contraindications
Hemodynamically significant heart disease	Severe anaemia
Restrictive lung disease	Unevaluated maternal cardiac arrhythmia
Incompetent cervix/cerclage	Chronic bronchitis
Multiple gestation at risk for premature labor	Poorly controlled type 1 diabetes
Persistent second or third trimester bleeding	Extreme morbid obesity

Absolute Contraindications	Relative Contraindications
Placenta praevia after 26 wk gestation	Extreme underweight (body mass index <12)
Premature labor during the current pregnancy	History of extremely sedentary lifestyle
Ruptured membranes	Intrauterine growth restriction in current pregnancy
Pregnancy induced hypertension	Poorly controlled hypertension/ preeclampsia Orthopedic limitations Poorly controlled seizure disorder Poorly controlled thyroid disease Heavy smoker

Source: Artal, R, and O'Toole, M: Guidelines of the American College of Obstetricians and Gynecologists for exercise during pregnancy and the post-partum period. *Br J Sports Med 37*:6–12, 2003.

ACOG Warning Signs to Terminate Exercise While Pregnant

- Vaginal bleeding
- Dyspnea before exertion
- Dizziness
- Headache
- Chest pain
- Muscle weakness
- Calf pain or swelling (need to rule out thrombophlebitis)
- Preterm labor
- Decreased fetal movement
- Amniotic fluid leakage

Sources:

American College of Obstetrician and Gynecologists (ACOG) Committee on Obstetric Practive. ACOG's committee opinion: Exercise during pregnancy and the postpartum period. No. 267, January 2002.

Artal, R, and O'Toole, M: Guidelines of the American College of Obstetricians and Gynecologists for exercise during pregnancy and the post-partum period. Br J Sports Med 37:6–12, 2003.

Signs and Symptoms of Preterm Labor (PTL)

- Uterine contractions every 10 min or more often.
- Clear, pink or brownish fluid (water) leaking from the vagina.
- The feeling that the baby is pushing down.
- A low, dull backache that is unresponsive to changes in posture.
- Menstrual-like cramps.
- Cramps with or without diarrhea.

Source:

Association of Women's Health, Obstetric and Neonatal Nurses (AWHONN)—Lifelines Patient: Preventing premature birth. www.awhonn.org/awhonn/content.do?name=02_Practice Resources/2H_PatientHandouts.htm.

WOMEN

⬤ TABLE 10.6 Classification of Hypertensive Disorders During Pregnancy

Disorder	Characteristics
Chronic hypertension	• Hypertension that is present and observable before pregnancy or that is diagnosed before the 20th wk of gestation. • Hypertension that is diagnosed for the first time during pregnancy and that does not resolve postpartum.
Preeclampsia-eclampsia	• A pregnancy-specific syndrome usually occuring after 20th wk of gestation. • Gestational blood pressure elevation accompanied by proteinuria. • May include symptoms of headache, blurred vision, abdominal pain, low platelet counts, or abnormal liver enzymes. • Eclampsia is the occurrence of seizures in a woman diagnosed with preeclampsia.
Preeclampsia superimposed on chronic hypertension	• Preeclampsia occurring in a woman who is already hypertensive. • Hypertension and no proteinuria early in pregnancy (<20 wk); new-onset proteinuria. • Hypertension and proteinuria before 20 wk gestation. • Sudden increase in hypertension in woman whose hypertension was previously well controlled. • Thrombocytopenia.
Gestational hypertension	• Blood pressure elevation detected for the first time after midpregnancy, without proteinuria. • Includes women with preeclampsia who have not manifested proteinuria. • A term usually used during pregnancy until a more specific diagnosis can be made postpartum.

Sources: *Working Group Report on High Blood Pressure in Pregnancy.* National Institutes of Health, Bethseda, MD, NIH Publication No. 00-3029, July 2000. and National High Blood Pressure Education Working Group Report on High Blood Pressure in Pregnancy. *Am J Obstet Gynecol 183*:S1–S22, 2000.

Labor and Delivery

The three stages of labor are *labor, delivery,* and *afterbirth.* The human child in utero from 3 mo to birth is referred to as the *fetus.* The inability of the fetus to descend through the pelvis in a timely manner is referred to as *dystocia.* Dystocia is one of the major reasons for medical intervention during labor and delivery.

TABLE 10.7 Stages of Labor and Delivery

Stage	Definition	Physical Activity	Therapeutic Intervention
Stage 1—Prelabor	The early labor period, or *latent phase*. Characterized by the initiation of regular uterine contractions (up to 15 sec, spaced 10–30 min apart) with dilation of the cervix to 3 cm. Accompanied by bloody mucous vaginal discharge, spontaneous rupture of membranes, and/or complete cervical effacement.	Walking, relaxing in a tub, meeting with family/friends, preparing light meals.	Exercises to facilitate fetal engagement into the pelvis and rotating through the inlet. If TENS being considered for lower back and perineal pain, placement of electrodes and instruction can be initiated.
Stage 1—Active Labor	Stage of labor in which cervical dilation is greater than 3 cm and progressing to 8 cm with contractions lasting up to 45 sec. Contraction intervals 5–10 min apart. Initial progression 1 cm/hr for 2 hr. Progression from 4 cm to full dilation should occur over a maximal 12-hr period.	Walking and movement are encouraged if medically cleared.	Positioning techniques, effleurage massage, heat and cold applications, warm bath, and breathing instructions for comfort and relaxation. Knee-to-chest, quadraped position, and rocking exercises to encourage rotation of fetus. TENS treatment can be started; results are mixed but no evidence of adverse effects on mother or fetus.
Stage 1—Transition	Characterized by cervix dilating from 8 to 10 cm with contractions lasting 90 sec at intervals 1–2 min. Cervix moves anteriorly and retracts around the fetal head during last 1–2 cm of dilation to allow for descent into vaginal canal.	Discouragement of forced pushing, despite the spontaneous urge to do so in this stage.	Pain relief and/or relaxation modalities such as TENS, massage, heat, breathing exercises, and counterpressure over lumbar and sacral areas.

(table continues on page 708)

WOMEN

WOMEN

TABLE 10.7 Stages of Labor and Delivery (continued)

Stage	Definition	Physical Activity	Therapeutic Intervention
Stage 2—Delivery	Complete cervical dilation (10 cm) with spontaneous efforts by the mother to expel the baby, ending with birth.		Possible changes in position to enhance engagement of fetus and spontaneous pushing: Kneeling, squatting, dangle legs over side of bed, or leaning forward while sitting. Oxytocin may be administered if spontaneous pushing does not occur. Arrested labor may result in primary cesarean section.
Stage 3—Afterbirth	Final stage of labor in which placenta, amniotic sac, and umbilical cord are expelled. Discharge from the uterus of blood, mucous, and tissue is referred to as the *lochia*.		Medical intervention may be needed to control hemorrhaging.

Source: Irion, JM, and Irion, GL (eds): *Women's Health in Physical Therapy.* Lippincott Williams & Wilkins, Philadelphia, 2010, pp 294–298.
TENS = Transcutaneous Electrical Nerve stimulation

The Bishop Score

The most commonly used methodology to evaluate cervical ripening is the Bishop score because it is simple and has the most predictive value. This score uses cervical dilation, effacement, consistency, position, and the station of the presenting part. A Bishop score of 5 or more is considered significant for cervical ripening and favorable for induction of labor. Calculation of the Bishop score is described in Table 10.8.

TABLE 10.8 The Bishop Score

	Score			
	0	**1**	**2**	**3**
Dilation (cm)	0	1–2	3–4	5–6
Effacement (%)	0–30	40–50	60–70	80
Station (cm)	–3	–2	–1	+1 to +2
Cervical consistency	Firm	Medium	Soft	
Cervix position	Posterior	Midposition	Anterior	

Source: Rai, J, and Schreiber, JR: *Cervical Ripening.* e-Medicine, WebMD, updated August 2008. http://emedicine.medscape.com/article/263311-overview

Postpartum

The postpartum (or *puerperium*) is the period during which the uterus repairs itself and returns to normal size—approximately the first 3 mo after childbirth. This is the period during which the generative organs usually return to normal and most of the mother's physical recovery takes place. The following table summarizes the postpartum changes of the lochia (vaginal discharge), uterus, and perineum.

WOMEN

WOMEN

TABLE 10.9 Postpartum Changes of the Lochia, Uterus, and Perineum

Location	First Hours After Birth	First Week After Birth	Second Week After Birth	Third Week to Third Month after Birth
Lochia	• Placenta separates from the uterus and is expelled.	• Vaginal discharge as the uterus heals. • For the first 3 days, the lochial flow will look much like a menstrual period; may contain clots. • From days 3 to 10, lochial flow turns pink.	• Lochial flow is made up of a small amount of blood, mucus, and white blood cells. • The color is pink or brown-tinged and continues until about day 10. • After day 10, the flow should become white or pale yellow.	• White or pale yellow lochial flow lasting from 2 to 8 wk. • Should not contain any blood or clots and should not have an odor. • If breastfeeding, the menstrual period will usually start again 1 to 3 mo after weaning. • If not breastfeeding, the menstrual period can return anywhere from 1 to 4 mo after the birth.
Uterus	• Needs to shrink back to its normal size.	• Should shrink about one finger width a day. • Some women will notice "afterbirth pains" that feel like menstrual cramps.	• By end of the second week, should no longer be able to feel the top of the uterus through the belly. • The "afterbirth pains" should cease.	• Should return close to its prepregnant size by the sixth week.
Perineum	• This area is often swollen and may have torn or undergone a surgical incision (episiotomy).	• Will probably still be swollen, and it may be uncomfortable for the first week.	• Swelling should be mostly gone by the end of the second week. • The area may still be uncomfortable if there was an episiotomy.	• If there is an episiotomy wound, it should heal by the end of the third week.

Source: Association of Women's Health, Obstetric and Neonatal Nurses (AWHONN): *Postpartum Changes: Taking Care of Yourself.* http://www.awhonn.org/awhonn/

Postpartum Warning Signs

The patient is advised to contact her health-care provider if any of the following symptoms appear:

- Fever higher than 100.4°F (38°C)
- Sharp pains in the abdomen, breast, or chest
- Blurred vision or dizziness
- Headache that does not go away
- Severe pain or burning sensation in the legs (this pain could be a sign of phlebitis)
- Foul smell or an unexpected change in the lochia; should not see bright-red bleeding or clots after the first postpartum week
- Localized swelling or tenderness in the breasts
- Burning or urgency upon urination; being unable to urinate
- Crying spells or mood swings that feel out of control
- Thoughts of harming oneself or the baby

Source:

Association of Women's Health, Obstetric and Neonatal Nurses (AWHONN): Postpartum Changes: Taking Care of Yourself. http://www.awhonn.org/awhonn/content.do?name=02_ PracticeResources/2H_PatientHandouts.htm.

Psychosocial Issues

Domestic Violence

Domestic violence encompasses physical, sexual, and psychological abuse, as well as social and economic intimidation and/or deprivation. Up to 23% of pregnant women in the United States seeking prenatal care are reported to be victims of domestic violence. Domestic violence is one of the most frequent causes of injury to women and crosses all racial, ethnic, socioeconomic, and age categories. Women between the ages of 17 and 28 years are at the greatest risk, followed by aging or disabled women. Warning signs that may alert the therapist to domestic violence, as well as the legal and ethical reporting requirements, are summarized below.

Reference:

Toomey, TC, et al: Relationship of sexual and physical abuse to pain description, coping, psychological distress, and health-care utilization in a chronic pain sample. Clin J Pain 11: 307–315, 1995.

Legal and Ethical Reporting Requirements for Domestic Violence

Physical therapists, occupational therapists, and other allied health professionals may be mandated to report suspected domestic violence. The law varies by state and the age and independent status of the person in question. Legal reporting requirements may not be stated explicitly in specific practice acts, but instead may appear in other laws, rules, or regulations. Allied health professionals are responsible for familiarizing themselves with the warning signs (see below) and reporting requirements in their state.

TABLE 10.10 Warning Signs of Domestic Violence

Domestic Abuse	Physical Violence	Isolation
Seems afraid or anxious to please partner.	Frequent injuries, with the excuse of "accidents."	Restricted from seeing family and friends.
Goes along with everything partner says and does.	Frequently misses work, school, or social occasions, without explanation.	Rarely goes out in public without their partner.
Checks in often with partner to report where she is and what she's doing.	Dresses in clothing designed to hide bruises or scars.	Has limited access to money, credit cards, or the car.
Receives frequent, harassing phone calls from partner.		
Talks about partner's temper, jealousy, or possessiveness.		
Very low self-esteem.		
Shows major personality changes.		
Depressed, anxious, or suicidal.		

Source: Domestic violence and abuse: Signs of abuse and abusive relationships. http://www.helpguide.org/mental/domestic_violence_abuse_types_signs_causes_effects.htm#warning

Postpartum Depression (PPD)

Postpartum depression (PPD) is defined by the American Psychiatric Association as a "non-psychotic depressive episode that begins in the postpartum period, includes at least two weeks of depressed mood or loss of interest in almost all activities, and at least four of the following symptoms: changes in appetite or weight, sleep, and psychomotor activity; decreased energy; feelings of worthlessness or guilt; difficulty thinking, concentrating, or making decisions; or recurrent thoughts of death or suicidal ideation, plans or attempts." PPD is classified as one of several postpartum mood disorders that include postpartum psychosis, bipolar II disorder, and the postpartum depression impostor. Although postpartum depression usually appears in the first 3 months' postpartum, it can occur any time during the first 12 months after delivery. Incidence rates for major and minor postpartum depression combined are estimated at up to 14.5%. The causes of PPD are complex and unknown. Contributing factors are listed below.

Reference:

American Psychiatric Association: Diagnostic and statistical manual of mental disorders, DSM-IV, ed. 4. American Psyciatric Association, Arlington, VA, 2000.

Contributing Factors for Postpartum Depression

- A steep and rapid drop of hormone levels after childbirth
- Feeling overwhelmed about one's new role as a mother
- Lack of support
- Marital strife
- Financial problems
- Physical or mental abuse
- Previous history of depression or anxiety

Source:

Beck, CT: AWHONN Symposium: Postpartum Mood and Anxiety Disorders: Case Studies, Research and Nursing Care. Washington, DC, 2008. http://www.awhonn.org/awhonn/content.do? name=02_PracticeResources/2H_PatientHandouts.htm.

WOMEN

ONCOLOGY

Introduction

Rehabilitation examination and intervention at the initiation of cancer treatment planning are becoming standards of cancer care. Specific education and attention by the rehabilitation therapist throughout the continuum of cancer prevention, treatment, survivorship, and palliative care are essential to effectively address the multitude of complex rehabilitative needs. An understanding of cancer epidemiology and co-morbid conditions leads to better comprehension of the prognosis for long-term survival, thus providing a framework to develop local and regional oncology-specific exercise promotion programs including the areas of cancer prevention, rehabilitation, palliative care, and hospice.

Epidemiology

Incidence

- As of 2012, slightly more than one out of three women and slightly less than one out of two men in the United States will develop cancer.
- According to the American Cancer Society, there are currently almost 12 million cancer survivors.
- Rapidly evolving diagnostic and treatment methods change the trend of cancer incidence, prevalence, and mortality.
- The online resources of the American Cancer Society provide a key source of up-to-date information on new cancer diagnosis, survival and mortality rates, as well as data ranked by state and global cancer trends.

Modifiable Risk Factors for Cancer Prevention

- Tobacco
- Obesity, lack of exercise, poor nutrition
- Ultraviolet radiation

ONCOL

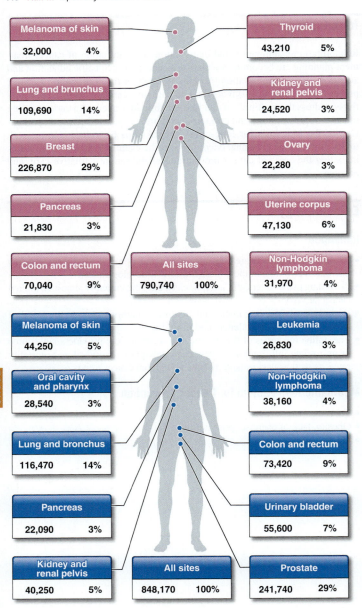

Melanoma of skin	
32,000	4%

Thyroid	
43,210	5%

Lung and brunchus	
109,690	14%

Kidney and renal pelvis	
24,520	3%

Breast	
226,870	29%

Ovary	
22,280	3%

Pancreas	
21,830	3%

Uterine corpus	
47,130	6%

Colon and rectum	
70,040	9%

All sites	
790,740	100%

Non-Hodgkin lymphoma	
31,970	4%

Melanoma of skin	
44,250	5%

Leukemia	
26,830	3%

Oral cavity and pharynx	
28,540	3%

Non-Hodgkin lymphoma	
38,160	4%

Lung and bronchus	
116,470	14%

Colon and rectum	
73,420	9%

Pancreas	
22,090	3%

Urinary bladder	
55,600	7%

Kidney and renal pelvis	
40,250	5%

All sites	
848,170	100%

Prostate	
241,740	29%

Ten leading cancer types for estimated new cancer cases by sex, United States, 2009.
Data from: Siegel, R, et al: Cancer statistics. *CA: A Cancer Journal for Clinicians,*
62:10–29. 2012.

Mortality

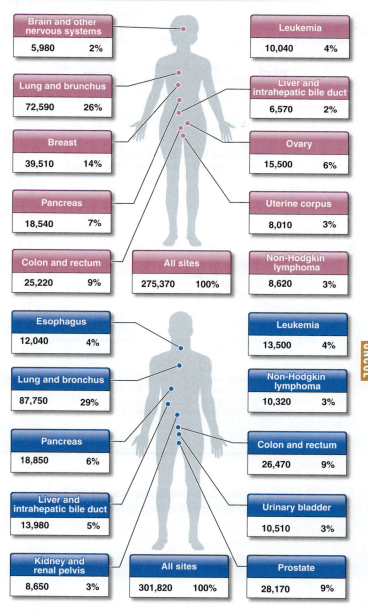

Brain and other nervous systems	
5,980	2%

Leukemia	
10,040	4%

Lung and brunchus	
72,590	26%

Liver and intrahepatic bile duct	
6,570	2%

Breast	
39,510	14%

Ovary	
15,500	6%

Pancreas	
18,540	7%

Uterine corpus	
8,010	3%

Colon and rectum	
25,220	9%

All sites	
275,370	100%

Non-Hodgkin lymphoma	
8,620	3%

Esophagus	
12,040	4%

Leukemia	
13,500	4%

Lung and bronchus	
87,750	29%

Non-Hodgkin lymphoma	
10,320	3%

Pancreas	
18,850	6%

Colon and rectum	
26,470	9%

Liver and intrahepatic bile duct	
13,980	5%

Urinary bladder	
10,510	3%

Kidney and renal pelvis	
8,650	3%

All sites	
301,820	100%

Prostate	
28,170	9%

ONCOL

Ten leading cancer types for estimated cancer deaths by sex, United States, 2009.
Data from: Siegel, R, et al: Cancer statistics. *CA: A Cancer Journal for Clinicians,*
62:10–29. 2012.

Survivorship

- Generally defined from the moment of cancer diagnosis.
- Many survivors have complex medical needs secondary to multiple co-morbidities in combination from the primary cancer, prior cancer treatments, and resultant sequelae after those treatments.
  - Often results in multisystem impairments with activity limitations.
  - Early and late side effects such as cancer-related fatigue and lymphedema may cause significant morbidity and should be promptly addressed in a holistic manner.
- Five-year survival rates for men and women of all ages are 67%.

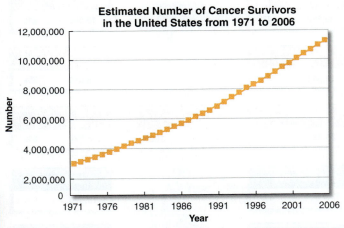

Estimated number of cancer survivors in the United States from 1971 to 2006. Based on data from: Horner, MJ, et al (eds): *SEER Cancer Statistics Review, 1975–2006, National Cancer Institute.* Bethesda, MD, http://seer.cancer.gov/csr/1975_2006/, based on November 2008 SEER data submission, posted to the SEER website, 2009. Accessed May 1, 2010.

Screening

American Cancer Society Screening Guidelines for the Early Detection of Cancer in Average-Risk Asymptomatic People

Individuals with a personal or family history or other risk factors should follow recommendations for individuals at increased risk.

Breast

- Breast self-examination (BSE) is an option for women starting around age 20 and women should discuss benefit/limitations of BSE with their provider.
- Clinical breast examination at least every 3 years for women in their 20s and 30s; annually for asymptomatic women age 40 and older.
- Annual mammography for women starting at age 40.

Colorectal

Men and women age 50 and older, any of the following options:

- Annual fecal occult blood test
- Annual fecal immunochemical test
- Stool DNA test (interval uncertain)
- Flexible sigmoidoscopy every 5 years
- Double-contrast barium enema every 5 years
- Colonoscopy every 10 years
- CT colonography every 5 years

Prostate

- Beginning at age 50, men who have at least a 10-year life expectancy should discuss the potential benefits and limitations of prostate cancer screening (prostate-specific antigen [PSA] blood test and the digital rectal examination) with their doctor.

Cervical

- Cervical cancer screening should begin about 3 years after vaginal intercourse begins, but no later than 21 years of age. Screening should be done annually with a conventional Pap test or every 2 years using a liquid-based Pap test.
- At or after age 30, women who have had three normal Pap test results in a row may be screened every 2 to 3 years with either Pap test alone, or every 3 years with an HPV DNA test plus a Pap test.
- Women 70 years of age or older who have had three or more normal Pap tests and no abnormal Pap tests in the past 10 years, or women who have had a total hysterectomy, may choose to stop cervical cancer screening.

Endometrial (uterine)

- At the time of menopause, all women at average risk should be informed about the risks and symptoms of endometrial cancer and report any unexpected bleeding or spotting to their doctors.

Cancer-Related Check-Up

- People age 20 or older should have a cancer-related check-up to include health counseling regarding risk factors and examinations for cancers of the thyroid, testicles, ovaries, lymph nodes, oral cavity, and skin during periodic health examinations.

Cancer Diagnosis

Hematological Cancers

Hematological cancers arise from blood and bone marrow and are characterized by immature and abnormal blood cells crowding out healthy cells, leading to anemia, infection, or bleeding. Hematological cancers (such as Hodgkin's and non-Hodgkin's lymphoma, leukemia, and myeloma) are diagnosed and staged by blood and bone marrow testing. These tests, and ultimately staging, vary depending on cancer type and phase (e.g., chronic myelogenous leukemia leading to chronic, accelerated, or blast phases).

Solid Tumors

Tumor Identification

A number of diagnostic tests are available to determine the cell of origin and thus the cancer type. This is important as the cell of origin (which is usually identifiable, e.g., rhabdomyosarcoma) thus determines the course of treatment.

TNM Cancer Staging (tumor, node, metastasis)

The T describes the primary tumor.

TX Primary tumor cannot be evaluated.
T0 No evidence of primary tumor.
Tis Carcinoma in situ (early cancer that has not spread to neighboring tissue).
T1–T4 Size and/or extent of the primary tumor.

ONCOL

The N describes cancer spread to lymph nodes.

NX Regional lymph nodes cannot be evaluated.
N0 No regional lymph node involvement (no cancer found in the lymph nodes).
N1–N3 Involvement of regional lymph nodes (number and/or extent of spread).

The M describes distant metastatic spread.

MX Distant metastasis cannot be evaluated.
M0 No distant metastasis (cancer has not spread to other parts of the body).
M1 Distant metastasis (cancer has spread to distant parts of the body).

- For example, a T1N2M0 cancer is a cancer with a T1 tumor, N2 involvement of the lymph nodes, and no metastasis.
- The original stage at time of diagnosis remains with the patient, even if the disease recurs or spreads later on (e.g., stage II breast cancer with metastasis to liver and bone).

Cancer Grading

- Surgical biopsy
- Pathologist review:
  - Surgical margins achieved (negative or positive—which determines the need for further resection)
  - Establishes if a tumor is benign or malignant

Tumor grading classifies the abnormality and thus aggressiveness of the cancer cells.

This provides information to predict patient prognosis and thus grading is one important aspect the oncologist uses to determine the appropriate course of treatment. The American Joint Commission on Cancer (AJCC) recommends the following grading system, and then each cancer type *has its own* further grading system. In general, grade 1 tumors resemble normal cells, are slower growing and are not as aggressive as a grade 3 or 4 tumor; a lower grade such as grade 1 has a better prognosis.

TABLE 11.1 AJCC Grading System

Grade	Differentiation	Assessment
GX	Grade cannot be assessed	Undetermined grade
G1	Well differentiated	Low grade
G2	Moderately differentiated	Intermediate grade
G3	Poorly differentiated	High grade
G4	Undifferentiated	High grade

For more information: American Joint Committee on Cancer: *AJCC Cancer Staging Manual*, ed. 7. Springer, New York, 2010.

Medical Management

Cancer treatment options may be the primary or secondary mode of treatment, and may be used for primary disease control or palliation (i.e., radiation for pain relief). Each option has its own specific side effects (beyond the malignancy effects on function), all of which can cause significant impairment and functional limitation. These options include the following:

- Surgery
- Chemotherapy
- Radiation
- Hormone therapy
- Immunotherapy (including monoclonal antibodies)

ONCOL

The following tables are examples of common oncological treatments with coinciding rehabilitation implications (not all inclusive) to provide appropriate red flags for safe intervention.

● TABLE 11.2 Surgery: Rehabilitation Implications

Mode	Potential Side Effects Affecting Rehabilitation
Side effects from treatment can be dose limiting or may cause the oncologist to change medical course of action; therefore, feedback by the rehabilitation therapist as part of the medical team is imperative. Note: This list is not all inclusive.	
Wide local excision	Musculoskeletal, scar tissue adhesion, local edema, pain
En-bloc resection	Loss of organ function, scar tissue adhesion, local edema, pain
Lymph node resection	Lymphedema, cellulitis risk, lymphatic cording
Amputation	Musculoskeletal, gait, phantom sensation/pain, scar tissue adhesion, local edema
Joint replacement	Musculoskeletal, range of motion, gait, scar tissue adhesion, local edema, pain
Joint fusion	Musculoskeletal, range of motion, gait, posture, psychological
Skin grafting	Donor site weakness, graft failure, wounds, scar tissue adhesion, local edema, pain, psychological
Reconstruction	Donor site weakness, wounds, scar tissue adhesion, local edema, pain, posture, psychological

● TABLE 11.3 Chemotherapy: Rehabilitation Implications

Common Agents	Potential Side Effects Affecting Rehabilitation
Side effects from treatment can be dose limiting or may cause the oncologist to change medical course of action; therefore, feedback by the rehabilitation therapist as part of the medical team is imperative. Note: This list is not all inclusive.	
Doxorubicin	Bone marrow suppression, cardiac toxicity (arrhythmia and/or congestive heart failure), peripheral edema, radiation recall
Busulfan	Bone marrow suppression, pulmonary and hepatic toxicity, fatigue, seizure, adrenal insufficiency, weakness, dizziness

ONCOL

Common Agents	Potential Side Effects Affecting Rehabilitation
Cyclophosphamide	Bone marrow suppression, cardiac toxicity, hemorrhagic cystitis, fatigue
Etoposide	Bone marrow suppression, hypotension, peripheral neuropathy, fatigue, unilateral edema or pain, radiation recall
Fludarabine	Bone marrow suppression, peripheral edema, tumor lysis syndrome, fatigue, central neurotoxicity, Stevens-Johnson syndrome, gastrointestinal bleeds, severe pulmonary toxicity, cardiac toxicity
Hydroxyurea	Bone marrow suppression, fatigue, radiation recall
Ifosfamide	Bone marrow suppression, hemorrhagic cystitis, central neurotoxicity
Methotrexate	Bone marrow suppression, renal toxicity, central neurotoxicity, acute chemical arachnoiditis, radiation recall
Paclitaxel	Bone marrow suppression, cardiac toxicity, peripheral neuropathy, arthralgia, myalgia, lower extremity edema, fatigue, radiation recall
Vincristine	Bone marrow suppression, peripheral neuropathy, bone or abdominal pain

ONCOL

■ TABLE 11.4 Radiation: Rehabilitation Implications

Mode	Potential Side Effects Affecting Rehabilitation
Side effects from treatment can be dose limiting or may cause the oncologist to change medical course of action; therefore, feedback by the rehabilitation therapist as part of the medical team is imperative. Note: This list is not all inclusive.	
External beam (including proton)	Tissue fibrosis, lymphedema, local edema, decreased range of motion, fatigue, bone marrow suppression, skin desquamation, infection, radiation recall
Internal (including seed implant/brachytherapy)	Tissue fibrosis, tissue atrophy, stenosis, lymphedema, local edema, decreased range of motion, fatigue, bladder/bowel dysfunction, incontinence, sexual dysfunction, impotence, radiation recall

TABLE 11.5 Hormone Therapy: Rehabilitation Implications

Common Examples	Potential Side Effects Affecting Rehabilitation
Side effects from treatment can be dose limiting or may cause the oncologist to change medical course of action; therefore, feedback by the rehabilitation therapist as part of the medical team is imperative. Note: This list is not all inclusive.	
Leuprolide	Muscle atrophy, fat-to-lean body ratio/weight gain/obesity, osteoporosis, diabetes
Anastrozole	Weakness, fatigue, difficulty breathing, headaches, arthritis, joint/bone/back pain, osteoporosis, fracture, infection, dizziness, peripheral edema, hypertension, deep venous thrombosis, myocardial infection, depression, anxiety
Letrozole	Joint pain, weakness, weight gain, insomnia
Capecitabine	Anemia, weakness, fatigue, hand/foot syndrome, depression, weight gain, insomnia
Trastuzumab	Pain, fatigue, weakness, arrhythmia, hypertension, heart failure, depression, insomnia
Paclitaxel	Bone marrow suppression, peripheral neuropathy
Orchiectomy	Erectile dysfunction, weight gain, mood swings, depression, fatigue, anemia, muscle atrophy, osteoporosis
Oophorectomy	Surgical menopause, cardiovascular disease, osteoporosis, psychological

ONCOL

TABLE 11.6 Immunotherapy: Rehabilitation Implications

Type	Potential Side Effects Affecting Rehabilitation
Side effects from treatment can be dose limiting or may cause the oncologist to change medical course of action; therefore, feedback by the rehabilitation therapist as part of the medical team is imperative. Note: This list is not all inclusive.	
Interferon: alpha, beta, gamma	Flu-like symptoms, fever/chills, headache, severe fatigue, orthostatic hypotension, peripheral edema, peripheral neuropathy of hands/feet
Interleukin II	Flu-like symptoms, fever/chills, headache, severe fatigue, orthostatic hypotension, peripheral edema, peripheral neuropathy of hands/feet
Monoclonal antibody	Flu-like symptoms, bone marrow suppression, fatigue, thrombus, hemorrhage, heart failure, myocardial infarct

● TABLE 11.7 Common Adverse Cancer Treatment Effects on Various Body Systems: Rehabilitation Implications

System/Process	Side Effects Which May Affect Rehabilitation Planning
	Side effects from treatment can be dose limiting or may cause the oncologist to change medical course of action; therefore, feedback by the rehabilitation therapist as part of the medical team is imperative. Note: This list is not all inclusive.
Immunology	Drug-related hemolysis
Auditory	Hearing loss, tinnitus
Bone marrow/blood	Thrombocytopenia, petechiae, anemia, leukopenia
Cardiac	Arrhythmia, cardiomyopathy, heart failure, hypertension
Coagulation	Hemorrhage, disseminated intravascular coagulation, thrombosis, embolism
Constitutional	Fever, fatigue, obesity/weight gain
Skin	Chemo or radiation dermatitis, rash, photosensitivity, graft-versus-host disease of skin and/or fascia (post-hematopoietic transplant), scleroderma
Endocrine	Diabetes, hypo/hyperthyroidism, adrenal insufficiency, osteoporosis
Gastrointestinal	Ascites, dehydration, graft versus host disease, xerostomia, mucositis, nausea, dysgeusia
Growth/development	Delayed growth or motor milestones, delayed bone growth
Hemorrhage	Petechiae, pulmonary/central nervous system/gastrointestinal bleed, hematoma
Hepatobiliary/pancreas	Cholecystitis, pancreatitis, liver failure, graft versus host disease
Infection	Cellulitis, sepsis, febrile neutropenia, respiratory syncytial virus, aspergillosis, methicillin-resistant staphylococcus aureus
Lymphatic	Metastatic or non metastatic lymphedema, lymphocele
Metabolic	Hyperbilirubinemia, hypoalbuminemia, peripheral edema, hypercholesterolemia

(table continues on page 726)

ONCOL

TABLE 11.7 Common Adverse Cancer Treatment Effects on Various Body Systems: Rehabilitation Implications (continued)

System/Process	Side Effects Which May Affect Rehabilitation Planning
Musculoskeletal	Muscle atrophy, steroid myopathy, seroma, cording, graft versus host disease of skin/fascia, rash, osteopenia. osteoporosis, fracture, fibrosis, arthralgia, myalgia
Neurology	Depression, psychosis, ataxia, brachial plexopathy, confusion, dizziness, cranial/motor/sensory neuropathy
Ocular	Cataracts, vitreous hemorrhage, diplopia, retinopathy, scleral edema, graft versus host disease
Pain	General, organ or bone specific, neurologic, musculoskeletal
Pulmonary	Atelectasis, aspiration, dyspnea, pneumonitis, pulmonary fibrosis, graft versus host disease
Renal	Bladder spasms, incontinence, renal failure
Genitourinary	Perforation, obstruction
Secondary malignancy	Secondary to cancer treatment, i.e., chest wall sarcoma post past chest radiation treatment or acute myeloid leukemia post past chemotherapy treatment
Sexuality/fertility	Infertility, gynecomastia, vaginal dryness or stenosis, graft versus host disease
Syndromes	Tumor lysis syndrome, Stevens-Johnson syndrome
Vascular	Phlebitis, thrombosis, embolism, peripheral edema

For more information: *NCI Common Terminology Criteria for Adverse Effects (CTCAE).* http://ctep.cancer.gov/protocolDevelopment/electronic_applications/docs/ctcaev3.pdf. Accessed March 30, 2010.

ONCOL

● TABLE 11.8 Commonly Used Antineoplastic Drugs

Drug	Mechanism of Action	Commonly Responsive Tumors	Toxicity and Comments
Antimetabolites: Folate Antagonists			
Methotrexate	Binds to dihydrofolate reductase and interferes with thymidylate synthesis	Acute lymphocytic leukemia Choriocarcinoma (women) Head and neck cancer Malignant lymphoma Osteogenic sarcoma Ovarian cancer	Mucosal ulceration Bone marrow suppression Increased toxicity with impaired renal function or ascitic fluid (with pooling of drug) Reversal of toxicity with leucovorin rescue at 24 h (10–20 mg q 6 h × 10 doses)
Pemetrexed	Inhibits thymidylate synthase	Lung cancer Mesothelioma Ovarian cancer	Bone marrow suppression Mucosal ulceration
Antimetabolites: Purine Antagonists			
Cladribine	Inhibits ribonucleotide reductase	Leukemia Lymphoma	Myelosuppression Immunosuppression
Clofarabine	Inhibits DNA synthesis	Acute lymphocytic leukemia refractory to at least 2 prior chemotherapy regimens	Myelosuppression Immunosuppression Nausea Diarrhea
Fludarabine	Terminates DNA synthesis and inhibits ribonucleotide reductase	Leukemia Lymphoma	Myelosuppression Immunosuppression Autoimmune reactions
6-Mercaptopurine	Blocks de novo purine synthesis	Acute leukemia	Myelosuppression Immunosuppression
Nelarabine		Leukemia Lymphoma	Myelosuppression Immunosuppression

(table continues on page 728)

ONCOL

⬤ TABLE 11.8 **Commonly Used Antineoplastic Drugs** (continued)

Drug	Mechanism of Action	Commonly Responsive Tumors	Toxicity and Comments
Pentostatin		Leukemia	Myelosuppression Immunosuppression Nausea Vomiting
Antimetabolites: Pyrimidine Antagonists			
Capecitabine	Inhibits thymidylate synthase	Breast cancer GI tumors	Mucositis Alopecia Myelosuppression Diarrhea Vomiting Hand or foot tenderness Ulceration
Cytarabine	Terminates chain when incorporated into DNA	Acute leukemia (especially nonlymphocytic) Lymphoma	Myelosuppression Nausea Vomiting Cerebellar toxicity (at high doses) Conjunctival toxicity (at high doses) Rash
5-Fluorouracil	Inhibits thymidylate synthase	Breast cancer GI tumors	Mucositis Alopecia Myelosuppression Diarrhea Vomiting
Gemcitabine	Terminates chain when incorporated into DNA and inhibits ribonucleotide reductase	Bladder cancer Lung cancer Pancreatic cancer	Myelosuppression Hemolytic-uremic syndrome
Hydroxyurea	Inhibits ribonucleotide reductase	Chronic myelocytic leukemia	Myelosuppression
Biological Response Modifiers			
Interferon-alfa	Has antiproliferative effect	Chronic myelocytic leukemia	Fatigue Fever Myalgias

Drug	Mechanism of Action	Commonly Responsive Tumors	Toxicity and Comments
		Hairy cell leukemia Kaposi's sarcoma Lymphomas Melanoma Renal cell cancer	Arthralgias Myelosuppression Nephrotic syndrome (rare)
Bleomycins Bleomycin	Causes DNA strands to break	Lymphoma Squamous cell cancer Testicular cancer	Anaphylaxis Chills and fever Rash Pulmonary fibrosis at dosage >200 mg/m^2 Requires renal excretion
DNA Alkylating Agents: Nitrosoureas Carmustine	Alkylates DNA with restricted uncoiling and replication of strands	Brain tumors Lymphoma	Myelosuppression Pulmonary toxicity (fibrosis)
Lomustine	Alkylates DNA with restricted uncoiling and replication of strands	Brain tumors (astrocytoma, glioblastoma)	Myelosuppression Pulmonary toxicity (delayed) Renal toxicity
DNA Cross-Linking Drugs and Alkylating Agents Bendamustine Chlorambucil Cyclophosphamide Ifosfamide Mechlorethamine (nitrogen mustard) Melphalan	Form adducts with DNA, causing DNA strands to break	Breast cancer Chronic lymphocytic leukemia Gliomas Hodgkin lymphoma Lymphoma Multiple myeloma Small cell lung cancer	Alopecia with high IV dosage Nausea Vomiting Myelosuppression Hemorrhagic cystitis (especially with cyclophosphamide and ifosfamide), which can be ameliorated with mesna

ONCOL

(table continues on page 730)

TABLE 11.8 Commonly Used Antineoplastic Drugs (continued)

Drug	Mechanism of Action	Commonly Responsive Tumors	Toxicity and Comments
		Testicular cancer	Mutagenesis Secondary leukemias Aspermia Permanent sterility (possible)
Dacarbazine	Form adducts with DNA	Melanoma	Neutropenia
Temozolomide		Malignant glioma	Nausea Vomiting Secondary leukemias
Procarbazine	Unclear	Hodgkin lymphoma	Neutropenia Nausea Vomiting Secondary leukemias
Enzymes Asparaginase	Depletes asparagine, on which leukemic cells depend	Acute lymphocytic leukemia	Acute anaphylaxis Hyperthermia Pancreatitis Hyperglycemia Hypofibrinogenemia
Hormones Bicalutamide			Decreased libido
Flutamide			Hot flushes Gynecomastia
Fulvestrant			Nausea Vomiting Constipation Diarrhea Abdominal pain Headache Back pain Hot flushes Pharyngitis
Leuprolide acetate	Inhibits go-nadotropin secretion	Prostate cancer	Hot flushes Decreased libido Irritation at injection site

ONCOL

Drug	Mechanism of Action	Commonly Responsive Tumors	Toxicity and Comments
Megestrol acetate	Progesterone agonist	Breast cancer Endometrial cancer	Weight gain Fluid retention
Tamoxifen	Binds to estrogen receptor	Breast cancer	Hot flushes Hypercalcemia Deep venous thrombosis
Hormones: Aromatase Inhibitors			
Anastrozole Exemestane Letrozole	Block conversion of androgen to estrogen	Breast cancer	Osteoporosis Hot flushes
Monoclonal Antibodies			
Alemtuzumab	Binds to B and T cells	Lymphomas	Immunosuppression
Bevacizumab	Binds to vascular endothelial growth factor	Colon cancer Renal cancer	Hypersensitivity Bleeding Hypertension
Gemtuzumab	Binds to CD33 on leukemic cells	Acute myelocytic leukemia	Myelosuppression
Ibritumomab Tiuxetan	Binds to CD20 on lymphoid cells	Lymphomas	Delivers radiation to cancer cells
Iodine-131 tositumomab	Binds to CD20 on lymphoid cells	Lymphomas	Myelosuppression Fever Rash
Rituximab	Binds to CD20 on B cells	B-cell lymphoma	Hypersensitivity Immunosuppression
Trastuzumab	Binds to HER2/neu receptor	Breast cancer	Hypersensitivity Cardiac toxicity

(table continues on page 732)

ONCOL

⬤ **TABLE 11.8 Commonly Used Antineoplastic Drugs** (continued)

Drug	Mechanism of Action	Commonly Responsive Tumors	Toxicity and Comments
Other Antibiotics			
Mitomycin	Inhibits DNA synthesis by acting as a bifunctional alkylator	Breast cancer Colon cancer Gastric adeno-carcinoma Lung cancer Transitional cell cancer of the bladder	Local extravasation causing tissue necrosis Myelosuppression, with leukopenia and thrombocy-topenia 4 to 6 wk after treatment Alopecia Lethargy Fever Hemolytic-uremic syndrome
Platinum Complexes			
Carboplatin	Establishes cross-links within and between DNA strands	Breast cancer Lung cancer Ovarian cancer	Myelosuppression Peripheral neuropathy
Cisplatin	Establishes cross-links within and between DNA strands	Bladder cancer Breast cancer Head and neck cancer Gastric cancer Lung cancer (especially small cell) Testicular cancer	Anemia Ototoxicity Nausea Vomiting Peripheral neuropathy Myelosuppression
Oxaliplatin	Establishes cross-links within and between DNA strands	Colon cancer	Myelosuppression Neuropathic throat pain Peripheral neuropathy
Proteasome Inhibitors			
Bortezomib	Inhibits proteasome functions	Multiple myeloma	Myelosuppression Diarrhea Nausea Constipation Peripheral neuropathy

ONCOL

Drug	Mechanism of Action	Commonly Responsive Tumors	Toxicity and Comments
Spindle Poison (from Plantae): Taxanes			
Docetaxel	Promotes assembly of microtubules	Breast cancer Head and neck cancer Lung cancer Ovarian cancer	Myelosuppression Alopecia Rash Fluid retention
Paclitaxel	Promotes assembly of microtubules	Bladder cancer Breast cancer Head and neck cancer Lung cancer Ovarian cancer	Myelosuppression Alopecia Myalgia Arthralgia Neuropathy
Spindle Poison (from Plantae): Vincas			
Vinblastine	Arrests mitosis by inhibiting polymerization of microtubules	Breast cancer Ewing's sarcoma Leukemia Lymphomas Testicular cancer	Alopecia Myelosuppression Peripheral neuropathy
Vincristine	Arrests mitosis by inhibiting polymerization of microtubules	Acute leukemia Lymphoma	Peripheral neuropathy Ileus Syndrome of inappropriate antidiuretic hormone secretion
Vinorelbine	Arrests mitosis by inhibiting polymerization of microtubules	Breast cancer Lung cancer	Myelosuppression Neuropathy
Topoisomerase Inhibitors: Anthracyclines			
Daunorubicin (daunomycin)	Inhibits topoisomerase II and causes DNA strands to break	Leukemia	Myelosuppression Cardiac toxicity at cumulative dosage > 1000 mg/m^2

(table continues on page 734)

ONCOL

⬤ **TABLE 11.8 Commonly Used Antineoplastic Drugs** (continued)

Drug	Mechanism of Action	Commonly Responsive Tumors	Toxicity and Comments
Doxorubicin	Inhibits topoisomerase II and causes DNA strands to break	Acute leukemia Breast cancer Lung cancer Lymphoma	Nausea Vomiting Alopecia Myelosuppression Cardiac toxicity at cumulative dosage >550 mg/m^2
Epirubicin	Inhibits topoisomerase II and causes DNA strands to break	Acute myelocytic leukemia Breast cancer Gastric cancer	Myelosuppression Cardiac toxicity at cumulative dosage > 1,000 mg/m^2
Topoisomerase Inhibitors: Camptothecins			
Irinotecan	Inhibits topoisomerase I	Colon cancer Lung cancer Rectal cancer	Diarrhea Myelosuppression Alopecia
Topotecan	Inhibits topoisomerase I	Ovarian cancer Small cell lung cancer	Myelosuppression
Topoisomerase Inhibitors: Podophyllotoxins			
Etoposide Teniposide	Inhibit topoisomerase II and cause DNA strands to break	Acute leukemia Hodgkin lymphoma Lymphoma Lung cancer (especially small cell) Testicular cancer	Nausea Vomiting Myelosuppression Peripheral neuropathy Increased toxicity in renal failure Neutropenia Cleared by liver and kidneys
Mitoxantrone	Inhibit topoisomerase II and cause DNA strands to break	Acute leukemia Lymphoma	Neutropenia Nausea Vomiting
Tyrosine Kinase Inhibitors			
Erlotinib Gefitinib	Inhibit epidermal growth factor receptor	Non–small cell lung cancer	Acne Diarrhea

ONCOL

Drug	Mechanism of Action	Commonly Responsive Tumors	Toxicity and Comments
Imatinib	Inhibits Bcr-Abl kinase and c-kit kinase	Chronic myelocytic leukemia GI stromal tumors	Leukopenia Hepatocellular toxicity Edema
Lapatinib	Inhibits Her2/neu activity	Breast cancer	Diarrhea Nausea Rash Vomiting Fatigue
Sorafenib	Inhibits intra-cellular and cell surface kinases (e.g., vascular endothelial growth factor receptors)	Hepatocellular cancer Renal cancer	Hypertension Proteinuria
Sunitinib	Inhibits receptor tyrosine kinases	GI stromal tumors Renal cancer	Hypertension Proteinuria

From: Porter, R (ed): *The Merck Manual of Diagnosis and Therapy.* Copyright 2009–2010 by Merck & Co., Inc., Whitehouse Station, NJ. http://www.merck.com/mmpe. Accessed May 1, 2010.

ONCOL

◗ TABLE 11.9 Frequently Used Combination Chemotherapy Regimens

Chemotherapeutic Regimen*	Components of Regimen	Primary Indication
ABVD	Doxorubicin (Adriamycin), bleomycin (Blenoxane), vinblastine (Velban), dacarbazine (DTIC)	Hodgkin's lymphoma
BEP	Bleomycin, etoposide, cisplatin (Platinol)	Germ cell tumors
CHOP	Cyclophosphamide (Cytoxan), doxorubicin,† vincristine (Oncovin), prednisone	Non-Hodgkin's lymphoma
CMF	Cyclophosphamide (Cytoxan), methotrexate, 5-fluorouracil	Breast cancer
COP	Cyclophosphamide (Cytoxan), vincristine (Oncovin), prednisone	Non-Hodgkin's lymphoma
FAC	5-Fluorouracil, doxorubicin (Adriamycin), Cyclophosphamide (Cytoxan)	Breast cancer
ICE	Ifosfamide, carboplatin, etoposide	Nonsmall cell lung cancer
MOPP	Mechlorethamine (Mustargen), vincristine (Oncovin), procarbazine, prednisone	Hodgkin's disease
VAD	Vincristine, doxorubicin (Adriamycin), dexamethasone	Multiple myeloma
VIP	Vincristine, ifosfamide, cisplatin (Platinol)	Germ cell tumors

From: Ciccone, CD: *Pharmacology in Rehabilitation,* ed. 4. FA Davis, Philadelphia, 2007, p 583, with permission.

*A few examples of commonly used regimens are listed here. Many other combinations are used clinically, and regimens are often tailored to the needs of each patient.

†The H in this regimen refers to hydroxyldaunorubicin, the chemical synonym for doxorubicin.

ONCOL

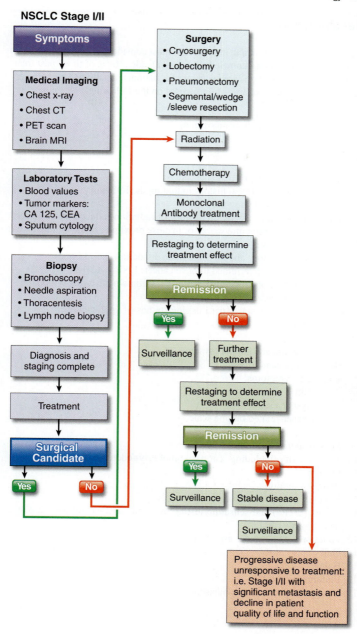

Diagnosis and treatment pathway. A patient might be referred to an oncologist specializing in lung cancer once symptoms are suspicious for cancer. The diagnosis and treatment pathway for a patient with non-small cell lung cancer (NSCLC) Stage I or II might look like this.

Rehabilitation

Appropriate examination and intervention must consider the cancer treatments received and incorporate knowledge of typical side effects of those past treatments. Some modifications are necessary for patients in palliative care. In general, though, a holistic examination focuses on the following:

1. Patient demographics
2. Anthropometrics/body composition
   a. Height
   b. Weight
   c. BMI
   d. Body fat percentage
3. Past medical and surgical history including the following:
   a. Specific chemotherapy agents
   b. Radiation dosage (including history of radiation-induced tissue fibrosis and/or joint contracture within or in close proximity to the radiated area)
   c. Surgical history:
      i. Include history about lymph node dissection (i.e., 12 nodes removed, 3 determined to have cancer: LND = +3/12)
      ii. History of post-operative cellulitis, seroma/hematoma, lymphatic cording, etc.
   d. Location of metastases per imaging studies (if applicable)
4. Medications
5. Laboratory values
6. Home situation and support systems
7. History of present illness:
   a. Current symptoms:
      i. Pain
      ii. Dyspnea scale
      iii. Cancer-related fatigue scale
8. Vital signs
9. Mental status/cognition
10. Skin integrity (including scar tissue mobility)/edema/lymphedema
11. Posture
12. Range of motion
13. Strength and coordination
14. Reflex (DTRs) and sensation testing including assessment for peripheral neuropathy
15. Functional and transfer assessment
16. Gait
17. Balance
18. Endurance
19. Functional performance measures

ONCOL

Functional Performance Scales/Performance Measures

Examples of scales and performance measures applicable to the oncology population include the following.

- Eastern Cooperative Oncology Group (ECOG) performance status. http://ecog.dfci.harvard.edu/general/perf_stat.html. Accessed January 28, 2012.
- Functional assessment of cancer therapy (FACT-G). http://www.facit.org/. Accessed January 28, 2012.
- Rate of perceived exertion and dyspnea symptom scales
- Six-minute walk test
- Fixed load submaximal patient testing
- Modified Bruce protocol treadmill test
- Timed up and go
- Forward reach
- Single limb stance

An example of important aspects of comprehensive rehabilitation examination and intervention for non–small cell lung cancer (NSCLC) stage I or II is the following:

Examination

Oncology-specific measures plus the following:

- Cardiopulmonary functional capacity assessment
- Radiation pneumonitis/pulmonary fibrosis/pericarditis impact (if applicable)
- Thoracotomy scar tissue mobility (if applicable) and thoracotomy pain assessment
- Rib excursion assessment
- Shoulder and thoracic range-of-motion assessment
- Peripheral neuropathy evaluation (history of paclitaxel); Semmes-Weinstein monofilament testing
- Functional assessment with/without supplemental oxygen (if applicable)

ONCOL

Rehabilitation Intervention Including Plan of Care

- Deep breathing and effective coughing exercise
- Scar tissue release, myofascial release at thoracotomy site (if applicable)
- Pain management at thoracotomy site (if applicable)
- Postural reeducation
- Cardiovascular exercise prescription
- Upper/core/lower extremity strengthening prescription
- Flexibility prescription
- Referral to oncology dietician
- Referral to smoking cessation program and/or oncology social worker/psychologist (if applicable)
- Referral to pulmonary rehabilitation program (if applicable)
- Discharge planning

Please note: These are only guidelines and appropriate exercise prescription may vary.

Use of Physical Agents and Modalities in Persons With Cancer

For additional information, see Section XVIII, Physical Agents.

TABLE 11.10 Uses of Physical Agents and Modalities in Persons with Cancer

Physical Agent	Contraindications	Effectiveness†
Superficial heating agents: hot packs, paraffin baths, infrared lamps, fluidotherapy, local immersion, monochromatic-infrared photo energy (MIRE)	• Over dysvascular tissue (after radiation therapy) and with people who are insensate to temperature or pain in application area. • Over areas of bleeding or hemorrhage (i.e., if there has been long-term corticosteroid therapy or chemotherapy) • Over an acute injury or inflammation • Presence of thrombophlebitis • Directly over a tumor • Over open wounds (except whirlpool at warm temperature)	• Heat and stretch may decrease pain and muscle spasm in abnormal tissue; modulates pain and facilitates relaxation (gating effect). • Not effective with deep cancer pain or bone pain (NSAIDs used).
Deep heating agents: diathermy, ultrasound, full-body immersion hydrotherapy Potential benefits	• Over growing epiphyses • Over areas of acute hemorrhage (long-term use of corticosteroids or NSAIDs) • Over acute injury or inflammation • Over insensitive skin; dysvascular or irradiated skin • Over tumors (unless trained in hyperthermia) • Over implants or devices, such as pacemakers or defibrillators, insulin pumps, morphine pumps, breast implants, plastic components, joint prosthetics-ultrasound over joint	• Acute stage—there is a cancer treatment used for tumor hyperthermia to kill tumor tissue, administered at greater than therapeutic doses. • Advanced cancer/terminal stage—not indicated over tumor: this will increase tumor growth, often increasing the severity of symptoms such as pain.

Physical Agent	Contraindications	Effectiveness†
	• Over reproductive organs; over lumbosacral, pelvic, and lumbar regions if pregnant	
Cryotherapy: cold packs, ice massage, cold hydrotherapy or baths, vapocoolant spray, cold compression	• Over dysvascular tissue (after radiation therapy) and with people who are insensate to temperature or pain in application area • When transient increase of blood pressure might be dangerous (monitor anyone with hypertension) • When wound healing is delayed • If nerve injury has occurred (applies especially to irradiation- or chemotherapy-induced nerve injury) • If Raynaud's disease or peripheral vascular disease is present (exacerbated by chemotherapy)	• Acute stage or advanced cancer—tumor treatment: supercooled at below therapeutic temperatures for local, superficial tumor destruction (e.g., liquid nitrogen for precancerous skin lesions). • Immediate post-chemotherapy cancer treatment—cold packs to head (cold cap) are suggested to reduce hair loss. • Chronic stage and cured or in remission—used for usual indications for cold therapy. • Occasionally selected by clients for pain relief; must be monitored by health or personal caregiver. • Treatment of pain in advanced cancer—not as acceptable to some for comfort care.
Mechanical agents: traction (sustained or intermittent, mechanical or manual, spinal or peripheral)	• Structural disease (tumor, infection) • Acute injury • Positive vertebral artery test • Positive alar ligament test	• Effective when there has not been previous radiation therapy to spine.
External compression: mechanical or manual Jobst pump, Lymphapress, Wright linear pump, garments, bandages	• Difficulty tolerating treatment (impaired circulation) • Phlebitis, deep vein thrombosis, thrombosis in area to be compressed	• Acute stage—may not be indicated. • Immediately after cancer treatment, advanced or terminal stage, chronic stage or cured—not

(table continues on page 742)

⬤ **TABLE 11.10 Uses of Physical Agents and Modalities in Persons with Cancer** (continued)

Physical Agent	Contraindications	Effectiveness†
	• Compression setting should not be greater than 45 mm Hg	indicated for lymphedema management unless cleared of cancer metastasis or recurrence or new cancer in region(s) to be treated.
Hydrotherapy with agitation (agitation and local immersion hydrotherapy)	• Depending on water temperature, same as for superficial heat and/or cold in region to be immersed • Agitation should be minimized with painful open lesions, severely traumatized tissue, or recent skin grafts • Risk of cross infection must be controlled, especially for immunocompromised clients	• Same as for superficial heat in region to be immersed.
Electrical stimulation: neuromuscular electrical nerve stimulation (and FES)	• If there is a potential for pathologic fracture in the area • Any type of implanted electronic device (pacemaker, insulin pump, morphine pump, defibrillator) • Severe cardiopulmonary insufficiency • Active phlebitis, deep vein thrombosis, thrombosis in area to be treated	• Wound healing HVPC or LIDC (microcurrent). • Strengthening. • Increased endurance.
TENS and electrical stimulation at acupuncture points	• Any type of implanted electronic device (pacemaker, insulin pump, morphine pump, defibrillator) • Not useful in control of generalized pain or deep bone pain	• Advantages over narcotic analgesics: few side effects, relatively inexpensive and easy to use. • Allows interpersonal interaction and is controlled by the client.

ONCOL

Physical Agent	Contraindications	Effectiveness†
	• Occasional allergic reactions to gel or adhesive • Decreased effectiveness over time	• During treatment (chemotherapy) is effective as an antiemetic for nausea and vomiting. • Immediately after treatment for postoperative pain and chronic pain control for 24 mo.

Modified from: Goodman, CC, and Fuller, KS: *Pathology: Implications for the Physical Therapist*, ed. 3. Saunders, St. Louis, MO, 2009, pp 381–382. Courtesy Lucinda Pfalzer, PT, PhD, University of Michigan, 2007. Used with permission of Lucinda Pfalzer.

FES = functional electrical stimulation; HVPC = high-voltage pulsed current; LIDC = low-intensity direct current; NSAIDs = nonsteroidal anti-inflammatory drugs; TENS = transcutaneous electrical nerve stimulation.

*Under investigation; some reports of adverse response (e.g., burns when used beyond recommended duration as a result of insensate, avascular conditions.

†Safe if cleared for possible cancer recurrence, metastasis, or new cancer in area or areas to be treated and if the sensation and circulation in the area or areas to be treated are not impaired.

TABLE 11.11 Risk for Physical Agent and Modality Use Based on Stage of Medical Management

Acute Stage

• Medical diagnosis and treatment for new or newly recurrent cancer.
• Potential for disseminated cancer until the medical diagnostic process is completed (except cases of local cancer).
• Stage I cancer: local disease, usually receives a local treatment (e.g., surgery and/or radiation therapy).
• Stage II cancer: option of local treatment (surgery and radiation therapy) without systemic therapy (e.g., chemotherapy); higher risk of metastases or recurrence.
• Stage III cancer: systemic therapy, often chemotherapy; the process of micrometastases is unlikely in someone responding to chemotherapy.

Risk: high risk; thermal agents should not be used during or in close time proximity to radiation or chemotherapy; general contraindications/precautions apply (e.g., insensate or dysvascular tissue with decreased sensation or decreased blood flow).

Subacute Stage

• Immediately after cancer treatment; may extend 6–12 mo depending on treatment intervention (e.g., surgery, chemotherapy, radiation); hormone therapy (e.g., tamoxifen or aromatase inhibitors for breast cancer) continues for 5 yr.
• Acute side effects or toxicities from treatment (e.g., radiation or chemotherapy) begin to subside.

(table continues on page 744)

ONCOL

TABLE 11.11 **Risk for Physical Agent and Modality Use Based on Stage of Medical Management** (continued)

Risk: high-risk; thermal agents should not be used during or in close time proximity to radiation and chemotherapy; general contraindications/precautions apply (e.g., insensate or dysvascular tissue with decreased sensation or decreased blood flow).

Chronic Stage
- Remission or recurrence may occur from 6–12 mo up to 5 yr or more after cancer treatment.
- Chronic states of cancer with risk of death for people living with cancer metastases or advanced disease.
- Risk of recurrence decreases over time so that the likelihood of recurrence diminishes the further the client is from the time of diagnosis and treatment.

Risk: Stage I*—no restrictions on use of physical agents or modalities in the absence of clinical signs or symptoms of recurrence or new cancer; client has had recent medical check-up including testing for cancer (e.g., bone scan, serum markers) that is negative; general contraindications/precautions apply (e.g., insensate or dysvascular tissue with decreased sensation or decreased blood flow).

Risk: Stage II*—moderate-to-low-risk group; same restrictions as stage I.

Risk: Stage III*—moderate-risk group; same restrictions as stage I.

Risk: Stage IV* (advanced)—high-risk group; caution should be taken over any painful area or mass; thermal agents should not be used during or in close proximity to radiation or chemotherapy; general contraindications/precautions apply.

Statistically Cured Stage
- Remission more than 5 yr after cancer treatment.
- Statistical risk of recurrence is minimal.
- Return to lifetime risk of cancer as an individual statistical measure.

Risk: low-risk group; no restrictions on use of physical agents or modalities in the absence of clinical signs or symptoms of potential recurrence or new cancer; general contraindications/precautions apply.

From: Goodman, CC, and Fuller, KS: *Pathology: Implications for the Physical Therapist,* ed. 3. Saunders, St. Louis, MO, 2009, p 383. Courtesy Lucinda Pfalzer, PT, PhD, University of Michigan, 2007. Used with permission of Lucinda Pfalzer.
*At the time of diagnosis.

ONCOL

Therapeutic Exercise

Appropriate intervention depends on results from a holistic patient examination and must take into consideration the various cancer treatment history, expected early and late side effects, and any plan for future cancer to develop a safe, comprehensive exercise program. Comprehensive exercise prescription *prior* to cancer treatment initiation is ideal. The following should routinely occur and be initiated as appropriate:

Post-Surgical Intervention

- Scar tissue restriction evaluation/treatment; teach patient/caregiver scar tissue release/myofascial release

- Pain (including phantom pain/sensation) reduction
- Cellulitis prevention education
- Lymphatic cording evaluation/treatment
- Radiation-induced fibrosis prevention/treatment education
- Local edema/peripheral edema management*
- Lymphedema risk reduction education
- Self–manual lymphatic drainage (MLD) education
- Baseline bilateral extremity girth measurements
- Lymphedema management†
- Safety and fatigue management
- Joint bracing
- Orthotic training
- Gait and balance training
- Weight management
- Full body comprehensive exercise prescription with emphasis on flexibility

Intervention Prior, During, or Post Other Cancer Treatment

- Scar tissue massage and myofascial release if restrictions remain or were not previously addressed
- Peripheral neuropathy management
- Radiation-induced fibrosis prevention/treatment education
- Local edema/peripheral edema management
- Lymphedema management
- Wound management
- Safety and fatigue management
- Orthotic training
- Gait and balance training
- Weight management
- Full body comprehensive exercise prescription

Palliative Intervention

The following rehabilitation needs for these patients are extensive and often neglected:

- Pain management
- Fatigue management
- Decubitus ulcer risk reduction education
- Peripheral edema management

---

*Peripheral edema of the lower extremities and/or genital area may be exacerbated by a number of medical factors including ascites, hypoalbuminemia, infusions/transfusions, or a weakened muscle pump action, which can cause fluid volume overload. Peripheral edema contributes to patient discomfort, fatigue, infection, fall risk, decreased mobility, and lower quality of life. Prompt rehabilitation intervention in each case is critical, regardless of patient prognosis.

†Lymphedema is a lifelong risk for any patient of any gender or age who undergoes lymph node resection of any amount and/or radiation; therefore, early post-operative, routine patient education is important to reduce this risk. Restricted scars may cause localized sluggish lymphatic flow. Skin breakdown and wounds can occur with poorly managed lymphedema and restricted scar tissue.

ONCOL

- Lymphedema management
- Wound management
- Equipment prescription
- Patient and caregiver functional mobility training
- Modified full body comprehensive exercise prescription with close monitoring

Exercise prescription should include slow, monitored, gently progressive exercise to avoid patient harm including loss of balance, fracture, and lymphedema risk. In general, for patients during treatment and post-treatment, slowly progressive weight training is recommended two times a week (beginning with low weight and low repetition), flexibility exercise at least two times a week, and cardiovascular training as summarized below with close monitoring of blood laboratory value results (until consistently normal).

Hematology and Blood Chemistry

Some comprehensive cancer centers, in conjunction with their rehabilitation department, may have established different laboratory values to determine when and how much exercise is safe. Treatment guidelines may vary depending on the duration of anemia and past medical and past functional history of the patient and therefore must be verified with the medical team. The following tables illustrate both a published and a clinical comprehensive cancer center guideline. **It is necessary to check hematological values prior to *each* rehabilitation treatment session as a standard of care** both during cancer treatment(s) and/or for as long as abnormal hematology values occur after treatment(s) to avoid adverse events and potentially serious patient harm.

TABLE 11.12 Exercise Guidelines Based on Blood Values

	Normal Values	No Exercise	Light Exercise	Regular Exercise
Hematocrit Women Men	37%–47% 40%–50%	<25%	>25%	>25%
Hemoglobin Women Men	12–16 g/dL 14–18 g/dL	<8 g/dL	8–10 g/dL	>10 g/dL
White blood cells	4,000– 10,000/mm^3	<500/mm^3	>500/mm^3	>500/mm^3
Platelets	200,000– 400,000/mm^3	<5,000/mm^3	5,000– 10,000/mm^3	10,000/mm^3

From: Sayre, RS, and Marcoux, BC: Exercise and autologous bone marrow transplants. *Clin Manage Phys Ther 12*(4):78–82, 1992.

ONCOL

TABLE 11.13 Seattle Cancer Care Alliance Hematological and Exercise Guidelines

	No Exercise	Gentle Seated Aerobic and Anti-Gravity Exercise,No Weights*	Aerobic and Resistive Exercise
Hematocrit	<25%	>25%	>25%
Hemoglobin	<8.5 g/dL	>8.5 g/dL	>8.5 g/dL
Platelets	<10,000/mm³	10,000–20,000/mm³	>20,000/mm³

Used with permission of the SCCA.
*No hand, machine weights, tubing, or bands. Patient must be monitored for signs/ symptoms of bleeding or anemia. If petechiae are present, exercise is usually suspended until platelet transfusion occurs, and ideally post-transfusion blood work is done.

Strength Training Prescription

Strength training must be carefully monitored for proper posture, technique and safety. If applicable, thorough assessment for fracture risk from osteoporosis and/or bony metastasis, loss of balance from peripheral neuropathy or contracture, and lymphedema risk is important; therefore, consultation with the medical team prior to prescribing strength training may be necessary.

TABLE 11.14 Seattle Cancer Care Alliance Guidelines for Strength Training*

	Initial Recommendation	Progression
Significant functional decline	• Back support. • Extra height added to chair (i.e., 4-in. foam cushion) for comfort and safety and to facilitate sit-to-stand transfers. • Anti-gravity exercise. • Slower progression for patients with risk of lymphedema. • Teach valsalva avoidance during exercise.	• Add standing exercise. • Remove foam cushion either partially (cut height in half) or fully for transfer training, lower extremity and gluteal strengthening. • Add dumbbell and cuff weights slowly in 1-lb increments. • Continue to progress as able with careful monitoring. Slower progression for patients with risk of lymphedema.
Moderate functional decline	• Back support. • Begin with 1-lb dumbbell and cuff weights and increase as able. Slower	• Eventually add weight machines and continue with free weights. • Add standing exercise.

(table continues on page 748)

TABLE 11.14 Seattle Cancer Care Alliance Guidelines for Strength Training* (continued)

	Initial Recommendation	Progression
	progression for patients with risk of lymphedema. • Teach valsalva avoidance during exercise.	• Continue to progress as able with careful monitoring. Slower progression for patients with risk of lymphedema.
Minimal functional decline	• Exercise with and without back support. • Weight machines and free weights. • Mixture of open and closed chain weight training. Slower progression for patients with risk of lymphedema. • Teach valsalva avoidance during exercise.	• Continue to progress as able with careful monitoring. Slower progression for patients with risk of lymphedema.
Maintenance of muscle mass (e.g. premorbid exercisers and athletes)	• Regular exercise program depending on hematologic values and the presence of central lines (port, Hickman, etc.). Slower progression for patients with risk of lymphedema. • Teach valsalva avoidance during exercise.	• Continue to progress as able with careful monitoring. Slower progression for patients with risk of lymphedema.

Used with permission of the SCCA.
*Recommend using strength-training methods other than tubing or bands, because resistance with tubing and bands is difficult to quantify.

Stretching Prescription

Flexibility exercise is of particular importance to this patient population. Premorbid inflexibility or joint stiffness is common and tends to worsen during treatment. Long appointment waiting times, surgery, and periods of prolonged sitting or sleeping may affect overall flexibility. Particular focus on areas of prior surgery or radiation (once completely healed) as well as shoulder, pectoral, psoas, hamstring, quadricep, gastrocnemius, and ankle stretching are helpful for most cancer patients. Patients who have had a diagnosis of radiation-induced fibrosis contracture, graft-versus-host disease of skin/fascia/joints, or scleroderma need to be on a 5 to 7 days/week stretching program. Particular attention should be focused on safe technique with reduction of joint compensation by the patient.

Aerobic/Cardiovascular Prescription

Cardiovascular exercise is an essential component of exercise for all cancer patients. The toxicity to the cardiopulmonary system from many of the modes of cancer treatments necessitates standard cardiovascular prescription in the oncology population. A mode that concurrently exercises both upper and lower extremities together, if possible, is ideal. Patients may have pre-morbid heart disease, chronic obstructive pulmonary disease, and/or diabetes, all of which affect exercise planning and require careful monitoring.

● **TABLE 11.15 Exercise Prescription for the Cancer Survivor**

According to the American College of Sports Medicine, evidence is lacking for precise recommendations regarding optimal components of exercise prescription for each cancer type. The following are general guidelines, and appropriate exercise prescription may vary for each individual cancer survivor.

Type of Exercise	Frequency	Intensity	Duration	Possible Activities
Aerobic	3–5 days/wk	40%–<60% oxygen uptake reserve or heart rate reserve	20–60 min per day, with accumulated shorter bouts if necessary	Prolonged, rhythmic activities using large muscle groups, such as walking, cycling, swimming
Resistance	2–3 days/wk with at least 48 hr between sessions	40%–60% one repetition, maximum	1–3 sets of 8–12 repetitions per exercise with an upper limit of 15 repetitions appropriate for deconditioned, fatigued, or frail individuals	Weights, resistance machines, or weight-bearing functional tasks (e.g., sit to stand) targeting all major muscle groups

(table continues on page 750)

ONCOL

TABLE 11.15 Exercise Prescription for the Cancer Survivor (continued)

Type of Exercise	Frequency	Intensity	Duration	Possible Activities
Flexibility	2–7 days/wk	Slow static stretching to the point of tension	4 repetitions of 10–30 sec per stretch	Stretching or range-of-motion exercises of all major muscle groups also addressing specific areas of joint or muscle restriction that may have results from treatment with steroids, radiation, or surgery

Modified from: *ACSM's Guidelines for Exercise Testing and Prescription*, ed. 8. Lippincott Williams & Wilkins, Philadelphia, 2009, p 231.

Oncology Emergencies

An oncology emergency occurs when a significant new symptom(s) appears that may indicate a new, undiagnosed secondary cancer, undiagnosed primary cancer recurrence affecting a major body system, or other medical emergency. Any new symptom(s) representative of the following concerns warrants an immediate referral back to the patient's physician.

I. **Hematological**
   a. Myelosuppression
   b. Disseminated intravascular coagulation (DIC)
II. **Obstruction**
   a. Spinal cord compression
   b. Superior vena cava syndrome
   c. Intestinal obstruction or perforation
   d. Third space syndrome
III. **Increased Pressure/Fluid Accumulation**
   a. Increased intracranial pressure
   b. Pericardial effusion/neoplastic cardiac tamponade
   c. Pleural effusion
   d. Peritoneal effusion: ascites
IV. **Metabolic**
   a. Hypercalcemia
   b. Syndrome of inappropriate antidiuretic hormone (SIADH)
   c. Tumor lysis syndrome
V. **Pathological Fracture**

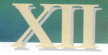

GENERAL MEDICINE

Common Laboratory Tests

TABLE 12.1 Laboratory Reference Values

Hematology and Coagulation

Analyte	Specimen*	Units Used at MGH	SI Units
Activated clotting time	WB	70–180 sec	70–180 sec
Activated protein C resistance (factor V Leiden)	P	Ratio >2.1	Not applicable
Alpha₂-antiplasmin	P	80–130%	0.80–1.30
Antiphospholipid-antibody panel			
Partial-thromboplastin time–lupus anticoagulant screen	P	Negative	Negative
Platelet-neutralization procedure	P	Negative	Negative
Dilute viper-venom screen	P	Negative	Negative
Anticardiolipin antibody	S		
IgG		0–15 GPL units	0–15 arbitrary units
IgM		0–15 MPL units	0–15 arbitrary units
Antithrombin III	P		
Antigenic		22–39 mg/dl	220–390 mg/liter
Functional		80–130%	0.8–1.30 U/liter
Anti-Xa assay (heparin assay)	P		
Unfractionated heparin		0.3–0.7 IU/ml	0.3–0.7 kIU/liter
Low-molecular-weight heparin		0.5–1.0 IU/ml	0.5–1.0 kIU/liter
Danaparoid		0.5–0.8 IU/ml	0.5–0.8 kIU/liter
Bleeding time		2.0–9.5 min	2.0–9.5 min
Carboxyhemoglobin	WB		
Nonsmoker		0–2.3%	0–0.023
Smoker		2.1–4.2%	0.021–0.042

Hematology and Coagulation

Analyte	Specimen*	Units Used at MGH	SI Units
Clot retraction	WB	50–100%/2 hr	0.50–1.00/2 hr
Cryofibrinogen	P	Negative	Negative
D-Dimer	P	<0.5 µg/ml	<0.5 mg/liter
Differential blood count	WB		
Neutrophils		40–70%	0.40–0.70
Band forms		0–10%	0–0.10
Lymphocytes		22–44%	0.22–0.44
Monocytes		4–11%	0.04–0.11
Eosinophils		0–8%	0–0.08
Basophils		0–3%	0–0.03
Erythrocyte count	WB		
Male		$4.50–5.90 \times 10^6/mm^3$	$4.50–5.90 \times 10^{12}/liter$
Female		$4.00–5.20 \times 10^6/mm^3$	$4.50–5.20 \times 10^{12}/liter$
Erythrocyte lifespan	WB		
Normal survival		120 days	120 days
Chromium labeled, half-life		25–35 days	25–35 days
Erythrocyte sedimentation rate	WB		
Female		1–25 mm/hr	1–25 mm/hr
Male		0–17 mm/hr	0–17 mm/hr
Factor II, prothrombin	P	60–140%	0.60–1.40
Factor V	P	60–140%	0.60–1.40
Factor VII	P	60–140%	0.60–1.40
Factor VIII	P	50–200%	0.50–2.00

(table continues on page 754)

GEN MED

GEN MED

TABLE 12.1 Laboratory Reference Values (continued)

Hematology and Coagulation

Analyte	Specimen*	Units Used at MGH	SI Units
Factor IX	P	60–140%	0.60–1.40
Factor X	P	60–140%	0.60–1.40
Factor XI	P	60–140%	0.60–1.40
Factor XII	P	60–140%	0.60–1.40
Factor XIII screen	P	No deficiency detected	Not applicable
Factor-inhibitor assay	S	<0.5 Bethesda unit	<0.5 Bethesda unit
Ferritin			
Male	P	30–300 ng/ml	30–300 μg/liter
Female	P	10–200 ng/ml	10–200 μg/liter
Fibrin and fibrinogen-degradation products	P	<2.5 μg/ml	<2.5 mg/liter
Fibrinogen	S, P	150–400 mg/dl	1.50–4.00 g/liter
Folate (folic acid)			
Normal		3.1–17.5 ng/ml	7.0–39.7 nmol/liter
Borderline deficient		2.2–3.0 ng/ml	5.0–6.8 nmol/liter
Deficient		<2.2 ng/ml	<5.0 nmol/liter
Excess		>17.5 ng/ml	>39.7 nmol/liter
Glucose-6-phosphate dehydrogenase, erythrocyte	WB	No gross deficiency	Not applicable
Ham's test (acidified serum test)	WB	Negative	Negative
Haptoglobin	S	16–199 mg/dl	0.16–1.99 g/liter
Hematocrit	WB		
Male		41.0–53.0%	0.41–0.53
Female		36.0–46.0%	0.36–0.46
Hemoglobin			
Plasma	P	1–5 mg/dl	0.01–0.05 g/liter

Hematology and Coagulation

Analyte	Specimen*	Units Used at MGH	SI Units
Whole blood			
Hemoglobin			
Male	WB	13.5–17.5 g/dl	8.4–10.9 mmol/liter
Female	WB	12.0–16.0 g/dl	7.4–9.9 mmol/liter
Hemoglobin electrophoresis	WB		
Hemoglobin A		95–98%	0.95–0.98
Hemoglobin A₂		1.5–3.5%	0.015–0.035
Hemoglobin F		0–2.0%	0–0.02
Hemoglobins other than A, A₂, or F		Absent	Absent
Heparin-induced thrombocytopenia antibody	P	Negative	Negative
Homocysteine	P	0–12 µmol/liter	0–12 µmol/liter
Iron	S	30–160 µg/dl	5.4–28.7 µmol/liter
Iron-binding capacity	S	228–428 µg/dl	40.8–76.7 µmol/liter
Leukocyte count (WBC)	WB	4.5–11.0 × 10³/mm³	4.5–11 × 10⁹/liter
Mean corpuscular hemoglobin (MCH)	WB	26.0–34.0 pg/cell	26.0–34.0 pg/cell
Mean corpuscular hemoglobin concentration (MCHC)	WB	31.0–37.0 g/dl	310–370 g/liter
Mean corpuscular volume (MCV)	WB	80–100 µm³	80–100 fl
Methemoglobin	WB	≤1% of total hemoglobin	
Osmotic fragility of erythrocytes	WB	No increased hemolysis as compared with normal control	Not applicable
Partial-thromboplastin time, activated	P	22.1–35.1 sec	22.1–35.1 sec
Plasminogen	P		
Antigenic		8.4–14.0 mg/dl	84–140 mg/liter
Functional		80–130%	0.80–1.30
Plasminogen activator inhibitor 1	P	4–43 ng/ml	4–43 µg/liter

(table continues on page 756)

GEN MED

TABLE 12.1 Laboratory Reference Values (continued)

Hematology and Coagulation

Analyte	Specimen*	Units Used at MGH	SI Units
Platelet aggregation	PRP	>65% aggregation in response to adenosine diphosphate, epinephrine, collagen, ristocetin, and arachidonic acid	Not applicable
Platelet count	WB	$150–350 \times 10^3/mm^3$	$150–350 \times 10^9/liter$
Prekallikrein assay	P	60–140%	0.60–1.40
Prekallikrein screen	P	Deficiency not detected	Not applicable
Protein C	P		
Total antigen		70–140%	0.70–1.40
Functional		70–140%	0.70–1.40
Protein S	P		
Total antigen		70–140%	0.70–1.40
Functional		70–140%	0.70–1.40
Free antigen		70–140%	0.70–1.40
Prothrombin-gene mutation G20210A	WB	Not present	Not applicable
Prothrombin time	P	11.1–13.1 sec	11.1–13.1 sec
Protoporphyrin, free erythrocyte	WB	$16–36 \mu g/dl$ red cells	$0.28–0.64 \mu mol/liter$ red cells
Red-cell distribution width	WB	11.5–14.5%	0.115–0.145
Reptilase time	P	16–24 sec	16–24 sec
Reticulocyte count	WB	0.5–2.5% red cells	0.005–0.025 red cells
Reticulocyte hemoglobin content	WB	>26 pg/cell	>26 pg/cell

Hematology and Coagulation

Analyte	Specimen*	Units Used at MGH	SI Units
Ristocetin cofactor (functional von Willebrand factor)	P		
Blood group O		75% mean of normal	0.75 mean of normal
Blood group A		105% mean of normal	1.05 mean of normal
Blood group B		115% mean of normal	1.15 mean of normal
Blood group AB		125% mean of normal	1.25 mean of normal
Schilling test, orally administered vitamin B_{12} excreted in urine	U	7–40%	Not applicable
Sickle-cell test	WB	Negative	Negative
Sucrose hemolysis	WB	<10%	<0.1
Thrombin time	P	16–24 sec	16–24 sec
Transferrin receptor	S, P	9.6–29.6 nmol/liter	9.6–29.6 nmol/liter
Viscosity	P	1.7–2.1	1.7–2.1
	S	1.4–1.8	1.4–1.8
Vitamin B_{12}	S, P		
Normal		>250 pg/ml	>185 pmol/liter
Borderline		125–250 pg/ml	92–185 pmol/liter
Deficient		<125 pg/ml	<92 pmol/liter
von Willebrand factor (vWF) antigen (factor VIII:R antigen)	P		
Blood group O		75% mean of normal	0.75 mean of normal
Blood group A		105% mean of normal	1.05 mean of normal
Blood group B		115% mean of normal	1.15 mean of normal
Blood group AB		125% mean of normal	1.25 mean of normal

(table continues on page 758)

TABLE 12.1 Laboratory Reference Values (continued)

Hematology and Coagulation

Analyte	Specimen*	Units Used at MGH	SI Units
von Willebrand factor multimers	P	Normal distribution	Normal distribution
White cells: see Leukocytes			

Immunology

Analyte	Specimen*	Units Used at MGH	SI Units
Autoantibodies			
Antiadrenal antibody	S	Negative at 1:10 dilution	Not applicable
Anti–double-stranded (native) DNA	S	Negative at 1:10 dilution	Not applicable
Antiglomerular basement membrane antibody	S		
Qualitative		Negative	Negative
Quantitative		<5 U/ml	<5 kU/liter
Antigranulocyte antibody	S	Negative	Not applicable
Anti–Jo-1 antibody	S	Negative	Not applicable
Anti-La antibody	S	Negative	Not applicable
Antimitochondrial antibody	S	Negative	Not applicable
Antineutrophil cytoplasmic autoantibody, cytoplasmic (c-ANCA)	S		
Qualitative		Negative	Negative
Quantitative (antibody to proteinase 3)		<2.8 U/ml	<2.8 kU/liter
Antineutrophil cytoplasmic autoantibody, perinuclear (p-ANCA)	S		
Qualitative		Negative	Negative
Quantitative (antibody to myeloperoxidase)		<1.4 U/ml	<1.4 kU/liter

Immunology

Analyte	Specimen*	Units Used at MGH	SI Units
Antinuclear antibody	S	Negative at 1:40 dilution	Not applicable
Antiparietal-cell antibody	S	Negative at 1:20 dilution	Not applicable
Anti-Ro antibody	S	Negative	Not applicable
Antiplatelet antibody	S	Negative	Not applicable
Anti-RNP antibody	S	Negative	Not applicable
Anti–Scl-70 antibody	S	Negative	Not applicable
Anti-Smith antibody	S	Negative	Not applicable
Antismooth-muscle antibody	S	Negative at 1:20 dilution	Not applicable
Antithyroglobulin	S	Negative	Not applicable
Antithyroid antibody	S	<0.3 IU/ml	<0.3 kIU/liter
Bence Jones protein	S	None detected	Not applicable
Qualitative	U	None detected in 50-fold concentrated specimen	Not applicable
Quantitative	U		
Kappa		<2.5 mg/dl	<0.03 g/liter
Lambda		<5.0 mg/dl	<0.05 g/liter
Beta$_2$-microglobulin	S	<0.27 mg/dl	<2.7 mg/liter
	U	<120 µg/day	<120 µg/day
C1-esterase–inhibitor protein	S		
Antigenic		12.4–24.5 mg/dl	0.12–0.25 g/liter
Functional		Present	Present

(table continues on page 760)

GEN MED

TABLE 12.1 Laboratory Reference Values (continued)

Immunology

Analyte	Specimen*	Units Used at MGH	SI Units
C-reactive protein	S		
Routine		0.08–3.10 mg/liter	0.08–3.10 mg/liter
High-sensitivity		0.02–8.00 mg/liter	0.02–8.00 mg/liter
Complement			
C3	S	86–184 mg/dl	0.86–1.84 g/liter
C4	S	20–58 mg/dl	0.20–0.58 g/liter
Total complement, enzyme immunoassay	S	63–145 U/ml	63–145 kU/liter
Factor B	S	17–42 mg/dl	0.17–0.42 g/liter
Cryoproteins	S	Negative	Not applicable
Immunofixation	S	Negative	Not applicable
Immunoglobulin			
IgA	S	60–309 mg/dl	0.60–3.09 g/liter
IgD	S	0–14 mg/dl	0–140 mg/liter
IgE	S	10–179 IU/ml	24–430 µg/liter
IgG	S	614–1,295 mg/dl	6.14–12.95 g/liter
IgG1	S	270–1,740 mg/dl	2.7–17.4 g/liter
IgG2	S	30–630 mg/dl	0.3–6.3 g/liter
IgG3	S	13–320 mg/dl	0.13–3.20 g/liter
IgG4	S	11–620 mg/dl	0.11–6.20 g/liter
IgM	S	53–334 mg/dl	0.53–3.34 g/liter
Joint-fluid crystal	JF	Negative	Not applicable
Joint-fluid mucin	JF	Only type I mucin present	Not applicable
LE-cell test	WB	Negative	Negative
Rheumatoid factor	S, JF	<30.0 IU/ml	<30 kIU/liter
Serum protein electrophoresis	S	Normal pattern	Not applicable

Clinical Chemistry

Analyte	Specimen*	Units Used at MGH	SI Units
Acetoacetate	P	<1 mg/dl	<100 μmol/liter
Albumin	S	3.5–5.5 g/dl	35–55 g/liter
Aldolase	S	0–6 U/liter	0–100 nkat/liter
Alpha₁-antitrypsin	S	85–213 mg/dl	0.8–2.1 g/liter
Alpha-fetoprotein	S	<15 ng/ml	<15 μg/liter
Aminotransferases			
Aspartate (AST, SGOT)		0–35 U/liter	0–0.58 μkat/liter
Alanine (ALT, SGPT)		0–35 U/liter	0–0.58 μkat/liter
Ammonia, as NH₃	P	10–80 μg/dl	6–47 μmol/liter
Amylase	S	60–180 U/liter	0.8–3.2 μkat/liter
Angiotensin-converting enzyme (ACE)	S	<40 U/liter	<670 nkat/liter
Anion gap	S	7–16 mmol/liter	7–16 mmol/liter
Apolipoprotein	S		
Apolipoprotein A-1		119–240 mg/dl	1.2–2.4 g/liter
Apolipoprotein B		52–163 mg/dl	0.52–1.63 g/liter
Apolipoprotein B:apolipoprotein A-1		0.35–0.98	0.35–0.98
Arterial blood gases, sea level	WB, arterial		
Bicarbonate (HCO₃⁻)		21–30 mEq/liter	21–28 mmol/liter
Partial pressure of carbon dioxide (PCO₂)		35–45 mm Hg	4.7–5.9 kPa
pH		7.38–7.44	7.38–7.44
Partial pressure of oxygen (PO₂)		80–100 mg Hg	11–13 kPa

(table continues on page 762)

GEN MED

GEN MED

TABLE 12.1 Laboratory Reference Values (continued)

Clinical Chemistry

Analyte	Specimen*	Units Used at MGH	SI Units
β-Hydroxybutyrate	P	<3 mg/dl	<300 μmol/liter
Beta$_2$-microglobulin	S	1.2–2.8 mg/liter	1.2–2.8 mg/liter
	U	≤200 μg/liter	≤200 μg/liter
	S		
Bilirubin			
Total		0.3–1.0 mg/dl	5.1–17.0 μmol/liter
Direct		0.1–0.3 mg/dl	1.7–5.1 μmol/liter
Indirect		0.2–0.7 mg/dl	3.4–12.0 μmol/liter
Brain-type natriuretic peptide (BNP)	P	<167 pg/ml (age- and sex-dependent)	<167 ng/liter (age- and sex-dependent)
Calcium	S	9.0–10.5 mg/dl	2.2–2.6 mmol/liter
Calcium, ionized	WB	4.5–5.6 mg/dl	1.1–1.4 mmol/liter
CA 15-3	S	0–30 U/ml	0–30 kU/liter
CA 19-9	S	0–37 U/ml	0–37 kU/liter
CA 27-29	S	0–32 U/ml	0–32 kU/liter
CA 125	S	0–35 U/ml	0–35 kU/liter
	S		
Calcitonin			
Male		3–26 pg/ml	3–26 ng/liter
Female		2–17 pg/ml	2–17 ng/liter
Carbon dioxide			
Content, sea level	P	21–30 mEq/liter	21–30 mmol/liter
Partial pressure (PCO$_2$), sea level	WB, arterial	35–45 mm Hg	4.7–5.9 kPa
Carbon monoxide content	WB	Symptoms with 20% saturation of hemoglobin	Symptoms with 20% saturation of hemoglobin

Clinical Chemistry

Analyte	Specimen*	Units Used at MGH	SI Units
Carcinoembryonic antigen (CEA)	S	0–3.4 ng/ml	0–3.4 µg/liter
Ceruloplasmin	S	27–37 mg/dl	270–370 mg/liter
Cholinesterase	S	5–12 U/ml	5–12 kU/liter
Chloride	S	98–106 mEq/liter	98–106 mmol/liter
Cholesterol	P		
Low-density lipoprotein (LDL) cholesterol			
Optimal		<100 mg/dl	<2.59 mmol/liter
Near or above normal		100–129 mg/dl	2.59–3.34 mmol/liter
Borderline high		130–159 mg/dl	3.36–4.11 mmol/liter
High		160–189 mg/dl	4.13–4.88 mmol/liter
Very high		≥190 mg/dl	≥4.91 mmol/liter
High-density lipoprotein (HDL) cholesterol			
Low		<40 mg/dl	<1.03 mmol/liter
High		≥60 mg/dl	≥1.55 mmol/liter
Total cholesterol			
Desirable		<200 mg/dl	<5.17 mmol/liter
Borderline high		200–239 mg/dl	5.17–6.18 mmol/liter
High		≥240 mg/dl	≥6.18 mmol/liter
Copper	S	70–140 µg/dl	11–22 µmol/liter
	U	3–35 µg/24 hr	0.047–0.55 µmol/24 hr
Coproporphyrins, types I and III	U	100–300 µg/24 hr	150–460 µmol/24 hr
C-peptide	S	0.5–2.0 ng/ml	0.17–0.66 nmol/liter

(table continues on page 764)

GEN MED

GEN MED

TABLE 12.1 Laboratory Reference Values (continued)

Clinical Chemistry

Analyte	Specimen*	Units Used at MGH	SI Units
Creatine kinase	S		
Total			
Female		40–150 U/liter	0.67–2.50 μkat/liter
Male		60–400 U/liter	1.00–6.67 μkat/liter
MB isoenzyme	S	0–7 ng/ml	0–7 μg/liter
Relative index†	S	Method-dependent	Method-dependent
Creatinine	S	<1.5 mg/dl	<133 μmol/liter
Erythropoietin	S	5–36 IU/liter	5–36 IU/liter
Fatty acids, free (nonesterified)	P	<8–25 mg/dl	0.28–0.89 mmol/liter
Fibrinogen and fibrinogen-degradation products: see under Hematology and Coagulation			
Folic acid	RC	150–450 ng/ml/cells	340–1,020 nmol/liter/ cells
γ-Glutamyltransferase	S	1–94 U/liter	1–94 U/liter
Glucose	P		
Fasting			
Normal		75–115 mg/dl	4.2–6.4 mmol/liter
Diabetes mellitus		>125 mg/dl	>7.0 mmol/liter
2 Hr postprandial	P	120 mg/dl	<6.7 mmol/liter
Hemoglobin A$_{1c}$	WB	3.8–6.4%	0.038–0.064 hemoglobin fraction
Homocysteine	P	4–12 μmol/liter	4–12 μmol/liter
Hydroxyproline	U	0–1.3 mg/24 hr	0–10 μmol/24 hr
Iron	S	50–150 μg/dl	9–27 μmol/liter

Clinical Chemistry

Analyte	Specimen*	Units Used at MGH	SI Units
Iron-binding capacity	S	250–370 µg/dl	45–66 µmol/liter
Iron-binding capacity, saturation	S	20–45%	0.2–0.45
Ketone (acetone)	S, U	Negative	Negative
Lactate	P, venous	5–15 mg/dl	0.6–1.7 mmol/liter
Lactate dehydrogenase	S	100–190 U/liter	1.7–3.2 µkat/liter
Lactate dehydrogenase isoenzymes	S		
Fraction 1 (of total)		14–26%	0.14–0.25
Fraction 2		29–39%	0.29–0.39
Fraction 3		20–26%	0.20–0.25
Fraction 4		8–16%	0.08–0.16
Fraction 5		6–16%	0.06–0.16
Lead (adult)	S	<10–20 µg/dl	<0.5–1 µmol/liter
Lipase	S	0–160 U/liter	0–2.66 µkat/liter
Lipids, triglyceride: *see* Triglycerides	S	0–30 mg/dl	0–300 mg/liter
Lipoprotein(a)	S	1.8–3.0 mg/dl	0.8–1.2 mmol/liter
Magnesium			
Mercury	WB	0.6–59 µg/liter	3.0–294 nmol/liter
	U, 24 hr	<20 µg/liter	<99.8 nmol/liter
Microalbumin	U		
24-hr		<20 mg/liter or <31 mg/24 hr	<0.02 g/liter or <0.031 g/24 hr
Spot, morning		<0.03 mg albumin/mg creatinine	<0.03 g albumin/g creatinine

(table continues on page 766)

GEN MED

GEN MED

TABLE 12.1 Laboratory Reference Values (continued)

Clinical Chemistry

Analyte	Specimen*	Units Used at MGH	SI Units
Myoglobin	S		
Male		19–92 µg/liter	19–92 µg/liter
Female		12–76 µg/liter	12–76 µg/liter
5'-Nucleotidase	S	0–11 U/liter	0.02–0.18 µkat/liter
Osmolality	S	285–295 mOsm/kg serum	285–295 mmol/kg
	P	water	serum water
	U	300–900 mOsm/kg	300–900 mmol/kg
Oxygen			
Content, sea level	WB, arterial	17–21 vol%	
	WB, venous (arm)	10–16 vol%	
Saturation, sea level	WB, arterial	97%	0.97 mol/mol
	WB, venous (arm)	60–85%	0.60–0.85 mol/mol
Partial pressure (PO$_2$)	WB	80–100 mm Hg	11–13 kPa
pH	WB	7.38–7.44	
Parathyroid hormone–related peptide	S	<1.3 pmol/liter	<1.3 pmol/liter
Phosphatase			
Acid	S	0–5.5 U/liter	0.90 nkat/liter
Alkaline	S	30–120 U/liter	0.5–2.0 nkat/liter
Phosphorus, inorganic	S	3–4.5 mg/dl	1.0–1.4 mmol/liter
Porphobilinogen	U	None	None

Clinical Chemistry

Analyte	Specimen*	Units Used at MGH	SI Units
Potassium	S	3.5–5.0 mEq/liter	3.5–5.0 mmol/liter
Prealbumin	S	19.5–35.8 mg/dl	195–358 mg/liter
Prostate-specific antigen (PSA)	S		
Female		<0.5 ng/ml	<0.5 µg/liter
Male			
≥40 yr		0–2.0 ng/ml	0–2.0 µg/liter
>40 yr		0–4.0 ng/ml	0–4.0 µg/liter
Prostate-specific antigen (PSA), free (men 45–75 yr with PSA values between 4 and 20 ng/ml)		>25% associated with benign prostatic hyperplasia	>0.25 associated with benign prostatic hyperplasia
Protein			
Total	S	5.5–8.0 g/dl	55–80 g/liter
Fractions	S		
Albumin		3.5–5.5 g/dl (50–60%)	35–55 g/liter
Alpha$_1$		0.2–0.4 g/dl (4.2–7.2%)	2–4 g/liter
Alpha$_2$		0.5–0.9 g/dl (6.8–12%)	5–9 g/liter
Beta		0.6–1.1 g/dl (9.3–15%)	6–11 g/liter
Gamma		0.7–1.7 g/dl (13–23%)	7–17 g/liter
Globulin		2.0–3.5 g/dl (40–50%)	20–35 g/liter
Pyruvate	P, venous	0.5–1.5 mg/dl	60–170 µmol/liter
Sodium	S	136–145 mEq/liter	136–145 mmol/liter
Transferrin	S	230–390 mg/dl	2.3–3.9 g/liter
Triglycerides	S	<160 mg/dl	<1.8 mmol/liter

(table continues on page 768)

GEN MED

TABLE 12.1 Laboratory Reference Values (continued)

Clinical Chemistry

Analyte	Specimen*	Units Used at MGH	SI Units
Troponin			
I	S	0–0.4 ng/ml	0–0.4 μg/liter
T	S	0–0.1 ng/ml	0–0.1 μg/liter
Urea nitrogen	S	10–20 mg/dl	3.6–7.1 mmol/liter
Uric acid	S		
Male		2.5–8.0 mg/dl	150–480 μmol/liter
Female		1.5–6.0 mg/dl	90–360 μmol/liter
Urobilinogen	U	1–3.5 mg/24 hr	1.7–5.9 μmol/24 hr
Vitamin A	S	20–100 μg/dl	0.7–3.5 μmol/liter
Vitamin B_1 (thiamine)	S	0–2 μg/dl	0–75 nmol/liter
Vitamin B_2 (riboflavin)	S	4–24 μg/dl	106–638 nmol/liter
Vitamin B_6	P	5–30 ng/ml	20–121 nmol/liter
Vitamin C (ascorbic acid)	S	0.4–1.0 mg/dl	23–57 μmol/liter
Vitamin D_3 (1,25-dihydroxyvitamin D)	S	25–45 pg/ml	60–108 pmol/liter
Vitamin D_3 (25-hydroxyvitamin D)	P	10–68 ng/ml	24.9–169.5 nmol/liter
Vitamin E	S	5–18 μg/ml	12–42 μmol/liter
Vitamin K	S	0.13–1.19 ng/ml	0.29–2.64 nmol/liter

Metabolic and Endocrine Tests

Analyte	Specimen*	Units Used at MGH	SI Units
Adrenocorticotropin (ACTH)	P	6.0–76.0 pg/ml	1.3–16.7 pmol/liter
Aldosterone	S, P		
Supine, normal-sodium diet		2–9 ng/dl	55–250 pmol/liter

Metabolic and Endocrine Tests

Analyte	Specimen*	Units Used at MGH	SI Units
Upright, normal-sodium diet	S, P	2–5 times supine value with normal-sodium diet	
Supine, low-sodium diet	S, P	2–5 times supine value with normal-sodium diet	
Random, low-sodium diet	U	2.3–21.0 µg/24 hr	6.38–58.25 nmol/24 hr
Androstenedione	S	50–250 ng/dl	1.75–8.73 nmol/liter
Cortisol			
Fasting, 8 a.m.–noon	S	5–25 µg/dl	138–690 nmol/liter
Noon–8 p.m.		5–15 µg/dl	138–414 nmol/liter
8 p.m.–8 a.m.		0–10 µg/dl	0–276 nmol/liter
Cortisol, free	U	20–70 µg/24 hr	55–193 nmol/24 hr
Dehydroepiandrosterone (DHEA)			
Male	S	180–1,250 ng/dl	6.24–41.6 nmol/liter
Female	S	130–980 ng/dl	4.5–34.0 nmol/liter
Dehydroepiandrosterone (DHEA) sulfate			
Male		10–619 µg/dl	100–6,190 µg/liter
Female (premenopausal)		12–535 µg/dl	120–5,350 µg/liter
Female (postmenopausal)		30–260 µg/dl	300–2,600 µg/liter
Deoxycorticosterone (DOC)	S	2–19 ng/dl	61–576 nmol/liter
11-Deoxycortisol (8 a.m.)	S	12–158 ng/dl	0.34–4.56 nmol/liter
Dopamine	P	<87 pg/ml	<475 pmol/liter
	U	65–400 µg/day	425–2,610 nmol/day

(table continues on page 770)

GEN MED

TABLE 12.1 Laboratory Reference Values (continued)

Metabolic and Endocrine Tests

Analyte	Specimen*	Units Used at MGH	SI Units
Epinephrine			
Supine (30 min)	P	<50 pg/ml	<273 pmol/liter
Sitting	P	<60 pg/ml	<328 pmol/liter
Standing (30 min)	P	<900 pg/ml	<4,914 pmol/liter
	U	0–20 µg/day	0–109 nmol/day
Estradiol	S, P		
Female			
Menstruating			
Follicular phase		<20–145 pg/ml	184–532 pmol/liter
Mid-cycle peak		112–443 pg/ml	411–1,626 pmol/liter
Luteal phase		<20–241 pg/ml	184–885 pmol/liter
Postmenopausal		<59 pg/ml	217 pmol/liter
Male		<20 pg/ml	184 pmol/liter
Estrone	S, P		
Female			
Menstruating			
Follicular phase		1.5–15.0 pg/ml	55–555 pmol/liter
Luteal phase		1.5–20.0 pg/ml	55–740 pmol/liter
Postmenopausal		1.5–5.5 pg/ml	55–204 pmol/liter
Male		1.5–6.5 pg/ml	55–240 pmol/liter

Metabolic and Endocrine Tests

Analyte	Specimen*	Units Used at MGH	SI Units
Follicle-stimulating hormone (FSH)	S, P		
Female			
Menstruating			
Follicular phase		3.0–20.0 mIU/ml	3.0–20.0 IU/liter
Ovulatory phase		9.0–26.0 mIU/ml	9.0–26.0 IU/liter
Luteal phase		1.0–12.0 mIU/ml	1.0–12.0 IU/liter
Postmenopausal		18.0–153.0 mIU/ml	18.0–153.0 IU/liter
Male		1.0–12.0 mIU/ml	1.0–12.0 IU/liter
Fructosamine	S	1.61–2.68 mmol/liter	1.61–2.68 mmol/liter
Gastrin	S	<100 pg/ml	<100 ng/liter
Glucagon	P	20–100 pg/ml	20–100 ng/liter
Growth hormone (resting)	S	0.5–17.0 ng/ml	0.5–17.0 µg/liter
Human chorionic gonadotropin (hCG) (nonpregnant women)	S	<5 mIU/ml	<5 IU/liter
17-Hydroxyprogesterone	S		
Male		5–250 ng/dl	0.15 nmol/liter
Female			
Menstruating			
Follicular phase		20–100 ng/dl	0.6–3.0 nmol/liter
Mid-cycle peak		100–250 ng/dl	3.0–7.5 nmol/liter
Luteal phase		100–500 ng/dl	3.0–15 nmol/liter
Postmenopausal		≤70 ng/dl	≤2.1 nmol/liter
5-Hydroxyindoleacetic acid (5-HIAA)	U	<6 mg/24 hr	<31 µmol/24 hr

(table continues on page 772)

GEN MED

GEN MED

TABLE 12.1 Laboratory Reference Values (continued)

Metabolic and Endocrine Tests

Analyte	Specimen*	Units Used at MGH	SI Units
Insulin	S, P	2–20 µU/ml	14.35–143.50 pmol/liter
17-Ketosteroids	U	3–12 mg/24 hr	10–42 µmol/24 hr
Luteinizing hormone (LH)	S, P		
Female			
Menstruating			
Follicular phase		2.0–15.0 mIU/ml	2.0–15.0 IU/liter
Ovulatory phase		22.0–105.0 mIU/ml	22.0–105.0 IU/liter
Luteal phase		0.6–19.0 mIU/ml	0.6–19.0 IU/liter
Postmenopausal		16.0–64.0 mIU/ml	16.0–64.0 IU/liter
Male		2.0–12.0 mIU/ml	2.0–12.0 IU/liter
Metanephrine	P	<0.5 nmol/liter	<0.5 nmol/liter
	U	0.05–1.20 µg/mg creatinine	0.03–0.69 mmol/mol creatinine
Norepinephrine	U	15–80 µg/24 hr	89–473 nmol/24 hr
Norepinephrine	P		
Supine (30 min)		<110–410 pg/ml	650–2,423 pmol/liter
Sitting		120–680 pg/ml	709–4,019 pmol/liter
Standing (30 min)		125–700 pg/ml	739–4,137 pmol/liter
Parathyroid hormone	S	10–60 pg/ml	10–60 ng/liter
Pregnanetriol	U	Age- and sex-dependent	Age- and sex-dependent
Progesterone	S, P		
Menstruating female			
Follicular		<0.2 ng/ml	<0.6 nmol/liter
Midluteal		3–20 ng/ml	9.54–63.6 nmol/liter
Male		<0.2–1.4 ng/ml	<0.60–4.45 nmol/liter

Metabolic and Endocrine Tests

Analyte	Specimen*	Units Used at MGH	SI Units
Prolactin	S		
Female		0–20 ng/ml	0–20 µg/liter
Male		0–15 ng/ml	0–15 µg/liter
Serotonin	WB	50–200 ng/ml	0.28–1.14 µmol/liter
	Platelets	125–500 ng/10⁹ platelets	0.7–2.8 amol/platelet
Sex hormone–binding globulin	S		
Male		13–71 nmol/liter	13–71 nmol/liter
Female		18–114 nmol/liter	18–114 nmol/liter
Somatostatin	P	<25 pg/ml	<25 ng/liter
Somatomedin C (insulin-like growth factor I [IGF-I])	S		
16–24 yr		182–780 ng/ml	182–780 µg/liter
25–39 yr		114–492 ng/ml	114–492 µg/liter
40–54 yr		90–360 ng/ml	90–360 µg/liter
>54 yr		71–290 ng/ml	71–290 µg/liter
Testosterone	S		
Total, morning			
Female		6–86 ng/dl	0.21–2.98 nmol/liter
Male		270–1,070 ng/dl	9.36–37.10 nmol/liter
Unbound, morning			
Female		0.2–3.1 pg/ml	6.9–107.5 pmol/liter
Male		12.0–40.0 pg/ml	416–1,387 pmol/liter

(table continues on page 774)

GEN MED

GEN MED

TABLE 12.1 Laboratory Reference Values (continued)

Metabolic and Endocrine Tests

Analyte	Specimen*	Units Used at MGH	SI Units
Thyroglobulin	S	0–60 ng/ml	0–60 µg/liter
Thyroid-binding globulin	S	16–24 µg/ml	206–309 nmol/liter
Thyroid-stimulating hormone	S	0.5–4.7 µU/ml	0.5–4.7 µU/liter
Thyroxine	S		
Total (T₄)		4.5–10.9 µg/dl	58–140 nmol/liter
Free (fT₄)		0.8–2.7 ng/dl	10.3–35.0 pmol/liter
Triiodothyronine	S		
Total (T₃)		60–181 ng/dl	0.92–2.78 nmol/liter
Free (fT₃)		1.4–4.4 pg/ml	0.22–6.78 pmol/liter
Vanillylmandelic acid (VMA)	U	0.15–1.20 mg/24 hr	7.6–37.9 µmol/24 hr
Vasoactive intestinal polypeptide (VIP)	P	<75 pg/ml	<75 ng/liter

Therapeutic Drug Monitoring and Toxicology

Drug	Therapeutic Level		Toxic Level	
	Units Used at MGH	SI Units	Units Used at MGH	SI Units
Acetaminophen	10–30 µg/ml	66–199 µmol/liter	>200 µg/ml	>1,324 µmol/liter
Amikacin				
Peak	25–35 µg/ml	43–60 µmol/liter	>35 µg/ml	>60 µmol/liter
Trough	4–8 µg/ml	6.8–13.7 µmol/liter	>10 µg/ml	>17 µmol/liter
Amitriptyline	120–250 ng/ml	433–903 nmol/liter	>500 ng/ml	>1,805 nmol/liter
Amphetamine	20–30 ng/ml	148–222 nmol/liter	>200 ng/ml	>1,480 nmol/liter

Therapeutic Drug Monitoring and Toxicology

Drug	Therapeutic Level		Toxic Level	
	Units Used at MGH	SI Units	Units Used at MGH	SI Units
Barbiturates, most short-acting			>20 mg/liter	>88 μmol/liter
Bromide			>1,250 μg/ml	>15.6 mmol/liter
Carbamazepine	6–12 μg/ml	26–51 μmol/liter	>15 μg/ml	>63 μmol/liter
Chlordiazepoxide	700–1,000 ng/ml	2.34–3.34 μmol/liter	>5,000 ng/ml	>16.7 μmol/liter
Clonazepam	15–60 ng/ml	48–190 nmol/liter	>80 ng/ml	>254 nmol/liter
Clozapine	200–350 ng/ml	0.6–1.0 μmol/liter		
Cocaine			>1,000 ng/ml	>3,300 nmol/liter
Cyclosporine	Varies with time after dose and type of transplantation, with ranges of 100–400 ng/ml	Varies with time after dose and type of transplantation, with ranges of 83–333 nmol/liter	Varies with time after dose and type of transplantation	Varies with time after dose and type of transplantation
Desipramine	75–300 ng/ml	281–1,125 nmol/liter	>400 ng/ml	>1,500 nmol/liter
Diazepam	100–1,000 ng/ml	0.35–3.51 μmol/liter	>5,000 ng/ml	>17.55 μmol/liter
Digoxin	0.8–2.0 ng/ml	1.0–2.6 nmol/liter	>2.5 ng/ml	>3.2 nmol/liter
Doxepin	30–150 ng/ml	107–537 nmol/liter	>500 ng/ml	>1790 nmol/liter
Ethanol			>300 mg/dl	>65 mmol/liter
Behavioral changes			>20 mg/dl	>4.3 mmol/liter
Clinical intoxication			>100 mg/dl	>1 g/liter
Ethosuximide	40–100 μg/ml	283–708 μmol/liter	>150 μg/ml	>1,062 μmol/liter
Flecainide	0.2–1.0 μg/ml	0.5–2.4 μmol/liter	>1.0 μg/ml	>2.4 μmol/liter

(table continues on page 776)

GEN MED

GEN MED

TABLE 12.1 Laboratory Reference Values (continued)

Therapeutic Drug Monitoring and Toxicology

Drug	Therapeutic Level		Toxic Level	
	Units Used at MGH	SI Units	Units Used at MGH	SI Units
Gentamicin				
Peak	8–10 µg/ml	16.7–20.9 µmol/liter	>10 µg/ml	>21.0 µmol/liter
Trough	<2–4 µg/ml	<4.2–8.4 µmol/liter	>4 µg/ml	>8.4 µmol/liter
Ibuprofen	10–50 µg/ml	49–243 µmol/liter	100–700 µg/ml	485–3,395 µmol/liter
Imipramine	125–250 ng/ml	446–893 nmol/liter	>500 ng/ml	>1,784 nmol/liter
Lidocaine	1.5–6.0 µg/ml	6.4–26 µmol/liter	6–8 µg/ml	26–34.2 µmol/liter
Central nervous system or cardiovascular depression				
Seizures, obtundation, decreased cardiac output			>8 µg/ml	>34.2 µmol/liter
Lithium	0.6–1.2 mEq/liter	0.6–1.2 nmol/liter	>2 mEq/liter	>2 mmol/liter
Methadone	100–400 ng/ml	0.32–1.29 µmol/liter	>2,000 ng/ml	>6.46 µmol/liter
Methotrexate	Variable	Variable		
1–2 wk after low dose			>9.1 ng/ml	>20 nmol/liter
48 hr after high dose			>227 ng/ml	>0.5 µmol/liter
Morphine	10–80 ng/ml	35–280 nmol/liter	>200 ng/ml	>700 nmol/liter
Nortriptyline	50–170 ng/ml	190–646 nmol/liter	>500 ng/ml	>1.9 µmol/liter
Phenobarbital	10–40 µg/ml	43–170 µmol/liter		
Slowness, ataxia, nystagmus			35–80 µg/ml	151–345 µmol/liter
Coma with reflexes			65–117 µg/ml	280–504 µmol/liter
Coma without reflexes			>100 µg/ml	>430 µmol/liter

Therapeutic Drug Monitoring and Toxicology

Drug	Therapeutic Level		Toxic Level	
	Units Used at MGH	SI Units	Units Used at MGH	SI Units
Phenytoin	10–20 μg/ml	40–79 μmol/liter	>20 μg/ml	>79 μmol/liter
Procainamide	4–10 μg/ml	17–42 μmol/liter	>10–12 μg/ml	>42–51 μmol/liter
Quinidine	2–5 μg/ml	6–15 μmol/liter	>6 μg/ml	>18 μmol/liter
Salicylates	150–300 μg/ml	1,086–2,172 μmol/liter	>300 μg/ml	>2,172 μmol/liter
Theophylline	8–20 μg/ml	44–111 μmol/liter	>20 μg/ml	>110 μmol/liter
Thiocyanate				
After nitroprusside infusion	6–29 μg/ml	103–499 μmol/liter	>120 μg/ml	>2,064 μmol/liter
Nonsmoker	1–4 μg/ml	17–69 μmol/liter		
Smoker	3–12 μg/ml	52–206 μmol/liter		
Tobramycin				
Peak	8–10 μg/ml	17–21 μmol/liter	>10 μg/ml	>21 μmol/liter
Trough	<4 μg/ml	<9 μmol/liter	>4 μg/ml	>9 μmol/liter
Valproic acid	50–150 μg/ml	347–1,040 μmol/liter	>150 μg/ml	>1,040 μmol/liter
Vancomycin				
Peak	18–26 μg/ml	12–18 μmol/liter	>80–100 μg/ml	>55–69 μmol/liter
Trough	5–10 μg/ml	3–7 μmol/liter		

(table continues on page 778)

GEN MED

TABLE 12.1 Laboratory Reference Values (continued)

Urine Analysis

Analyte	Units Used at MGH	SI Units
Acidity, titratable	20–40 mEq/24 hr	20–40 mmol/24 hr
Ammonia	30–50 mEq/24 hr	30–50 mmol/24 hr
Amylase	4–400 U/liter	0.07–7.67 nkat/liter
Amylase:creatinine clearance ratio‡	1–5	1–5
Calcium (with dietary calcium 10 mEq/24 hr or 200 mg/24 hr)	<300 mg/24 hr	<7.5 mmol/24 hr
Creatine, as creatinine		
Female	<100 mg/24 hr	<760 µmol/24 hr
Male	<50 mg/24 hr	<380 µmol/24 hr
Creatinine	1.0–1.6 g/24 hr	8.8–14 mmol/24 hr
Eosinophils	<100 eosinophils/ml	<100 eosinophils/ml
Glucose, true (oxidase method)	50–300 mg/24 hr	0.3–1.7 mmol/24 hr
Microalbumin	0–2.0 mg/dl	0–0.02 g/liter
Oxalate	2–60 mg/24 hr	228–684 µmol/24 hr
pH	5.0–9.0	5.0–9.0
Phosphate (phosphorus)	400–1,300 mg/24 hr (varies with intake)	12.9–42.0 mmol/24 hr (varies with intake)
Potassium	25–100 mEq/24 hr (varies with intake)	25–100 mmol/24 hr (varies with intake)
Protein	<150 mg/24 hr	<0.15 g/24 hr
Sediment		
Bacteria	Negative	Negative
Bladder cells	Negative	Negative

Urine Analysis

Analyte	Units Used at MGH	SI Units
Broad casts	Negative	Negative
Crystals	Negative	Negative
Epithelial-cell casts	Negative	Negative
Granular casts	Negative	Negative
Hyaline casts	0–5/low-power field	0–5/low-power field
Red-cell casts	Negative	Negative
Red cells	0–2/high-power field	0–2/high-power field
Squamous cells	Negative	Negative
Tubular cells	Negative	Negative
Waxy casts	Negative	Negative
White cells	0–2/high-power field	0–2/high-power field
White-cell casts	Negative	Negative
Sodium	100–260 mEq/24 hr (varies with intake)	100–260 mmol/24 hr (varies with intake)
Specific gravity	1.001–1.035	1.001–1.035
Urea nitrogen	6–17 g/24 hr	214–607 mmol/24 hr
Uric acid (with normal diet)	250–800 mg/24 hr	1.49–4.76 mmol/24 hr

(table continues on page 780)

GEN MED

TABLE 12.1 Laboratory Reference Values (continued)

Microbiology

Specimen	Routinely Cultured For	Also Reported	Normal Flora
Throat	Group A beta-hemolytic strepto-cocci, pyogenic groups C and G betahemolytic streptococci, *Arcanobacterium haemolyticum*	If complete throat culture is re-quested: *Haemophilus influen-zae, Staphylococcus aureus, Streptococcus pneumoniae, Neisseria meningitidis,* and yeast	Alpha-hemolytic streptococci, non-hemolytic streptococci, diph-theroids, coagulase-negative staphylococci, saprophytic neisseria
Sputum	Pneumococci, *H. Influenzae*, beta-hemolytic streptococci, *Staph. aureus, Moraxella (Branhamella) catarrhalis*, gram-negative bacilli	Presence or absence of normal throat flora	Little or no normal throat flora, if specimen carefully collected
Urine	Aerobic bacteria and yeast: "abundant" if >10^5 colony-forming units/ml, "moderate" if 10^4–10^5 colony-forming units/ml	"Few" if 10^3–10^4 colony-forming units/ml, "rare" if 10^2–10^3 colony-forming units/ml (either may indi-cate clinically significant bacteriuria if accompanied by pyuria, clinical symptoms, or both)	No mixed bacterial species (i.e., not more than one of the following: lactobacilli, non-beta-hemolytic streptococci, diphtheroids, coagulase-negative staphylococci, or *Gardnerella vaginalis*) if speci-men carefully collected
Blood	Aerobic bacteria, anaerobic bacteria, yeasts		None: common contaminants: aero-bic diphtheroids, anaerobic diph-theroids, coagulase-negative staphylococci
Cerebrospinal fluid and other fluids	Aerobic bacteria, anaerobic bacteria, yeasts (including cryptococcus)	Any organism isolated	None

Microbiology

Specimen	Routinely Cultured For	Also Reported	Normal Flora
Stool	Enteric pathogens: salmonella, shigella, campylobacter, plesiomonas, and aeromonas when predominant	Moderate or abundant yeast or *Staph. aureus*; presence or absence of normal gram-negative enteric flora; if special cultures requested, yersinia, *Vibrio cholerae, V. Parahemolyticus, V. Parahemolyticus,* or hemorrhagic strains of *Escherichia coli* (O157)	Enterobacteriaceae, streptococci, pseudomonas, small numbers of staphylococci and yeast (and anaerobes that are not routinely cultured)
Wounds	Aerobic bacteria, anaerobic bacteria, yeasts	Yeasts and enteric gram-negative rods if present in large numbers	
Cervical or vaginal	Gonococci, group A beta-hemolytic streptococci, pyogenic groups C and G beta-hemolytic streptococci, *Staph. aureus* (Gram's stain for diagnosis of bacterial vaginosis according to Nugent score)		

From Kratz, A, et al: Normal reference laboratory values. *N Engl J Med 351:*1548–1563, 2004, with permission

* WB denotes whole blood, P plasma, S serum, PRP platelet-rich plasma, U urine, and JF joint fluid, and RC red cells.
† The creatine kinase relative index is calculated as [MB isoenzyme (in nanograms per milliliter)÷total creatine kinase (in units per liter)]×100.
‡ The amylase:creatinine clearance ratio is calculated as [amylase clearance÷creatinine clearance]×100.

GEN MED

TABLE 12.2 Common Laboratory Tests and Their Disease Associations

Laboratory Test	Increase	Decrease
Acid phosphatase	Prostatic carcinoma, postprostatic massage, prostatitis, myocardial infarction, excess platelet destruction, bone disease, liver disease	
Alanine aminotrans-ferase (ALT or SGPT)	Hepatitis, cirrhosis, liver metastases, obstructive jaundice, infectious mononucleosis, hepatic congestion, pancreatitis, renal disease, ethanol ingestion	Pyridoxine (vitamin B_6) deficiency
Albumin	Dehydration, diabetes insipidus	Overhydration, malnu-trition, malabsorption, nephrosis, hepatic failure, burns, multiple myeloma, meta-static carcinomas
Alkaline phosphatase	Bone growth, bone metas-tases, Paget's disease, rickets, healing fracture, hyperparathyroidism, hepatic disease, obstructive jaundice, hepatic metastases, pulmonary infarction, heart failure, pregnancy	Pernicious anemia, hypoparathyroidism, hypophosphatasia
α-Fetoprotein	Hepatoma, testicular tumor, hepatitis	
Amylase	Pancreatitis, GI obstruc-tion, mesenteric throm-bosis and infarction, macroamylasemia, parotitis, mumps, renal disease, ruptured tubal pregnancy, lung carci-noma, acute ethanol ingestion, postoperative abdominal surgery	Marked pancreatic destruction

GEN MED

Laboratory Test	Increase	Decrease
Aspartate amino-transferase (AST or SGOT)	Myocardial infarction, heart failure, myocarditis, pericarditis, myositis, muscular dystrophy, trauma, hepatic disease, pancreatitis, renal infarct, eclampsia, neoplasia, cerebral damage, seizures, hemolysis, ethanol intake	Pyridoxine (vitamin B_6) deficiency, terminal stage of liver disease
B-type natriuretic peptide	Heart failure, acute coronary syndromes, pulmonary hypertension, valvular heart disease	
Bilirubin	Hepatic disease, obstructive jaundice, hemolytic anemia, pulmonary infarct, Gilbert's disease, Dubin-Johnson syndrome, neonatal jaundice	
Calcium	Hyperparathyroidism, bone metastases, myeloma, sarcoidosis, hyperthyroidism, hypervitaminosis D, malignancy without bone metastases, milk-alkali syndrome	Hypoparathyroidism, renal failure, malabsorption, pancreatitis, hypoalbuminemia, vitamin D deficiency, overhydration
Cholesterol	Hyperlipidemia (dyslipidemia), hypothyroidism, obstructive jaundice, nephrosis, diabetes mellitus, pancreatitis, pregnancy, familial factors, steroid use	Hyperthyroidism, infection, malnutrition, heart failure, malignancies, severe liver damage (due to chemicals, drugs, hepatitis)
HDL cholesterol	Vigorous exercise, increased clearance of triglyceride (VLDL), moderate ethanol consumption, insulin, estrogens	Dyslipidemia, starvation, obesity, cigarette smoking, diabetes mellitus, hypothyroidism, liver disease, nephrosis, uremia

GEN MED

(table continues on page 784)

◼ TABLE 12.2 Common Laboratory Tests and Their Disease Associations (continued)

Laboratory Test	Increase	Decrease
C-Reactive protein	Infection, myocardial infarction, oral contraceptives, pregnancy, rheumatoid arthritis, inflammatory bowel disease, other inflammatory states	
Creatine kinase	Myocardial infarction, muscle disease, burns, chest trauma, collagen-vascular disease, meningitis, drugs (e.g., lovastatin), burns, status epilepticus, brain infarction, hyperthermia, postoperative increase	
Creatinine	Renal failure, urinary obstruction, dehydration, hyperthyroidism, diet, muscle disease	Aging
Glucose	Diabetes mellitus, IV glucose, thiazides, corticosteroids, pheochromocytoma, hyperthyroidism, Cushing's syndrome, acromegaly, brain damage, hepatic disease, nephrosis, hemochromatosis, stress (e.g., emotion, burns, shock, anesthesia), acute or chronic pancreatitis, Wernicke's encephalopathy (vitamin B_1 deficiency), epinephrine, estrogens, ethanol, phenytoin, propranolol, chronic hyper-vitaminosis A	Excess insulin, insulinoma, Addison's disease, myxedema, hepatic failure, malabsorption, pancreatitis, glucagon deficiency, extrapancreatic tumors, early diabetes mellitus, postgastrectomy, autonomic nervous system disorders, idiopathic leucine sensitivity, enzyme diseases (von Gierke's disease, fructose intolerance), oral hypoglycemic medications (factitious), malnutrition, alcoholism
Glycosylated Hemoglobin or hemoglobin A1c	Diabetes mellitus, iron deficiency anemia, alcoholism, and hypertriglyceridemia	Hemolytic anemia, chronic renal failure, insulinoma, hemoglobin S, C, D disease

GEN MED

Laboratory Test	Increase	Decrease
Lactate dehydrogenase (LDH)	Myocardial infarction, pulmonary infarction, hemolytic anemia, pernicious anemia, leukemia, lymphoma, other malignancies, hepatic disease, renal infarction, seizures, cerebral damage, trauma, sprue	
Lipase	Same as amylase (except not in parotitis, mumps), macroamylasemia	
Magnesium	Renal disease, excess Mg (IV or PO)	Diarrhea, malabsorption, renal tubular acidosis, acute tubular necrosis, chronic glomerulonephritis, drugs (diuretics, antibiotics), aldosteronism, hyperthyroidism, hypercalcemia, uncontrolled diabetes, nutritional deficit
Phosphorus	Renal failure, hypoparathyroidism, diabetic acidosis, acromegaly, hyperthyroidism, high phosphate intake (IV or PO), vitamin D intoxication, lactic acidosis, cell lysis, leukemia, volume contraction, spurious, prolonged refrigeration of sample, heparin sodium contamination, hyperbilirubinemia, hyperlipidemia, dysproteinemia	Hyperparathyroidism, osteomalacia, rickets, Fanconi's syndrome, cirrhosis, hypokalemia, excess IV glucose, respiratory alkalosis, dietary deprivation, P-binding antacid, alcoholism, gout, hemodialysis, renal failure, hypoparathyroidism, diabetic acidosis, acromegaly, hyperthyroidism, high phosphate intake (IV or PO), vitamin D intoxication, lactic acidosis, cell lysis, leukemia, volume contraction, spurious, prolonged refrigeration of sample, heparin sodium contamination, hyperbilirubinemia, hyperlipidemia, dysproteinemia

GEN MED

(table continues on page 786)

TABLE 12.2 Common Laboratory Tests and Their Disease Associations (continued)

Laboratory Test	Increase	Decrease
Potassium	Hyperkalemic acidosis, diabetic acidosis, hypoadrenalism, hereditary hyperkalemia, hemolysis, myoglobinuria, K-retaining diuretic, ACE inhibitors, large exogenous K load, renal tubular defect, thrombocytosis	Cirrhosis, malnutrition, vomiting, metabolic alkalosis, diarrhea, nephrosis, diuretics, hyperadrenalism, familial periodic paralysis, ectopic ACTH excess, β-hydroxylase deficiency
Sedimentation rate or erythrocyte sedimentation rate	Infection, inflammatory states, collagen vascular disease, myocardial infarction, hyperthyroidism and hypothyroidism	Sickle cell disease, steroids
Sodium	Dehydration, diabetes insipidus, excessive salt ingestion, diabetes mellitus with diuresis, diuretic phase of acute tubular necrosis, hypercalcemic nephropathy with diuresis, "essential" hypernatremia due to hypothalamic lesions	Excess antidiuretic hormone, nephrosis, hypoadrenalism, myxedema, heart failure, diarrhea, vomiting, diabetic acidosis, diuretics, adrenocortical insufficiency, spurious (serum osmolality is normal or increased—avoid by using direct-reading potentiometry with ion-selective electrode); hyperlipidemia (serum Na decreases by 1 mmol/L per every 4.6 g/L increase in lipid), hyperglycemia (serum Na decreases 3 mEq/L per every 100 mg/dL increase of serum glucose), mannitol, hyperproteinemia (e.g., multiple myeloma)
Total protein	Multiple myeloma, myxedema, lupus, sarcoidosis, diabetes insipidus, dehydration, collagen disease	Burns, cirrhosis, malnutrition, nephrosis, malabsorption, overhydration, GI protein loss

GEN MED

Laboratory Test	Increase	Decrease
Triglyceride	Nephrosis, cholestasis, pancreatitis, cirrhosis, diabetes mellitus, hepatitis, dietary excess, hereditary	Malnutrition
Urea nitrogen	Renal disease, dehydration, GI bleeding, leukemia, heart failure, shock, postrenal azotemia, any obstruction of urinary tract (BUN:creatinine >10:1), acute myocardial infarction	Hepatic failure, overhydration, pregnancy, acromegaly, diet, IV feedings only
Uric acid	Gout, renal failure, diuretic therapy, leukemia, lymphoma, polycythemia, acidosis, psoriasis, hypothyroidism, eclampsia, multiple myeloma, pernicious anemia, tissue necrosis, inflammation, 25% of relatives of patients with gout, cancer chemotherapy (e.g., nitrogen mustards, vincristine, mercaptopurine), hemolytic anemia, sickle cell anemia, high-protein weight-reduction diet, lead poisoning, Lesch-Nyhan syndrome, polycystic kidneys, calcinosis universalis and circumscripta, hypoparathyroidism, sarcoidosis, elevated serum triglycerides	Uricosuric drugs, allopurinol, Wilson's disease, large doses of vitamin C, Fanconi's syndrome, xanthinuria

Based on: *Ferri's Clinical Advisor 2012.* Copyright 2011, Mosby, an imprint of Elsevier Inc.

ACE = angiotensin converting enzyme; ACTH = adrenocorticotropin; BUN = blood urea nitrogen; HDL = high-density lipoprotein

GEN MED

GEN MED

TABLE 12.3 Urine and Blood Changes in Electrolytes, pH, and Volume in Various Conditions

Condition	Blood Sodium	Potassium	Bicarbonate	Chloride	Volume
Acute Renal Failure	D	I	D	I	I
Chronic Renal Failure	D	N or D	D	D or N	V
Renal Tubular Acidosis	D	D	D	I	D
Thiazide Administration	D	D	D	D	D
Diabetic Acidosis	D	N or I	D	D	D
Diabetes Insipidus	N or I	N	N	I	D
Adrenal Cortical	D	I	N or D	D	D
Primary Aldosteronism	I	D	I	D	N
Salicylate Intoxication	N	N or D	D	I	N
Malabsorption	D	D	N or D	N	D
Starvation	N	D	D	N	N or D
Dehydration	I	N	N or D	I	D
Pyloric Obstruction	D	D	I	D	D
Diarrhea	D	D	D	D	D
Excessive Sweating	D	N	N	D	N
Congestive Heart Failure	N or D	N	N	D	I
Pulmonary Emphysema	N	N	I	D	N or 5I

Measurement	Urine Sodium	Potassium	pH	Volume
Acute Renal Failure	D	D	N or I	D
Chronic Renal Failure	I	I	I	V*
Renal Tubular Acidosis	I	I	I	I
Thiazide Administration	I	I	N or I	I
Diabetic Acidosis	I	I	D	I
Diabetes Insipidus	N	N	N	I
Adrenal Cortical	I	N or D	N or I	N or D
Primary Aldosteronism	D	N or I	N or D	I
Salicylate Intoxication	I	N or I	I	N
Malabsorption	N or I	D	N or D	N
Starvation	D	I or N	D	I
Dehydration	I	I	D	D
Pyloric Obstruction	D	N	I	D
Diarrhea	D	N or D	D	D
Excessive Sweating	D	N	N	N
Congestive Heart Failure	D	N	N	D
Pulmonary Emphysema	D	N	D	N

As appearing in *The Merck Manual*, ed. 16. Merck & Co., Rahway, NJ, 1992, p 2579. Based on Wallach, J: *Interpretation of Diagnostic Tests*. ed. 4. Little, Brown, Boston, 1986, with permission.

N = normal; D = decreased; I = increased; V = variable.

*Usually increased.

GEN MED

Infectious Disease

Bacterial Infections & Antimicrobial Therapy

● TABLE 12.4 Types of Bacteria

Type	Principal Features	Common Examples
Gram-positive bacilli	Generally rod shaped; retain color when treated by Gram's method of staining	*Bacillus anthracis, Clostridium tetani*
Gram-negative bacilli	Rod shaped; do not retain color of Gram's method	*Escherichia coli, Klebsiella pneumoniae, Pseudomonas aeruginosa*
Gram-positive cocci	Generally spherical or ovoid in shape; retain color of Gram's method	*Staphylococcus aureus, Streptococcus pneumoniae*
Gram-negative cocci	Spherical or ovoid; do not retain color of Gram's method	*Neisseria gonorrhoeae* (gonococcus), *Neisseria meningitidis* (meningococcus)
Acid-fast bacilli	Rod shaped; retain color of certain stains even when treated with acid	*Mycobacterium leprae, Mycobacterium tuberculosis*
Spirochetes	Slender, spiral shape; able to move about without flagella (intrinsic locomotor ability)	Lyme disease agent; *Treponema pallidum* (syphilis)
Actinomycetes	Thin filaments that stain positively by Gram's method	*Actinomyces israelii; Nocandia*
Others Mycoplasmas	Spherical; lack the rigid, highly structured cell wall found in most bacteria	*Mycoplasma pneumoniae*
Rickettsias	Small, gram-negative bacteria	*Rickettsia typhi, Rickettsia rickettsii*

From: Ciccone, CD: *Pharmacology in Rehabilitation*, ed. 3. FA Davis, Philadelphia, 2002, p 539, with permission.

● TABLE 12.5 Treatment of Common Infections Caused by Gram-Positive Bacilli

Bacillus	Disease	Primary Agent(s)	Alternative Agent(s)
Bacillus anthracis	Anthrax; pneumonia	Penicillin G	Doxycycline, erythromycin; a tetracycline; a cephalosporin; chloramphenicol
Clostridium difficile	Antibiotic-associated colitis	Metronidazole	Vancomycin
Clostridium perfringens	Gas gangrene	Penicillin G	A cephalosporin; clindamycin; doxycycline, imipenem; chloramphenicol
Clostridium tetani	Tetanus	Penicillin G, vancomycin	Clindamycin, doxycycline
Corynebacterium diphtheriae	Pharyngitis; laryngotra-cheitis; pneumonia; other local lesions	Erythromycin	A cephalosporin; clindamycin; rifampin
Corynebacterium species	Endocarditis; infections in various other tissues	Penicillin G ± an amino-glycoside; vancomycin	Rifampin + penicillin G; ampicillin-sulbactam
Erysipelothrix rhusiopathiae	Erysipeloid	Penicillin G	Chloramphenicol; doxycycline; erythromycin
Listeria monocyto-genes	Bacteremia; meningitis	Ampicillin or penicillin G ± gentamicin	Trimethoprim-sulfamethoxazole; chloramphenicol; erythromycin

Based on: Gilbert, D, et al: *The Sanford Guide to Antimicrobial Therapy*, ed. 41. Antimicrobial Therapy Inc., Sperryville, VA, 2011.

GEN MED

◼ **TABLE 12.6 Treatment of Common Infections Caused by Gram-Negative Bacilli**

Bacillus	Disease	Primary Agent(s)	Alternative Agent(s)
Acinetobacter	Infections in various tissues; hospital-acquired infections	An aminogly-coside; imipenem	A cephalosporin, trimethoprim-sulfanethoxazole
Brucella	Brucellosis	Doxycycline + gentamicin; doxycycline + rifampin; trimethoprim + rifampin	Chloramphenicol; trimethoprim-sulfamethoxazole ± gentamicin
Calymmato-bacterium granulomatis	Granuloma inguinale	Doxycycline	Trimethoprim-sulfamethoxazole
Campylobacter fetus	Bacteremia; endocarditis; meningitis	Ampicillin; gentamicin	Ceftriaxone; chloramphenicol; ciprofloxacin or ofloxacin; imipenem
Campylobacter jejuni	Enteritis	Ciprofloxacin or ofloxacin	Azithromycin or clarithromycin; clindamycin; erythromycin
Enterobacter species	Urinary tract and other infections	An aminogly-coside; imipenem	Ciproflozacin or ofloxacin; a broad spectrum penicillin; trimethoprim-sulfamethoxazole
Escherichia coli	Bacteremia; urinary tract infections; infections in other tissues	Ampicillinan ± an aminogly-coside; a cephalosporin; ciprofloxacin ofloxacin; trimethoprim-sulfamethoxa-zole	An aminoglycoside, aztreonam; doxycycline; nitrofurantoin; a penicillin + a penicllinase inhibitor
Flavobacterium meningosep-ticum	Meningitis	Vancomycin	Trimethoprim-sulfamethoxazole; rifampin

GEN MED

Bacillus	Disease	Primary Agent(s)	Alternative Agent(s)
Francisella tularensis	Tularemia	Gentamicin or streptomycin	Chloramphenicol; ciprofloxacin; doxycycline
Fusobacterium nucleatum	Empyema; genital infections; gingivitis; lung abscesses; ulcerative pharyngitis	Penicillin G; clindamycin	Cefoxitin; a cephalosporin; metronidazole; chloramphenicol; erythromycin; doxycycline
Haemophilus ducreyi	Chancroid	Ceftriaxone; erythromycin; trimethoprim-sulfamethoxazole	Ciprofloxacin; doxycycline; a sulfonamide
Haemophilus influenzae	Epiglottitis, meningitis	Ceftriaxone or cefotaxime; chloramphenicol	Ampicillin-sulbactam; trimethoprim-sulfamethoxazole
Haemophilus influenzae	Otitis media; pneumonia, sinusitis	Amoxicillin-clavulanate; trimethoprim-sulfamethoxazole	Amoxicillin or ampicillin; azithromycin; cefuroxime; ciprofloxacin
Klebsiella pneumoniae	Pneumonia; urinary tract infection	A cephalosporin ± an aminoglycoside	Ciprofloxacin or ofloxacin; mezlocillin or piperacillin; aztreonam; trimethoprim-sulfamethoxazole; a penicillin + a penicillinase inhibitor imipenem
Legionella pneumophila	Legionnaires' disease	Erythromycin ± rifampin	Azithromycin or clarithromycin; ciprofloxacin; trimethoprim-sulfamethoxazole
Pasteurella multocida	Abscesses; bacteremia; meningitis; wound infections (animal bites)	Penicillin G; amoxicillin-clavulanate	A cephalosporin-doxycycline

(table continues on page 794)

GEN MED

⬤ TABLE 12.6 Treatment of Common Infections Caused by Gram-Negative Bacilli (continued)

Bacillus	Disease	Primary Agent(s)	Alternative Agent(s)
Proteus mirabilis	Urinary tract and other infections	Ampicillin or amoxicillin	An aminoglycoside; a cephalosporin; ciprofloxacin or ofloxacin
Proteus, other species	Urinary tract and other infections	An aminoglycoside; a cephalosporin	Aztreonam; imipenem; penicillin + a beta-lactamase inhibitor
Pseudomonas aeruginosa	Urinary tract infection	Ceftazidime; ciprofloxacin or ofloxacin; a broad-spectrum penicillin	An aminoglycoside; aztreonam; imipenem or meropenem
Pseudomonas aeruginosa	Bacteremia; pneumonia	A broad-spectrum penicillin ± an aminoglycoside	Ciprofloxacin + broad-spectrum penicillin or an aminoglycoside; ceftazidime + an aminoglycoside; aztreonam + an aminoglycoside; imipenem + aminoglycoside
Pseudomonas mallei	Glanders	Streptomycin + tetracycline	Streptomycin + chloramphenicol
Pseudomonas pseudomallei	Melioidosis	Ceftazidime of ceftriaxone; trimethoprim-sulfamethoxazole	Chloramphenicol; imipenem
Salmonella	Acute gastroenteritis	Ciprofloxacin or norfloxacin	Ampicillin; trimethoprim-sulfamethoxazole
Salmonella	Bacteremia; paratyphoid fever; typhoid fever	Ceftriaxone; ciprofloxacin or ofloxacin; trimethoprim-sulfamethoxazole	Ampicillin; chloramphenicol

GEN MED

Bacillus	Disease	Primary Agent(s)	Alternative Agent(s)
Serratia	Various opportunistic and hospital-acquired infections	Cefoxitin, cefotetan, or third-generation cephalosporin; imipenem; a broad-spectrum penicillin + an aminoglycoside	Aztreonam; piperacillin-tazobactam or ticarcillin-clavulanate
Shigella	Acute gastroenteritis	Ciprofloxacin or norfloxacin	Ampicillin; trimethoprim-sulfamethoxazole
Streptobacillus moniliformis	Abscesses; bacteremia; endocarditis	Penicillin G	Streptomycin; a tetracycline; chloramphenicol; erythromycin
Vibrio cholerae	Cholera	Ciprofloxacin or ofloxacin; doxycycline	Chloramphenicol; trimethoprim-sulfamethoxazole
Yersinia enterocolitica	Sepsis, yersiniosis	An aminoglycoside; chloramphenicol; trimethoprim-sulfamethoxazole	A cephalosporin; ciprofloxacin or ofloxacin
Yersinia pestis	Plague	Streptomycin ± a tetracycline	Chloramphenicol; ciprofloxacin; ofloxacin

GEN MED

Based on: Gilbert, D, et al: *The Sanford Guide to Antimicrobial Therapy,* ed. 41. Antimicrobial Therapy Inc., Sperryville, VA, 2011.

TABLE 12.7 Treatment of Common Infections Caused by Gram-Positive and Gram-Negative Cocci

Gram-Positive Coccus	Disease	Primary Agent(s)	Alternative Agent(s)
Enterococcus	Endocarditis or other serious infections (bacteremia)	Gentamicin + penicillin G or ampicillin	Vancomycin + gentamicin
Enterococcus	Urinary tract infection	Ampicillin or penicillin	Ciprofloxacin; vancomycin
Staphylococcus aureus	Abscesses; bacteremia; endocarditis; osteomyelitis; pneumonia		A cephalosporin; clindamycin; erythromycin; other combinations
Streptococcus agalactiae (group B)	Meningitis; bacteremia; endocarditis	Ampicillin or penicillin G ± an aminoglycoside	A cephalosporin; chloramphenicol; vancomycin
Streptococcus bovis	Bacteremia; endocarditis	Penicillin G ± gentamicin	Ceftriaxone; vancomycin
Streptococcus pneumoniae	Arthritis; otitis; pneumonia; sinusitis	If penicillin sensitive: amoxicillin; penicillin. If penicillin resistant: ceftriaxone or cefotaxime; penicillin (large doses); vancomycin	A cephalosporin; chloramphenicol; clindamycin; trimethoprim-sulfamethoxazole; a macrolide
Streptococcus pyogenes (group A)	Bacteremia; cellulitis; pharyngitis; pneumonia; scarlet fever; other local and systemic infections	amoxicillin; penicillin	A cephalosporin; clindamycin; erythromycin; vancomycin

GEN MED

Gram-Positive Coccus	Disease	Primary Agent(s)	Alternative Agent(s)
Streptococcus (anaerobic species)	Bacteremia; brain and other abscesses; endocarditis; sinusitis	Penicillin G	A cephalosporin; clindamycin; chloramphenicol; erythromycin
Streptococcus (*viridans* group)	Bacteremia; endocarditis	Penicillin G ± gentamicin	A ceftriaxone; vancomycin
Moraxella catarrhalis	Otitis; pneumonia; sinusitis	Amoxicillin + clavulanate; ampicillin + sulbactam; trimethoprim-sulfamethoxazole	A cephalosporin; ciprofloxacin; erythromycin; tetracycline
Neisseria gonorrhoeae (gonococcus)	Arthritis-dermatitis syndrome; genital infections	If penicillin sensitive: ampicillin or amoxicillin + probenecid; penicillin G. If penicillinase producing: cefixime or ceftriaxone	Cefixime, cefoxitin or ceftriaxone; doxycycline; trimethoprim-sulfamethoxazole; ciprofloxacin or ofloxacin; erythromycin; spectinomycin
Neisseria meningitidis (meningococcus)	Meningitis	Penicillin G	Cefotaxime or ceftriaxone; chloramphenicol

Based on: Gilbert, D, et al: *The Sanford Guide to Antimicrobial Therapy,* ed. 41. Antimicrobial Therapy Inc., Sperryville, VA, 2011.

GEN MED

TABLE 12.8 Treatment of Infections Caused by Acid-Fast Bacilli, Spirochetes, Actinomycetes, and Other Microorganisms

Microorganism	Disease	Primary Agent(s)	Alternative Agent(s)
Acid-Fast Bacilli			
Mycobacterium avium intracellulare	Disseminated diseases in AIDS	Clarithromycin + ethambutol ± clofazimine ± ciprofloxacin	Amikacin; rifabutin; rifampin
Mycobacterium leprae	Leprosy	Dapsone + rifampin	Clofazimine, ofloxacin
Mycobacterium tuberculosis	Pulmonary, renal, meningeal, and other tuberculosis infections	Isoniazid + rifampin + pyrazinamide + ethambutol	Various combinations of the primary drugs ± streptomycin
Spirochetes			
Treponema pallidum	Syphilis	Penicillin G	Ceftriaxone; doxycycline
Treponema pertenue	Yaws	Penicillin G; streptomycin	Doxycycline
Leptospira	Meningitis, Weil's disease	Penicillin G	Doxycycline
Borrelia burgdorferi	Lyme disease	Stage 1: doxycycline Stage 2: ceftriaxone	Stage 1: amoxicillin; azithromycin or clarithromycin; ceftriaxone Stage 2: penicillin G; tetracycline
Borrelia recurrentis	Relapsing fever	Doxycycline	Erythromycin; penicillin G
Actinomycetes			
Actinomyces israelii	Cervicofacial, abdominal, thoracic, and other lesions	Penicillin G or ampicillin	Doxycyclin; erythromycin

GEN MED

Microorganism	Disease	Primary Agent(s)	Alternative Agent(s)
Actinomycetes			
Nocardia asteroides	Brain abscesses; pulmonary and other lesions	A sulfonamide; trimethoprim-sulfamethoxazole	Amikacin; amoxicillin-clavulanate; ceftriaxone; minocycline ± a sulfonamide
Other Microorganisms			
Chlamydia psittaci	Ornithosis	Doxycycline	Chloramphenicol
Chlamydia pneumoniae	Pneumonia	Doxycycline	Azithromycin or clarithromycin; erythromycin
Chlamydia trachomatis	Blennorrhea; lymphogranuloma venereum; nonspecific urethritis trachoma	Doxycycline	Azithromycin; erythromycin; a sulfonamide
Mycoplasma pneumoniae	"Atypical" pneumonia	Erythromycin; doxycycline	Azithromycin or clarithromycin
Pneumocystis carinii	Pneumonia (in impaired host)	Trimethoprim-sulfamethoxazole	Mild moderate disease: atovaquone; clindamycin-primaquine; trimethoprim-dapsone. Moderate severe disease: clindamycin-primaquine; pentamidine; trimetrexate
Rickettsia	Q fever; rickettsialpox; Rocky Mountain spotted fever; typhus fever, other diseases	Doxycycline	Chloramphenicol
Ureaplasma urealyticum	Nonspecific urethritis	Doxycycline	Erythromycin

Based on: Gilbert, D, et al: *The Sanford Guide to Antimicrobial Therapy,* ed. 41. Antimicrobial Therapy Inc., Sperryville, VA, 2011.

GEN MED

TABLE 12.9 Drugs That Inhibit Bacterial Cell Membrane Synthesis

Penicillins	Cephalosporins	Other Agents	Penicillin and Beta-Lactamase Combinations
Natural penicillins	First-generation	Aztreonam	Ampicillin and
Penicillin G	cephalosporins	(Azactam)	clavulanate
(Bicillin,	Cefadroxil (Duricef)	Bacitracin	(Augmentin)
Wycillin, many	Cefazolin (Ancef,	(Bacitracin	Ampicillin and
others)	Kefzol)	ointment)	sulbactam
Penicillin V	Cephalexin (Keflex,	Colistin (Coly-	(Unasyn)
(Beepen-VK, V-	Keftab)	Mycin S)	Piperacillin
Cillin K, others)	Cephalothin	Cycloserine	and tazobac-
Penicillinase-	(Keflin)	(Seromycin)	tam (Zosyn)
resistant	Cephapirin (Cefadyl)	Imipenem/	Ticarcillin and
penicillins	Cephradine (Velosef)	cilastatin	clavulanate
Cloxacillin	Second-generation	(Primaxin)	(Timentin)
(Cloxapen,	cephalosporins	Meropenem	
Tegopen)	Cefaclor (Ceclor)	(Merrem	
Dicloxacillin	Cefonicid (Monocid)	I.V.)	
(Dycill, Dynapen,	Cefamandole	Polymyxin B	
Pathocil)	(Mandol)	(generic)	
Nafcillin (Unipen)	Cefoxitin (Mefoxin)	Vancomycin	
Methicillin	Cefotetan (Cefotan)	(Vancocin)	
(Staphcillin)	Cefprozil (Cefzil)		
Oxacillin	Cefuroxime (Ceftin,		
(Bactocill,	Kefurox, Zinacef)		
Prostaphilin)	Third-generation		
Aminopenicillins	cephalosporins		
Amoxicillin	Cefixime (Suprax)		
(Amoxil, Poly-	Cefoperazone		
mox, others)	(Cefobid)		
Ampicillin	Cefotaxime		
(Omnipen, Poly-	(Claforan)		
cillin, others)	Cefpodoxime (Vantin)		
Bacampicillin	Ceftazidime (Fortaz,		
(Spectrobid)	Tazicef, others)		
Extended-spectrum	Ceftibuten (Cedax)		
penicillins	Ceftizoxime (Cefizox)		
Carbenicillin	Ceftriaxone (Ro-		
(Geocillin,	cephin)		
Geopen,	Moxalactam		
Pyopen)	(Moxam)		
Mezlocillin	Fourth-generation		
(Mezlin)	cephalosporins		
Piperacillin	Cefepime (Maxipime)		
(Pipracil)			
Ticarcillin (Ticar)			

From: Ciccone, CD: *Pharmacology in Rehabilitation,* ed. 3. FA Davis, Philadelphia, 2002, p 545, with permission. Hardman, JG, et al: *Goodman and Gillman's the Pharmacological Basis of Therapeutics,* ed. 9, McGraw-Hill, New York, p 1033, permission granted by McGraw-Hill.

GEN MED

🔵 TABLE 12.10 Drugs Used to Inhibit Bacterial Protein Synthesis

Aminoglycosides	Erythromycins	Tetracyclines	Other Agents
Amikacin (Amikin)	Erythromycin (ERYC, E-Mycin, others)	Demeclocycline (Declomycin)	Chloramphenicol (Chloromycetin)
Gentamicin (Garamycin)	Erythromycin estolate (Ilosone)	Doxycycline (Mono-dox, Vibramycin, others)	Clindamycin (Cleocin)
Kanamycin (Kantrex)	Erythromycin ethylsuccinate (E.E.S., EryPed)	Minocycline (Minocin)	Ethionamide (Trecator-SC)
Neomycin (generic)	Erythromycin gluceptate (Ilotycin)	Oxytetracycline (Terramycin)	Lincomycin (Lincocin, Lincorex)
Netilmicin (Netromycin)	Erythromycin lactobionate (Erythrocin)	Tetracycline (Achromycin V, others)	
Streptomycin (generic)	Erythromycin stearate (Erythrocin, Erythrocot, others)		
Tobramycin (Nebcin)			

From: Ciccone, CD: *Pharmacology in Rehabilitation,* ed. 3. FA Davis, Philadelphia, 2002, p 554, with permission

🔵 TABLE 12.11 Drugs Used to Inhibit Bacterial DNA/RNA Synthesis and Function

Fluoroquinolones	Sulfonamides	Others
Ciprofloxacin (Cipro)	Sulfacytine (Renoquid)	Aminosalicylic acid (Tubasal)
Enoxacin (Penetrex)	Sulfadiazine (Silvadene)	Clofazimine (Lamprene)
Grepafloxacin (Raxar)	Sulfamethizole (Thiosulfil Forte)	Dapsone (Avlosulfon)
Lomefloxacin (Maxaquin)	Sulfamethoxazole (Gantanol, Urobak)	Ethambutol (Myambutol)
Levofloxacin (Levaquin)	Sulfisoxazole (Gantrisin)	Metronidazole (Flagyl, Protostat, others)
Norfloxacin (Noroxin)		Rifampin (Rifadin, Rimactane)
Ofloxacin (Floxin)		Trimethoprim (Proloprim, Trimpex)
Sparfloxacin (Zagam)		

From: Ciccone, CD: *Pharmacology in Rehabilitation,* ed. 3. FA Davis, Philadelphia, 2002, p 558, with permission.

GEN MED

Viruses

TABLE 12.12 Common Viruses Affecting Humans

Family	Virus	Related Infections
DNA Viruses Adenoviridae	Adenovirus, types 1–33	Respiratory tract and eye infections
Hepatitis B	Hepatitis B virus	Hepatitis B
Herpesviridae	Cytomegalovirus	Cytomegalic inclusion disease (i.e., widespread involvement of virtually any organ, especially the brain, liver, lung, kidney, and intestine)
	Epstein-Barr virus	Infectious mononucleosis
	Herpes simplex, types 1 and 2	Local infections of oral, genital, and other mucocutaneous areas; systemic infections
	Varicella-zoster virus	Chickenpox; herpes zoster (shingles); other systemic infections
Poxviridae	Smallpox virus	Smallpox
RNA Viruses Coronaviridae	Coronavirus	Upper respiratory tract infection
Flaviviridae	Hepatitis C virus	Hepatitis C
Orthomyxoviridae	Influenza virus, types A and B	Influenza
Paramyxoviridae	Measles virus Mumps virus Respiratory syncytial virus	Measles Mumps Respiratory tract infection in children
Picornaviridae	Hepatitis A virus Polioviruses Rhinovirus, types 1–89	Hepatitis A Poliomyelitis Common cold
Retroviridae	Human immunodeficiency virus (HIV)	AIDS

Family	Virus	Related Infections
Rhabdoviridae	Rabies virus	Rabies
Togaviridae	Alphavirus Rubella virus	Encephalitis Rubella

Based on: Gilbert, D, et al: *The Sanford Guide to Antimicrobial Therapy,* ed. 41.
  Antimicrobial Therapy Inc., Sperryville, VA, 2011.
AIDS = acquired immunodeficiency syndrome.

Methods of Disease Transmission

■ TABLE 12.13 Methods of Transmission of Some Common Communicable Diseases

Disease	How Agent Leaves the Body	How Organisms May Be Transmitted	Method of Entry Into the Body
Acquired immuno-deficiency syndrome (AIDS)	Blood, semen, or other body fluids, including breast milk	Inoculation by use of con-taminated needles or by direct contact so that infected body fluids can enter the body	Transplacentally to embryo or fetus Nursing at breast
Cholera	Excreta from intestinal tract	As in typhoid fever	As in typhoid fever
Diphtheria	Sputum and discharges from nose and throat Skin lesions	Direct contact Droplet infection from patient coughing Hands of nurse Articles used by and about patient	Through mouth to throat or nose to throat
Gonococcal disease	Lesions Discharges from infected mucous membranes	Direct contact as in sexual intercourse Towels, bath-tubs, toilets, etc.	Directly onto mucous membrane Through breaks in membrane

(table continues on page 804)

GEN MED

TABLE 12.13 **Methods of Transmission of Some Common Communicable Diseases** (continued)

Disease	How Agent Leaves the Body	How Organisms May Be Transmitted	Method of Entry Into the Body
		Hands of infected persons soiled with their own discharges Hands of attendant	
Hepatitis A, viral	Feces	As in typhoid fever	As in typhoid fever, rarely by blood transfusion
Hepatitis B, viral and delta hepatitis	Blood and serum-derived fluids, including semen and vaginal fluids	Contact with blood and body fluids	Transfusion Exposure to body fluids including during hetero- or homosexual intercourse
Hepatitis C	Blood	Transfusion Parenteral drug use Laboratory exposure to blood Health-care workers exposed to blood, e.g., dentists and their assistants, and clinical and laboratory staff	Infected blood Contaminated needles
Hookworm	Feces	Direct contact with soil polluted with feces Eggs in feces hatch in sandy soil Feces may also contaminate food	Larvae enter through breaks in skin, especially skin of feet, and after devious passage through the body settle in the intestine

Disease	How Agent Leaves the Body	How Organisms May Be Transmitted	Method of Entry Into the Body
Influenza	As in pneumonia	As in pneumonia	As in pneumonia
Leprosy	Uncertain, may be from lesions Bacilli found in nodules that may break down, forming lesions	Uncertain, probably nasal discharges of untreated patients	Uncertain, probably via upper respiratory tract and broken skin
Measles (rubella)	As in streptococcal sore throat	As in streptococcal sore throat	As in streptococcal sore throat
Meningitis, meningococcal	Discharges from nose and throat	Direct contact Hands of nurse or attendant Articles used by and about patient Flies	Mouth and nose
Mumps	Discharges from infected glands and mouth	Direct contact with persons affected	Mouth and nose
Ophthalmia neonatorum (gonococcal infection of eyes of newborn)	Purulent discharges from the eye	Direct contact with infected areas as vagina of infected mother during birth Other infected babies Hands of doctor or nurse Linens	Directly on the conjunctiva
Pneumonia	Sputum and discharges from nose and throat	Direct contact Hands of nurse	Through mouth and nose to lungs

GEN MED

(table continues on page 806)

TABLE 12.13 Methods of Transmission of Some Common Communicable Diseases (continued)

Disease	How Agent Leaves the Body	How Organisms May Be Transmitted	Method of Entry Into the Body
Poliomyelitis	Discharges from nose and throat, and via feces	Direct contact Hands of nurse or attendant Rarely in milk	Through mouth and nose
Rubeola	Secretions from nose and throat Airborne spread is possible	Droplet spread from nose or throat by direct contact with nasal or throat secretions	Through mouth and nose
Streptococcal sore throat	Discharges from nose and throat Skin lesions	Direct contact Hands of nurse Articles used by and about patient	Through mouth and nose
Syphilis	Infected tissues Lesions Blood Transfer through placenta to fetus	Direct contact Kissing or sexual intercourse Contaminated needles and syringes	Directly into blood and tissues through breaks in skin or membrane Contaminated needles and syringes
Tetanus	Excreta from infected herbivorous animals and man	Soil, especially that with manure or feces in it Dust, etc. Articles used about stables	Directly into bloodstream through wounds (organism is an anaerobe and prefers deep, incised wound)
Trachoma	Discharges from infected eyes	Direct contact Hands, towels, handkerchiefs	Directly on conjunctiva
Tuberculosis, bovine		Milk from infected cow	As in tuberculosis, human

Disease	How Agent Leaves the Body	How Organisms May Be Transmitted	Method of Entry Into the Body
Tuberculosis, human	Sputum Lesions Feces	Direct contact such as kissing Droplet infection from a person coughing with mouth uncovered Sputum from mouth to fingers, thence to food and other things Soiled dressings	Through mouth to lungs and intestines From intestines via lymph channels to lymph vessels and to tissues
Typhoid fever	Feces and urine	Direct contact with food, water, articles, or insects contaminated with feces, or urine from patients	Through mouth via infected food or water and thence to intestinal tract
Whooping cough	Discharges from respiratory tract	Direct contact with persons affected	Mouth and nose

From: Thomas, CL (ed): *Taber's Cyclopedic Medical Dictionary*, ed. 17. FA Davis, Philadelphia, 1993, pp 426–428, with permission.

GEN MED

Precautions

Universal

The single most important measure to control transmission of pathogens is to treat all human blood and other potentially infectious materials AS IF THEY WERE infectious. Application of this approach is referred to as *universal precautions. Blood and certain body fluids from all acute care patients should be considered as potentially infectious materials.* These fluids cause *contamination,* defined in the standard as "the presence or the reasonably anticipated presence of blood or other potentially infectious materials on an item or surface."

OSHA Bloodborne Pathogens Standard

Some of the key components of the OSHA standard are summarized below.

Who Is Covered?

Employees who may be occupationally exposed to blood (human blood, blood products, or blood components) and other potentially infectious materials, such as saliva in dental procedures, semen, vaginal secretions; cerebrospinal, synovial, pleural, pericardial, peritoneal, and amniotic fluids; body fluids visibly contaminated with blood; unfixed human tissues or organs; HIV-containing cell or tissue cultures; and HIV- or HBV-containing culture mediums.

Occupational exposure means a "reasonably anticipated skin, eye, mucous membrane, or parenteral contact with blood or other potentially infectious materials that may result from the performance of the employee's duties."

Federal OSHA authority extends to all private sector employers with one or more employees, as well as federal civilian employees. In addition, many states administer their own occupational safety and health programs through plans approved under section 18(b) of the OSH Act.

The Exposure Control Plan

A written exposure control plan is necessary for the safety and health of workers. At a minimum, the plan must include the following:

- Identify job classifications where there is exposure to blood or other potentially infectious materials.
- Explain the protective measures currently in effect in the acute care facility and/or a schedule and methods of compliance to be implemented, including hepatitis B vaccination and post-exposure follow-up procedures; how hazards are communicated to employees; personal protective equipment; housekeeping; and record-keeping.
- Establish procedures for evaluating the circumstances of an exposure incident.

The written exposure control plan must be available to workers and OSHA representatives and updated at least annually or whenever changes in procedures create new occupational exposures.

Who Has Occupational Exposure?

The exposure determination must be based on the definition of occupational exposure without regard to personal protective clothing and equipment. Where all employees are occupationally exposed, it is not necessary to list specific work tasks. Where only some of the employees have exposure, specific tasks and procedures causing exposure must be listed. When employees with occupational exposure have been identified, the next step is to communicate the hazards of the exposure to the employees.

Communicating Hazards to Employees

The initial training for current employees must be scheduled within 90 days of the effective date of the bloodborne pathogens standard, at no cost to the employee, and during working hours. Training also is required for new workers at the time of their initial assignment to tasks with occupational exposure or when job tasks change, causing occupational exposure, and annually thereafter. In addition to communicating hazards to employees and providing training to identify and control hazards, other preventive measures also must be taken to ensure employee protection.

Preventive Measures

Preventive measures such as hepatitis B vaccination, universal precautions, engineering controls, safe work practices, personal protective equipment, and housekeeping measures help reduce the risks of occupational exposure.

Methods of Control

Engineering and Work Practice Controls

Engineering controls isolate or remove the hazard from employees and are used in conjunction with work practices. Personal protective equipment also shall be used when occupational exposure to bloodborne pathogens remains even after instituting these controls. Some engineering controls that apply to acute care facilities and are required by the standard include the following:

1. Use puncture-resistant, leak-proof containers, color-coded red or labeled, according to the standard to discard contaminated items such as needles, broken glass, scalpels, or other items that could cause a cut or puncture wound.
2. Use puncture-resistant, leak-proof containers, color-coded red or labeled, to store contaminated reusable sharps until they are properly reprocessed.
3. Store and process reusable contaminated sharps in a way that ensures safe handling. For example, use a mechanical device to retrieve used instruments from soaking pans in decontamination areas.
4. Use puncture-resistant, leak-proof containers to collect, handle, process, store, transport, or ship blood specimens and potentially infectious materials. Label these specimens if shipped outside the facility. Labeling is not required when specimens are handled by employees trained to use universal precautions with all specimens and when these specimens are kept within the facility.

Similarly, *work practice controls* reduce the likelihood of exposure by altering the manner in which the task is performed. All procedures shall minimize splashing, spraying, splattering, and generation of droplets. Work practice requirements include the following:

1. Wash hands when gloves are removed and as soon as possible after contact with blood or other potentially infectious materials.
2. Provide and make available a mechanism for immediate eye irrigation, in the event of an exposure incident.
3. Do not bend, recap, or remove contaminated needles unless required to do so by specific medical procedures or the employer can demonstrate that no alternative is feasible. In these instances, use mechanical means such as forceps, or a one-handed technique to recap or remove contaminated needles.
4. Do not shear or break contaminated needles.
5. Discard contaminated needles and sharp instruments in puncture-resistant, leak-proof, red or biohazard-labeled containers that are accessible, maintained upright, and not allowed to be overfilled.
6. Do not eat, drink, smoke, apply cosmetics, or handle contact lenses in areas of potential occupational exposure. (Note: use of hand lotions is acceptable.)
7. Do not store food or drink in refrigerators or on shelves where blood or potentially infectious materials are present.

GEN MED

8. Use red, or affix biohazard labels to, containers to store, transport, or ship blood or other potentially infectious materials, such as laboratory specimens.
9. Do not use mouth pipetting to suction blood or other potentially infectious materials; it is prohibited.

Personal Protective Equipment

Personal protective equipment is specialized clothing or equipment used by employees to protect against direct exposure to blood or other potentially infectious materials. Protective equipment must not allow blood or other potentially infectious materials to pass through to workers' clothing, skin, or mucous membranes. Such equipment includes, but is not limited to, gloves, gowns, laboratory coats, face shields or masks, and eye protection.

The employer also must ensure that employees observe the following precautions for safely handling and using personal protective equipment:

1. Remove all personal protective equipment immediately following contamination and on leaving the work area, and place in an appropriately designated area or container for storing, washing, decontaminating, or discarding.
2. Wear appropriate gloves when contact with blood, mucous membranes, nonintact skin, or potentially infectious materials is anticipated; when performing vascular access procedures; and when handling or touching contaminated items or surfaces.
3. Provide hypoallergenic gloves, liners, or powderless gloves or other alternatives to employees who need them.
4. Replace disposable, single-use gloves as soon as possible when contaminated, or if torn, punctured, or barrier function is compromised.
5. Do not reuse disposable (single-use) gloves.
6. Decontaminate reusable (utility) gloves after each use and discard if they show signs of cracking, peeling, tearing, puncturing, deteriorating, or failing to provide a protective barrier.
7. Use full face shields or face masks with eye protection, goggles, or eyeglasses with side shields when splashes of blood and other bodily fluids may occur and when contamination of the eyes, nose, or mouth can be anticipated (e.g., during invasive and surgical procedures).
8. Also wear surgical caps or hoods and/or shoe covers or boots when gross contamination may occur, such as during surgery and autopsy procedures.

Housekeeping Procedures

Equipment. The employer must ensure a clean and sanitary workplace. Contaminated work surfaces must be decontaminated with a disinfectant on completion of procedures or when contaminated by splashes, spills, or contact with blood; other potentially infectious materials; and at the end of the work shift. Surfaces and equipment protected with plastic wrap, foil, or other nonabsorbent materials must be inspected frequently for contamination; and these protective coverings must be changed when found to be contaminated. Waste cans and pails must be inspected and decontaminated on a regularly scheduled basis. Broken glass should be cleaned up with a brush or tongs; never pick up broken glass with hands, even when wearing gloves.

Waste. Waste removed from the facility is regulated by local and state laws. Special precautions are necessary when disposing of contaminated sharps and other contaminated waste, and include the following:

1. Dispose of contaminated sharps in closable, puncture-resistant, leak-proof, red or biohazard-labeled containers.
2. Place other regulated waste in closable, leak-proof, red or biohazard-labeled bags or containers. If outside contamination of the regulated waste container occurs, place it in a second container that is closable, leak-proof, and appropriately labeled.

Laundry. The following requirements should be met with respect to contaminated laundry:

1. Bag contaminated laundry as soon as it is removed and store in a designated area or container.
2. Use red laundry bags or those marked with the biohazard symbol unless universal precautions are in effect in the facility and all employees recognize the bags as contaminated and have been trained in handling the bags.
3. Clearly mark laundry sent off site for cleaning by placing it in red bags or bags clearly marked with the orange biohazard symbol; use leak-proof bags to prevent soak-through.
4. Wear gloves or other protective equipment when handling contaminated laundry.

Definition of an Exposure Incident

An *exposure incident* is the specific eye, mouth, or other mucous membrane, non-intact skin, or parenteral contact with blood or other potentially infectious materials that results from the performance of an employee's duties. An example of an exposure incident is a puncture from a contaminated sharp.

Evaluation and Action When an Exposure Incident Occurs

When evaluating an exposure incident, immediate assessment and confidentiality are critical issues. Employees should immediately report exposure incidents to enable timely medical evaluation and follow-up by a health-care professional as well as a prompt request by the employer for testing of the source individual's blood for HIV and HBV. The *source individual* is any patient whose blood or body fluids are the source of an exposure incident to the employee.

At the time of the exposure incident, the exposed employee must be directed to a health-care professional. The employer must provide the health-care professional with a copy of the bloodborne pathogens standard; a description of the employee's job duties as he/she relates to the incident; a report of the specific exposure, including route of exposure; relevant employee medical records, including hepatitis B vaccination status; and results of the source individual's blood tests, if available. At that time, a baseline blood sample should be drawn from the employee, if he/she consents. If the employee elects to delay HIV testing of the sample, the health-care professional must preserve the employee's blood sample for at least 90 days.

Testing the source individual's blood does not need to be repeated if the source individual is known to be infectious for HIV or HBV; and testing cannot be done in most states without written consent. The results of the source individual's blood tests are confidential. As soon as possible, however, the test results of the source individual's blood must be made available to the exposed employee through consultation with the health-care professional.

Following post-exposure evaluation, the health-care professional will provide a written opinion to the employer. This opinion is limited to a statement that the employee has been informed of the results of the evaluation and told of the need, if any, for any further evaluation or treatment. The employer must provide a copy of the written opinion to the employee within 15 days. This is the only information shared with the employer following an exposure incident; all other employee medical records are confidential.

Record-Keeping

There are two types of records required by the bloodborne pathogens standard: medical and training.

A *medical record* must be established for each employee with occupational exposure. This record is confidential and separate from other personnel records. This record may be kept on site or may be retained by the health-care professional who provides services to employees. The medical record contains the employee's name, social security number, hepatitis B vaccination status, including the dates of vaccination and the written opinion of the health-care professional regarding the hepatitis B vaccination. If an occupational exposure occurs, reports are added to the medical record to document the incident and the results of testing following the incident. The post-evaluation written opinion of the health-care professional is also part of the medical record. The medical record also must document what information has been provided to the health-care provider. Medical records must be maintained 30 years past the last date of employment of the employee. Emphasis is on confidentiality of medical records. No medical record or part of a medical record should be disclosed without direct, written consent of the employee or as required by law.

Training Records

A *training record* is used to document each training session. Training records are to be kept for 3 years, and must include the date, content outline, trainer's name and qualifications, and names and job titles of all persons attending the training sessions.

Based on:

United States Department of Labor: OSHA Standards—Bloodborne Pathogens, OSHA 1910.1030. Web site accessed September 24, 2011.

Isolation Precautions for Hospitals

Guidelines for Isolation Precautions

Category IA Recommendations

Implementation strongly recommended for all hospitals. The recommendations are strongly supported by well-designed experimental, clinical, or epidemiological studies.

Category IB Recommendations

Implementation strongly recommended for all hospitals and viewed as effective by experts in the field and a consensus of HICPAC. The recommendations are supported by some experimental, clinical, or epidemiological studies and strong theoretical rationale.

Category 1C Recommendations

Required for implementation and supported by suggestive clinical or epidemiological studies or a theoretical rationale.

Category II Recommendations

Suggested for implementation in many hospitals. Recommendations may be supported by suggestive clinical or epidemiological studies, a strong theoretical rationale, or definitive studies applicable to some but not all hospitals.

GEN MED

TABLE 12.14 Guidelines for Isolation Precautions

Type of Precaution	Description	Indication	Classification of the Recommendation
Standard Precautions	The primary strategy for successful nosocomial infection control. Synthesizes the major features of Universal (blood and body fluid) Precautions and Body Substance Isolation	For the care of all patients receiving care in health-care settings regardless of diagnosis or presumed infection status.	IB
Hand washing	Plain (nonantimicrobial) soap for routine hand washing. Antimicrobial agent or a waterless antiseptic agent for specific circumstances (e.g., control of outbreaks or hyperendemic infections). After touching blood, body fluids, secretions, excretions, and contaminated items. After removal of gloves and between patient contacts. It may be necessary to wash hands between tasks and procedures on the same patient to prevent cross-contamination of different body sites.	As per Standard Precautions	IB, II
Gloves	Clean nonsterile gloves. When touching blood, body fluids, secretions, excretions, and contaminated items. When touching mucous membranes and nonintact skin. Change gloves between tasks and procedures on the same patient after contact with material that may contain a high concentration of microorganisms.	As per Standard Precautions	IB

Type of Precaution	Description	Indication	Classification of the Recommendation
	Remove gloves promptly after use, before touching noncontaminated items and environmental surfaces, and before going to another patient, and wash hands immediately to avoid transfer of microorganisms to other patients or environments.		
Mask, eye protection, face shield	Mask and eye protection or a face shield to protect mucous membranes of the eyes, nose, and mouth.	As per Standard Precautions and during procedures and patient-care activities that are likely to generate splashes or sprays of blood, body fluids, secretions, and excretions.	IB
Gown	Clean, nonsterile gown to protect skin and to prevent soiling of clothing. Select a gown that is appropriate for the activity and amount of fluid likely to be encountered. Remove a soiled gown as promptly as possible, and wash hands to avoid transfer of microorganisms to other patients or environments.	As per Standard Precautions and during procedures and patient-care activities that are likely to generate splashes or sprays of blood, body fluids, secretions, or excretions.	IB

(table continues on page 816)

GEN MED

GEN MED

TABLE 12.14 Guidelines for Isolation Precautions (continued)

Type of Precaution	Description	Indication	Classification of the Recommendation
Patient-care equipment	Used patient-care equipment soiled with blood, body fluids, secretions, and excretions is handled in a manner that prevents skin and mucous membrane exposure, contamination of clothing, and transfer of microorganisms to patients and others. Ensure that reusable equipment is not used for the care of another patient until it has been cleaned and reprocessed appropriately. Ensure that single-use items are discarded properly.	As per Standard Precautions	IB
Environmental control	Ensure that the hospital has adequate procedures for the routine care, cleaning, and disinfection of environmental surfaces, beds, bed rails, bedside equipment, and other frequently touched surfaces and ensure that these procedures are being followed.	As per Standard Precautions	IB
Linen	Used linen soiled with blood, body fluids, secretions, and excretions is handled in a manner that prevents skin and mucous membrane exposure, contamination of clothing, and transfer of microorganisms to other patients and environments.	As per Standard Precautions	IB

Type of Precaution	Description	Indication	Classification of the Recommendation
Occupational health and bloodborne pathogens	Proper use and disposable procedures are followed to prevent injuries when using needles, scalpels, and other sharp instruments or devices, or when cleaning used instruments. Never recap used needles, or otherwise manipulate them using both hands, or use any other technique that involves directing the point of a needle toward any part of the body; rather, use either a one-handed "scoop" technique or a mechanical device designed for holding the needle sheath. Do not remove used needles from disposable syringes by hand, and do not bend, break, or otherwise manipulate used needles by hand. Place used disposable syringes and needles, scalpel blades, and other sharp items in appropriate puncture-resistant containers, which are located as close as practical to the area in which the items were used, and place reusable syringes and needles in a puncture-resistant container for transport to the reprocessing area. Mouthpieces, resuscitation bags, or other ventilation devices are used as an alternative to mouth-to-mouth resuscitation methods in areas where the need for resuscitation is predictable.	As per Standard Precautions	IB

(table continues on page 818)

GEN MED

GEN MED

TABLE 12.14 Guidelines for Isolation Precautions (continued)

Type of Precaution	Description	Indication	Classification of the Recommendation
Patient placement	Private-room placement for patients who may contaminate their environment. If a private room is not available, consult with infection control professionals regarding patient placement or other alternatives.	For patients who do not (or cannot be expected to) assist in maintaining appropriate hygiene or environmental control.	IB
	Respiratory hygiene/cough etiquette (source containment of infectious respiratory secretions in symptomatic patients, beginning at initial point of encounter, e.g., triage and reception areas in emergency departments and physician offices)	Instruct symptomatic persons to cover mouth/nose when sneezing/coughing; use tissues and dispose in no-touch receptacle; observe hand hygiene after soiling of hands with respiratory secretions; wear surgical mask if tolerated or maintain spatial separation, >3 feet if possible.	
Airborne Precautions	Used in addition to Standard Precautions to reduce the risk of airborne transmission of infectious agents.	For patients known or suspected to be infected with microorganisms transmitted by airborne droplets (5 μ or smaller) traveling in air currents within a room or over a long distance.	IB

Type of Precaution	Description	Indication	Classification of the Recommendation
Patient placement	Private room with monitored negative air pressure, six to twelve air changes per hour. Appropriate discharge of air outdoors or monitored high-efficiency filtration of room air before the air is circulated to other areas in the hospital. Patient confined to room with door closed. When a private room is not available, place the patient in a room with a patient who has active infection with the same microorganism, unless otherwise recommended, but with no other infection. When a private room is not available and cohorting is not desirable, consultation with infection control professionals is advised before patient placement.	As per Airborne Precautions	IB
Respiratory protection	Respiratory protection is worn for patients known or suspected of infectious pulmonary tuberculosis. Susceptible persons should not enter the room of patients known or suspected to have measles (rubeola) or varicella (chickenpox) if other immune caregivers are available. If susceptible persons must enter the room of a patient known or suspected to have measles (rubeola) or varicella, they should wear respiratory protection. Persons immune to measles (rubeola) or varicella need not wear respiratory protection.	As per Airborne Precautions	IB

(table continues on page 820)

TABLE 12.14 Guidelines for Isolation Precautions (continued)

Type of Precaution	Description	Indication	Classification of the Recommendation
Patient transport	Patient transport and movement should be limited to essential purposes only; patient is masked when transported out of room.	As per Airborne Precautions	IB
Droplet Precautions	Used in addition to Standard Precautions to reduce the risk of droplet transmission of infectious microorganisms.	Patients known or suspected of being infected with microorganisms transmitted by droplets larger than 5 μ generated by the patient during coughing, sneezing, talking, or direct contact with conjunctivae or mucous membranes of the nose or mouth.	IB
Patient placement	Private room, or if unavailable, in a room with cohort infected with the same microorganism. When a private room is not available and cohorting is not achievable, maintain spatial separation of at least 3 ft between the infected patient and other patients and visitors. Special air handling and ventilation are not necessary, and the door may remain open. Never recap used needles, or otherwise manipulate them using both hands, or use any other technique that involves directing the point of a needle toward any part of the body; rather, use either a one-handed "scoop" technique or a mechanical device designed for holding the needle sheath.	As per Droplet Precautions	IB

Type of Precaution	Description	Indication	Classification of the Recommendation
	Do not remove used needles from disposable syringes by hand, and do not bend, break, or otherwise manipulate used needles by hand. Place used disposable syringes and needles, scalpel blades, and other sharp items in appropriate puncture-resistant containers, which are located as close as practical to the area in which the items were used, and place reusable syringes and needles in a puncture-resistant container for transport to the re-processing area. Mouthpieces, resuscitation bags, or other ventilation devices are used as an alternative to mouth-to-mouth resuscitation methods in areas where the need for resuscitation is predictable.		
Patient placement	Private-room placement for patients who may contaminate their environment. If a private room is not available, consult with infection control professionals regarding patient placement or other alternatives.	For patients who do not (or cannot be expected to) assist in maintaining appropriate hygiene or environmental control.	IB
Mask	In addition to Standard Precautions, wear a mask when working within 3 ft of the patient. (Logistically, some hospitals may want to implement the wearing of a mask to enter the room.)	As per Droplet Precautions	IB

(table continues on page 822)

GEN MED

GEN MED

TABLE 12.14 Guidelines for Isolation Precautions (continued)

Type of Precaution	Description	Indication	Classification of the Recommendation
Patient transport	Patient transport should be limited to essential purposes only; patient is masked when transported out of room.	As per Droplet Precautions	IB
Contact Precautions	Used in addition to Standard Precautions to reduce the risk of transmission of microorganisms by direct or indirect contact (e.g., skin to skin or skin to object).	Patients known or suspected to be infected or colonized with epidemiologically important microorganisms that can be transmitted by direct contact with the patient or indirect contact (touching) with environmental surfaces or patient-care items in the patient's environment.	IB
Patient placement	Private room, or if unavailable, in a room with a cohort infected with the same microorganism. When a private room is not available and cohorting is not achievable, consider the epidemiology of the microorganism and the patient population when determining patient placement. Consultation with infection control professionals is advised before patient placement.	As per Contact Precautions	IB

Type of Precaution	Description	Indication	Classification of the Recommendation
Gloves and hand washing	Wear gloves (clean, nonsterile gloves are adequate) when entering the room. During the course of providing care for a patient, change gloves after having contact with infective material that may contain high concentrations of microorganisms (fecal material and wound drainage). Remove gloves before leaving the patient's environment and wash hands immediately with an antimicrobial agent or a waterless antiseptic agent. After glove removal and hand washing, ensure that hands do not touch potentially contaminated environmental surfaces or items in the patient's room to avoid transfer of microorganisms to other patients or environments.	As per Contact Precautions	IB
Gown	Gown is worn before entering room and removed before leaving the room. After gown removal, ensure that clothing does not contact potentially contaminated environmental surfaces to avoid transfer of microorganisms to other patients or environments.	As per Contact Precautions and if you anticipate that your clothing will have substantial contact with the patient, environmental surfaces, or items in the patient's room, or if the patient is incontinent or has diarrhea, an ileostomy, a colostomy, or wound drainage not contained by a dressing.	IB

(table continues on page 824)

GEN MED

GEN MED

TABLE 12.14 Guidelines for Isolation Precautions (continued)

Type of Precaution	Description	Indication	Classification of the Recommendation
Patient transport	Transport limited to essential purposes. If the patient is transported out of the room, ensure that precautions are maintained to minimize the risk of transmission of microorganisms to other patients and contamination of environmental surfaces or equipment.	As per Contact Precautions	IB
Environmental control	Daily cleaning of patient-care items, bedside equipment, and frequently touched surfaces.	As per Contact Precautions	IB
Patient-care equipment	Noncritical patient-care equipment and items such as stethoscopes, sphygmomanometers, commodes, and thermometers are used for a single patient (or cohort of patients infected or colonized with the pathogen requiring precautions) when possible. If use of common equipment or items is unavoidable, then adequately clean and disinfect them before use for another patient.	As per Contact Precautions	IB

Based on: Siegel, JD, et al; the Healthcare Infection Control Practices Advisory Committee: *2007 Guideline for Isolation Precautions: Preventing Transmission of Infectious Agents in Healthcare Settings*. http://www.cdc.gov/incidod/dhqp/pdf/isolation2007/pdf.

Synopsis of Types of Precautions as in Draft Guidelines and Patients Requiring the Precautions

Standard Precautions

Use standard precautions for the care of all patients.

Airborne Precautions

In addition to standard precautions, use airborne precautions for patients known or suspected to have serious illnesses transmitted by airborne droplets. Examples of such illnesses are measles, varicella (including disseminated zoster), and tuberculosis.

Droplet Precautions

In addition to standard precautions, use droplet precautions for patients known or suspected to have serious illnesses transmitted by large particle droplets. Examples of such illnesses include the following:

1. Invasive *Haemophilus influenzae* type b, including meningitis, pneumonia, epiglottitis, and sepsis.
2. Invasive *Neisseria meningitidis*, including meningitis, pneumonia, and sepsis.
3. Invasive multidrug-resistant *Streptococcus pneumoniae,* including meningitis, pneumonia, sinusitis, and otitis media.
4. Other serious bacterial respiratory infections spread by droplet transmission, including the following:
   a. Diphtheria (pharyngeal)
   b. *Mycoplasma* pneumonia
   c. Pneumonic plague
   d. Streptococcal pharyngitis, pneumonia, or scarlet fever in infants and young children
5. Serious viral infections spread by droplet transmission, including adenovirus, influenza, mumps, parvovirus B19, rubella.

Contact Precautions

In addition to standard precautions, use contact precautions for patients known or suspected to have serious illnesses easily transmitted by direct patient contact or by contact with items in the patient's environment. Examples of such illnesses include the following:

1. Gastrointestinal, respiratory, skin, or wound infections or colonization with multidrug-resistant bacteria judged by infection control programs to be of special clinical epidemiologic significance based on current state, regional, or national recommendations.
2. Enteric infections with a low infectious dose or prolonged environmental survival, including *Clostridium difficile,* for diapered or incontinent patients, enterohemorrhagic *Escherichia coli* O157:H7, *Shigella,* hepatitis A, or rotavirus.
3. Respiratory syncytial virus, parainfluenza virus, or enteroviral infections in infants and young children.
4. Skin infections that are highly contagious or that may occur on dry skin, including diphtheria (cutaneous), herpes simplex (neonatal or mucocutaneous), impetigo, major (noncontaminated) abscesses, cellulitis, or decubiti, pediculosis, scabies, staphylococcal furunculosis in infants and young

GEN MED

children, staphylococcal scaled skin syndrome, zoster (disseminated or in the immunocompromised host)
5. Viral hemorrhagic conjunctivitis
6. Viral hemorrhagic fevers (Lassa fever or Marburg virus)

TABLE 12.15 Clinical Syndromes or Conditions Warranting Precautions to Prevent Transmission of Pathogens (Pending Confirmation of Diagnosis)

Clinical Syndrome or Condition	Potential Pathogens	Types of Precautions
Diarrhea Acute diarrhea with a likely infectious cause in an incontinent or diapered patient.	Enteric pathogens	Contact precautions
Diarrhea in an adult with a history of broad spectrum or long-term antibiotics	*Clostridium difficile*	Contact precautions
Meningitis	*Neisseria meningitidis*	Droplet precautions
Respiratory Infections Cough, fever, or upper lobe pulmonary infiltrate in an HIV-negative patient and in patients with a low risk for HIV infection	*Mycobacterium tuberculosis*	Airborne precautions
Cough, fever, or pulmonary infiltrate in any lung location in an HIV-infected patient and in patients at high risk for HIV infection	*Mycobacterium tuberculosis*	Airborne precautions
Paroxysmal or severe persistent cough during periods of pertussis activity	*Bordetella pertussis*	Droplet precautions
Respiratory infections, particularly bronchiolitis and croup, in infants and young children	Respiratory syncytial parainfluenza virus	Contact precautions
Risk of Multidrug-Resistant		
Microorganisms	Resistant bacteria	Contact precautions
History of infection or colonization with multidrug-resistant organisms		

GEN MED

Clinical Syndrome or Condition	Potential Pathogens	Types of Precautions
Skin, wound, or urinary tract infection in a patient with a recent hospital or nursing home stay in a facility where multidrug-resistant organisms are prevalent	Resistant bacteria	Contact precautions
Skin or Wound Infection Abscess or draining wound that cannot be covered	*Staphylococcus aureus,* group A *streptococcus*	Contact precautions

Based on: Siegel, JD, Rhinehart E, Jackson M, Chiarello L, et al: The Healthcare Infection Control Practices Advisory Committee. *2007 Guideline for Isolation Precautions: Preventing Transmission of Infectious Agents in Healthcare Settings.* http://www.cdc.gov/incidod/dhqp/pdf/isolation2007/pdf.

TABLE 12.16 Methods of Disinfection

Method	Concentration or Temperature	Use	Limitations
Moist Heat Autoclaving – (steam)	250°–270°F (121°–132°C)	Sterilize instruments not harmed by heat and water pressure.	Moisture will not permeate some materials. Cannot be used for heat-sensitive items.
Boiling water	212°F (100°C)	Kill non-spore-forming pathogenic organisms.	Does not kill spores. Probably not effective against hepatitis virus.
Radiation Ultraviolet light Ionizing		Air and surface disinfection. Sterilize medicines, some plastics, sutures, and biologicals.	Penetrates poorly. Harmful to unprotected skin and eyes. Expensive. May alter the medicine or material.
Filtration, membrane Fiberglass filters		Water purification. Air disinfection.	Slow and expensive. Only cleans incoming air; does not prevent recontamination.

(table continues on page 828)

GEN MED

◖ TABLE 12.16 Methods of Disinfection (continued)

Method	Concentration or Temperature	Use	Limitations
Physical Cleaning Ultrasonic		Disinfect instruments.	Aids in cleaning but not effective alone.
Washing		Disinfect hands and surfaces.	Does not remove all organisms.
Chemicals Alcohols Chlorines	70%–90%	Skin degerming.	Sometimes irritating. Does not kill spores.
	100–200 ppm	Water disinfection. Food surface sanitization.	Inactivated by inorganic matter. Does not kill spores. Ineffective at certain pH values.
Iodines, tincture	2%	Skin degerming.	Not sporicidal. Sometimes irritating.
Iodines, iodophors	74–450 ppm	General disinfectant.	Not sporicidal.
Phenols	1%–4%	General disinfectant.	Ineffective against some bacteria.
Quaternary ammonia compounds, tincture	0.1%	Skin degerming.	Neutralized by soap. Not sporicidal.
Quaternary ammonia compounds, aqueous	Diluted 1 part : 750 parts	General disinfectant.	May be incompatible with some water. Ineffective against some bacteria.
Mercurials	0.1%	Skin degerming.	Slow acting. May be irritating.
Formaldehyde (formalin)	5%	Drastic disinfection.	Irritating, corrosive.

GEN MED

Method	Concentration or Temperature	Use	Limitations
Glutaraldehyde	2%	Instrument sterilization.	Irritates mucous membranes. Unstable.
Germicidal soaps (hexachlorophene)	2%–3%	Skin degerming.	Bacteriostatic rather than bactericidal.
Gaseous Ethylene oxide	450 mg/L of air	Sterilization of heat-sensitive materials or those that must be kept dry.	Temperature, lengthy time, risks to employees, humidity critical. Treated materials need to air for varying periods of time (depending on composition) following treatment.
Formaldehyde gas		Fumigation. Sterilization of heat-sensitive materials.	Irritating, corrosive, toxic.
Hydrogen peroxide gas plasma		Materials that can tolerate high heat and humidity.	
Peracetic acid sterilization	35% peracetic acid	Used primarily for endoscopes.	

Based on: Rutala, WA, and Weber D; Healthcare Infection Control Practices Advisory Committee (HICPAC): *Guideline for Disinfection and Sterilization in Healthcare Facilities.* 2008. http://www.cdc.gov/ncidod/gl_environinfection.html. Accessed September 24, 2011.
ppm = parts per million.

Based on:

Siegel, JD, et al: The Healthcare Infection Control Practices Advisory Committee: 2007 Guideline for Isolation Precautions: Preventing Transmission of Infectious Agents in Healthcare Settings. http://www.cdc.gov/incidod/dhqp/pdf/isolation2007/pdf.

GEN MED

GEN MED

Drug Abuse

TABLE 12.17 Commonly Abused Drugs

Drug(s)	Classification/Action	Route/Method of Administration	Effect Desired by User	Principal Adverse Effects
Alcohol	Sedative-hypnotic	Oral, from various beverages (wine, beer, other alcoholic drinks)	Euphoria; relaxed inhibitions; decreased anxiety; sense of escape	Physical dependence; impaired motor skills; chronic degenerative changes in brain, liver, and other organs
Barbiturates Nembutal Seconal Others	Sedative-hypnotic	Oral or injected (IM, IV)	Relaxation and a sense of calmness; drowsiness	Physical dependence; possible death from overdose; behavior changes (irritability, psychosis) following prolonged use
Benzodiazepines Valium Librium Others	Similar to barbiturates	Similar to barbiturates	Similar to barbiturates	Similar to barbiturates
Caffeine	CNS stimulant	Oral, from coffee, tea, other beverages	Increased alertness; decreased fatigue; improved work capacity	Sleep disturbances; irritability; nervousness; cardiac arrhythmias
Methamphetamine Amphetamine Cocaine	CNS stimulant (when taken systemically)	"Snorted" (absorbed via nasal mucosa); smoked (in crystalline form); injected	Euphoria; excitement; feelings of intense pleasure and well-being	Physical dependence; acute CNS and cardiac toxicity; profound mood swings

Drug(s)	Classification/Action	Route/Method of Administration	Effect Desired by User	Principal Adverse Effects
Cannabinoids Hashish Marijuana	Psychoactive drugs with mixed (stimulant and depressant) activity	Smoked; possible oral ingestion	Initial response: euphoria, excitement, increased perception; later response: relaxation, stupor, dreamlike state	Possible endocrine changes (decreased testosterone in males) and changes in respiratory function in heavy use; similar to chronic cigarette smoking
Narcotics Demerol Morphine Heroin Others	Natural and synthetic opioids; analgesics	Oral or injected (IM, IV)	Relaxation; euphoria; feelings of tranquility; prevent onset of opiate withdrawal	Physical dependence; respiratory depression; high potential for death due to overdose
Nicotine	CNS toxin: produces variable effects via somatic and autonomic nervous system interaction	Smoked or absorbed from tobacco products (cigarettes, cigars, chewing tobacco)	Relaxation; calming effect; decreased irritability	Physical dependence; possible carcinogen; associated with pathological changes in respiratory function during long-term tobacco use

(table continues on page 832)

GEN MED

TABLE 12.17 Commonly Abused Drugs (continued)

Drug(s)	Classification/Action	Route/Method of Administration	Effect Desired by User	Principal Adverse Effects
Psychedelics LSD Mescaline Phencyclidine (PCP) Psilocybin MDMA (Ecstasy)	Hallucinogens	Oral; may also be smoked or inhaled	Altered perception and insight; distorted senses; disinhibition	Severe hallucinations; panic reaction; acute psychotic reactions
Anabolic Androgenic steroids		Oral, injected	Improved strength and endurance; enhanced performance	Hypertension, hepatoxicity, cardiomyopathy, acne, feminization and masculinization, mood disorders and hyperlipidemia

Based on: Weiss, RD: Drug abuse and dependence. In Goldman, L, and Shafer, AI (eds): *Goldman's Cecil Medicine,* ed. 24. Elsevier Saunders, Philadelphia, 2011.
CNS = central nervous system; LSD = lysergic acid diethylamide.

Diabetes Mellitus

TABLE 12.18 General Characteristics of Types 1 and 2 Diabetes Mellitus

Characteristic	Type 1	Type 2
Age at onset	Most commonly <30 yr	Most commonly >30 yr
Associated obesity	No	Very common
Propensity to ketoacidosis requiring insulin treatment for control	Yes	No
Plasma levels of endogenous insulin	Extremely low to undetectable	Variable; may be low, normal, or elevated depending on degree of insulin resistance and insulin secretory defect
Twin concordance	≤50%	>90%
Associated with specific HLA-D antigens	Yes	No
Islet cell antibodies at diagnosis	Yes	No
Islet pathology	Insulitis, selective loss of most β cells	Smaller, normal-appearing islets; amyloid (amylin) deposition common
Prone to develop diabetic complications (retinopathy, nephropathy, neuropathy, atherosclerotic cardiovascular disease)	Yes	Yes
Hyperglycemia responds to oral antihyperglycemic drugs	No	Yes, initially in many patients

Based on: Merck Manual Online, http://www.merckmanuals.com/professional/endocrine_and_metabolic_disorders/diabetes_mellitus_and_disorders_of_carbohydrate_metabolism/diabetes_mellitus_dm.html, accessed September 24, 2011, with permission.

TABLE 12.19 Onset, Peak, and Duration of Action of Human Insulin Preparations*

Insulin Preparation	Onset of Action	Peak Action	Duration of Action
Rapid-acting Lispro, aspart, glulisine†	5–15 min	45–75 min	3–5 hr
Short-acting Regular†	30–60 min	2–4 hr	6–8 hr
Intermediate-acting NPH‡	About 2 hr 3–4 hr	4–12 hr 8–12 hr	18–26 hr 12–18 hr
Long-acting	4–8 hr	10–16 hr	16–20 hr
Glargine	1–2 hr	No peak	24 hr
Detemir	1–2 hr	No peak	14–24 hr
Premixed 70% NPH/30% regular	30–60 min	Dual (NPH & R)	10–16 hr
50% NPH/50% regular	30–60 min	Dual (NPH & R)	10–16 hr
75% NPL/25% lispro	5–15 min	Dual (NPL & lispro)	10–16 hr
70% NPA/30% aspart	5–15 min	Dual (NPA & aspart)	10–16 hr

Based on: Merck Manual Online, http://www.merckmanuals.com/professional/endocrine_and_metabolic_disorders/diabetes_mellitus_and_disorders_of_carbohydrate_metabolism/diabetes_mellitus_dm.html, accessed September 24, 2011, with permission.

NPA = neutral protamine; NPH = neutral protamine Hagedorn; NPL = neutral protamine lispro.

*Times are approximate, assume subcutaneous administration, and may vary with injection technique and factors influencing absorption.

† Lispro and aspart are also available in premixed forms with intermediate-acting insulins.

‡ NPH also exists in premixed form (NPH/regular).

TABLE 12.20 Characteristics of Oral Antihyperglycemics

Generic Name	Daily Dosage	Duration of Action (h)	Comments
Insulin Secretagogues **Sulfonylureas**			Augment pancreatic β-cell insulin secretion Can be used alone or in combination with other oral drugs and insulin. Major adverse effects are hypoglycemia and possible weight gain
1st-Generation			
Acctohexamide	250 mg once/day–750 mg bid	12–24	
Chlorpropamide	100 mg once/day–750 mg once/day	24–36	Chlorpropamide may cause hyponatremia and flushing after alcohol ingestion
Tolbutamide	250 mg once/day–1500 mg bid	12	
Tolazamide	100 mg once/day–500 mg bid	14–16	
2nd-Generation			
Glyburide, regular-release	1.25 mg once/day–10 mg bid	12–24	No evidence of increased effectiveness of doses above 10 mg/day for glipizide and glyburide
Glyburide, micronized	0.75 mg once/day–6 mg bid	12–24	
Glipizide, regular-release	2.5 mg once/day–20 mg bid	12–24	
Glipizide, extended-release	2.5-20 mg once/day	24	
Glimepiride	1–8 mg once/day	24	
Short-acting insulin secretagogues			
Nateglinide	60–120 mg tid with meals	3–4	
Repaglinide	0.5–4 mg tid with meals	3–4	

(table continues on page 836)

GEN MED

● TABLE 12.20 Characteristics of Oral Antihyperglycemics (continued)

Generic Name	Daily Dosage	Duration of Action (h)	Comments
Insulin Sensitizers **Biguanides**			
Melformin, regular-release	500 mg once/day–1250 mg bid	6–10	Augments suppression of hepatic glucose production by insulin Can be used alone or in combination with other oral drugs and insulin
Metformin, extended-release	500 mg–2 g once/day	24	Major adverse effects: lactic acidosis (rare); contraindicated in at-risk patients, including those with renal insufficiency, heart failure, metabolic acidosis, hypoxia, alcoholism, and dehydration Does not cause hypoglycemia Other adverse effect: GI distress (diarrhea, nausea, pain): vitamin B_{12} malabsorption Potentiates weight loss
Thiazolidinediones Pioglitazone	15–45 mg once/day	24	Major adverse effects: weight gain, fluid retention, anemia (mild) Rosiglitazone may increase low-density lipoprotein cholesterol Hepatotoxicity is rare, but liver function monitoring is required
Rosiglitazone	2–8 mg once/day	24	

Generic Name	Daily Dosage	Duration of Action (h)	Comments
Intestinal Enzyme Inhibitors			
α-Glucosidase inhibitors			
Acarbose	25–100 mg tid with meals	6–10	Applied as monotherapy or combination therapy with other oral drugs or insulin to decrease post-prandial plasma glucose levels
Miglitol	25-100 mg tid with meals	6–10	Must be taken with the first bite of meal
			GI adverse effects (flatulence, diarrhea, bloating) common but may decrease over time
			Start with small dose (25 mg/day) and gradually titrate over several weeks.

Reprinted with permission, from Porter, R (ed): *The Merck Manual of Diagnosis and Therapy*, 19th ed. Copyright (2011) by Merck & Co., Inc., Whitehouse Station, NJ. http://www.merck.com/mmpe. Accessed September 24, 2011.

🔸 TABLE 12.21 Diabetic and Hypoglycemic Comas

	Diabetic Coma	Hypoglycemic Coma
Onset	Gradual	Often sudden
History	Often of acute infection in a diabetic or insufficient insulin intake. Previous history of diabetes may be absent.	Recent insulin injection, inadequate meal, or excessive exercise after insulin
Skin	Flushed, dry	Pale, sweating
Tongue	Dry or furred	Moist

(table continues on page 838)

🔴 **TABLE 12.21 Diabetic and Hypoglycemic Comas** (continued)

	Diabetic Coma	Hypoglycemic Coma
Breath	Smell of acetone	Acetone odor rare
Thirst	Intense	Absent
Respiration	Deep (air hunger) (Kussmaul)	Shallow
Vomiting	Common	Rare
Pulse	Rapid, feeble	Full and bounding
Eyeball tension	Low	Normal
Urine	Sugar and acetone present	No sugar or acetone, unless bladder has not been emptied for some hours
Blood sugar	Raised (over 200 mg/dL)	Subnormal (20–50 mg/dL)
Blood pressure	Low	Normal
Abdominal pain	Common and often acute	Absent

From: Thomas, CL (ed): *Taber's Cyclopedic Medical Dictionary,* ed. 17. FA Davis, Philadelphia, 1993, p 424, with permission.

GEN MED

Organ Transplantation

Organ transplantation is the transfer of an organ from one body to another to replace a damaged or failing organ with a working one. Organ donors can either be living or deceased. Autograph is the transplant of tissue to the same person, which can occur with skin grafts or stem cells in bone marrow transplantation. Allograft occurs when transplanting a tissue or organ between nonidentical members of the same species. The recipient's immune system will identify the organ as foreign (leading to rejection of the organ), so the recipient must take anti-rejection, or immunosuppressive medications. Xenotransplantation is the transplant of an organ/tissue from one species to another and has not been successfully applied to humans.

Under contract with the U.S. Department of Health and Human Services' Health Services & Resources Administration (HRSA), the United Network for Organ Sharing (UNOS) maintains a centralized computer network linking all organ procurement organizations and transplant centers. This computer network is accessible 24 hours a day, 7 days a week, with organ placement specialists in the UNOS Organ Center always available to answer questions.

Major Organs Transplanted

TABLE 12.22 Major Organs Transplanted

Organ	Body System	Living	Deceased
Heart	Thoracic		✓
Lung	Thoracic	✓	✓
Liver	Abdominal	✓	✓
Kidney	Abdominal	✓	✓
Pancreas	Abdominal	✓*	✓
Intestine	Abdominal		✓

*Donors have been found to have an increased risk of developing diabetes, so living donor pancreas transplants are now rarely performed.

Process of Organ Transplantation

Step 1: **Patient is referred to transplant center that evaluates his/her candidacy**

Kidney and pancreas transplant position determined by waiting time; all other organs determined by medical urgency

Step 2: **Identification of deceased donor organ**

UNOS computerized system matches available organ(s) with potential recipients, the order of which is determined by organ allocation policies, which include: blood type, length of time in waiting list, immune status, illness severity, and distance between potential recipient and donor

Step 3: **Organ Offer**

Patient at the top of the list must be healthy enough and ready for surgery immediately

Successful cross match, a blood test which measures compatibility between donor and recipient, ensures the organ is not rejected by the recipient's immune system

Step 4: **Transplant**

Contingent on success of steps 1 through 3.

The recovered organs are stored in a cold preservation solution during transport

Based on:
http://www.unos.org/inthenews/factsheets.asp.

Compatibility Testing

antibody screen: An antibody is a protein substance made by the body's immune system in response to an antigen. Exposure to human leukocyte antigens (HLA) can occur through blood transfusions, pregnancy, virus, and previous transplant(s). Often a panel of reactive antibodies (PRA) is performed to determine how sensitive a potential transplant recipient will

GEN MED

be to having antibodies to a potential donor. In this test, the potential recipient's serum is mixed with a panel of known HLA. The percent of reactivity to this panel determines the PRA.

crossmatching: A blood test to see if the potential recipient will have an immune response to and reject the donor organ. If the crossmatch is "positive" from the recipient's antibodies to the donor, then the donor and recipient are incompatible. If the crossmatch is "negative," then the transplant may proceed. Crossmatching is routinely performed before all transplants.

> **Based on:**
>
> *Danovich, GM (ed): Handbook of Kidney Transplantation, ed. 5. Lippincott Williams & Wilkins, Philadelphia, 2004.*

Living Donation

Organs and tissues can be made available on a voluntary basis from living donors. They can include kidneys, lungs, and liver.

Single kidney. This is the most frequent type of living organ donation. If the potential donor passes the medical workup, then there is little risk in living with one kidney because the remaining kidney compensates to do the work of both kidneys

Liver. Individuals can donate segments of the liver, which has the ability to regenerate the segment that was donated and regain full function.

Lung. Individuals can donate lobes of the lung. Lung lobes do not regenerate.

Possible advantages: Living donation eliminates the recipient's need for placement on the national waiting list. Transplant surgery can be scheduled at a mutually agreed-on time rather than performed as an emergency operation. Transplants from living donors are often more successful, due to the decreased time the organ is out of the body and the decreased rate of delay in functioning of the organ after transplant. Perhaps the most important aspect of living donation is the psychological benefit. The recipient can experience positive feelings knowing that the gift came from a loved one or a caring stranger. The donor experiences the satisfaction of knowing that he or she has contributed to the improved health of the recipient.

Qualifications for Living Donors

To qualify as a living donor, an individual must be physically fit; in good general health; and free from high blood pressure, diabetes, cancer, kidney disease, and heart disease. Individuals considered for living donation are usually between 18 and 60 years of age. Gender and race are not factors in determining a successful match.

The living donor must first undergo a blood test to determine blood type compatibility with the recipient.

Donor Evaluation

If the donor and recipient have compatible blood types, the donor undergoes an evaluation that includes the following:

1. History and physical examination by a psychiatrist/psychologist, transplant physician, transplant surgeon, social worker, and donor advocate (usually a

hospital employee who is not part of the transplant department, or a previous organ donor).

2. Laboratory evaluation to assess his/her kidney function, electrolytes, liver function tests, cholesterol profile, red blood cell count, white blood cell cout, platelet count, and blood clotting ability.
3. Twenty-four-hour urine collection, which is a more accurate measure of kidney function. This can also assess for possible protein in the urine.
4. Imaging studies. Includes chest x-ray, EKG to screen for heart and lung disease; abdominal CT scan with contrast to evaluate the abdominal organs, specifically looking at the blood flow to and from the kidneys. Often the potential donor will have more than one artery and/or renal vein. This is not a contraindication to transplant, but useful for the donor surgeon to know prior to surgery.*

*Based on:
http://www.unos.org/inTheNews/factSheets.asp.

TABLE 12.23 **Common Immunosuppressive Drugs**

| | | Primary Indications* | |
Generic Name	Trade Name(s)	Prevention or Treatment of Transplant Rejection	Diseases With an Autoimmune Response
Antibodies	Names vary according to specific lymphocyte targets	Bone marrow, other organ transplants	Idiopathic thrombocytic purpura, other hemolytic disorders
Azathioprine	Imuran	Kidney, heart, liver, pancreas	Rheumatoid arthritis, inflammatory bowel disease, myasthenia gravis, systemic lupus erythematosus (SLE), others
Cyclophosphamide	Cytoxan, Neosar	Bone marrow, other organ transplants	Rheumatoid arthritis, multiple sclerosis, SLE, dematomyositis, glomerulonephritis, hematologic disorders

(table continues on page 842)

● TABLE 12.23 Common Immunosuppressive Drugs (continued)

Generic Name	Trade Name(s)	Primary Indications*	
		Prevention or Treatment of Transplant Rejection	Diseases With an Autoimmune Response
Cyclosporine	Neoral, Sandimmune	Kidney, liver, heart, lung, pancreas, bone marrow	Psoriasis, rheumatoid arthritis, nephrotic syndrome
Glucocorticoids	See list of glucocorticoids used as immunosuppressive drugs	Heart, kidney, liver, bone marrow	Multiple sclerosis, rheumatoid arthritis, SLE, inflammatory bowel disease, hemolytic disorders, others
Methotrexate	Folex, Mexate, Rheumatrex	—	Rheumatoid arthritis, psoriasis
Mycophenolate mofetil	CellCept	Heart, Kidney	—
Sirolimus	Rapamune	Kidney, heart, liver	Rheumatoid arthritis, psoriasis, SLE
Sulfasalazine	Azulfidine, others	—	Rheumatoid arthritis, inflammatory bowel disease
Tacrolimus	Prograf	Liver, kidney heart, lung pancreas	Uveitis

From: Ciccone, CD: *Pharmacology in Rehabilitation*, ed. 3. FA Davis, 2002, p 637, with permission.
*Indications vary considerably and many indications listed here are not in the U.S. product labeling for each drug; optimal use of these drugs alone or in combination with each other continues to be investigated.
SLE = systemic lupus erythematosus.

TABLE 12.24 Glucocorticoids Used as Immunosuppressive Drugs

Betamethasone (Celestone)	Methylprednisolone (Medrol)
Corticotropin (Acthar)	Prednisolone (Pediapred, Predate, others)
Cortisone (Cortone)	Prednisone (Deltasone, others)
Dexamethasone (Decadron, others)	Triamcinolone (Aristocort)
Hydrocortisone (Cortef)	

From: Ciccone, CD: *Pharmacology in Rehabilitation,* ed. 3. FA Davis, Philadelphia, 2002, p 639, with permission.
Common trade names are shown in parentheses.

TABLE 12.25 Systemic Effects of Organ Failures Associated With Organ Transplants

Decreased peripheral oxygenation
Hypertension
Pulmonary congestion
Poor diaphragmatic excursion
Limited chest wall compliance
Anemia
Increased release of calcium ions from bone
Increased risk of infection
Muscle degradation and fiber loss
Peripheral neuropathies
Altered abdominal mechanics
Generalized muscle weakness and deconditioning

TABLE 12.26 Common Side Effects of Drugs Frequently Used in Transplantation

Steroids
Increased serum cholesterol
Mood swings
Weight gain
Hyperglycemia
Muscle weakness
Loss of connective tissue compliance
Bruising

Cyclosporine
Nephrotoxicity
Gingival hyperplasia
Hirsutism
Hypertension
Disease of central nervous system white matter (usually transient)
Tremors

TABLE 12.27 Symptoms Commonly Associated With Transplants

Liver Transplants
Fragile skin continuity
Easy bruising and bleeding
Encephalopathy
Weak abdominal musculature
Poor breathing patterns
Low back pain

Renal Transplants
Orthostatic hypotension (due to antihypertensive medication)
Osteopenia, osteodystrophy
Hypoglycemia (diabetics)
Hypertension
Muscle fiber loss
Weak abdominal musculature

Heart and Heart-Lung Transplants
Delayed heart rate response to exercise-deprived hearts (requires at least 5 min for circulating catecholamines to increase heart rate; requires at least 10 min to resorb and return to resting heart rate after cessation of exercise)
Two heart beats (in heterotopic transplants)
Decreased shoulder range of motion
Muscle weakness
Pulmonary congestion
Loss of endurance

Bone Marrow Transplants
Pancytopenia
Sensitive skin (from graft-versus-host disease)
Nausea

GEN MED

TABLE 12.28 Blood Types

Recipient's Blood Type	Donor's Blood Type
O	O
A	A or O
B	B or O
AB	A, B, AB or O

Hyperthyroidism and Hypothyroidism

Common Symptoms and Signs of Hyperthyroidism

- Palpitations
- Heat intolerance
- Nervousness
- Insomnia
- Breathlessness
- Increased bowel movements
- Light or absent menstrual periods
- Fatigue
- Fast heart rate
- Trembling hands
- Weight loss
- Muscle weakness
- Warm moist skin
- Hair loss
- Staring gaze

Symptoms are those problems noted by the patient. Signs refer to objective observations and measures detected, usually by a physician. For instance, a patient may express the symptom of "feeling hot." A physician will touch the patient's skin and note that the skin is warm and moist, recorded as a sign.

Based on:
http://www.endocrineweb.com/hyper1.html. *Accessed January 4, 2010.*

Common Symptoms and Signs of Hypothyroidism

- Fatigue
- Weakness
- Weight gain or increased difficulty losing weight
- Coarse, dry hair
- Dry, rough pale skin
- Hair loss
- Cold intolerance (patient can't tolerate cold temperatures in the same manner as those around him/her)
- Muscle cramps and frequent muscle aches
- Constipation
- Depression
- Irritability
- Memory loss
- Abnormal menstrual cycles
- Decreased libido

Each individual patient may have any number of these symptoms, and they will vary with the severity of the thyroid hormone deficiency and the length of time the body has been deprived of the proper amount of hormone.

Based on:
http://www.endocrineweb.com/hypo1.html. *Accessed January 4, 2010.*

TABLE 12.29 Primary Symptoms of Hyperthyroidism and Hypothyroidism

Hyperthyroidism	Hypothyroidism
Nervousness	Lethargy/slow cerebration
Weight loss	Weight gain (in adult hypothyroidism)
Diarrhea	Constipation
Tachycardia	Bradycardia
Insomnia	Sleepiness
Increased appetite	Anorexia
Heat intolerance	Cold intolerance
Oligomenorrhea	Menorrhagia
Muscle wasting	Weakness
Goiter	Dry, coarse skin
Exophthalmos	Facial edema

Based on: Kuhn, MA: Thyroid and parathyroid glands. In Kuhn, MA (ed): *Pharmacotherapeutics: A Nursing Process Approach,* ed. 3. FA Davis, Philadelphia, p 981, 1994.

AIDS and HIV

TABLE 12.30 Estimates of Risk of Acquiring HIV Infection by Portals of Entry

Entry Site	Type of Risk	Risk Virus Gets to Entry Site	Risk Virus Enters	Risk Inoculated
Conjunctiva	Random	Moderate	Moderate	Very low*
Oral mucosa	Random	Moderate	Moderate	Low*
Nasal mucosa	Random	Low	Low	Very low*
Lower respiratory	Low	Very low	Very low	Very low
Anus	High	Very high	Very high	Very high
Skin, intact	Low	Very low	Very low	Very low
Skin, broken	High	Low	High	High

Entry Site	Type of Risk	Risk Virus Gets to Entry Site	Risk Virus Enters	Risk Inoculated
Sexual: Vagina	Choice	Low	Low	Medium
Penis	Choice	High	Low	Low
Ulcers (STD)	Choice	High	High	Very high
Blood: Products	Choice	High	High	High
Shared needles	Choice	High	High	Very high
Accidental needle	Accident	Low	High	Low
Traumatic wound	Accident	Modest	High	High
Perinatal	Accident	High	High	High

STD = sexually transmitted disease.
*Based on data summarized in Recommendations for prevention of HIV transmission in health-care settings. *MMWR 36*:3S, 1987; and Update: Universal precautions for prevention of transmission of HIV, hepatitis B virus, and other bloodborne pathogens in health-care settings. *MMWR 37*:377, 1988. Adapted from Hopp, JW, and Rogers, EA: *AIDS and the Allied Health Professions.* FA Davis, Philadelphia, 1989, p 68.

● **TABLE 12.31 Estimates of Risk of Acquiring HIV Infection by Portals of Exit**

Portal of Exit	Virus Content	Potential for Spread	Chance to Be Inoculated
Respiratory Nasal:		Efficient	Very low
Sputum	Very low	Efficient	Very low
Saliva	Very low	Inefficient	Very low
Tears	Low	Dependent	Very low
GI: Vomitus	Very low	Dependent	Very low
Stool	Very low	Dependent	Very low
Urine	Very low	Inefficient	Very low
Sweat	Very low	Inefficient	Very low

(table continues on page 848)

GEN MED

TABLE 12.31 Estimates of Risk of Acquiring HIV Infection by Portals of Exit (continued)

Portal of Exit	Virus Content	Potential for Spread	Chance to Be Inoculated
Skin fomites	Very low	Inefficient	Very low
Intact skin	Very low	Dependent	Low
Broken skin	Low	Dependent	Med-high
Bleeding wound	High	Efficient	Very high
Sexual: Ejaculate	Very high	Efficient	Low-mod
Vaginal secretions	Moderate	Efficient	Very high
Purulent	Very high	Efficient	Very high
Blood: Transfusion	Very high	Efficient	Very high
Shared needles	High	Efficient	Low
Accidental needle	Low	Inefficient	Very low
Body fluids (usually blood tinged): Cerebrospinal fluid	Low	Inefficient	Very low
Synovial fluid	Low	Inefficient	Very low
Pleural fluid	Very low	Inefficient	Very low
Peritoneal fluid	Very low	Inefficient	Very low
Pericardial fluid	Very low	Inefficient	Very low
Amniotic fluid	Low	Efficient	Very high
Perinatal:	High	Dependent	Low
Breast milk	Low	Unknown	Low

Based on data summarized in Recommendations for prevention of HIV transmission in health-care settings. *MMWR 36*:3S, 1987; and Update: Universal precautions for prevention of transmission of HIV, hepatitis B virus, and other bloodborne pathogens in health-care settings. *MMWR 37*:377, 1988. Adapted from Hopp, JW, and Rogers, EA: *AIDS and the Allied Health Professions*. FA Davis, Philadelphia, 1989, p 66.
GI = gastrointestinal.

GEN MED

TABLE 12.32 Common Manifestations of HIV Infection by Organ System

Syndrome	Cause	Diagnostic Evaluation	Treatment	Symptoms/ Comments
Neurologic				
Mild to severe dementia Cognitive impairment with or without motor deficits	Direct virus-induced brain damage	HIV RNA level in CSF CT or MRI to check for brain atrophy (nonspecific)	Antiretroviral drugs, which may reverse damage and improve function	Does not always progress to AIDS dementia
Ascending paralysis	Guillain-Barré syndrome or CMV polyradiculopathy	Spinal cord MRI CSF testing	Treatment of CMV polyradiculopathy Supportive care for Guillain-Barré syndrome	Neutrophilic pleocytosis due to CMV polyradiculopathy
Acute or subacute focal encephalitis	*Toxoplasma gondii*	CT or MRI to check for ring-enhancing lesions, especially near basal ganglia Antibody testing of CSF (sensitive but not specific) Response to empiric antiviral treatment Brain biopsy (rarely indicated)	Pyrimethamine, folinic acid, sulfadiazine, and possibly trimethoprim/sulfamethoxazole (clindamycin if allergic to sulfa)	Prophylaxis with clindamycin and pyrimethamine or trimethoprim/sulfamethoxazole (as for *Pneumocystis* pneumonia) indicated for patients with a CD4 count of <200/μL and previous toxoplasmosis or positive antibodies *(table continues on page 850)*

TABLE 12.32 Common Manifestations of HIV Infection by Organ System (continued)

Syndrome	Cause	Diagnostic Evaluation	Treatment	Symptoms/ Comments
Subacute encephalitis	CMV Less often, herpes simplex virus or varicella-zoster virus	CSF PCR Response to treatment	Antiviral drugs	With CMV, often delirium, cranial nerve palsies, myoclonus, seizures, and progressively impaired consciousness at presentation Often responds rapidly to treatment
Myelitis or polyradiculopathy	CMV	Spinal cord MRI CSF PCR	Antiviral drugs	Simulates Guillain-Barré syndrome
Progressive encephalitis of white matter only	Progressive multifocal leukoencephalopathy of HIV	Brain MRI CSF testing	Antiretroviral drugs	Usually fatal within a few months May respond to antiretroviral drugs
Subacute meningitis	*Cryptococcus, Histoplasma,* or *Mycobacterium tuberculosis*	CT or MRI CSF stains and cultures	Treatment of cause	Good outcomes if patients are treated early
Peripheral neuropathy	Direct effects of HIV or CMV or antiviral toxicity	History Sensory and motor testing	Treatment of cause or withdrawal of toxic drugs	Very common Not quickly reversible

Syndrome	Cause	Diagnostic Evaluation	Treatment	Symptoms/Comments
Ophthalmologic Retinitis	CMV	Direct retinoscopy	Specific anti-CMV drugs	Requires examination by specialist
Cardiac Cardiomyopathy	Direct viral damage to cardiac myocytes	Echocardiography	Antiretroviral drugs	Symptoms of heart failure
Renal Nephrotic syndrome or renal insufficiency	Direct viral damage resulting in focal glomerulosclerosis	Renal biopsy	Antiretroviral drugs or ACE inhibitors possibly useful	Increased incidence in African Americans and patients with a low CD4 count
Oral Oral candidiasis	Immunosuppression by HIV	Examination	Systemic antifungals	Possibly painless in early stages
Intraoral ulcers	Herpes simplex virus or aphthous stomatitis			May be severe and result in undernutrition

(table continues on page 852)

GEN MED

TABLE 12.32 Common Manifestations of HIV Infection by Organ System (continued)

Syndrome	Cause	Diagnostic Evaluation	Treatment	Symptoms/ Comments
Periodontal disease	Mixed oral bacterial flora	Examination	Improved hygiene and nutrition Antibiotics	May be severe, with bleeding, swelling, and tooth loss
Painless intraoral mass	Kaposi's sarcoma or lymphoma	Biopsy	Treatment of cause	—
Painless white filiform patches on the sides of the tongue (oral hairy leukoplakia)	Epstein-Barr virus	Examination	Acyclovir	Usually asymptomatic
GI Esophagitis	Candidiasis, CMV or herpes simplex virus	Esophagoscopy with biopsy or ulcers	Treatment of cause	Dysphagia, anorexia
Gastroenteritis or colitis	Intestinal *Salmonella*, MAC, *Cryptosporidium*, CMV, *Microsporidia*, *Isospora belli*, or *Clostridium difficile*	Cultures and stains of stools or biopsy, but determination of cause possibly difficult	Supportive treatment of cause and symptoms	Diarrhea, weight loss, abdominal cramping

Syndrome	Cause	Diagnostic Evaluation	Treatment	Symptoms/ Comments
Cholecystitis or cholangitis	CMV of *Cryptosporidium*	Ultrasonography or endoscopy	Treatment of CMV Antiretrovirals for *Cryptosporidium*	Possibly pain or obstruction
Anal, rectal, and perirectal lesions	Herpes simplex virus, human papillomavirus, or and cancer Possibly multiple causes	Examination Gram staining and culture Biopsy	Treatment of cause	High incidence in homosexual men
Hepatocellular damage due to hepatitis viruses, oportunistic infections, or antivirul toxicity	TB, MAC, CMV, or peliosis (bartonel-losis) Chronic hepatitis B or C, worsened by HIV	Differentiation from hepati-tis due to antiretroviral or other drugs Liver biopsy sometimes necessary	Treatment of cause	Symptoms of hepatitis (eg. anorexia, nausea, vomiting, jaundice)
Skin				
Herpes zoster	Varicella-zoster virus	Clinical evaluation	Acyslovir or related drugs	Common Possible prodrome of mild to severe pain or tingling before skin lesions

(table continues on page 854)

GEN MED

GEN MED

TABLE 12.32 Common Manifestations of HIV Infection by Organ System (continued)

Syndrome	Cause	Diagnostic Evaluation	Treatment	Symptoms/ Comments
Herpes simplex ulcers	Herpes simplex virus	Usually clinical evaluation	Antiviral drugs if lesions are severe, extensive, persistent, or disseminated	Atypical lesions of herpes simplex that are extensive, severe, or persistent
Scabies	*Sarcoptes scabiei*			Possibly severe hyperkeratotic lesions
Violaceous or red papules or nodules	Kaposi's sarcoma or bartonellosis	Biopsy	Treatment of cause	—
Centrally umbilicated skill lesions	Cryptococosis or molluscum contagiosum			May be the presenting sign of cryptococcemia
Pulmonary Subacute (occasionally acute) pneumonia	Mycobacteria, fungi such as *P. jiroveci*, *C. neoformans*, *H. capsulatum*, *Coccidioides immities*, or *Aspergillus*	Pulse oximetry Chest x-ray Skin tests (sometimes false-negative because of anergy) Bronchoscopy sometimes necessary	Treatment of cause	Possibly cough, tachypnea, and chest discomfort at presentation Mild hypoxia or increased alveolar-arterial O_2 gradient possible occurring before evidence of pneumonia on x-ray

Syndrome	Cause	Diagnostic Evaluation	Treatment	Symptoms/ Comments
Acute (occasionally subacute) pneumonia	Typical bacterial pathogens or Haemophilus, Pseudomonas, Nocardia, or Rhodococcus	In patients with known or suspected HIV and pneumonia, exclusion of opportunistic or unusual pathogens	Treatment of cause	Possibly cough, tachypnea, and chest discomfort at presentation
Tracheobronchitis	Candida or herpes simplex virus	—	Treatment of cause	Possibly cough, tachypnea, and chest discomfort at presentation
Subacute or chronic pneumonia or mediastinal adenopathy	Kaposi's sarcoma or B-cell lymphoma	Chest CT Bronchoscopy	Treatment of cause	Possibly cough, tachypnea, and chest discomfort at presentation
Systemic Systemic septicemia from disseminated opportunistic infections	M. tuberculosis, MAC, or H. capsulatum	Blood cultures Bone marrow examination	Treatment of cause	—
Gynecologic Vaginal candidiastis	Candida			Possibly increased in severity or recurrent

(table continues on page 856)

GEN MED

TABLE 12.32 Common Manifestations of HIV Infection by Organ System (continued)

Syndrome	Cause	Diagnostic Evaluation	Treatment	Symptoms/ Comments
Pelvic inflammatory disease	*Neisseria gonorrhorae, Chlanydia trachomatis,* and other usual pathogens			Possibly increased in severity, atypical, and difficult to treat
Hematologic Anemia	Multifactorial: HIV-induced bone marrow suppression Immune-mediated peripheral destruction Anemia of chronic disease Infections, particularly human parvovirus B-19, disseminated MAC, or histoplasmosis Cancers	For parvovirus, bone marrow examination (to check for multinucleated erythroblasts) or serum PCR	Treatment of cause Transfusion as needed Erythropoietin for anemia due to antineoplastic drugs or zidovudine if severity warrants transfusion and erythropoietin level is <500 mU/L IVIG for parvovirus	With parvovirus, sometimes acute severe anemia

Syndrome	Cause	Diagnostic Evaluation	Treatment	Symptoms/ Comments
Thrombocytopenia	Immune thrombocytopenia, drug toxicity, HIV-induced marrow suppression, immunemediated peripheral destruction, infections, or cancer	CBC, clotting tests, PTT, peripheral smear, bone marrow biopsy, or von Willebrand's factor measurement	Antiretroviral drugs IVIG for bleeding or preoperatively Possibly anti-Rho (D) IgG, vincristine, danazol, or interferon If severe and intractable, splenectomy	Often asymptomatic and may occur in otherwise asymptomatic HIV infection
Neutropenia	HIV-induced bone marrow suppression, immunemediated peripheral destruction, infections, cancer, or drug toxicity		For severe neutropenia (<500/µL) plus fever, immediate broad-spectrum antibiotics If drug-induced, granulocyte or granulocyte-macrophage colony-stimulating factors	—

CMV= cytomegalovirus; IVIG= IV immune globulin; MAC= *Mycobacterium avium complex*.
Reprinted with permission, from Porter, R (ed): *The Merck Manual of Diagnosis and Therapy*, 19th ed. Copyright (2011) by Merck & Co., Inc., Whitehouse Station, NJ. http://www.merck.com/mmpe. Accessed September 24, 2011.

TABLE 12.33 Antietroviral Drugs

Generic Name	Abbreviation	Usual Adult Dose (Oral)	Adverse Effects*
Entry (Fusion) Inhibitors			
Enfuvirtide	T-20	90 mg sc bid	Hypersensitivity reaction, local injection site reactions
Mariviroc (CCR5 inhibitor)	—	150–600 mg bid, depending on other drugs used	Myocardial ischemia or infarction
Vieriviroc† (CCR5 inhibitor)	—		
Integrase Inhibitors			
Raltegravir	—	400 mg bid	None
Non-Nucleoside Reverse Transcriptase Inhibitors	Rash (occasionally severe or life threatening), liver dysfunction		
Delavirdine	DLV	400 mg q 8 h	Inhibits cytochrome P-450 metabolism of indinavir Possibly serious effects if delavirdine is given with certain nonsedating antihistamines, sedative hypnotics, antiarrhythmics, Ca channel blockers, ergot alkaloid preparations, amphetamines, or cisapride
Efavirenz	EFV	600 mg at bedtime	CNS symptoms, false positive cannabinoid test results, excessive blood levels if the drug is taken after fatty meals
Etravirine		200 mg q 12 h	Skin rashes
Nevirapine	NVP	200 mg once/day for 2 wk, then 200 mg bid	Increased cytochrome P-450, reducing levels of protease inhibitors

GEN MED

Generic Name	Abbreviation	Usual Adult Dose (Oral)	Adverse Effects*
Nucleoside Reverse Transcriptase Inhibitors	Lactic acidosis, liver damage		
Abacavir	ABC	300 mg bid	Severe hypersensitivity reactions (especially during rechallenge), anorexia, nausea, vomiting
Didanosine	ddI	400 mg once/day or 200 mg bid if ≥60 kg 250 mg once/day or 125 mg bid if <60 kg	Peripheral neuropathy,[‡] pancreatitis,[§] diarrhea
Emtricitabine	FTC	200 mg once/day	Minimal: skin hyperpigmentation
Lamivudine	3TC	150 mg bid or 300 mg once/day	Peripheral neuropathy, rarely pancreatitis
Stavudine	d4T	40 mg bid if ≥60 kg 30 mg bid if <60 kg	Peripheral neuropathy, rarely pancreatitis, fat redistribution with lipoafrophy of face and extremities
Zalcitabine	ddC	0.75 mg tid	Peripheral neuropathy, pancreatitis,[§] oral ulcers
Zidovudine	ZDV, AZT	300 mg bid	Anemia and leukopenia,[Π] rarely pancreatitis, myositis
Nucleotide Reverse Transcriptase Inhibitor			
Tenofovir	TDF	300 mg once/day	Increased levels of ddI; otherwise minimal

(table continues on page 860)

GEN MED

◼ TABLE 12.33 **Antietroviral Drugs** (continued)

Generic Name	Abbreviation	Usual Adult Dose (Oral)	Adverse Effects*
Protease Inhibitors#		Nausea, vomiting, diarrhea, abdominal discomfort, increased plasma glucose and hypercholesterolemia (common), increased abdominal fat, liver dysfunction, bleeding tendency (particularly in hemophiliacs)	
Amprenavir	APV	1,200 mg bid with food	Rash
Atazanavir	ATV	400 mg once/day	Hyperbilirubinemia
Darunavir	—	600 mg bid, taken with ritonavir 100 mg bid and with food	Severe rash, fever
Fosamprenavir	None	1,400 mg bid	Rash
Indinavir	IND	800 mg tid on an empty stomach (600 mg for patients taking DLV; should not be given with ddI)	Kidney stones, occasionally obstructive (patients should ingest 1,300 mL of fluid daily); cross-resistance with other protease inhibitors, especially ritonavir
Lopinavir	LPV	400 mg q 12 h (in fixed combination with 100 mg ritonavir) with food	Altered taste, circumoral paresthesias
Nelfinavir	NLF	1,250 mg bid with food	
Ritonavir	RIT	600 mg bid with food	Altered taste, circumoral paresthesias Possibly decreased incidence and severity of adverse effects with dose reduction

Generic Name	Abbreviation	Usual Adult Dose (Oral)	Adverse Effects*
Saquinavir	SQV	1,200 mg tid, within 2 hr of a meal (trough levels and efficacy possibly increased when used with ritonavir)	
Tipranavir	TPV	500 mg with ritonavir 100 mg bid	Hepatitis

Reprinted with permission, from Porter, R (ed): *The Merck Manual of Diagnosis and Therapy*, 19th ed. Copyright (2011) by Merck & Co., Inc., Whitehouse Station, NJ. http://www.merck.com/mmpe. Accessed September 24, 2011.

*All classes of antiretroviral drugs may contribute to chronic metabolic adverse effects, which include elevated cholesterol and triglycerides, insulin resistance, and centripetal redistribution of body fat. Adverse effects listed for drug class can occur when any drug in that class is used.

†Vieriviroc is under study; it may be effective for patients who do not respond to enfuvirtide and other antiretrovirals.

‡Peripheral neuropathy may be reversible when the drug is stopped, and symptomatic treatment provides partial relief.

§If symptoms of pancreatitis (e.g., nausea, vomiting, back and abdominal pain) occur, ddI or ddC must be immediately stopped until pancreatitis is confirmed or excluded.

ⁿAnemia can be treated with transfusions or other drugs such as erythropoietin; leukopenia can be treated with colony-stimulating factor (granulocyte colony-stimulating factor or granulocyte-macrophage colony-stimulating factor).

#All are metabolized by the cytochrome P-450 system, creating potential for many drug interactions.

TABLE 12.34 Drug Treatment of Opportunistic Infections in Patients With AIDS

Organism	Type of Infection	Drug Treatment*
Viral Infections Cytomegalovirus	Pneumonia; hepatitis; chorioretinitis; involvement of many other organs	Foscarnet, ganciclovir
Herpes simplex	Unusually severe vesicular and necrotizing lesions of mucocutaneous areas (mouth, pharynx) and GI tract	Acyclovir, famciclovir, or valacyclovir

(table continues on page 862)

TABLE 12.34 Drug Treatment of Opportunistic Infections in Patients With AIDS (continued)

Organism	Type of Infection	Drug Treatment*
Varicella-zoster	Painful, vesicular eruption of skin according to dermatomal boundaries (shingles)	Acyclovir, famciclovir, or valacyclovir
Bacterial Infections Mycobacterium avium complex	Involvement of bone marrow, reticuloendothelial tissues	Clarithromycin plus ethambutol; rifabutin
Mycobacterium tuberculosis	Tuberculosis	Isoniazid plus pyridoxine; rifampin (if isoniazid resistant)
Salmonella	Enterocolitis and bacteremia	Ciprofloxacin or trimethoprim
Fungal Infections Candida	Inflammatory lesions in oropharyngeal region and esophagus	Oral infections: clotrimazole, fluconazole, or nystatin; esophageal infections: fluconazole or ketoconazole
Coccidioides	Primarily affects lungs but may disseminate to other tissues	Amphotericin B
Cryptococcus	Meningoencephalitis	Amphotericin B ± fluocytosine, followed by fluconazole
Histoplasma capsulatum	Affects various tissues including lungs, lymphatics and mucocutaneous tissues; also causes blood dyscrasias (anemias, leukopenia)	Amphotericin B or itraconazole
Protozoal Infections *Pneumocystis carinii*	Pneumonia	Trimethoprim-sulfamethoxazole, pentamidine, or atovaquone

GEN MED

Organism	Type of Infection	Drug Treatment*
Toxoplasma	CNS infections (cerebral degeneration, meningoencephalitis)	Pyrimethamine plus sulfadiazine

From Ciccone, CD: *Pharmacology in Rehabilitation,* ed. 3. FA Davis, Philadelphia, 2002, p 585, with permission.

CNS = central nervous system.

*Choice of specific drugs varies according to disease status, presence of other infections, and so forth. Pharmacotherapeutic rationale is also changing constantly as new agents are developed and tested.

Signs and Symptoms of AIDS Dementia Complex

Early Signs of Dementia
- Impaired cognition (mild to moderate)
- Leg monoparesis
- Leg paraparesis
- Motor-verbal slowness
- Normal mental status
- Pyramidal tract signs
- Tremor

Late Signs of Dementia
- Ataxia
- Dementia (moderate to severe)
- Hemiparesis
- Hypertonia
- Incontinence
- Mutism
- Myoclonus
- Organic psychosis (persistent and nonpersistent)
- Paraparesis
- Quadraparesis
- Seizures

Based on:

Hart, M, and Rogers, EA: *Acquired immunodeficiency syndrome. In Fletcher, GF, et al (eds): Contemporary Clinical Perspectives. Lea & Febiger, Philadelphia, 1992, p 345.*

HIV and AIDS Glossary

acquired immunodeficiency syndrome (AIDS): The most severe manifestation of infection with the human immunodeficiency virus (HIV). The Centers for Disease Control and Prevention (CDC) list numerous opportunistic infections and neoplasms (cancers) that, in the presence of HIV infection, constitute an AIDS diagnosis. In addition, a CD4+ T-cell count below 200/mm^3 in the presence of HIV infection constitutes an AIDS diagnosis. The period between infection with HIV and the onset of AIDS averages 10 years in the United States. People with AIDS often suffer infections of

GEN MED

the lungs, brain, eyes, and other organs, and frequently suffer debilitating weight loss, diarrhea, and a type of cancer called Kaposi's sarcoma. Even with treatment, most people with AIDS die within 2 years of developing infections or cancers that take advantage of their weakened immune systems.

acute HIV infection: As related to HIV infection: Once the virus enters the body, HIV infects a large number of CD4+ T cells and replicates rapidly. During this acute or primary phase of infection, the blood contains many viral particles that spread throughout the body, seeding themselves in various organs, particularly the lymphoid tissues.

AIDS Bibliography: The National Library of Medicine (NLM) publishes the monthly *AIDS Bibliography,* which includes all citations from the AIDSLINE database. The *AIDS Bibliography* is available from the Superintendent of Documents (telephone: 202-783-3238).

AIDSDRUGS: An online database service administered by the NLM, with references to drugs undergoing testing against AIDS, AIDS-related complex, and related opportunistic infections.

AIDSKNOWLEDGE base: Full-text electronic database on AIDS, available in print as well as in electronic form, produced and maintained by physicians and other health-care professionals. The database is edited by P. T. Cohen (San Francisco General Hospital), Merle Sande, and Paul Volberding.

AIDSLINE: An online database service administered by the NLM, with citations and abstracts covering the published scientific and medical literature on AIDS and related topics.

AIDSTRIALS: An online database service administered by the NLM, with information about clinical trials of agents under evaluation against HIV infection, AIDS, and related opportunistic infections.

AZT: Azidothymidine (also called zidovudine or ZDV; the Burroughs-Wellcome trade name is Retrovir). One of the first drugs used against HIV infection, AZT is a nucleoside analogue that suppresses replication of HIV.

B lymphocytes (B cells): One of the two major classes of lymphocytes. During infections, these cells are transformed into plasma cells that produce large quantities of antibody directed at specific pathogens. This transformation occurs through interactions with various types of T cells and other components of the immune system. In persons with AIDS, the functional ability of both the B and the T lymphocytes is damaged, with the T lymphocytes being the principal site of infection by the HIV virus. See *T cells.*

CD4 (T4) or CD4+ cells: (1) White blood cells killed or disabled during HIV infection. These cells normally orchestrate the immune response, signaling other cells in the immune system to perform their special functions. Also known as helper T cells. (2) HIV's preferred targets are cells that have a docking molecule called cluster designation 4 (CD4) on their surfaces. Cells with this molecule are known as CD4-positive (or CD4+) cells. Destruction of CD4+ lymphocytes is the major cause of the immunodeficiency observed in AIDS, and decreasing CD4+ lymphocyte levels appear to be the best indicator of morbidity in these patients. Although CD4 counts fall, the total T-cell level remains fairly constant through the course of HIV disease, owing to a concomitant increase in the CD8+ cells. The ratio of CD4+ to CD8+ cells is therefore an important measure of disease progression.

CD8 (T8) cells: A protein embedded in the cell surface of suppressor T lymphocytes. Also called cytotoxic T cells.

CDC National AIDS Clearinghouse (CDC NAC): The CDC's comprehensive reference, referral, and publication distribution service for HIV and AIDS information. The clearinghouse works in partnership with national, regional, state, and local organizations that develop and deliver HIV prevention programs and services.

DDC: Dideoxycytidine (zalcitabine, HIVID), a nucleoside analogue drug that inhibits the replication of HIV.

DDI: Dideoxyinosine (didanosine, Videx), a nucleoside analogue drug that inhibits the replication of HIV.

d4T: d4T is a dideoxynucleoside pyrimidine analogue (2′3′-didehydro-3′-deoxythymidine). Like other nucleoside analogues, d4T inhibits HIV replication by inducing premature viral DNA chain termination. d4T has been approved for patients with advanced HIV infection intolerant to or failing other antiretroviral drugs. Also known as Stavudine and Zerit.

ELISA: Enzyme-linked immunosorbent assay, a laboratory test to determine the presence of antibodies to HIV in the blood. A positive ELISA test generally is confirmed by the western blot test.

GP41: Glycoprotein 41, a protein embedded in the outer envelope of HIV. Plays a key role in HIV's infection of CD4+ T cells by facilitating the fusion of the viral and the cell membranes.

GP120: Glycoprotein 120, a protein that protrudes from the surface of HIV and binds to CD4+ T cells.

GP160: Glycoprotein 160, a precursor of HIV envelope proteins gp41 and gp120.

helper T cells: See *CD4 (T4) or CD4+cells.*

HIV disease: An infectious disease characterized by a gradual deterioration of immune function. During the course of infection, crucial immune cells called CD4+ T cells are disabled and killed, and their numbers progressively decline. CD4+ T cells play a crucial role in the immune response, signaling other cells in the immune system to perform their special functions.

human immunodeficiency virus type 1 (HIV-1): (1) The retrovirus isolated and recognized as the etiologic (i.e., causing or contributing to the cause of a disease) agent of AIDS. HIV-1 is classified as a lentivirus in a subgroup of retroviruses. See also *lentivirus; retrovirus.* (2) Most viruses and all bacteria, plants, and animals have genetic codes made up of DNA, which uses RNA to build specific proteins. The genetic material of a retrovirus such as HIV is the RNA itself. HIV inserts its own RNA into the host cell's DNA, preventing the host cell from carrying out its natural functions and turning it into an HIV virus factory.

human immunodeficiency virus type 2 (HIV-2): A virus closely related to HIV-1 that has been found to cause immune suppression. Most common in Africa.

immune thrombocytopenic purpura (ITP): Also called idiopathic immune thrombocytopenic purpura. A condition in which the body produces antibodies against the platelets in the blood, which are cells responsible for blood clotting. ITP is very common in HIV-infected people.

immunocompetent: (1) Capable of developing an immune response. (2) Possessing a normal immune system.

immunodeficiency: A deficiency of immune response or a disorder characterized by deficient immune response; classified as antibody (B cell), cellular (T cell), combined deficiency, or phagocytic dysfunction disorders.

GEN MED

immunogen: A substance, also called an antigen, capable of provoking an immune response.

immunosuppression: A state of the body in which the immune system is damaged and does not perform its normal functions. Immunosuppression may be induced by drugs or result from certain disease processes, such as HIV infection.

interferon: A general term used to describe a family of 20 to 25 proteins that cause a cell to become resistant to a wide variety of viruses. They are produced by cells infected by almost any virus.

interleukin-2 (IL-2): One of a family of molecules that controls the growth and function of many types of lymphocytes. IL-2 is an immune system protein produced in the body by T cells. It has potent effects on the proliferation, differentiation, and activity of a number of immune system cells, including T cells, B cells, and natural killer cells. Commercially, IL-2 is produced by recombinant DNA technology and is approved by the FDA for the treatment of metastatic renal (i.e., kidney) cell cancer. Studies have shown that in the test tube, addition of IL-2 can improve some of the immunologic functions that are abnormal in HIV-infected patients. In addition, IL-2 is a growth factor for T cells, causing them to increase in number. In a clinical study with IL-2, it was found that in a small number of HIV-infected patients, IL-2 boosted levels of CD4+ T cells (i.e., the infection-fighting white blood cells normally destroyed during HIV infection) for more than 2 years, a far longer time than typically seen with currently available anti-HIV drugs.

lymphadenopathy syndrome (LAS): Swollen, firm, and possibly tender lymph nodes. The cause may range from an infection such as HIV, the flu, mononucleosis, or lymphoma (cancer of the lymph nodes).

lymphocyte: A white blood cell. Present in the blood, lymph, and lymphoid tissue.

natural killer cells (NK cells): A type of lymphocyte that does not carry the markers to be B cells or T cells. Like cytotoxic T cells, they attack and kill tumor cells and protect against a wide variety of infectious microbes. They are "natural" killers because they do not need additional stimulation or need to recognize a specific antigen to attack and kill. Persons with immunodeficiencies such as those caused by HIV infection have a decrease in NK cell activity.

p24: (1) Within the envelope of the HIV virus is a bullet-shaped core made of another protein, p24, that surrounds the viral RNA. (2) The p24 antigen test looks for the presence of this protein in a patient's blood. (3) A positive result for the p24 antigen suggests active HIV replication. p24 found in the peripheral blood is thought to also correlate with the amount of virus in the peripheral blood. It is believed that there are measurable levels of p24 when first infected with the virus after which there is a strong antibody response to p24 in early disease. Low or unmeasureable levels of p24 may indicate that the virus is in a dormant stage. Spikes in p24 levels may indicate that HIV has begun active replication.

protease inhibitors: HIV protease is an aspartyl enzyme essential to the replicative life cycle of HIV. The three-dimensional molecular structure of the HIV protease has been fully determined. Pharmaceutical developers are therefore able to rationally design compounds to inhibit it and thus interfere with replication of the virus. In the United States, five peptide-based protease inhibitors (saquinavir, Roche; A–80987, ABT–538, Abbott Laboratories; L735,524, Merck; KNI–272, NCI) are in clinical development. All compounds inhibit HIV-1 in vitro in nanomolar concentrations. In Europe, two peptide-based compounds (ABT–987, Abbott Laboratories; AG–1343, Agouron Pharmaceuticals, Inc.) are currently in development.

regulatory genes: As related to HIV: Three regulatory HIV genes—tat, rev, and nef—and three so-called auxiliary genes—vif, vpr, and vpu—contain information for the production of proteins that control (i.e., regulate) the virus's ability to infect a cell, produce new copies of the virus, or cause disease.

regulatory T cells: T cells that direct other immune cells to perform special functions. The chief regulatory cell, the CD4+ T cell or helper T cell, is HIV's chief target.

retrovirus: HIV and other viruses that carry their genetic material in the form of RNA and that have the enzyme reverse transcriptase. Like all viruses, HIV can replicate only inside cells, commandeering the cell's machinery to reproduce. Like other retroviruses, HIV uses the enzyme called reverse transcriptase to convert its RNA into DNA, which is then integrated into the host cell DNA.

Ryan White CARE Act: The Ryan White Comprehensive AIDS Resources Emergency (CARE) Act of 1990 represents the largest dollar investment made by Congress to date specifically for the provision of services for people with HIV infection. The purpose of the act is "to improve the quality and availability of care for individuals and families with HIV disease."

suppressor T cells (T8, CD8): Subset of T cells that halt antibody production and other immune responses.

surrogate marker: A substitute; a person or thing that replaces another. In HIV disease, the number of CD4+ T cells and CD8+ cells is a surrogate immunologic marker of disease progression.

T cells (T lymphocytes): A thymus-derived white blood cell that participates in a variety of cell-mediated immune reactions. Three fundamentally different types of T cells are recognized: helper, killer, and suppressor (each has many subdivisions). T lymphocytes are CD3+ and can be separated into the CD4+ T helper cells and the CD8+ cytotoxic/suppressor cells.

tat: One of the regulatory genes of the HIV virus. Three HIV regulatory genes—tat, rev, and nef—and three so-called auxiliary genes—vif, vpr, and vpu—contain information necessary for the production of proteins that control the virus's ability to infect a cell, produce new copies of the virus, or cause disease. The tat gene is thought to enhance virus replication.

3TC: Also known as lamivudine, 3TC is composed of the (—) enantiomer of the racemic mixture 2′-deoxy-3′-thiacytidine. Like other nucleoside analogues, 3TC inhibits HIV replication through viral DNA chain termination. It has been used in clinical trials in combination with AZT.

viral burden (viral load): The amount of HIV virus in the circulating blood. Monitoring a person's viral burden is important because of the apparent correlation between the amount of virus in the blood and the severity of the disease: sicker patients generally have more virus than those with less advanced disease. A new, sensitive, rapid test—called the branched DNA

GEN MED

assay for HIV-1 infection—can be used to monitor the HIV viral burden. In the future, this procedure may help clinicians to decide when to give anti-HIV therapy. It may also help investigators determine more quickly if experimental HIV therapies are effective.

viral core: (1) Typically a virus contains an RNA or DNA core of genetic material surrounded by a protein coat. See also *deoxyribonucleic acid; ribonucleic acid.* (2) As related to HIV: Within HIV's envelope is a bullet-shaped core made of another protein, p24, that surrounds the viral RNA. Each strand of HIV RNA contains the virus's nine genes. Three of these—gag, pol, and env—are structural genes that contain information needed to make structural proteins. The env gene, for example, codes for gp160, a protein that is later broken down to gp120 and gp41.

viral envelope: As related to HIV: HIV is spherical in shape with a diameter of 1/10,000 of a millimeter. The outer coat, or envelope, is composed of two layers of fatlike molecules called lipids, taken from the membranes of human cells. Embedded in the envelope are numerous cellular proteins, as well as mushroom-shaped HIV proteins that protrude from the surface. Each mushroom is thought to consist of a cap made of four glycoprotein molecules called gp120, and a stem consisting of four gp41 molecules embedded in the envelope. The virus uses these proteins to attach to and infect cells.

virus: Organism composed mainly of nucleic acid within a protein coat, ranging in size from 100 to 2,000 Å (unit of length; 1 Å is equal to 10^{-10} m); they can be seen only with an electron microscope. During the stage of their life cycle when they are free and infectious, viruses do not carry out the usual functions of living cells, such as respiration and growth; however, when they enter a living plant, animal, or bacterial cell, they make use of the host cell's chemical energy and protein- and nucleic-acid–synthesizing ability to replicate themselves. Viral nucleic acids are single- or double-stranded and may be DNA or RNA. After viral components are made by the infected host cell, virus particles are released; the host cell is often dissolved. Some viruses do not kill cells but transform them into a cancerous state; some cause illness and then seem to disappear, while remaining latent and later causing another, sometimes much more severe, form of disease. Viruses known to cause cancer in animals are suspected of also causing cancer in humans. Viruses also cause measles, mumps, yellow fever, poliomyelitis, influenza, and the common cold. Some viral infections can be treated with drugs.

wasting syndrome: The HIV wasting syndrome involves involuntary weight loss of 10% of baseline body weight plus either chronic diarrhea (two loose stools per day for more than 30 days) or chronic weakness and documented fever (for 30 days or more, intermittent or constant) in the absence of a concurrent illness or condition other than HIV infection that would explain the findings.

GEN MED

Based on:
CDC RT National AIDS Clearinghouse: Glossary of HIV/AIDS-Related Terms, Publication #B037, June 1995. CDC National AIDS Clearinghouse publications can be obtained by contacting the CDC National AIDS Clearinghouse at (800)458-5231.

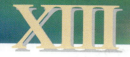

GENETICS

GENET

TABLE 13.1 Example Genes Associated With Exercise Performance

Gene Symbol	Full Name Biological Function(s)	Factor of Interest	OMIM Number	Gene Map Locus	Clinical Relevance	For More Information
ACE	Angiotensin I–Converting Enzyme ACE plays an important role in the conversion of angiotensin I into angiotensin II, a potent vasopressor.	Muscle mechanical efficiency	106180	17q23	Response to aerobic exercise training is dependent on ACE genotype.	Williams, AG, and Rayson, MP. Nature 403:614–615, 2000.
ACTN3	Alpha-Actinin-3 ACTN3 regulates the expression of the actin-binding protein alpha-actinin and is expressed in type 2 (fast) skeletal muscle fibers.	Muscle force generating capacity	102574	11q13-q14	The ACTN3 577R allele provides an advantage for power and sprint activities. ACTN3 R577X genotype influences the response to strength training in older adults.	Yang, N, et al: Am J Hum Genetics 73:627–631, 2003. Delmonico, MJ, et al: J Gerontol 62A(2): 206–212, 2007.

Gene Symbol	Full Name Biological Function(s)	Factor of Interest	OMIM Number	Gene Map Locus	Clinical Relevance	For More Information
APOE	Apolipoprotein E *APOE* is involved in lipid transport and metabolism. There are three alleles (variants) of this gene (*APOE2*, *APOE3*, and *APOE4*).	High-density lipoprotein cholesterol (HDL-C)	107741	19q13.2	**Ethnicity interacts with *E2/3* genotype at the *APOE* gene locus to influence response to endurance training.**	*Obisesan, TO. et al: Metabolism 57: 1669–1676, 2008.*
					Physical activity participation may counteract the potentially deleterious effects of the *APOE4* genotype on lipid profiles.	*Bernstein, MS, et al: Arterioscler Thromb Vasc Bio 22(1):133–140, 2002.*

Based on: National Center for Biotechnology Information, National Library of Medicine (Bethesda, MD): Entrez Gene. http://www.ncbi.nlm.nih.gov/sites/entrez?db=gene. Accessed May 29, 2009. McKusick-Nathans Institute of Genetic Medicine, Johns Hopkins University (Baltimore, MD), and National Center for Biotechnology Information, National Library of Medicine (Bethesda, MD): Online Mendelian Inheritance in Man, OMIM (TM) http://www.ncbi.nlm.nih.gov/omim/. Accessed May 21, 2009. OMIM is a compendium of human genes and genetic phenotypes.

GENET

GENET

■ **TABLE 13.2 Example Genes Associated With Musculoskeletal Conditions**

Gene Symbol	Full Name Biological Function(s)	Disease	OMIM Number	Gene Map Locus	Clinical Relevance	For More Information
COL9A2	Collagen, Type IX, Alpha-2; Trp 2 Allele *COL9A2* encodes one of the three alpha chains of type IX collagen, the major component of hyaline cartilage.	Intervertebral disc degeneration	120260	1p33–p32.2	The Trp2 allele of *COL9A2* is a risk factor for the development and severity of intervertebral disc degeneration.	*Jim, JJT, et al: Spine 30(24):2735–2742, 2005.*
IL1B	Interleukin 1-Beta This member of the interleukin 1 cytokine family is an important mediator of the acute inflammatory response.	Rotator cuff lesions with shoulder stiffness	147720	2q14	Shoulder stiffness is associated with increased *IL1B* expression and with greater myofibroblast recruitment into the subacromial bursa in rotator cuff lesions.	*Ko JY, et al: J Orthop Surg Res 26(8):1090–1097, 2008.*

Gene Symbol	Full Name Biological Function(s)	Disease	OMIM Number	Gene Map Locus	Clinical Relevance	For More Information
LRP5	Low-density lipoprotein Receptor-Related Protein 5 LRP5 has been implicated in bone mass accrual.	Osteoporosis	603506	11q13.4	**Bone density is associated with common variants in LRP5.**	van Meurs, JBJ, et al: JAMA 299(11): 1277–1290, 2008.
GDF5	Growth Differentiation Factor 5 The protein encoded by this gene is a member of the transforming growth factor-beta superfamily and is closely related to the sub-family of bone morphogenetic proteins.	Osteoarthritis	601146	20q11.2	**Genetic variation in the regulatory region of GDF5 is associated with susceptibility to osteoarthritis.**	Chapman, K, et al: Hum Mol Genet 17(10):1497–1504, 2008.

Based on: National Center for Biotechnology Information, National Library of Medicine (Bethesda, MD): Entrez Gene. http://www.ncbi.nlm.nih.gov/sites/entrez?db=gene. Accessed May 29, 2009. McKusick-Nathans Institute of Genetic Medicine, Johns Hopkins University (Baltimore, MD), and National Center for Biotechnology Information, National Library of Medicine (Bethesda, MD): Online Mendelian Inheritance in Man, OMIM (TM). http://www.ncbi.nlm.nih.gov/omim/. Accessed May 21, 2009. OMIM is a compendium of human genes and genetic phenotypes.

GENET

TABLE 13.3 Example Genes Associated With Neurological Conditions

Gene Symbol	Full Name Biological Function(s)	Disease	OMIM Number	Gene Map Locus	Clinical Relevance	For More Information
PARK2	Parkinson's Disease 2; Autosomal Recessive Juvenile Parkin, an E3 ubiquitin ligase, is involved in the degradation of cellular proteins.	Parkinson's Disease (PD)	600116 602544	6q25.2– q27	*Parkin* mutations are frequent in individuals with early-onset PD.	Lücking, CB, et al: N Engl J Med 342(21): 1560–1567, 2000.
APOE	Apolipoprotein E *APOE* is involved in lipid transport and metabolism. *APOE* also plays a key role in the maintenance and repair of neurons.	Alzheimer's Disease (AD) Traumatic Brain Injury (TBI)	107741	19q13.2	Physical activity may modify risk for dementia in *APOE4* carriers. *APOE4* may be a genetic risk factor for poor outcome after TBI.	Kivipelto, M, et al: J Cell Mol Med 12(6B): 2762–2771, 2008. Zhou, W, et al: J Neuro-trauma 25:279–290, 2008.

GENET

Gene Symbol	Full Name Biological Function(s)	Disease	OMIM Number	Gene Map Locus	Clinical Relevance	For More Information
HLA-DRB1	Major Histocompatibility Complex, Class II, DR BETA-1 Class II human leukocyte antigen molecules of the major histocompatibility complex are cell surface proteins that function to present foreign antigens to T cells.	Multiple Sclerosis (MS)	142857 See also 126200	6p21.3	The *HLA-DRB1*1501* allele increases disease severity in multiple sclerosis.	Okuda, DT, et al: Brain 132:250–259, 2009.

Based on: National Center for Biotechnology Information, National Library of Medicine (Bethesda, MD): Entrez Gene. http://www.ncbi.nlm.nih.gov/sites/entrez?db=gene. Accessed May 29, 2009. McKusick-Nathans Institute of Genetic Medicine, Johns Hopkins University (Baltimore, MD), and National Center for Biotechnology Information, National Library of Medicine (Bethesda, MD): Online Mendelian Inheritance in Man, OMIM (TM). http://www.ncbi.nlm.nih.gov/omim/. Accessed May 21, 2009. OMIM is a compendium of human genes and genetic phenotypes.

GENET

TABLE 13.4 Example Genes Associated With Cardiopulmonary Conditions

Gene Symbol	Full Name Biological Function(s)	Disease	OMIM Number	Gene Map Locus	Clinical Relevance	For More Information
LTBP4	Latent Transforming Growth Factor-Beta-Binding Protein 4 *LTBP4* has been linked to the development of emphysema in a mouse model.	Chronic Obstructive Pulmonary Disease (COPD)	604710	19q13.1–q13.2	Single nucleotide polymorphisms in *LTBP4* are associated with physical performance, exercise tolerance, and walking endurance in people with COPD.	*Hersh, CP, et al : Ame J Respir Crit Care Med 173:977–984, 2006.*
ADRB1 B1AR	Beta-1-Adrenergic Receptor *B1AR* mediates the effects of the hormone epinephrine and the neurotransmitter norepinephrine on the heart.	Congestive Heart Failure	109630	10q24-q26	Polymorphisms in *B1AR* may be determinants of exercise capacity in people with congestive heart failure.	*Wagoner, LE, et al: Am Heart J 144(5): 840–846, 2002.*

GENET

Gene Symbol	Full Name Biological Function(s)	Disease	OMIM Number	Gene Map Locus	Clinical Relevance	For More Information
ACE	Angiotensin I-Converting Enzyme See Table 14.1 for function	Essential hypertension	106180	17q23	**Regression of left ventricular hypertrophy in people with the ACE DD genotype is relatively resistant to ACE inhibitors.**	*Kohno, M, et al: Am J Med 106:544–549, 1999.*
EDN1	Endothelin 1 Endothelin-1, one of three isoforms of human endothelin, is a potent vasoconstrictor peptide produced by vascular endothelial cells.	Hypertension (HTN)	131240	6p24-p23	**The effect of EDN1 genotype on blood pressure is modulated by cardiorespiratory fitness levels or physical activity.**	*Rankinen, T, et al: Hypertension 50: 1120–1125, 2007.*

Based on: National Center for Biotechnology Information, National Library of Medicine (Bethesda, MD): Entrez Gene. http://www.ncbi.nlm.nih.gov/sites/entrez?db=gene. Accessed May 29, 2009. McKusick-Nathans Institute of Genetic Medicine, Johns Hopkins University (Baltimore, MD), and National Center for Biotechnology Information, National Library of Medicine (Bethesda, MD): Online Mendelian Inheritance in Man, OMIM (TM). http://www.ncbi.nlm.nih.gov/omim/. Accessed May 21, 2009. OMIM is a compendium of human genes and genetic phenotypes.

GENET

GENET

TABLE 13.5 Example Genes Associated With Common Chronic Conditions

Gene Symbol	Full Name Biological Function(s)	Disease	OMIM Number	Gene Map Locus	Clinical Relevance	For More Information
TCF7L2	Transcription Factor 7—Like 2 *TCL7L2* has been implicated in blood glucose homeostasis.	Type 2 Diabetes	602228	10q25.3	**Common variants in the transcription factor gene *TCL7L2* are associated with an increased risk of progression to diabetes in people with impaired glucose tolerance.**	*Florez, JC, et al : New Eng J Med 355(3):241–250, 2006.*
LEP	Leptin *LEP* encodes the protein leptin that is secreted by white adipocytes, and plays a major role in regulating body weight and adipose mass.	Obesity	164160	7q31.3	**Reductions in risk for obesity in females are associated with variation in *LEP* and *MC4R*.**	*Hart Sailors, ML, et al: Diabetes, Obes Metab 9:548–557, 2007.*
MC4R	Melanocortin 4 Receptor This gene is associated with the central control of feeding and energy balance.		155541	18q22		

Based on: National Center for Biotechnology Information, National Library of Medicine (Bethesda, MD): Entrez Gene. http://www.ncbi.nlm.nih.gov/sites/entrez?db=gene. Accessed May 29, 2009. Online Mendelian Inheritance in Man, OMIM (TM). McKusick-Nathans Institute of Genetic Medicine, Johns Hopkins University (Baltimore, MD), and National Center for Biotechnology Information, National Library of Medicine (Bethesda, MD): Online Mendelian Inheritance in Man, OMIM (TM). http://www.ncbi.nlm.nih.gov/omim/. Accessed May 21, 2009. OMIM is a compendium of human genes and genetic phenotypes.

TABLE 13.6 Example Genes Associated With Pediatric Conditions

Below are selected genes that have been implicated in conditions affecting children that are believed to be multifactorial in origin. Refer to O'Keefe (2006) for a more inclusive overview of chromosomal, single gene, and mitochondrial pediatric disorders.

Gene Symbol	Full Name / Biological Function(s)	Disease	OMIM Number	Gene Map Locus	Clinical Relevance	For More Information
ACE	Angiotensin 1–Converting Enzyme See Table 14.1 for function	Infant growth	106180	17q23	**ACE genotype is associated with birth weight and growth in the first year of life.** **ACE genotype is associated with health status of preterm infants.**	Hindmarsh, PC, et al: Ann Hum Genet 71:176–184, 2006. Harding, D, et al: J Pedatr 143: 746–749, 2003.
LRP5	Low Density Lipoprotein Receptor-Related Protein 5 LRP5 has been implicated in bone mass accrual.	Bone mineral density	603506	11q13.4	**LRP5 polymorphisms influence skeletal development in prepubertal and early pubertal children.**	Koay, MA, et al: Calcif Tissue Int 81:1–9, 2007.

(table continues on page 880)

GENET

TABLE 13.6 Example Genes Associated With Pediatric Conditions (continued)

Gene Symbol	Full Name Biological Function(s)	Disease	OMIM Number	Gene Map Locus	Clinical Relevance	For More Information
ORMDL3	ORM1-Like Protein 3 *ORMDL3* is a member of a gene family that encodes transmembrane proteins of the endoplasmic reticulum.	Asthma	610075	17q21.1	**Genetic variants at the *ORMDL3* locus on chromosome 17 are associated with asthma in children.**	*Bisgaard, H, et al: Am J Respir Crit Care Med 179: 179–185, 2009.*

Based on: National Center for Biotechnology Information, National Library of Medicine (Bethesda, MD): Entrez Gene. http://www.ncbi.nlm.nih.gov/sites/entrez?db=gene. Accessed May 29, 2009. O'Keefe, JA: Genomics and genetic syndromes affecting movement. In Campbell, SK, Vander Linden, DW, and Palisano, RJ (eds): *Physical Therapy for Children.* Saunders, St. Louis, MO, 2006. McKusick-Nathans Institute of Genetic Medicine, Johns Hopkins University (Baltimore, MD), and National Center for Biotechnology Information, National Library of Medicine (Bethesda, MD): Online Mendelian Inheritance in Man, OMIM (TM). http://www.ncbi.nlm.nih.gov/omim/. Accessed May 21, 2009. OMIM is a compendium of human genes and genetic phenotypes.

GENET

🔵 TABLE 13.7 Overview of Personalized Medicine and Tools to Assess Disease Risk

Tool	Implications for Health Care	For More Information
Personalized medicine	Personalized medicine employs new methods of molecular analysis to better manage a patient's disease or risk of developing a disease by helping physicians and patients choose the most optimal medical management approaches given a patient's genetic and environmental risk profile. These approaches include genetic screening to more precisely diagnose a disease or help physicians best select the type and dose of medication for a subgroup of patients.	*Adapted from the Personalized Medicine Coalition.* http://www.personalizedmedicinecoalition.org/about/aboutpmc.php. *Accessed June 21, 2009.* Feero, WG, et al: JAMA 299:1351–1352, 2008.
Genetic testing	Genetic markers for rare disorders as well as many common chronic diseases (such as for diabetes, heart disease, and several common types of cancer) are currently available.	*Feero, WG, et al: JAMA 299:1351–1352, 2008.*
	GeneTests' Web site is a publicly funded medical genetics information resource developed for physicians, other health-care providers, and researchers. GeneTests provides educational materials and a voluntary listing of genetics clinics that provide genetic evaluation and genetic counseling.	http://www.ncbi.nlm.nih.gov/sites/genetests/. Accessed June 21, 2009
	Additional information on genetic testing and finding a genetic counselor can be found at the website for the **National Society of Genetics Counselors.**	*National Society of Genetics Counselors.* http://www.nsgc.org/. *Accessed June 21, 2009*
Family history	http://familyhistory.hhs.gov/ **My Family Health Portrait** is the Web-based tool from National Human Genome Research Institute and the U.S. Surgeon General's Family History Initiative that helps an individual create a family tree of his/her own health history that can be printed and shared with family members or a	*My family health portrait. Courtesy: National Human Genome Research Institute, National Institutes of Health.* http://www.genome.gov/17516481. *Accessed May 29, 2009*

(table continues on page 882)

GENET

● TABLE 13.7 Overview of Personalized Medicine and Tools to Assess Disease Risk (continued)

Tool	Implications for Health Care	For More Information
	doctor. By tracking one's family health history an individual, along with his/her doctor, can better predict the risk of developing certain disorders. The **National Society of Genetics Counselors** website provides instructions on taking a family history.	*Family History Tool. National Society of Genetics Counselors.* http://www. nsgc.org/consumer/ familytree/index. cfm. *Accessed May 29, 2009*

● TABLE 13.8 Existing Federal Anti-Discrimination Legislation and Genomic Applications

Title	Description
Genetic Information Nondiscrimination Act (GINA)	The Genetic Information Nondiscrimination Act of 2008, also referred to as GINA, is a federal law that prohibits discrimination in health coverage and employment based on genetic information. GINA generally prohibits health insurers or health plan administrators from requesting or requiring genetic information of an individual or the individual's family members, or using it for decisions regarding coverage, rates, or preexisting conditions. The law also prohibits most employers from using genetic information for hiring, firing, or promotion decisions, and for any decisions regarding terms of employment.
Health Insurance Portability and Accountability Act (HIPAA) National Standards to Protect Patients' Personal Medical Records 2002	This regulation protects medical records and other personal health information maintained by health-care providers, hospitals, health plans, health insurers, and health-care clearinghouses. These standards are not specific to genetics; rather, they are sweeping regulations governing all personal health information.

GENET

Title	Description
Health Insurance Portability and Accountability Act of 1996 (HIPAA)	Federal Policy Recommendations Including HIPAA: • Applies to employer-based and commercially issued group health insurance only. HIPAA is the only federal law that directly addresses the issue of genetic discrimination. There is no similar law applying to private individuals seeking health insurance in the individual market. • Prohibits group health plans from using any health status–related factor, including genetic information, as a basis for denying or limiting eligibility for coverage or for increasing premiums. • States explicitly that genetic information in the absence of a current diagnosis of illness shall not be considered a preexisting condition.
Americans with Disabilities Act of 1990 (ADA)	Title I of the Americans with Disabilities Act (ADA), and similar disability-based antidiscrimination laws such as the Rehabilitation Act of 1973, do not explicitly address genetic information, but they do provide some protections in the workplace. • Prohibits discrimination against a person who is regarded as having a disability; protects individuals with symptomatic genetic disabilities; does not protect against discrimination based on unexpressed genetic conditions; does not protect potential workers from requirements or requests to provide genetic information to their employers after a conditional offer of employment. In March 1995, the Equal Employment Opportunity Commission (EEOC) issued an interpretation of the ADA. According to the interpretation: • Entities that discriminate on the basis of genetic predisposition are treating the individuals as having impairments, which would make such individuals covered by the ADA. • The ADA does not cover unaffected carriers of recessive and X-linked disorders or individuals who genetic testing or family history may identify as being at high risk of developing late-onset genetic disorders.

GENET

Modified: Courtesy of the National Human Genome Research Institute, National Institutes of Health. http://www.genome.gov/10002077. Accessed June 21, 2009.

⬤ TABLE 13.9 **Timeline of Milestones in Genetics**

Year	Milestone
2008	**Genetic Information Nondiscrimination Act (GINA)** The Genetic Information Nondiscrimination Act of 2008, also referred to as GINA, is a new federal law that prohibits discrimination in health coverage and employment based on genetic information. President Bush signed the act into federal law on May 21, 2008.
2006	**Initiatives to Establish the Genetic and Environmental Causes of Common Diseases Launched** • The Genes and Environment Initiative (GEI) was announced in early 2006 in order to analyze genetic variation among people with specific diseases and to develop new technology to monitor environmental exposures that interact with genetic variations leading to disease. • The Genetic Association Information Network (GAIN) is a public/private partnership that began with a donation from Pfizer Global Research & Development, New London, CT designed to support a series of genomic studies to determine the genetic contributions to five common diseases.
2005	**HapMap Project Completed** The International HapMap Consortium published a catalog of human genetic variation that is expected to help speed the identification of genes associated with common diseases such as asthma, cancer, diabetes, and heart disease. While the Human Genome Project (HGP) focused on the DNA sequence from a single individual, the HapMap project focused on variation in the genome and on human populations. The $138 million project was a 3-year collaboration between more than 200 researchers from Canada, China, Japan, Nigeria and the United States. The new paper described the completion of a Phase I HapMap that contains more than 1 million markers of genetic variation. At the time of the publication, the consortium was nearing completion of a Phase II HapMap that would contain more than 3 million genetic markers.
2004	**Surgeon General Stresses Importance of Family History** U.S. Surgeon General Richard H. Carmona announced that Thanksgiving Day would also mark National Family History Day. Since many families gather together for the Thanksgiving holiday, it is an ideal time for family members to share information about their family's health history. Even in our age of modern medicine, family histories remain vital to the prevention, diagnosis, and treatment of disease. To help families compile their health histories, the Surgeon General unveiled a free Web-based tool called "My Family Health Portrait." Families can use it to organize their health information and to produce a handout that they can share with family members or take to a doctor's office. Health-care professionals have long recognized that many common diseases such as heart disease and cancer tend to run in families. Using My Family Health Portrait is an easy and efficient way for families and health-care workers to use health histories to identify diseases for which a family may be at increased risk. This information can be used to design a personalized health plan for an individual that takes such predispositions into account.

GENET

Year	Milestone

2003 **Human Genome Project Completed**

The International Human Genome Sequencing Consortium announced the successful completion of the Human Genome Project more than two years ahead of schedule and under budget. The primary goal of the project was to produce a reference sequence of the human genome. The finished sequence announced by the international consortium covers 99 percent of the genome and is accurate to 99.99 percent.

2001 **First Draft of the Human Genome Sequence Released**

The Human Genome Project international consortium published a first draft and initial analysis of the human genome sequence. The draft sequence covered more than 90 percent of the human genome. One surprise is that the estimated number of genes was lower than expected, just 30,000–35,000. (The final genome sequence produced in 2003 has further lowered this estimate to the 20,000–25,000 range). The sequence data was immediately and freely released to the world. Researchers can access the data through public databases on the Internet and can use the information without restriction.

2000 **Working Draft**

In June 2000, rapid acceleration in the pace of DNA sequencing resulted in the compilation of a "working draft" of DNA sequence that covered more than 90 percent of the human genome.
Free Access to Genomic Information

In March 2000, U.S. President Clinton and U.K. Prime Minister Tony Blair stated that raw, fundamental data about human genome sequence and its variations should be freely available.

1999 **Chromosome 22**

In December 1999, the HGP completed the first finished, full-length sequence of a human chromosome—chromosome 22.

1998 **HGP Map Included 30,000 Human Genes**

In October 1998, HGP researchers released a gene map that included 30,000 human genes, estimated to represent approximately one-third of the total human genes.

1996 **Human Gene Map Created**

Scientists created a map showing the locations of ESTs (expressed sequence tags) representing fragments of more than 16,000 genes from throughout the genome.

(table continues on page 886)

GENET

TABLE 13.9 Timeline of Milestones in Genetics (continued)

Year	Milestone
1990	**ELSI Founded** Ethical, Legal and Social Implications (ELSI) programs founded at NIH and DOE was established as an integral part of the HGP. The ELSI Program was designed to identify, analyze, and address the ethical, legal, and social implications of human genetics research at the same time that the basic scientific issues are being studied. The NIH's National Human Genome Research Institute (NHGRI) committed 5 percent of its annual research budget to study ELSI issues. **Launch of the Human Genome Project** The Human Genome Project officially began in 1990. Beginning in December 1984, the U.S. Department of Energy (DOE), National Institutes of Health (NIH) and international groups had sponsored meetings to consider the feasibility and usefulness of mapping and sequencing the human genome.
1983	**PCR Invented** PCR—the polymerase chain reaction—is a technique for amplifying DNA that dramatically boosted the pace of genetic research. In a matter of a few hours, PCR can make billions of copies of a specific segment of DNA. The 1993 Nobel Prize in Chemistry was given for the invention of PCR. **First Disease Gene Mapped** A genetic marker linked to Huntington disease was found on chromosome 4 in 1983, making Huntington disease, or HD, the first genetic disease mapped using DNA polymorphisms. HD is inherited as an autosomal dominant disease.
1959	**Chromosome Abnormalities Identified** Professor Jerome Lejeune and his colleagues discovered that Down syndrome, first classified by J. L. H. Down in 1866, is caused by trisomy 21—that is, having three instead of two copies of chromosome 21. The extra copies of the genes on chromosome 21 affect the development of the brain and body.
1955	**46 Human Chromosomes** Joe Hin Tjio, NIH researcher, defined 46 as the exact number of human chromosomes
1953	**DNA Double Helix** Francis Crick and James Watson described the double helix structure of DNA. By the time Watson and Crick turned their attention to solving the chemical structure of DNA, DNA was known to have the following attributes: • DNA is made of nucleotides, chemical building blocks made of three parts: a phosphate group that is linked to a deoxyribose sugar, which is in turn linked to one of four nitrogenous bases—adenine (A), cytosine (C), guanine (G), or thymine (T). Nucleotides are linked in series into a chain, with phosphate and sugar groups alternating. Phoebus Levene had determined these chemical characteristics.

GENET

Year	Milestone

- In the DNA of any given type of cell, the amount of adenine approximately equals the amount of thymine, while the amount of cytosine approximately equals the amount of guanine. Erwin Chargaff had shown this in 1949.
- X-ray diffraction patterns obtained by Rosalind Franklin and Maurice Wilkins, revealed great symmetry and consistency in the structure of DNA and gave important clues about its dimensions.

1941 One Gene, One Enzyme

George Beadle and Edward Tatum, through experiments on the red bread mold *Neurospora crassa*, showed that genes act by regulating distinct chemical events—affirming the "one gene, one enzyme" hypothesis.

1911 Fruit Flies Illuminate the Chromosome Theory

Using fruit flies as a model organism, Thomas Hunt Morgan and his group at Columbia University showed that genes, strung on chromosomes, are the units of heredity.

1902 Chromosome Theory of Heredity

Walter Sutton, a graduate student in E. B. Wilson's lab at Columbia University, observed that in the process of cell division, called meiosis, that produces sperm and egg cells, each sperm or egg receives only one chromosome of each type. (In other parts of the body, cells have two chromosomes of each type, one inherited from each parent.) The segregation pattern of chromosomes during meiosis matched the segregation patterns of Mendel's genes.

1879 Mitosis Observed

Walter Flemming described chromosome behavior during animal cell division.

1869 DNA First Isolated

Friedrich Miescher isolates DNA for the first time.

1865 Mendel's Peas

Gregor Mendel describes his experiments with peas showing that heredity is transmitted in discrete units.

GENET

Modified: Courtesy of the National Human Genome Research Institute, National Institutes of Health. Website: http://www.genome.gov/25019887 (accessed 11/3/09).

IV

Resources for Practice

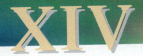
KINESIOLOGY, BIOMECHANICS, AND GAIT

Terminology

Kinesiology is broadly defined as the scientific study of human movement that encompasses anatomical, physiological, and mechanical concepts. Although most kinesiological analysis in clinical practice is qualitative in nature (i.e., one's knowledge of functional anatomy and physiology forms the basis for movement analysis), quantitative approaches to describing motion characteristics (*kinematics*) and identifying the causes of movement (*kinetics*) will also be considered in this section. These latter approaches to evaluating human movement are further expanded in the field of *biomechanics*.

Muscle Considerations

Types of Muscle Contractions

When excitation-contraction coupling occurs in skeletal muscle, actinomyosin is formed. A *muscle contraction* is defined as the formation of the cross-bridges between actin and myosin contractile proteins, resulting in the actin filaments being pulled toward the middle of the sarcomere. Depending on the relationship of the external load (resistance) to the tension generated, there may or may not be sliding of the actin filaments with a resultant shortening of the distance between z lines. The following contraction types are based on whether there is shortening of the whole muscle when excitation-contraction coupling occurs:

concentric contraction: There is a shortening of the sarcomeres, leading to a decrease in the length of the whole muscle. In practice, this means that joint rotation occurs and the limb segment moves in the direction of the muscle tension vector.

isometric contraction: There is a shortening of the sarcomeres to take up any slack in the muscle or connective tissue, and there is no observable change in the length of the whole muscle. In practice, this means that no joint rotation occurs and the limb segment does not move.

eccentric contraction: There is a lengthening of the sarcomeres leading to an increase in the length of the whole muscle. In practice this means that joint rotation occurs and the limb segment moves in the direction opposite to the muscle tension vector.

   Note: Eccentric muscle action can generate the greatest amount of torque through a given range of motion, followed by isometric, and concentric muscle contractions.

Force Relationships in Different Types of Muscle Contractions
Length-Tension Relationship
The magnitude of force produced by a muscle is related to the length of the muscle relative to its resting state as described in the figure on the following page.

KINES

🔵 TABLE 14.1 Three Types of Contractions Relative to Muscle Length

Type of Contraction	Muscle Length	Forces	Function	Mechanical Work
Concentric	Shortened	$M_m > M_r$	Acceleration	Positive ($W = F[+D]$)
Isometric	Same	$M_m = M_r$	Fixation	Zero (no change in length)
Eccentric	Lengthened	$M_m < M_r$	Deceleration	Negative ($W = F[-D]$)

M_r: Resistance moment. This is due to the weight of the limb segment and any load applied to that segment.
M_m: Rotary moment of the muscular force. This is the rotary component that is resolved from the tensile force created when a muscle contracts.
W = work.
F = force.
D = distance.
Source: Komi, PV: The stretch-shortening cycle and human power output. In Jones, NL, et al (eds): *Human Muscle Power*. Human Kinetics, Champaign, IL, 1986, pp 27–39.

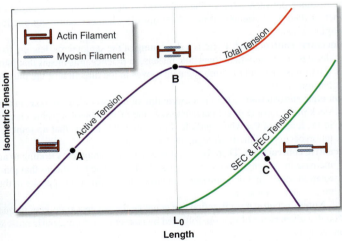

The ability of the muscle to develop active isometric muscle tension (purple curve) is impaired when the muscle is in the shortened state (A) (because actin and myosin filaments are maximally overlapped) and the elongated state (C) (when cross-bridges are pulled apart). The greatest active tension can be developed when the muscle length is slightly greater than the resting state, L_o (B). Note however that the Total Tension (red curve) increases beyond position (B) because the passive series elastic (SEC) and parallel elastic (PEC) components contribute to tension development (green curve). *Adapted from: Hamill and Knutzen, Biomechanical Basis of Human Movement, ed. 2. Lippincott & Williams, Baltimore, 2003, p 80.*

Force-Velocity Relationship

The relationship between force and velocity is different for eccentric, isometric, and concentric muscle actions. Maximum *power* (force X velocity) during concentric muscle action (a desirable goal when training some athletes) can be achieved at the point in the curve that corresponds to approximately one-third of maximum force and velocity .

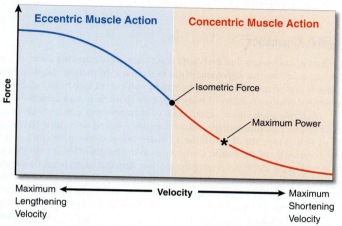

For concentric muscle actions (*right*) the force increases as the maximum shortening velocity decreases. Maximal power is indicated as an * on the curve. Maximal (isometric) force is achieved when the maximum shortening velocity is zero. For eccentric muscle actions (*left*) the force-velocity relationship is opposite to that in concentric action. When an external force (e.g., from gravity, antagonist muscle, or external load) exceeds the isometric maximum force, the muscle is lengthened as it tries to control the movement of the load. During this period of eccentric muscle action, muscle force generation increases as the velocity of muscle lengthening increases (only until the muscle can no longer control the movement of the load). *Adapted from: Hamill and Knutzen, Biomechanical Basis of Human Movement, ed. 2. Lippincott & Williams, Baltimore, 2003, p 81.*

Body Kinematics

KINES

Kinematics is the the study of the spatial and temporal components of body movement. Kinematic analysis may be qualitative or quantitative. Kinematics is used to describe spatial (3D) movement and includes measurement of body position, velocity and acceleration of body segments, joint angles, as well as angular velocity and acceleration. It excludes the study of forces that cause movement. Kinematics is further categorized as either *linear kinematics* or *angular kinematics*. Each of these subsets of kinematics is critical to understanding human movement because when an individual moves, body segments generally undergo both translation and rotation.

Linear Kinematics

A subset of kinematics that deals with describing motion in a straight line or curvilinear path (*translational* motion).

Quantification: some measurements can be expressed entirely by their magnitude (e.g., mass, distance, volume, speed) and are called *scalar* quantities; other measurements are expressed by magnitude and direction (e.g., velocity and acceleration) and are called *vector* quantities.

Angular Kinematics

A subset of kinematics that deals with describing angular motion about an *axis of rotation;* a line that is perpendicular to the plane of motion. Angular kinematics is critical to understanding human movement because nearly all human movement involves rotation of body segments about their joint centers.

Quantification: three scalar units of measurement can be used to describe angular motion: *degrees* (most common—based on a circle having an arc of 360°); number of *revolutions* (where one revolution equals a single 360° rotation); and the *radian* (rad), equal to the length of the arc divided by the radius of the circle describing the motion. Angular speed is another scalar quantity and is expressed as the angular distance traveled per unit time (°/s). There are numerous vector quantities used in describing angular kinematics; the most commonly used are *angular velocity* (omega symbol ω or °/s) and *angular acceleration* (alpha symbol α or either °/s^2 or rad/s^2). Other angular motion vectors used primarily in biomechanics are *tangential velocity* (V_T) and *tangential acceleration* (a_T), which are perpendicular to the radius of motion, and *centripetal velocity* (V_C) and *centripetal acceleration* (a_C), which are at right angles to their tangential components and directed toward the center of rotation.

In kinematics and biomechanics certain activities, such as locomotion, are cyclic (repetitive). In these instances *angle-angle diagrams* are used to represent the relationship between two angles during the movement (i.e., one angle is used for the x-axis and the other angle for the y-axis). In these diagrams, one angle is usually a *relative angle* (angle between two segments, such as the knee angle) and the other angle is usually relative to a reference frame (such as a thigh angle). Because these are two-dimensional plots, time must be indicated as marks placed on the curves at equal time intervals.

Kinematic Measurement Tools

The measurement systems used to quantify kinematic variables can be described categorically into exoskeletal, stereometric, and accelerometry systems.
exoskeletal systems: Instruments attached to the body for the purpose of body kinematic measurement. The following are among the most commonly used in kinesiological studies:
  • **electrogoniometers:** devices attached to the body to measure the angle between joint segments. Electrogoniometers are used primarily as a low-cost means of providing kinematic measurement during gait or other relatively slowly moving activities. There are two basic types:

Earlier versions use *rotational potentiometers* positioned over the approximate joint center—rotation of the potentiometer results in voltages that are linearly proportional to the angular displacement.

More recent *flexible electrogoniometers* use a flexible strain-gauged cable that is attached to the two body segments adjacent to the joint to be analyzed. The output signal is proportional to the angle of reciprocal orientation of the two bases in one plane only, and is insensitive to cable torsion and path.

- **foot switches:** electromechanical devices attached to the exterior of the shoe or as part of an insole, typically at the heel and toe, to measure temporal gait parameters.

stereometric systems: Camera and marker-based systems that provide high-resolution 3D reconstruction of the position and movement of body segments, relative to a *global coordinate system*. These systems have wide applicability to sports and other field locations and attain high spatial resolution and accuracy. Two categories are described:

- **stereophotogrammetric system:** A method of 3D measurement using photographic images and/or patterns of electromagnetic radiant energy for recording and digital acquisition of kinematic data. The 3D coordinate value of a point in space (referred to as the *global coordinate* of the point) is reconstructed from coordinate projections from at least two planes, where each plane is defined by an *internal* or *local coordinate system* derived from a camera in the system. Historically, high-speed photographic cameras have been used (16 mm and 35 mm) with speeds of 50 to 100 frames per second for gait and sports applications. These systems typically require extensive offline analysis, including film development and manual digitization, which can be a source of error. As a result they are being replaced in popularity by optoelectronic systems

- **optoelectronic system:** A method that relies on specialized markers and cameras interfaced with computers to facilitate automatic digitization of the camera image. They include video-kinematic systems with passive (reflective) or active (light emitting) markers. Passive markers are typically spherical or circular in shape, and can be stroboscopically illuminated (from the camera) by means of a group of infrared light emitting diodes (IRLEDs). Other types of systems include those with active coded body markers, such as IRLEDs that are position-sensitive, arrays of active marker sensors, or mirror assemblies that scan the markers. The significant advantage of these systems is that they provide automatic digitization.

accelerometer systems: Devices that measure acceleration. These systems are either *piezoelectric* (i.e., they convert mechanical forces exerted on a piezolectric material into voltages proportional to acceleration), or, in the case of more recent technology, are constructed of *small micro electro-mechanical systems (MEMS)*, where sensing elements are integrated with ultra low noise electronics. *Linear (uni-axial) accelerometers* provide an output signal (voltage) that is proportional to the acceleration of the sensor in one direction. *Bi-* or *tri-axial accelerometers* provide accelerometer measurements for two or three mutually perpendicular axes, respectively.

- When an accelerometer is placed on selective points of the body, the velocity and acceleration of these points can be calculated through numerical integration, when initial conditions are known.

KINES

- Low-pass filtering of accelerometer data can be used to extract the relative orientation of the sensor with respect to the gravity vector (*inclinometry*).

Source:

Medved, V: *Measurement of Human Locomotion.* CRC Press, Boca Raton, FL, 2001.

Standards for Reporting Kinematic Data

The Standardization and Terminology Committee of the International Society of Biomechanics (ISB) has provided recommendations for standardization in the reporting of kinematic data (refer to Wu, G, and Cavanagh, PR: ISB recommendations for standardization in the reporting of kinematic data. *J Biomechanics* 28(10), 1257–1261, 1995). The following recommendations were intended as a framework on which future progress can be made, and only a sample of these recommendations is provided here.

Convention for Global Reference Frame and Segmental Local Center of Mass Reference Frame

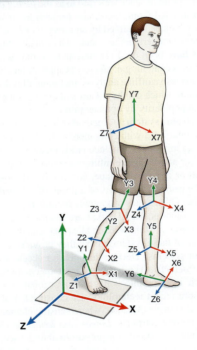

Adapted from:

Medved, V: *Measurement of Human Locomotion.* CRC Press, Boca Raton, FL, 2001, p 37.

Convention for Specification of Orientation of a Segment With Respect to the Global Reference Frame

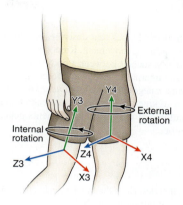

Adapted from:
Medved, V: Measurement of Human Locomotion. CRC Press, Boca Raton, FL, 2001, p 238.

Convention for Specification of the Relative Orientation of the Body Segments With Respect to One Another (example is for a joint coordinate system of the knee)

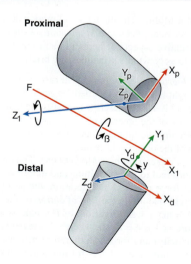

Adapted from:

Medved, V: Measurement of Human Locomotion. CRC Press, Boca Raton, FL, 2001, p 240.

Body Kinetics

Kinetics is a branch of mechanics that describes the forces and moments of force that are developed during movement. Kinetic measurements include those that take place externally, such as between a body and its environment, as well as those that take place internally, such as the forces and moments acting on a joint. Kinetics is further categorized as either *linear kinetics* or *angular kinetics*. Each of these subsets of kinetics is critical to understanding human movement because when an individual moves, body segments generally undergo both translation and rotation.

Linear Kinetics

A subset of kinetics that describes the mechanical causes of translatory motion (i.e., in a straight line or curvilinear path).

Quantification: the basis for the understanding of the kinetics of linear motion is force. *Force* is a vector quantity defined as any interaction (a push or pull) between two objects that can cause an object to accelerate. Units of force are expressed in newtons (N), for the International System (SI) of measurement, although force can also be expressed for comparison purposes in kinesiology and biomechanics as the ratio of force to body weight or body mass. Refer to Kinesiological Terms for a list of the many different kinds of forces described in linear kinetics.

Newton's Laws of Motion. The three laws of motion described by Sir Isaac Newton in his famous book, *Principia Mathematica* (1687), form the corner-stone for the quantitative aspects of human kinetics and biomechanics. The laws, also referred to as Newton's principles, are briefly described:

First Law (Law of Inertia): A body remains at rest or continues to move uniformly in a straight line, unless that body is acted on by a force. The term *inertia* of an object is used to describe its resistance to motion; it is directly related to the mass of the object (i.e., the greater the mass, the greater the inertia). To overcome the inertia of an object, a net external force greater than the inertia of the object is necessary.

Second Law (Law of Acceleration or Momentum): The change in motion of a body is proportional to the magnitude and duration of the force acting on it. If the net force produces acceleration, the accelerated object will travel in a straight line along the *line of action* of the force. This law is expressed as $F = \text{mass} \times \text{acceleration}$; or $F = ma$. Newton's second law can also be expressed as $F = dp/dt$, where p is the *momentum* of an object ($p = \text{mass} \times \text{velocity}$) and force can therefore be considered as the time rate of change of momentum. Units for momentum are kilogram-meters per second (kgm/s).

Third Law (Law of Action-Reaction): Action and reaction are equal: therefore, any force acting on one body will be counteracted by an equal and opposite force. This law dictates that forces never act in isolation but always in pairs.

Analyses Using Newton's Laws of Motion.

Numerous linear kinematic analyses are possible in kinesiology and biomechanics. These analyses can be categorized as describing the effects of forces applied a) at an instance in time; b) over a period of time; and c) applied over a distance.

Effect of Force at an Instance in Time: This effect is analyzed for *static* conditions (when the system is at rest or moving at a constant velocity) or for *dynamic* conditions (when the acceleration of the system is non-zero). Free body diagrams (see description below) are commonly used in conjunction with static analysis whereas *inverse dynamics* is used to calculate forces based on the acceleration of the objects. These analyses are typically applied to studying gait, exercise, sports activities, and materials-handling tasks such as lifting.

Effect of Force Applied Over Time: This effect is most commonly analyzed to describe *impulse-momentum relationships*, such as the analysis of ground reaction forces from a force platform during walking, running, or jumping. (see Kinetic Measurement System below in this section).

Effect of Force Applied Over a Distance: Used to describe *mechanical work* (the product of the magnitude of force applied against an object and the distance the object moves while the force is applied; or $W = F \times d$). If a force acts on an object and does not cause the object to move, no mechanical work is done. The most commonly used units of work are the newton-meter (Nm) and the joule (J); where 1 Nm = 1 J. A common application in kinesiology and biomechanics is the study of the pressure distribution pattern of the foot during walking and running (e.g., to evaluate running shoes, orthotics, or pathology).

Note: Work done per unit time is referred to as *power*, an important measure in kinesiological and biomechanical studies when analyzing muscle dynamics. Power has units of Watts (W). *Energy* is the capacity to do work, and is usually described in the metric unit joule (J). There are two basic kinds of mechanical energy:

Kinetic Energy (KE): The energy resulting from motion. Linear kinetic energy is expressed as $KE = \frac{1}{2} mv^2$ where **m** is the mass of the object and **v** is the velocity.

Potential Energy (PE): The stored energy describing the capacity to do work due to the position of the object relative to gravity or to its form (also termed *strain energy (SE),* where the force required to deform an object is stored as potential energy). Potential energy related to position is described mathematically as $PE = mgh$ where **m** is the mass of the object, **g** is acceleration due to gravity, and **h** is the height of the object. Potential energy related to deformation is described mathematically as $SE = \frac{1}{2} k \times \Delta x$ where k is a proportionality constant and Δx is the distance over which the object was deformed. Muscles, ligaments, and tendons are studied in this manner because they store strain energy and release it to aid in human movement.

KINES

Angular Kinetics

A subset of kinetics that describes the mechanical causes of angular motion.

Quantification: The fundamental measure of angular kinetics is *torque (T)* or *moment of force,* which is defined as the tendency of a force to produce a rotation about a specific axis. Torque is mathematically derived by $T = F \times r$ where F is the applied force and r is the perpendicular distance from the line of action of the force to the centor of rotation (*moment arm*). Units are typically expressed as newton-meters (nm). Torque measurements are used throughout kinesiology because muscles typically insert at a distance from the joint axis, thereby producing a torque. The *center of mass (COM)* is a theoretical point located in or outside of the body, in which the sum of the torques equal zero. In biomechanics, the center of mass determination for the human body is estimated by calculating the COM for each of the body segments and combining them—a procedure known as the *segmental method.* Center of mass determinations are used throughout the field of kinesiology, as for example in describing the angular kinetics of locomotion, postural stability, and sports activities.

Note: Newton's Laws of Motion, described previously as the basis for linear kinetics, also forms the basis for describing the forces causing angular movement or equilibrium. Therefore, each linear quantity and relationship previously described (see Linear Kinetics) has a corresponding angular analogue. For example, the angular analogue of force is *torque*, the angular analogue of mass is *moment of inertia*, and the the angular analogue of acceleration is *angular acceleration*. These analogue measures are simply substituted into the linear algorithms to derive their angular counterpart. This rule applies for all of the relationships described previously for static and dynamic analysis, angular impulse-momentum relationship, angular power, angular work, and rotational kinetic and potential energy.

Free Body Diagram for Kinetic Analysis.
Because the analysis of human movement typically takes into consideration a number of linear reactive forces as well as moments of forces acting on the body, a simplified *free body diagram* drawing, such as a stick figure or outline of the body, is used showing the vector representations of these forces and their points of application.

Kinetic Measurement Systems

Data acquired from motion capture systems can be analyzed using inverse dynamics to calculate kinetic data. Other more direct kinetic measurement systems use *ground reaction force platforms* or *pressure distribution systems.*

ground reaction force platforms: Devices that measure the total force vector (F_x, F_y, F_z) that results from contact between the subject's body (e.g., the foot) and the floor during locomotion. These devices can provide the moment of force vector (M_x, M_y, M_z) as well as planar coordinate values (X and Y) of the *center of pressure*, which are displayed as time curves. Force platforms are commonly used for locomotion studies, clinical gait analysis, and assessment of postural stability. Force measurement is derived most commonly from either *strain gauge* or *piezoelectric* transducers.

• *Measurement Parameters:*

Kinetic data from ground reaction force platforms are typically in the form of time-dependent curves where the individual F_x, F_y, F_z components of the force are plotted separately as a time series, and pathology is identified by comparison to well-established norms. Other, more specialized signal representations are used, such as *vector diagrams* and *stabilograms.*

Vector Diagram: a spatiotemporal sequence of component ground reaction force vectors in the sagittal (i.e., F_z and F_x) and frontal (i.e., F_z and F_y) planes. The vector patterns produced by changes in direction, amplitude, and location of the force vectors during locomotion provide a graphic representation of locomotion that can be used to identify pathological gait.

Stabilogram: a spatiotemporal sequence (i.e., trajectory) of the calculated *center of pressure* (COP) in the support plane (i.e., the plane defined by the force platform surface) derived from ground reaction force and torque data as a measure of postural stability. A stabilogram is typically acquired during "quiet" standing to estimate postural sway. Stability can be inferred by comparing the trajectory of the COP (e.g., its area and pattern of movement) with respect to the subject's base of support. Stabilograms are also used to assess *dynamic postural stability* using specialized platforms in which the base of support is briefly rotated or shifted to momentarily perturb the subject. Dynamic stability is assessed with respect to the ability of the subject to recover postural equilibrium.

pressure distribution measurement systems: Systems that measure pressure distribution for the purpose of studying the dynamic contact between the foot and the ground. These systems have been developed with either sensors embedded in the footwear (such as in the sole of the shoe), or sensors installed in a removable insole, or as sensors embedded in an instrumented walkway. The majority of these systems measure only the vertical pressure component. The primary advantages of these systems are that they provide spatially precise information and they allow measurement of many strides. One disadvantage is that their measurements are typically less accurate than those derived from force platforms.

Kinesiological Electromyography

In addition to its use as a diagnostic tool for neuromuscular disorders (see Clinical Electromyography, p. 305), electromyography can be used as a kinesiological tool to quantify muscle function during specific activities. *Electromyography* is the study of the electrical activity that is produced when a muscle contracts. The *electromyographic (EMG) signal* is the spatial and temporal summation of the *motor unit action potentials* that are within the detection zone of a sensor (see Neurology Section p. 305). The *electromyogram* is a voltage-time plot of the EMG signal after it has been detected and conditioned by the EMG acquisition system. The figure on p. 902 provides a schematic of the EMG signal detected from the surface of the skin, with the underlying motor unit action potential signal sources propagating along the muscle fibers.

KINES

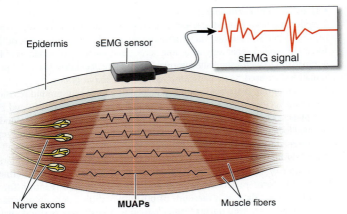

Epidermis sEMG sensor

sEMG signal

Nerve axons **MUAPs** Muscle fibers

Derivation of the surface electromyographic (sEMG) signal.

EMG Acquisition

To record the EMG signal, a *signal acquisition system* is needed that includes a *sensor* and *signal conditioning* hardware/software.

EMG Sensors

Surface EMG (sEMG) sensors are most often used for kinesiological studies and biofeedback therapy. The sensor is placed on the skin over the muscle of interest. The sEMG sensor is typically applied as a *differential pair* (two contacts on the skin); either in the form of one encapsulated sensor containing both contacts at a fixed distance apart, or as two separate sensors containing one contact each that are separated by a distance selected by the user. sEMG sensors with fixed contact surfaces are typically encapsulated with the conditioning amplifiers contained within the sensor (referred to as an *active* sEMG sensor) and are re-usable. In contrast, the non-fixed sensor pairs may be disposable without signal conditioning circuitry as part of the sensor (referred to as a *passive* EMG sensor). See the figure on the following page for examples of sEMG sensors.

Fine-wire EMG sensors are a type of indwelling EMG sensor in the form of a pair of insulated fine wires with hooked exposed tips that are inserted into the muscle belly using a hypodermic needle. The needle is withdrawn, leaving the wires embedded in the muscle during the recording period. The wires are removed by pulling them carefully from the muscle tissue and disposing of them. Sterilization procedures are used to prevent infection, and caution must be observed to prevent trauma to blood vessels and nerves by the needle.

All sEMG and fine-wire sensors are used in conjunction with a *ground reference electrode* that is typically placed on the skin over a bony prominence.

KINES

Recent advancements in sEMG sensor technology have resulted in *wireless sensors* that transmits the sEMG signal directly from the sensor through the air via a carrier frequency, where it is received by either a body-worn transceiver or a base station. These sensors allow freedom of movement without the constraint of wires in contact with the body or the need to tether the subject to a computer workstation. These advantages are particularly useful when monitoring dynamic activities such as sports or exercise.

Advantages/Disadvantages.

sEMG sensors are noninvasive, can provide signals from a relatively large portion of the muscle, and can be easily configured as multi-sensor systems for analyzing more than one muscle group at the same time. Their primary disadvantages are that they are limited to recording superficial muscle groups and may not provide adequate spatial resolution when recording from relatively small muscle groups that are in close proximity to one another. Active sEMG sensors have the advantage of requiring less skin preparation and are less susceptible to external noise sources (such as artifacts produced by movement of recording leads) compared to passive sEMG sensors. Fine-wire electrodes have the advantage of recording from deep muscles. Because they have a smaller detection zone than sEMG sensors, they also provide better spatial resolution for isolated recordings from small muscle groups in close proximity to one another.

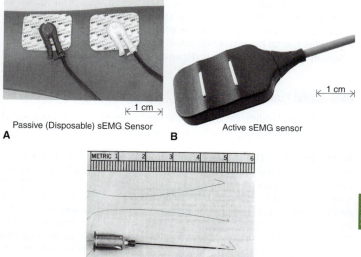

Passive (Disposable) sEMG Sensor
A

Active sEMG sensor
B

Fine-wire (Invasive) EMG sensor
C

Types of electromyographic sensors. From: Portney, LG, Roy, SH, and Echternach, JL: Electromyography and nerve conduction velocity tests. In O'Sullivan, SB, and Schmitz, TJ (eds): Physical Rehabilitation, ed. 5, FA Davis, Philadelphia, 2006, pp 275–276, with permission.

sEMG Sensor Placement: To fully understand the guidelines for placement of the sEMG sensor, it is recommended that the intended user understand the many intrinsic and extrinsic factors that influence the fidelity of the sEMG signal. These factors are beyond the scope of this Handbook and are discussed in the resources listed below.

Guidelines

- Prior to placement of the sensor, prepare the skin by shaving it of excessive hair and wiping it with an alcohol pad. For passive sensors, the skin may need mild sanding with a fine abrasive to reduce skin resistance (note: sanding is typically not needed for active sensors, although repeated tape peels to the skin is recommended).
- The sensor contacts should be aligned in parallel to the direction of the muscle fibers.
- The sensor should be located in the midline of the muscle belly away from its lateral borders to minimize contamination of the EMG signal by propagated signals from neighboring muscle groups (referred to as *EMG crosstalk*).
- Avoid placement of sensor on tendonous regions of the muscle or innervation zone.
- When using sensors that do not have fixed sensor contacts, the contact separations should be maintained at a fixed distance apart during and between recording periods (note: a separation of 1 cm is recommended for most applications, although ranges from 0.5 to 2.0 cm can be found in the literature).
- The sensor should be adhered to the skin using a hypoallergenic medical-grade tape or insert to minimize skin irritation.
- Once the general location for the sensor is determined, preliminary contractions of the muscle should be performed to ensure signal quality.

EMG Signal Conditioning

The EMG signal is differentially amplified and filtered prior to being sampled and stored on a computer workstation for processing.

Amplification. The sEMG signals being detected by the sensor at the surface of the skin are relatively small (from 5 µV to 1–10 mV) and it is recommended that they be amplified to match the input range of the computer workstations that are typically in a much higher 1- to 10-V range, depending on the manufacturer. Because the human body acts as an antenna, thereby attracting electromagnetic energy from the environment, differential amplification is needed to subtract this unwanted signal interference from the two contact surfaces of the sensor, leaving just the desired composite muscle action potential signal.

Filtering. Even with the use of state-of-the-art acquisition equipment and adherence to recommended guidelines for recording the sEMG signal, there will be unwanted signal contaminants (referred to as signal *artifact* or *noise*) that can be attenuated by conditioning the signal using *bandpass filters* that are typically provided as part of the differential amplifier. The sEMG signal has signal components from the motor unit action potentials that occupy a specific range of frequencies or *bandwidth* (from DC-500 Hz for most sEMG recordings). The unwanted artifacts or signal contaminants are present either at the low frequency portion of the sEMG signal spectrum (DC-20 Hz; resulting from *movement artifact* caused by disturbances between the sensor-skin interface) or at the high frequency portion of the sEMG spectrum (typically above 400 Hz; resulting from electronic noise inherent in the recording equipment). Therefore, a bandpass filter set at 20 to 450 Hz will allow only those signal components between 20 and 450 Hz to "pass" through the amplifier to the output stages by filtering out signal sources below 20 Hz or above 450 Hz.

EMG Signal Processing

Sampling and Storage. Historically, prior to the availability of digital technologies and PC workstations, the sEMG signal was viewed on an oscilloscope and either stored on an FM tape recorder or printed directly to a pen or chart recorder for later analysis. Currently, the procedure has changed considerably, and most kinesiological studies digitize and store the EMG signals using a PC workstation that consists of a personal computer that is configured with an analogue to digital (A/D or A-to-D) processing card and acquisition software. The fidelity of the resultant signal is dependent in part on the digitization process that converts the analogue signal (continuous time series of voltages) to discrete data points sampled at a specified frequency using the A/D card. The following rules should be observed when processing and storing the sEMG signal using a PC workstation:

- Set the sampling rate to at least twice the maximal frequency content of the sEMG signal. Typically, sEMG signal content is below 500 Hz and therefore a minimal sampling rate of 1,000 Hz should be used. Undersampling the signal will distort the sEMG waveforms and thereby invalidate the results.
- The gain of the amplifier should be set to maximize the sEMG signal amplitude so that it matches the amplitude range of the A/D card. Most cards for sEMG acquisition systems can be set to either ±1V, ±5V, or ±10V.
  - Setting the gain too high so that the output voltage of the sEMG signal exceeds the maximal range of the A/D card will result in unwanted distortion of the sEMG waveform by clipping of the signal.
  - Setting the gain too low so that the output voltage of the sEMG signal is an order of magnitude lower than the maximal range will result in poor resolution of the sEMG waveform, thereby losing possibly useful informational content of the signal.
- A/D cards should be selected to provide ample signal resolution to differentiate the EMG signal from the baseline noise. For example, with a typical sEMG baseline noise of ±5 μV, it is necessary to digitize the signal with enough bits so that even the faintest EMG activity can be appreciably resolved. A 16-bit A/D system set at ±5 V has a resolution of 0.153 μV for a system with a gain of 1,000. This means that the recorded noise can be resolved with at least 5 bits (i.e., 32 quantization steps). This leaves ample resolution for identifying EMG activity, which will be decidedly larger than the baseline level. A/D cards of at least 12 bits are recommended, providing that the gain is adequate as in the example.

Temporal Processing of the Electromyographic (EMG) Signal: Once the signal is sampled and stored, further processing is done in software to extract kinesiologically useful information based on changes either in the amplitude or frequency content of the signal as a function of contraction duration.

Amplitude Parameters of the sEMG Signal

Amplitude parameters of the EMG signal are most widely used for kinesiological studies. Depending on the task being monitored and the recording procedures, changes in the amplitude of the EMG signal can be used to derive information related to the timing of muscle activity, the relative force contribution, or the presence of specific involuntary movement disorders. Because the sEMG signal appears to have a complex appearance characterized by unpredictable deviations in voltage from positive to negative values of different magnitude, post-processing of the *raw signal* waveform is commonly practiced to derive amplitude parameters that simplify the representation of the amplitude content of the signal. Some of the most common amplitude parameters of the signal are described below, followed by illustrations in the figure on the following page.

full-wave rectified: The negative voltages are transposed to positive values; equivalent to providing the absolute value of the EMG signal. Because simple averaging of the positive and negative voltages of the signal does not provide useful information, rectification of the signal is commonly used before further signal conditioning (such as moving averages or integration) is conducted.

average rectified value (ARV) or mean rectified value (MRV): The time average of the full-wave rectified EMG signal over a specified period of time. The shorter this time interval, the less smooth this averaged value will appear. By taking the average of randomly varying values of the EMG signal, the larger fluctuations in the signal are removed.

linear envelope: Low-pass filtering of the full-wave rectified signal produces a linear envelope of the signal. It is a type of moving average that follows the trend of the EMG signal and closely resembles the shape of the muscle tension curve. This form of signal conditioning is often incorrectly confused with integration.

moving average: A digital moving-average where the mean of the rectified EMG is calculated over a defined time interval or "window." The shorter this time interval, the less smooth this average value will be. To obtain the time-varying average of a complete EMG record, it is necessary to shift the time window forward by an amount (T) less than or equal to the time equivalent of the window. For typical applications, a value of T ranging from 100 to 200 ms is recommended. Normally the average is calculated for the middle of the window because it does not introduce a lag in its output; special forms of weighting (exponential, triangular, etc.) can also be applied.

integrated EMG (iEMG or IEMG): A widely used procedure in electromyography that is frequently confused with signal averaging techniques or linear envelope detection. The correct interpretation of integration is purely mathematical and means "area under the curve"; the correct units are millivolt-seconds (mV•s) or microvolt-seconds (μV•s). There are many methods of integrating the EMG; three common procedures are illustrated and described.

- **integration over the contraction:** The simplest form of integration starts at some preset time and continues for the remaining time of the muscle activity.
- **resetting of the integrated signal:** The integrated signal is reset to 0 at regular intervals of time during the muscle activity, usually from 50 to 200 ms (the time should be specified). Such a scheme yields a series of peaks that represents the trend of the EMG amplitude with time (similar to a moving average). The sum of all the peaks in any given contraction should equal the integrated EMG over that contraction.
- **integrating with voltage level reset:** The integration begins before the contraction. If the muscle activity is high, the integrator rapidly charges up to the reset level; if low activity occurs, the integrator takes longer to reach reset. Thus the activity level is reflected in the frequency of resets.

root-mean-square (RMS): The RMS is an electronic average representing the square root of the average of the squares of the current or voltage; RMS provides a nearly instantaneous output of the power of the EMG signal. It is one of the most commonly used amplitude parameters of the sEMG signal because of its advantages in providing an estimate of muscle force.

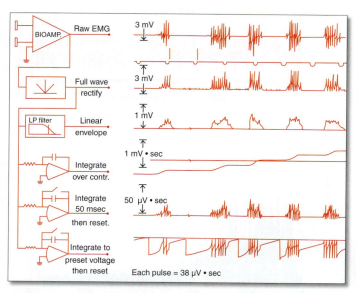

Illustration of the raw EMG signal and several methods of processing the raw signal to extract amplitude measurements. *From: Winter, DA: Biomechanics of Human Movement. Wiley, New York, 1979, p 140, with permission.*

Frequency Parameters of the sEMG Signal

These parameters of the sEMG signal are most widely used in kinesiological studies for monitoring *localized muscle fatigue* (fatigue that takes place as a result of physiological processes distal to the myoneural junction). During an isometric contraction sustained at a constant force level that impedes both the delivery of oxygenated blood to the muscle and the removal of metabolic by-products, there is progressive loss in the force generating capacity of the muscle that is paralleled by changes to the sEMG signal. These *myoelectric manifestations of fatigue* consist of an increase in the low-frequency content of the sEMG signal and a decrease in the high frequency content of the signal.

- The amount of shift in the distribution of the signal power toward the lower frequency end of the sEMG signal frequency spectrum can be continuously monitored as a decrease in either the *mean* or *median* frequency of the sEMG signal.
- A myoelectric fatigue index is typically derived by calculating either the mean or median value of the EMG power density spectrum for a specified time window (typically 250 or 500 ms) that is shifted in time during the contraction period.
- Dynamic (nonisometric or nonisotonic) contractions are not typically amenable to this analysis technique without the use of specialized signal processing procedures such as time-frequency transformations or wavelet analysis.

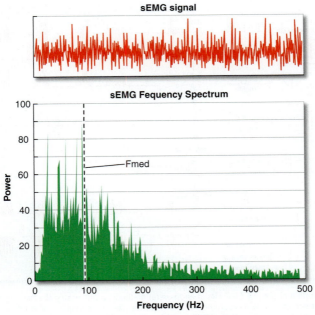

Frequency spectrum (power density spectrum) of sEMG signal.

Normal and Pathological Gait

Gait Terminology

gait cycle: Nomenclature used to describe the spatial and temporal divisions of the gait cycle is based on events beginning with the first foot contact of the reference extremity with the ground and ending when the same extremity reestablishes contact with the ground. The following figure shows these divisions as percentages of the gait cycle. The *stride* is depicted as the interval in the gait cycle between two sequential initial contacts with the same foot (i.e., two *steps*). A *step* is the interval between initial contact with one foot and then the other foot (e.g., right to left). Support times during stance are divided into phases of *double (limb) support* (weight-bearing is shared by both lower extremities) and *single (limb) support* (weight-bearing is on one lower extremity). The *swing phase* is that portion of the gait cycle when the reference extremity is not in contact with the ground. Similar terminology is used when describing the distance measurements of the gait cycle (e.g., *step length* and *stride length*).

phases of gait: Stance can be further divided into *heel strike, midstance,* and *deceleration* phases. Swing can be further divided into *acceleration, midswing,* and *deceleration* phases.

KINES

Divisions of the Gait Cycle

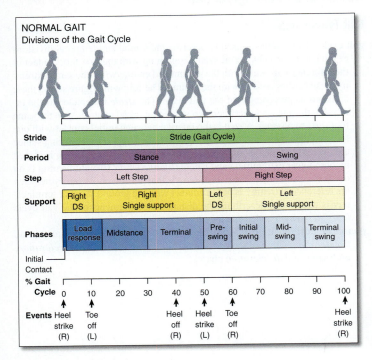

Divisions of the gait cycle.

Rancho Los Amigos Nomenclature for Describing Gait: The Los Amigos Research and Education Institute (LAREI) of the Rancho Los Amigos National Rehabilitation Center has developed an alternate functional terminology for describing the phases of gait, which are summarized with respect to the more traditional measures in Table 14.2.

TABLE 14.2 Terms Used to Describe Gait for Observational Analysis

Traditional	Rancho Los Amigos
Stance Phase	
Heel strike: The beginning of the stance phase when the heel contacts the ground.	*Initial contact*: The beginning of the stance phase when the heel or another part of the foot contacts the ground.

KINES

Traditional	Rancho Los Amigos
Stance Phase	
Foot flat: The portion of the stance phase that occurs immediately after *Heel strike:* When the sole of the foot contacts the floor.	*Loading response*: The portion of the first double support period of stance phase from initial contact until the contralateral extremity leaves the ground.
Midstance: The point at which the body passes directly over the reference extremity.	*Midstance*: The portion of the single limb support that begins when the contralateral extremity leaves the ground and ends when the body is directly over the supporting limb.
Heel-off: The point following midstance at which time the heel of the reference extremity leaves the ground.	*Terminal stance*: The last portion of single limb support that begins with heel rise and continues until the contralateral extremity contacts the ground.
Toe-off: The point after heel-off when only the toe of the reference extremity is in contact with the ground.	*Preswing*: The beginning of the second double-support period from the initial contact of the contralateral extremity to lift-off of the reference extremity.
Swing Phase	
Acceleration: The beginning portion of swing from the moment the toe of the reference extremity leaves the ground to the point when the reference extremity is directly under the body.	*Initial swing*: The portion of swing from the point when the reference extremity leaves the ground to maximum knee flexion of the same extremity.
Midswing: Portion of the swing phase when the reference extremity passes directly below the body. Midswing extends from the end of acceleration to the beginning of deceleration.	*Midswing*: Portion of the swing phase from maximum knee flexion of the reference extremity to a vertical tibial position.
Deceleration: The portion of the swing phase when the reference extremity is decelerating in preparation for heel strike.	*Terminal swing*: The portion of the swing phase from a vertical position of the tibia of the reference extremity to just prior to initial contact.

KINES

From: O'Sullivan, SB, and Schmitz, TJ: *Physical Rehabilitation,* ed. 5. FA Davis, Philadelphia, 2006, p 321, with permission.

From:

Norkin, CC: Examination of gait. In O'Sullivan, SB, and Schmitz, TJ (eds): Physical Rehabilitation, ed. 5. FA Davis, Philadelphia, 2006, p 321.

Muscles Controlling Gait

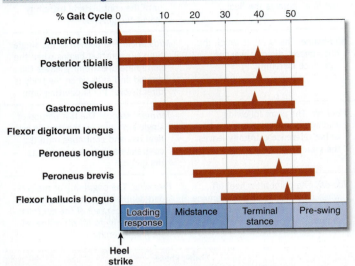

Muscle sequence controlling the foot during stance. *From: Perry, J: Gait Analysis: Normal and Pathological Function. Slack, Thorofare, NJ, 1992, p 163, with permission.*

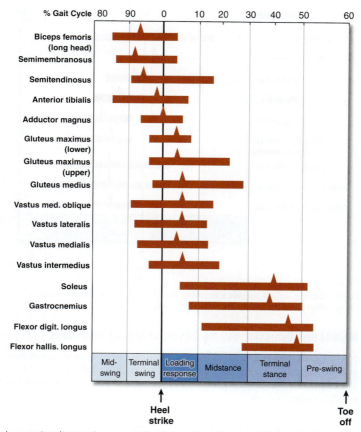

Lower extremity muscle sequence for stance. *From: Perry, J: Gait Analysis: Normal and Pathological Function. Slack, Thorofare, NJ, 1992, p 163, with permission.*

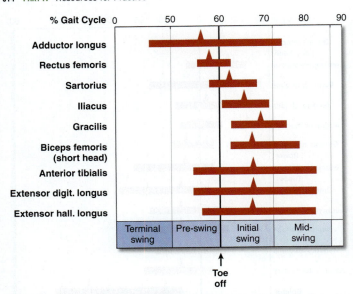

Lower extremity muscle sequence for swing. *From: Perry, J: Gait Analysis: Normal and Pathological Function. Slack, Thorofare, NJ, 1992, p 163, with permission.*

Normal Gait Dynamics and the Effects of Muscle Weakness

Normal joint motion and the functional contributions of muscles controlling gait are summarized for joints of the lower extremity in Tables 14.3 to 14.8. The tables also summarize common results of isolated muscle weaknesses and possible compensations.

TABLE 14.3 Ankle and Foot Gait Analysis: Stance Phase—Sagittal Plane

Portion of Phase	Normal Motion	Normal Moment	Normal Muscle Action	Result of Weakness	Possible Compensation
Heel strike to foot flat	0°–15° plantar flexion	Plantar flexion	Pretibial group acts eccentrically to oppose plantar flexion moment; thereby prevents foot slap by controlling plantar flexion.	Lack of ability to oppose the plantar flexion moment causes the foot to slap the floor.	To avoid foot slap and to eliminate the plantar flexion moment, the foot may be placed flat on the floor or placed with the toes first at initial contact.
Foot flat through midstance	15° plantar flexion to 10° dorsiflexion	Plantar flexion to dorsiflexion	Gastrocnemius and soleus act eccentrically to oppose the dorsiflexion moment and to control tibial advance.	Excessive dorsiflexion and uncontrolled tibial advance.	To avoid excessive dorsiflexion, the ankle may be maintained in plantar flexion.
Midstance to heel-off	10°–15° dorsiflexion	Dorsiflexion	Gastrocnemius and soleus contract eccentrically to oppose the dorsiflexion moment and control tibial advance.	Excessive dorsiflexion and uncontrolled forward motion of tibia.	The ankle may be maintained in plantar flexion. If the foot is flat on the floor, the dorsiflexion moment is eliminated and a step-to gait is produced.

(table continues on page 916)

KINES

TABLE 14.3 Ankle and Foot Gait Analysis: Stance Phase—Sagittal Plane (continued)

Portion of Phase	Normal Motion	Normal Moment	Normal Muscle Action	Result of Weakness	Possible Compensation
Heel-off to toe-off	15° dorsiflexion to 20° plantar flexion	Dorsiflexion	Gastrocnemius, soleus, peroneus brevis, peroneus longus, flexor hallucis longus contract to plantar flex the foot.	No roll-off. Decreased contralateral step.	Whole foot is lifted off the ground.

From: O'Sullivan, SB, and Schmitz, TJ: *Physical Rehabilitation: Assessment and Treatment*, ed 5. FA Davis, Philadelphia, 2006, p 322.

KINES

TABLE 14.4 Ankle and Foot Gait Analysis: Swing Phase—Sagittal Plane

Portion of Phase	Normal Motion	Normal Moment	Normal Muscle Action	Result of Weakness	Possible Compensation
Acceleration to midswing	Dorsiflexion to neutral	None	Dorsiflexors contract to bring the ankle into neutral and to prevent the toes from dragging on the floor.	Footdrop and/or toe dragging.	Hip and knee flexion may be increased to prevent toe drag, or the hip may be hiked or circumducted. Sometimes vaulting on the contralateral limb may occur.
Midswing to deceleration	Neutral	None	Dorsiflexion	Footdrop and/or toe dragging.	Hip and knee flexion may be increased to prevent toe drag. The swing leg may be circumducted, or vaulting may occur on the contralateral side.

From: O'Sullivan, SB, and Schmitz, TJ: *Physical Rehabilitation*, ed 5. FA Davis, Philadelphia, 2006, p 322.

KINES

TABLE 14.5 Knee Gait Analysis: Stance Phase—Sagittal Plane

Portion of Phase	Angular Motion	Normal Moment	Normal Muscle Activity	Result of Weakness	Possible Compensation
Heel strike to foot flat	Flexion 0°–15°	Flexion	Quadriceps contracts initially to hold the knee in extension and then eccentrically to oppose the flexion moment and to control the amount of flexion.	Excessive knee flexion because the quadriceps cannot oppose the flexion moment.	Plantar flexion at ankle so that foot flat instead of heel strike occurs. Plantar flexion eliminates the flexion moment. Trunk leans forward to eliminate the flexion moment at the knee.
Foot flat through midstance	Extension 15°–5°	Flexion to extension	Quadriceps contracts in early part, and then no activity is required.	Excessive knee flexion initially.	Same as above in early part of midstance. No compensation required in later part of phase.
Midstance to heel-off	5° flexion to 0° (neutral)	Flexion to extension	No activity is required.		None is required.
Heel-off to toe-off	0°–40° flexion	Extension to flexion	Quadriceps is required to control amount of knee flexion.		

From: O'Sullivan, SB, and Schmitz, TJ: *Physical Rehabilitation*, ed 5. FA Davis, Philadelphia, 2006, p 323.

⬤ TABLE 14.6 Knee Gait Analysis: Swing Phase—Sagittal Plane

Portion of Phase	Angular Motion	Normal Muscle Activity	Result of Weakness	Possible Compensation
Acceleration to midswing	40°–60° flexion	Little or no activity in quadriceps; biceps femoris (short head), gracilis, and sartorius contract concentrically.	Inadequate knee flexion.	Increased hip flexion, circumduction, or hiking.
Midswing	60°–30° extension			
Deceleration	30°–0° extension	Quadriceps contracts concentrically to stabilize knee in extension in preparation for heel strike.	Inadequate knee extension.	

From: O'Sullivan, SB, and Schmitz, TJ: *Physical Rehabilitation,* ed. 5. FA Davis, Philadelphia, 2006, p 323.

KINES

KINES

TABLE 14.7 Hip Gait Analysis: Stance Phase—Sagittal Plane

Portion of Phase	Angular Motion	Normal Moment	Normal Muscle Activity	Result of Weakness	Possible Compensation
Heel strike to foot flat	30° flexion	Flexion	Erector spinae, gluteus maximus, hamstrings.	Excessive hip flexion and anterior pelvic tilt owing to inability to counteract flexion moment.	Trunk leans backward to prevent excessive hip flexion and to eliminate the hip flexion moment.
Foot flat through midstance	30° flexion to 5° (neutral)	Flexion to extension	Gluteus maximus at beginning of period to oppose flexion moment; then activity ceases as moment changes from flexion to extension.	At the beginning of the period, excessive hip flexion and anterior pelvic tilt due to inability to counteract flexion moment.	May lean trunk backward at beginning to prevent excessive hip flexion; once the flexion moment changes to an extension moment, compensatory action not required.
Midstance to heel-off		Extension	No activity	None.	None required.
Heel-off to toe-off	10° extension to neutral	Extension	Iliopsoas, adductor, magnus, and adductor longus.	Undetermined.	Undetermined.

From O'Sullivan, SB, and Schmitz, TJ: *Physical Rehabilitation*, ed 5. FA Davis, Philadelphia, 2006, p 324.

TABLE 14. 8 Hip Gait Analysis: Swing Phase—Sagittal Plane

Portion of Phase	Angular Motion	Normal Moment	Normal Muscle Activity	Result of Weakness	Possible Compensation
Acceleration to midswing	20°–30° flexion	None	Hip flexor activity to initiate swing: iliopsoas, rectus femoris, gracilis, sartorius, tensor fasciae latae.	Diminished hip flexion, causing an inability to initiate the normal forward movement of the extremity and to raise the foot off the floor.	Circumduction and/or hip hiking may be used to bring the leg forward and to raise the foot high enough to clear the floor.
Midswing to deceleration	30° flexion to neutral	None	Hamstrings	A lack of control of the swinging leg; inability to place limb in position for heel strike.	

From: O'Sullivan, SB, and Schmitz, TJ: *Physical Rehabilitation*, ed. 5. FA Davis, Philadelphia, 2006, p 324.

KINES

From:

Norkin, CC: Examination of gait. In O'Sullivan, SB, and Schmitz, TJ: Physical Rehabilitation,
ed. 5. Philadelphia, FA Davis, 2006, pp 322–324.

Common Gait Deviations

🔴 TABLE 14.9 Common Deviations, Ankle and Foot Stance Phase—Sagittal Plane

Portion of Phase	Deviation	Description	Possible Causes	Analysis
Initial contact	Foot slap	At heel strike, forefoot slaps the ground.	Weak or flaccid dorsiflexors; or recipricol inhibition of dorsiflexors.	Test for muscle weakness of dorsiflexors. Look for steppage gait (excessive hip and knee flexion) in swing phase.
	Toes first	Toes contact ground instead of heel. A tip-toe posture may be maintained throughout the phase, or the heel may contact the ground.	Leg length discrepancy; contracted heel cord; plantar flexion contraction; spasticity of plantar flexors; flaccidity of dorsiflexor; painful heel.	Compare leg lengths and look for hip and/or knee flexion contractures. Analyze muscle tone and timing of activity in plantar flexors. Check for pain in heel.
	Foot flat	Entire foot contacts the ground at heel strike.	Excessive fixed dorsiflexion; flaccid or weak dorsiflexors; neonatal/proprioceptive walking.	Check range of motion at ankle. Check for hyperextension at the knee and persistence of immature gait pattern.

Portion of Phase	Deviation	Description	Possible Causes	Analysis
Midstance	Excessive positional plantar flexion	Tibia does not advance to neutral from 10° plantar flexion.	No eccentric contraction of plantar flexors; could be due to flaccidity/ weakness in plantarflexors; surgical overrelease, rupture, or contracture of Achilles tendon.	Check for spastic or weak quadriceps; hyperextension at the knee; hip hyperextension; backward- or forward-leaning trunk. Check for weakness in plantar flexors or rupture of Achilles tendon.
	Heel lift in mid-stance	Heel does not contact ground in midstance.	Spasticity of plantar flexors.	Check for spasticity of plantar flexors, quadriceps, hip flexors, and adductors.
	Excessive positional dorsiflexion	Tibia advances too rapidly over the foot, creating a greater than normal amount of dorsiflexion.	Inability of plantar flexors to control tibial advance; knee flexion or hip flexion contractures.	Look at ankle muscles, knee and hip flexors, range of motion, and position of trunk.
	Toe clawing	Toes flex and "grab" floor.	Plantar grasp reflex that is only partially integrated; positive supporting reflex; spastic toe flexors.	Check plantar grasp reflex, positive supporting reflexes, and range of motion of toes.

(table continues on page 924)

KINES

🔴 **TABLE 14.9** **Common Deviations, Ankle and Foot Stance Phase—Sagittal Plane** (continued)

Portion of Phase	Deviation	Description	Possible Causes	Analysis
Push-off (heel-off to toe-off)	No roll-off	Insufficient transfer of weight from lateral heel to medial forefoot.	Mechanical fixation of ankle and foot. Flaccidity or inhibition of plantar flexors, inverters, and toe flexors. Rigidity/cocontraction of plantar flexors and dorsiflexors; pain in forefoot.	Check range of motion at ankle and foot. Check muscle function and tone at ankle. Look at dissociation between posterior foot and forefoot.

From O'Sullivan, SB, and Schmitz, TJ: *Physical Rehabilitation,* ed. 5. FA Davis, Philadelphia, 2006, p 328.

🔴 **TABLE 14.10** **Common Deviations, Ankle and Foot Swing Phase—Sagittal Plane**

Portion of Phase	Deviation	Description	Possible Causes	Analysis
Swing	Toe drag	Insufficient dorsiflexion (and toe extension) so that forefoot and toes do not clear floor.	Flaccidity or weakness of dorsiflexors and toe extensors. Spasticity of plantar flexors. Inadequate knee or hip flexion.	Check for ankle, hip, and knee range of motion. Check for strength and muscle tone at hip, knee, and ankle.
	Varus	Foot excessively inverted.	Spasticity of invertors. Flaccidity or weakness of dorsiflexors and evertors. Extensor pattern.	Check for muscle tone of invertors and plantar flexors. Check strength of dorsiflexors and evertors. Check for extensor pattern of the lower extremity.

From: O'Sullivan, SB, and Schmitz, TJ: *Physical Rehabilitation,* ed. 5. FA Davis, Philadelphia, 2006, p 329.

KINES

TABLE 14.11 Common Deviations, Knee Stance Phase—Sagittal Plane

Portion of Phase	Deviation	Description	Possible Causes	Analysis
Initial contact (heel strike)	Excessive knee flexion	Knee flexes or buckles rather than extends as foot contacts ground.	Painful knee; spasticity of knee flexors or weak or flaccid quadriceps; short leg on contralateral side.	Check for pain at knee; tone of knee flexors; strength of knee extensors; leg lengths; anterior pelvic tilt.
Foot flat	Knee hyper-extension (genu recurvatum)	A greater-than-normal extension at the knee.	Flaccid/weak quadriceps and soleus compensated for by pull of gluteus maximus; spasticity of quadriceps; accommodation to a fixed ankle plantar flexion deformity.	Check strength and muscle tone of knee and ankle flexors, and range of motion at ankle.
Midstance	Knee hyper-extension (genu recurvatum)	During single limb support, tibia remains behind ankle mortise as body weight moves over foot; ankle is plantar flexed.	Same as above.	Same as above
Push-off (heel-off to toe-off)	Excessive knee flexion	Knee flexes to more than 40° during push-off.	Center of gravity is unusually far forward of pelvis. Could be due to rigid trunk, knee/hip flexion contractures; flexion-withdrawal reflex; dominance of flexion synergy in middle of recovery from stroke.	Look at trunk posture, knee and hip range of motion, and flexor synergy.
	Limited knee flexion	The normal amount of knee flexion (40°) does not occur.	Spastic/overactive quadriceps and/or plantar flexors.	Examine tone of hip, knee, and ankle muscles.

From O'Sullivan, SB, and Schmitz, TJ: *Physical Rehabilitation*, ed. 5. FA Davis, Philadelphia, 2006, p 329. CVA = cerebrovascular accident.

KINES

TABLE 14.12 Common Deviations, Knee Swing Phase—Sagittal Plane

Portion of Phase	Deviation	Description	Possible Causes	Analysis
Accelerating to midswing	Excessive knee flexion	Knee flexes more than 65°.	Diminished pre-swing knee flexion, flexor-withdrawal reflex, dysmetria.	Look at reflexes of hip, knee, and ankle muscles; test for reflexes and dysmetria.
	Limited knee flexion	Knee does not flex to 65°.	Pain in knee, diminished range of knee motion, extensor spasticity; circumduction at the hip.	Assess for pain in knee and knee range of motion. Test reflexes at knee and hip.

From O'Sullivan, SB, and Schmitz, TJ: *Physical Rehabilitation,* ed. 5. FA Davis, Philadelphia, 2006, p 330.

TABLE 14.13 Common Deviations, Hip Stance Phase—Sagittal Plane

Portion of Phase	Deviation	Description	Possible Causes	Analysis
Heel strike to foot flat	Excessive flexion	Flexion exceeds 30°.	Hip and/or knee flexion contractures. Knee flexion caused by weak soleus and quadriceps. Hyper-reflexivity of hip flexors.	Check hip and knee range of motion and force of soleus and quadriceps. Check tone of hip flexors.
Heel strike to foot flat	Limited hip flexion	Hip flexion does not attain 30°.	Weakness of hip flexors. Limited range of hip flexion. Gluteus maximus weakness.	Check strength of hip flexors and extensors. Analyze range of hip motion.
Foot flat to midstance	Limited hip extension	The hip does not attain a neutral position.	Hip flexion contracture; spasticity of hip flexors.	Check hip range of motion and tone of hip muscles.
	Internal rotation	An internally rotated position of the extremity.	Hyper-reflexive internal rotators; weakness of external rotators; excessive forward rotation of opposite pelvis.	Check tone of internal rotators and strength of external rotators. Measure range of motion of both hip joints.
	External rotation	An externally rotated position of the extremity.	Excessive backward rotation of opposite pelvis.	Assess range of motion at both hip joints.
	Abduction	An abducted position of the extremity.	Contracture of the gluteus medius. Trunk lateral lean over the ipsilateral hip.	Check for abduction pattern.
	Adduction	An adducted position of the lower extremity.	Spasticity of hip flexors and adductors such as seen in spastic diplegia. Pelvic drop to contralateral side.	Assess tone of hip flexors and adductors. Test strength of hip abductors.

From O'Sullivan, SB, and Schmitz, TJ: *Physical Rehabilitation*, ed. 5. FA Davis Philadelphia, 2006, p 330.

KINES

TABLE 14.14 Common Deviations, Hip Swing Phase—Sagittal Plane

Portion of Phase	Deviation	Description	Possible Causes	Analysis
Swing	Circumduction	A lateral circular movement of the entire lower extremity consisting of abduction, external rotation, adduction, and internal rotation.	A compensation for weak hip flexors or the inability to shorten the leg so that it can clear the floor.	Check strength of hip flexors, knee flexors, and ankle dorsiflexors. Check range of motion in hip flexion, knee flexion, and ankle dorsiflexion. Check for extensor pattern.
	Hip hiking	Shortening of the swing leg by action of the quadratus lumborum muscle.	A compensation for lack of knee flexion and/or ankle dorsiflexion. May also be a compensation for extensor spasticity of swing leg.	Check force and range of motion at knee, hip, and ankle. Also check muscle tone at knee and ankle.
	Excessive hip flexion	Flexion greater than 20°–30°.	Attempt to shorten extremity in presence of footdrop. Flexor pattern.	Check strength and range of motion at ankle and foot. Check for flexor pattern.

From: O'Sullivan, SB, and Schmitz, TJ: *Physical Rehabilitation*, ed. 5. FA Davis, Philadelphia, 2006, p 331.

KINES

TABLE 14.15 Common Deviations, Trunk Stance Phase—Sagittal Plane

Portion of Phase	Deviation	Description	Possible Causes	Analysis
Stance	Lateral trunk lean	A lean of the trunk over the stance extremity (gluteus medius gait/Trendelenburg gait).	A weak or paralyzed gluteus medius in the stance side cannot prevent a drop of the pelvis on the swing side. A trunk lean over the stance leg helps compensate for the weak muscle. A lateral trunk lean also may be used to reduce force on hip if a patient has a painful hip.	Check force of gluteus medius and assess for pain in the hip.
	Backward trunk lean	A backward learning of the trunk, resulting in hyperextension at the hip (gluteus maximus gait).	Weakness or paralysis of the gluteus maximus muscle on the stance leg. Anteriorly rotated pelvis.	Check for strength of hip extensors. Check pelvic position.
	Forward trunk lean	A forward leaning of the trunk, resulting in hip flexion.	Compensation for quadriceps weakness. The forward lean eliminates the flexion moment at the knee. Hip and knee flexion contractures.	Check strength of quadriceps.
		A forward flexion of the upper trunk.	Posteriorly rotated pelvis.	Check pelvic position.

From: O'Sullivan, SB, and Schmitz, TJ: *Physical Rehabilitation*, ed. 5. FA Davis, Philadelphia, 2006, p 331.

From:

Norkin, CC: Examination of gait. In O'Sullivan, SB, and Schmitz, TJ: *Physical Rehabilitation,*
ed. 5. Philadelphia, FA Davis, 2006, pp 322–324.

Terms Used to Describe Common Gait Deviations

Gait deviations take on many forms, and their etiologies may be complex. The
list below is not meant to be all inclusive. Only the most common patterns are
listed, and only the most common etiologies for those patterns are noted.

antalgic gait (painful gait): Avoidance of weight-bearing on the affected side,
shortening of the stance phase, and an attempt to unload the limb as much
as possible. In addition, the painful region is often supported by one hand,
while the other arm is outstretched. This pattern is often the result of pain
caused by injury to the hip, knee, ankle, or foot.

arthrogenic gait: Elevation of the pelvis and circumduction of the leg on the
involved side with exaggerated plantar flexion of the opposite ankle. This
pattern is often due to stiffness, laxity, or deformity of the hip or knee and
is often seen with fusion of these joints or after the recent removal of a cylin-
der cast.

ataxic gait: This gait may take two forms, depending on the pathology.

- **spinal ataxia:** A gait deviation that is characterized by the patient walking
with a broad base and throwing out the feet, which come down first on the
heel and then on the toes with a slapping sound or "double tap." It is characteristic for patients to watch their feet while walking. In milder cases,
the gait may appear near normal with the eyes open, but when the patient
is asked to walk with eyes closed, the patient staggers, becomes unsteady,
and may be unable to walk. This gait is thought to result from the disruption of sensory pathways in the central nervous system, as occurs with
tabes dorsalis or multiple sclerosis.

- **cerebellar ataxia:** A gait deviation that is equally severe when the patient
walks with eyes open or closed. The gait is wide based, unsteady, and irregular. The patient staggers and is unable to walk tandem or to follow a
straight line. This form of ataxia occurs with cerebellar lesions. If the disease is localized to one hemisphere, there is persistent deviation or swaying
toward the affected side.

calcaneous gait: See *gastrocnemius-soleus gait.*

crouch gait: Bilateral impairment typified by excessive hip and knee flexion,
excessive plantar flexion, and anterior pelvic tilt. A characteristic gait of
children with diplegia, quadriplegia, or paraplegia.

digitigrade: Walking on toes (see *equinus gait*).

dorsiflexor: See *footdrop gait.*

dystrophic (penguin) gait: There is a pronounced waddling element to this
gait. The patient rolls the hips from side to side during the stance phase of
every forward step to shift the weight of the body. There is an exaggerated
lumbar lordosis while walking or standing. It usually presents as a difficulty
in running or climbing stairs. This gait is encountered in various myopathies
and is most typical of muscular dystrophy.

equinus gait: Excessive plantar flexion usually associated with fixed ankle
deformity, contracture, or extensor hyperactivity (see *digitigrade*).

KINES

flaccid gait: See *hemiplegic gait.*

footdrop (dorsiflexor or steppage) gait: The patient lifts the knee high and slaps the foot to the ground on advancing to the involved side. This gait is typical of patients with weak or paralyzed dorsiflexor muscles.

gastrocnemius-soleus (calcaneus) gait: This deviation is demonstrated best when the patient walks up an incline. At push-off, the heel does not come off the ground, and the affected side lags compared to the other side. This gait results from weakness to the gastrocnemius and/or the soleus muscles.

genu recurvatum gait: Excessive knee extension (hyperextension) during the stance phase of gait.

gluteus maximus (hip extensor) gait: A lurching gait characterized by a posterior thrust of the thorax at heel strike to maintain hip extension of the stance leg. The knee is tightly extended in midstance, which slightly elevates the hip on that side. This gait usually results from weakness to the gluteus maximus muscle.

gluteus medius (Trendelenburg) gait: In the uncompensated gluteus medius limp, the pelvis dips more when the unaffected limb is in swing phase and there is an apparent lateral protrusion of the stance hip; if necessary, the patient may use a steppage gait to clear the swing leg. The gluteus medius gait commonly occurs owing to weakness of the gluteus medius muscle or with congenital dislocations of the hip or with coxa vara. If the gluteus medius is absent or extremely weak, a compensated gait appears where the patient shifts the trunk to the affected side during the stance phase.

hemiplegic or hemiparetic (flaccid) gait: The patient swings the paretic leg outward and ahead in circle (circumduction) or pushes it ahead. Heel strike is often missing, and the patient strikes with the forefoot. This gait is present when one leg is shorter than the other or with a deformity in one of the bones of the leg.

hip extensor gait: See *gluteus maximus gait.*

painful gait: See *antalgic gait.*

Parkinsonian gait: This is a highly stereotypical gait in which the patient has impoverished movement of the lower limb. There is generalized lack of extension at the ankle, knee, hip, and trunk. Diminished step length and a loss of reciprocal arm swing are noted. Patients have trouble initiating movement, and this results in a slow and shuffling gait characterized by small steps. Because patients with parkinsonism often exhibit flexed postures, their centers of gravity project forward, causing a festinating gait. The patients, in an attempt to regain their balance, take many small steps rapidly. The rapid stepping causes the patients to increase their walking speed. In some cases patients will break into a run and can stop their forward progression only when they run into an object. Less common than the forward propulsive gait pattern is a retropulsive pattern that occurs when patients lose their balance in a backward direction (retropulsion is more common in patients with cerebellar lesions).

penguin gait: See *dystrophic gait.*

plantigrade: Simultaneous floor contact by the forefoot and heel.

scissors gait: Excessive hip adduction during swing causing the swing limb to cross the stance limb.

steppage gait: See *footdrop gait.*

KINES

stiff-knee gait: Failure of the knee to flex during stance and swing phase of gait.

Trendelenburg gait: See *gluteus medius gait*.

unguligrade: Tip-toe walking.

Crutch-Walking Gait

four-point gait: One crutch is advanced in this gait pattern, followed by advancement of the opposite lower extremity. Only one leg or crutch is off the floor at a time, leaving three points for support making this a very stable and safe gait. This gait can be used for the patient who is able to move his legs alternately but who has poor balance or is not able to bear full weight bilaterally without the support of crutches.

partial-weight-bearing gait: See *three-point gait*.

swing-through gait: Both crutches are moved forward together, and the lower extremities are then swung forward to a position beyond the crutches. This gait is often used by paraplegic patients who are unable to move their legs alternately.

swing-to gait: Both crutches are moved forward together, and the lower extremities are then swung forward to a position between the crutches. This gait is often used by paraplegic patients who are unable to move their legs alternately.

three-point gait: Both crutches are moved forward with the affected limb. This non-weight-bearing gait can be used if the patient has one normal lower limb that can tolerate full weight-bearing. For example, this mode of crutch walking is used after hip or knee operations. A modified three-point gait is the partial-weight-bearing gait during which the affected extremity is allowed to bear some weight when both crutches are on the ground.

two-point gait: A modification of the four-point gait. The right crutch and left leg move together, and the left crutch and right leg move together. It is close to the natural rhythm of walking.

Based on:

O'Sullivan, SB, and Schmitz, TJ: *Physical Rehabilitation: Assessment and Treatment, ed. 3. FA Davis, Philadelphia, 1994, pp 268–269, with permission.*

Techniques Used to Climb Stairs While Using Assistive Devices

The sequences presented here describe stair-climbing techniques without the use of a railing. When a secure railing is available, the patient should be instructed to use it always.

I. Cane
   A. Ascending
   1. The unaffected lower extremity leads up.
   2. The cane and affected lower extremity follow.
   B. Descending
   1. The affected lower extremity and cane lead down.
   2. The unaffected lower extremity follows.

II. Crutches: three-point gait (non-weight-bearing gait)

    A. Ascending

        1. The patient is positioned close to the foot of the stairs. The involved lower extremity is held back to prevent "catching" on the lip of the stairs.

        2. The patient pushes down firmly on both handpieces of the crutches and leads up with the unaffected lower extremity.

        3. The crutches are brought up to the stair that the unaffected lower extremity is now on.

    B. Descending

        1. The patient stands close to the edge of the stair such that the toes protrude slightly over the top. The involved lower extremity is held forward over the lower stair.

        2. Both crutches are moved down *together* to the *front* half of the next step.

        3. The patient pushes down firmly on both handpieces and lowers the unaffected lower extremity to the step that the crutches are now on.

III. Crutches: partial-weight-bearing gait

    A. Ascending

        1. The patient is positioned close to the foot of the stairs.

        2. The patient pushes down on both handpieces of the crutches and distributes weight partially on the crutches and partially on the affected lower extremity while the unaffected lower extremity leads up.

        3. The involved lower extremity and crutches are then brought up together.

    B. Descending

        1. The patient stands close to the edge of the stair such that the toes protrude slightly over top of the stair.

        2. Both crutches are moved down *together* to the *front* half of the next step. The affected lower extremity is then lowered (depending on patient skill, these may be combined). **Note:** When crutches are not in floor contact, greater weight must be shifted to the uninvolved lower extremity to maintain a partial-weight-bearing status.

        3. The uninvolved lower extremity is lowered to the step the crutches are now on.

IV. Crutches: two- and four-point gait

    A. Ascending

        1. The patient is positioned close to the foot of the stairs.

        2. The right lower extremity is moved up and then the left lower extremity.

        3. The right crutch is moved up and then the left crutch is moved up (patients with adequate balance may find it easier to move the crutches up together).

    B. Descending

        1. The patient stands close to the edge of the stair.

        2. The right crutch is moved down and then the left (may be combined).

        3. The right lower extremity is moved down and then to the left.

KINES

From:

O'Sullivan, SB, and Schmitz, TJ: *Physical Rehabilitation: Assessment and Treatment, ed. 3.* FA Davis, Philadelphia, 1994, p 273, with permission.

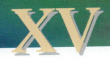

Prosthetics

Terminology

People with amputations (also known as amputees) have a wide variety of responses to the loss of limb(s). The terms *patient, wearer,* and *amputee* will be used synonymously throughout this chapter. Persons who are born with a congenital limb deficiency (also referred to as *limb difference*) may possess concerns when labeled as an amputee because, technically, no body portion was amputated. The term *stump* has been associated with negative connotations and should be avoided. Health-care professionals are encouraged to refer to the person's remaining body region after an amputation as the *residual limb* (RL) to encourage patient acceptance versus disdain.

A *prosthesis* is an artificial limb. *Prostheses* are more than one artificial limb. *Prosthetic* is an adjective, not a noun. Hence someone may wear one prosthesis or two prostheses but they do not wear a prosthetic—they wear a prosthetic leg, prosthetic arm, or a prosthetic device. *Prosthetics* refers to the profession associated with making artificial limbs and the knowledge base contained therein. *Prosthetists* are the allied health-care practitioners who practice the art and science of making prostheses.

Prosthetists' Education and Credentialing

Prosthetists are far more than artificial limb makers and dispensers of devices. They must evaluate patients, generate and implement comprehensive treatment plans, and then follow up with those treatment plans. As a result, prosthetic education is moving to reflect the expansion of knowledge necessary for one to be a competent practitioner. As of 2012, the minimum educational requirement for clinical training in Prosthetics (and Orthotics) will be a master's degree. The highest level of national certification in Prosthetics (and Orthotics) is awarded through the American Board for Certification in Prosthetics, Orthotics and Pedorthics (ABC). After the student completes his/her primary training in Prosthetics (and Orthotics), a year of post-graduate residency training in the discipline (Prosthetics or Orthotics) is required to sit for the ABC National Board examination (there are separate examination tracks for each discipline). The Scope of Practice for Prosthetists, Orthotists and Pedorthists as well as a listing of states requiring licensure can be accessed on the ABC Web site (http://www.abcop.org).

Epidemiology of Amputation in the United States

Based on data from the Healthcare Cost and Utilization Project from 1988 to 1996, Dillingham reported that 82.0% of amputations were the result of dysvascular causes, 16.4% were from trauma, 0.9% were from cancer, and 0.8% were from congenital presentations. Furthermore, from the period 1988 to 1996, dysvascular amputation rates increased 26.9%, traumatic amputations decreased 50.2%, amputations secondary to cancer decreased 42.6%, and congenital deficiencies remained the same. The ratio of major lower limb amputations (those at or proximal to the ankle) to major upper limb amputations (those at or proximal to the wrist) is about 40:1.

PROSTH

Reference:
Dillingham, TR, Pezzin, LE, and MacKenzie, EJ: Limb amputation and limb deficiency: Epidemiology and recent trends in the United States. South Med J 95(8):875–883, 2002.

Rehabilitation Planning for People With Amputations

When a person requires a limb amputation, it is a life-altering event. To set appropriate goals and develop treatment plans for rehabilitation, nine distinct phases of amputation rehabilitation have been identified. These phases apply to both lower and upper limb amputations (Table 15.1). It is crucial to have the patient meet a prosthetist as soon as possible. Do not wait until the residual limb is healed and ready for fitting.

● TABLE 15.1 **Amputation Rehabilitation Phases**

Phase	Description	Goals
1. Pre-operative	The period prior to amputation	Assessment of body condition; patient education about impending residual limb pain, phantom pain, and phantom sensations; discussion of surgical level, post-operative prosthetic plans, and process for adaptation
2. Amputation with surgical reconstruction	The amputation procedure	Provide reconstruction to create a viable residual limb that will facilitate successful prosthetic fitting and rehabilitation, if the patient is a candidate
3. Acute post-operative	The period from surgical closure of the amputation to patent wound closure	Wound healing, pain control, emotional support, strengthening, and range-of-motion maintenance
4. Pre-prosthetic	The period from wound closure to prosthetic prescription	Residual limb shaping, residual limb care, edema management, soft tissue mobility, adhesion prevention, desensitization, strength and range-of-motion maintenance, core strengthening, balance, and postural control
5. Prosthetic prescription and fabrication	The period from prosthetic prescription to completion of a prosthesis	Determining candidacy for prosthetic rehabilitation, creation of the prosthesis, modification to the initial prescription if necessary

Phase	Description	Goals
6. Prosthetic training	The period from delivery of the prosthesis until rehabilitation goals are met	Increased static and dynamic use of the prosthesis and increased wearing time of the prosthesis; short-, medium-, and long-term goal setting; independent donning and doffing; care and maintenance of the prosthesis
7. Community reintegration	Reentering society and community and returning to those feasible activities deemed important	Resumption of roles and responsibilities in the family and community, regaining emotional equilibrium and healthy coping strategies, pursuit of recreational activities
8. Vocational rehabilitation	Return to meaningful employment (if that is a client goal)	Assessment and planning for future vocational activities; need for further education, training or job modification, and accommodations
9. Functional follow-up	Lifelong phase of rehabilitation, which aims to meet the changing needs of the wearer	Lifelong prosthetic; functional, medical, emotional support; regular assessment of functional level; and prosthetic problem solving

Adapted from: Meier, RH, and Esquenazi, A: Rehabilitation planning for the upper extremity amputee. In Meier, RH, and Atkins, DJ (eds): *Functional Restoration of Adults and Children with Upper Extremity Amputation.* Demos, New York, 2004.

PROSTH

Classification Systems for Congenital Limb Deficiencies

In 1961, Frantz and O'Rahilly developed a classification system for congenital deficiencies that is still in use today in some clinics (see figure below).

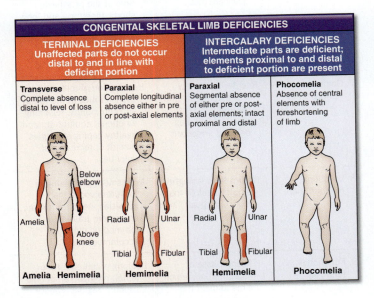

CONGENITAL SKELETAL LIMB DEFICIENCIES			
TERMINAL DEFICIENCIES Unaffected parts do not occur distal to and in line with deficient portion		**INTERCALARY DEFICIENCIES** Intermediate parts are deficient; elements proximal to and distal to deficient portion are present	
Transverse Complete absence distal to level of loss	**Paraxial** Complete longitudinal absence either in pre or post-axial elements	**Paraxial** Segmental absence of either pre or post-axial elements; intact proximal and distal	**Phocomelia** Absence of central elements with foreshortening of limb
Amelia / Below elbow / Above knee	Radial / Ulnar / Tibial / Fibular	Radial / Ulnar / Tibial / Fibular	
Amelia Hemimelia	**Hemimelia**	**Hemimelia**	**Phocomelia**

Reference:

Meier, RH, and Esquenazi, A: Rehabilitation planning for the upper extremity amputee. In Meier, RH, and Atkins, DJ (eds): Functional Restoration of Adults and Children with Upper Extremity Amputation, Demos, New York, 2004, pp 55–61.

Adapted from:

Hall, CB, Brooks, MD, and Dennis, JF: Congenital skeletal deficiencies of the extremeties: Classification and fundamentals of treatment. JAMA 181:591, 1962.

In 1989 an International Standards Organization (ISO) standard was adopted (ISO 8548-1, Method of Describing Limb Deficiencies Present at Birth) to facilitate scientific communication through clarification of the language. In the ISO system, all congenital limb deficiencies are categorized as either *transverse* or *longitudinal*. Transverse deficiencies through the long bones (thigh, leg, arm, and forearm) are described by naming the affected limb segment and the approximate location (i.e., a right short below the elbow deficiency is classified as a *transverse deficiency right forearm upper third*). Refer to the figure on p. 939 for a schematic representation of ISO Classification of Transverse Congenital Deficiencies.

Reference:

Frantz and O'Rahilly classification system from Hall, CB, Brooks, MD, and Dennis, JF: Congenital skeletal deficiencies of the extremities; classification and fundamentals of treatment. JAMA 181:591, 1962, with permission.

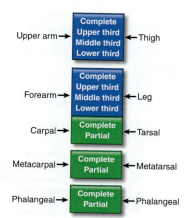

Schematic representation of ISO Classification of Transverse Congenital Deficiencies. *Adapted from: Day, HJB: The ISO/ISPO classification of congenital limb deficiency. Prosthet Orthot Int 15(2):67–69, 1991.*

Any congenital presentation in which the affected level is not transverse is a longitudinal deficiency. These deficiencies are characterized by limb segments being affected through their long axis, and as a result distal anatomy will be present. Longitudinal deficiencies are named from proximal to distal, listing bones or segments and whether the segments are totally or partially absent.

For example, an infant presents to the clinic with a lower limb anomaly in which a portion of the child's right fibula is missing but retains the ankle and foot anatomy. The classification of this child's limb anomaly would be *longitudinal deficiency of the right fibula, partial.* In the event the fibula was completely absent including the lateral tarsal bones, the metatarsals, and phalanges of the second through fifth rays, the limb anomaly would be classified as *longitudinal deficiency of the right fibula, complete, tarsus, partial, ray 2–5 complete.*

Graphic representations of the longitudinal deficiencies for the lower and upper limbs as classified by the ISO classification system can be found in the figure on p. 940.

Prosthetics in rehabilitation

(A) The ISO classification system for upper limb congenital limb deficiency. (B) An example of a lower limb longitudinal congenital limb deficiency. The shaded areas represents missing segments. *Adapted from: Day, HJB: The ISO/ISPO classification of congenital limb deficiency. Prosthet Orthot Int 15(2):67–69, 1991.*

Pediatric Prosthetic Rehabilitation

Children with congenital limb deficiencies will adapt better to a missing limb than a child who requires a sudden amputation as a result of trauma or tumor. Children with acquired amputations through long bones are at risk for bony overgrowth. As a result of growth, children in grade school often require a new prosthesis every 12 to 18 months, but teenagers may require a new one every 18 to 24 months. The role the parents play in successful prosthetic rehabilitation and the child's ultimate acceptance of their body image is critical.

Lower Limb Amputation Levels, Functional Levels, and Patient Evaluation

Levels of Lower Limb Acquired Amputations

For classification purposes, a major lower limb amputation may involve structures through the ankle joint (Symes amputation) or structures proximal to the ankle joint (see the figure on p. 941). Minor lower limb amputations are those distal to the ankle and include toe amputations, ray amputations, transmetatarsal amputations, Lisfranc amputation (metatarsal disarticulation), Chopart amputation (through the calcaneo-cuboid talo-navicular joints), and Boyd/Pirogoff amputation (calcaneous is transected and anchored to the cut distal tibia).

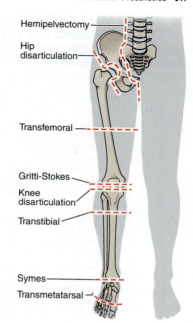

Hemipelvectomy

Hip
disarticulation

Transfemoral

Gritti-Stokes

Knee
disarticulation

Transtibial

Symes

Transmetatarsal

Lower limb amputation levels. *Adapted
from: Thomson, A., Skinner, A., and
Piercy, J.: Tidy's Physiotherapy, ed. 12.
Butterworth-Heinemann, Boston, 1991,
p 261.*

Medicare Functional Classification Levels (MFCL or K Levels)

In 1995, the Centers for Medicare & Medicaid Services adopted a functional
classification system designed to ensure consistency in documentation so that
lower limb prosthetic components were appropriately matched to the prosthetic
wearer's functional capabilities. The Medicare Functional Classification Levels
(MFCL) uses "K" levels to classify a potential wearer of a prosthesis based on
the person's predicted ability to attain a functional state within a reasonable
period of time. The person's potential functional ability is based on the reasonable expectations of the prosthetist and ordering physician. The required documentation by Medicare for certain prosthetic components (feet, ankles, and
knees) is dependent on the wearer's K level.

PROSTH

TABLE 15.2 Medicare Guidelines: Functional Classification of Patients with a Prosthesis

K Level	Descriptor
K0	Does not have the ability or potential to ambulate or transfer safely with or without assistance and a prosthesis does not enhance their quality of life or mobility.
K1	Has the ability or potential to use a prosthesis for transfers or ambulation on level surfaces at fixed cadence. Typical of the limited and unlimited household ambulator.
K2	Has the ability or potential for ambulation with the ability to traverse low-level environmental barriers such as curbs, stairs, or uneven surfaces. Typical of the limited community ambulator.
K3	Has the ability or potential for ambulation with variable cadence. Typical of the community ambulator who has the ability to traverse most environmental barriers and may have vocational, therapeutic, or exercise activity that demands prosthetic utilization beyond simple locomotion.
K4	Has the ability or potential for prosthetic ambulation that exceeds basic ambulation skills, exhibiting high impact, stress, or energy levels. Typical of the prosthetic demands of the child, active adult, or athlete.

From: *DMERC Medicare Advisory Bulletin*. DMERC, Columbia, SC, December 1994, pp 94–214.

Patient Evaluation for Lower Limb Prosthetic Rehabilitation

For a prosthetist to generate a treatment plan for someone with an amputation, he/she must conduct a thorough history and physical. Table 15.3 provides an overview of the topics that must be investigated for the prosthetist to develop an appropriate treatment plan.

TABLE 15.3 Relevant Patient History/Evaluation for Lower Limb Amputations

Topics	Aspects to Explore
Chief complaint	1. Primary reason for seeking prosthetic rehabilitation
Amputation history	1. Cause/level of amputation 2. Date of amputation 3. Dates/causes of revisions
Short-/medium-/long-term goals	1. Short: 1–2 mo 2. Medium: next 6 mo 3. Long: 1 yr, 5 yr, 10 yr
Employment/work/leisure	1. Current and prior work 2. Community activities

PROSTH

Topics	Aspects to Explore
	3. Recreational pursuits 4. Hobbies 5. Exercise
Social history	1. Cultural beliefs and behaviors 2. Family and caregiver resources 3. Family role 4. Social interactions, activities, and support systems 5. Isolation
General health status	1. Perception of general health
Living environment	1. Assistive devices 2. Adaptive equipment 3. Home environment (architectural barriers; safety rails; stairs; other hazards, such as small rugs, unsturdy rails) 4. Discharge destination (if relevant)
Social health habits	1. Smoking 2. Alcohol 3. Drug abuse 4. Physical fitness/exercise
Medical/surgical history	1. Prior hospitalizations 2. Prior sugeries 3. Pre-existing medical conditions 4. Other health related conditions
Current and prior functional status	1. Preamputation mobility, self-care, home management, ADL, and IADL 2. Preamputation mobility, work and community/leisure activities 3. Current mobility, self-care, home management, ADL, and IADL 4. Current mobility, work and community/leisure activities
Medications	1. Current prescription medications 2. Current over-the-counter medications 3. Current supplements, homeopathic, other medications
Systems review	1. General, skin, eyes, ears, nose, throat, cardiovascular, respiratory, gastrointestinal, musculoskeletal, neurological, psychological, cognitive, allergic
Psychological	1. Emotional status (depression, denial, anger, cooperativeness, enthusiasm) 2. Motivation

(table continues on page 944)

PROSTH

● TABLE 15.3 Relevant Patient History/Evaluation for Lower Limb Amputations (continued)

Topics	Aspects to Explore
Pain Cognitive	1. Residual limb pain 2. Phantom pain/phantom sensations 3. Other pain 4. Sleep (quality, amount, day/night, naps) 5. Mental status (alert, senile, intelligent, limited ability to understand) 6. Memory 7. Learning capacity
Activities of daily living	1. Transfers (bed to wheelchair, to toilet, to tub, to automobile; independent, dependent) 2. Ambulatory status (with crutches, walker; type of gait; independent, dependent) 3. Self-care (independent, dependent; includes residual limb care)
Hand dexterity	1. No limitations 2. Limitations present that would impede donning/doffing of a prosthesis and/or residual limb care 3. Hand dominance
Post-operative management modalities (see Table 16.6)	1. Soft dressings (elastic shrinker, elastic bandage, medicated bandage [Unna's paste]) 2. Rigid dressings (removable or nonremoveable; plaster or thermoplastic) 3. Independent, dependent with post-operative protocol 4. Physical therapy (duration, type)
Prior prosthesis	1. Type 2. Components 3. Likes/dislikes 4. Gait deviations
Footwear	1. Is similar in heel height to the shoe in which the prosthesis was originally aligned (unless the foot has an adjustable heel height) 2. Fit with appropriately designed foot orthosis, particularly if person possesses impaired protective sensation and/or possesses joint deformities and/or requires load alteration

Adapted from: Sanders, GT: *Lower Limb Amputations: A Guide to Rehabilitation*. FA Davis, Philadelphia, 1986, p 373.

ADL = activities of daily living; IADL = instrumental activities of daily living.

PROSTH

Residual Limb Evaluation

Prior to palpating someone's residual limb, *always* ask permission and inquire if areas exist on the person's limb(s) that are especially sensitive to touch.

● TABLE 15.4 Residual Limb Evaluations for Persons With Lower Limb Amputations

Item to Be Evaluated	Observe For
Skin	1. Scar (location; healed, unhealed; adherent, mobile; invaginated, flat, thickened, keloid; from other surgery or a burn) 2. Open lesions (size, shape, exudate) 3. Moisture (moist, dry, crusting) 4. Sensibility (absent, diminished, hypersensitive to touch or pressure) 5. Grafts (location, type, degree of healing) 6. Dermatologic lesions (psoriasis, eczema, acne vulgaris, dermatitis, boils, epidermis cysts, foliculitis) 7. Redundant tissue
Residuum lengths	1. Bone length: Transtibial from medial tibial plateau or mid-patellar tendon to distal end of tibia (compress soft tissue). In transfemoral from distal ischium to distal end of femur (compress soft tissue) 2. Residual limb length: Transtibial from medial tibial plateau or mid-patellar tendon to distal end of residual limb (do not compress soft tissue). In transfemoral from distal ischium to distal end of residual limb (do not compress soft tissue)
Shape	1. Transtibial: Cylindrical, conical, or bulbous. May have prominent triangular corners at the suture line known as "dog-ears" post-operatively 2. Transfemoral: Cylindrical, conical, or bulbous. May have "dog-ears" post-operatively. May have medial adductor roll from previous poorly fit socket
Vascularity (both limbs if cause of amputation is vascular disease)	1. Pulses (femoral, popliteal, dorsalis pedis, posterior tibial) 2. Color (cyanotic, redness) 3. Temperature (cool, warm) 4. Edema (circumference measurements, pitting) 5. Pain (in dependent position, throbbing, claudication) 6. Trophic changes (shininess, dryness, loss of hair)

(table continues on page 946)

PROSTH

⬤ **TABLE 15.4** **Residual Limb Evaluations for Persons With Lower Limb Amputations** (continued)

Item to Be Evaluated	Observe For
Neurological	1. Sensibility (light touch; pressure; joint proprioception; Semmes-Weinstein; two-point discrimination, both limbs) 2. Neuroma (location, tenderness) 3. Phantom pains: "pins and needles," throbbing, burning, stabbing, electrical shock; duration, triggers, and reliefs 4. Phantom sensations: toes/foot/leg still present and movable but does not cause pain (i.e., still able to "move it") 5. Residual limb pain: post-operative, prosthesis induced
Range of motion (both legs)	1. Hips (flexion, abduction, or external rotation contracture) 2. Knee (flexion contracture) 3. Ankle (plantar flexion contracture)
Strength	1. Major muscle groups; adaptation must be made for shortened lever arm

Based on: Sanders, GT: *Lower Limb Amputations: A Guide to Rehabilitation.* FA Davis, Philadelphia, 1986, p 373.

Lower Limb Post-Operative Prosthetic Protocols

Goals for Post-Operative Management

Post-operative protocols range from conservative to aggressive approaches and require varying levels of skill on the part of the practitioner and the rehabilitation team providing treatment. Regardless of the modality, the goals of post-operative management are contained in Table 15.5.

⬤ **TABLE 15.5 Goals for Post-Operative Management**

Contracture prevention	Early ambulation	Bed mobility & transfers
Pain management	RL protection	Fall prevention
Emotional care	RL activity	Trunk stability
Post-operative edema reduction	Volume change accommodation	Distal end loading, desensitization, & weight-bearing

RL = residual limb.

PROSTH

Post-Operative Modalities

Post-operative management modalities, indications, contraindications, advantages, and disadvantages are found in Table 15.6.

● **TABLE 15.6 Post-Operative Modalities, Indications, Contraindications, Advantages, and Disadvantages**

Modality	Description	Indications	Contraindications	Advantages	Disadvantages
Ace wrap	• 4- or 6-in. elastic bandage • Optimally applied at the time of closure • Applied with a figure-eight pattern • Greater compression distally than proximally • Transfemoral levels require two 6-in. bandages sewn together and anchored around the waist	Any amputation	Need for protection from falls	• Fair edema control • Ease of access to the wound • Very inexpensive	• Difficult to properly apply • Difficult to maintain even compression • Difficult for patient to self-don • No contracture prevention • No RL protection from falls • Falls off (TF mainly)
Shrinker	• Elastic compression socks • Available in sizes based on RL length and circumferences • Some designs are folded to increase compression	Any amputation (preferably with sutures/staples removed)	A suture line with staples may catch when donning Need for protection from falls	• Good edema control • Access to the wound • Inexpensive • Ease of application • Even compression • Self-suspending	• May stress suture line • More painful to don than an Ace wrap • No RL protection from falls

(table continues on page 948)

PROSTH

PROSTH

TABLE 15.6 Post-Operative Modalities, Indications, Contraindications, Advantages, and Disadvantages (continued)

Modality	Description	Indications	Contraindications	Advantages	Disadvantages
	• Transfemoral designs have waist belts incorporated • Are ordered from a prosthetist				• Some fall prevention • Requires experience for application • Limited wound access
Unna's paste	• Usually made immediately after wound closure • Made of zinc oxide, glycerin, calamine, & gelatin-impregnated gauze • Dries to a leathery consistency in 24 hr	Any amputation	Need for protection from falls	• Good edema control • Inexpensive	
Nonremovable rigid dressing	• Made of plaster of Paris or resin-impregnated fiber • Consist of thick socks, padding, and a rigid outer structure • Suspended by a waist belt • Designed not to be removed for 7–10 days • Transtibial designs extend to mid-thigh to prevent knee contractures	RL protection needed Wound access is not required	Those with high risk of infection Poorly developed rehabilitation team	• Best edema control • TT: Contracture prevention • RL protection from falls	• Limited wound access • Heavy • Requires informed team for management • Requires close monitoring • Requires removal and reapplication in 7–10 days

Modality	Description	Indications	Contraindications	Advantages	Disadvantages
Removable rigid dressings	• Made of plaster of Paris, resin-impregnated fiber, or thermoplastics • Worn over socks • Suspended by a waist belt or cuff strap • Removable for wound inspection	RL protection needed Wound access is needed	Questionable capabilities to manage socks & dressing Poorly developed rehabilitation team	• Very good edema control • Wound is accessible • Compression is adjustable with socks • RL protection from falls • TT: Contracture prevention	• Requires patient's ability to manage socks • Some do not offer contracture prevention • Bulky
Immediate post-operative prosthesis	• Consist of a rigid dressing upon which a removable pylon and foot have been installed • Transfemoral designs usually contain a locking knee component • Foot/pylon may be retained in therapy treatment area to prevent patient unauthorized ambulation • Touchdown weight-bearing *only* (not >20 lb) • IPOPs made from nonremovable rigid dressing need to be removed after 7–10 days	Those indicated for aggressive rehabilitation Are cognizant, motivated, and compliant	Questionable ambulators Potential healing complications Those who will have very good follow-up care Poorly developed rehabilitation team	• Best edema control • Early return to ambulation • Early discharge/return to previous lifestyle • Psychological benefits • Residual limb shaping • TT: Contracture prevention • RL protection from falls • Lower overall hospital expense by early discharge	• Risk for complications • Requires close monitoring and an informed rehabilitation team • Requires removal and reapplication in 7–10 days (nonremovable designs) • Cost • Bulky

(table continues on page 950)

PROSTH

PROSTH

TABLE 15.6 Post-Operative Modalities, Indications, Contraindications, Advantages, and Disadvantages (continued)

Modality	Description	Indications	Contraindications	Advantages	Disadvantages
Prefabricated pneumatic post-operative prostheses	• Consist of pneumatic bladders inside a thermoplastic socket designed to allow for edema control and socket cushioning • Ordered by size • Have foot (and knee for transfemoral) attachment • Suspended by a waist belt	Those indicated for aggressive rehabilitation Are cognizant, motivated, and compliant	Questionable ambulators Potential healing complications Those who will have very good follow-up care Poorly developed rehabilitation team	• Best edema control • Early return to ambulation • Early discharge/return to previous lifestyle • Psychological benefits • Residual limb shaping • TT: Contracture prevention • RL protection from falls • Lower overall hospital expense by early discharge	• Risk for complications • Requires close monitoring and an informed rehabilitation team • Cost • Bulky

CAUTION: For nonremovable rigid dressings and Immediate Post-Op Prostheses (IPOPs) made with nonremovable rigid dressings, the person's suture line will not be accessible. With removable devices, the person's residual limb is exposed to potential complications due to donning and doffing of the prosthesis. Therefore, all rehabilitation personnel need to be aware of problem symptoms that require immediate removal/discontinuation of the post-operative prosthesis protocols. These are included in Table 15.7.

TABLE 15.7 Signs/Symptoms Indicating Discontinuation of Post-Operative Protocols

Signs	Symptoms
Drainage through the cast	Fever
Sharp localized pain in the residual limb	Significant pistoning of the limb in the cast/socket
Physician requires wound access	The unmistakable scent of infection

Lower Limb Prosthetics (LLP)

Prostheses for the lower limb are categorized according to their purpose and are roughly prescribed relative to their application since the time of amputation. The three types of lower limb prostheses include post-operative prosthesis, preparatory or temporary prosthesis, and definitive prosthesis (Table 15.8).

TABLE 15.8 Types of Lower Limb Prostheses

Type of Prosthesis	Description
Post-operative prosthesis	• Fit either in the operating room or within the first week after amputation • Utilized only the first few weeks after amputation • Not every amputee receives a post-operative prosthesis
Preparatory or temporary prosthesis	• Fit when distal circumference is = or < proximal circumference (not bulbous), usually around 6 wk after amputation • Utilized for up to 1–2 yr • May require a socket replacement to address significant edema reduction
Definitive prosthesis (not permanent)	• Fit when RL has stabilized • Should last a number of years • May require socket replacement to reflect RL changes

PROSTH

LLP Structure

Lower limb prostheses fall into one of two categories of basic structure: exoskeletal or endoskeletal (see figure on p. 953). The vast majority of prostheses in most developed nations are endoskeletal.

● TABLE 15.9 Lower Limb Prosthetic Structure

Prosthetic Structure	Description	Advantages	Disadvantages
Exoskeletal	• Strength and aesthetics of the prosthesis are created by a laminated external shell	• Highly durable and low maintenance	• No post-fabrication modification • Heavier than endoskeletal designs • Limited component availability
Endoskeletal	• Strength is from internal pylons that connect the foot/ankle to the socket (in TT applications) or to the prosthetic knee (in TF applications) • Aesthetics are established through a shaped foam cover that is then covered by an elastic "skin" or fabric hosiery • Outer foam cover/skin is optional if wearer prefers to utilize prosthesis without a cover	• Ease of post-fabrication adjustments • Modularity of the system allows for components to be readily interchanged • Soft feel of the prosthesis • Realism of the outer skins	• Durability of the outer foam cover and skins is limited

PROSTH

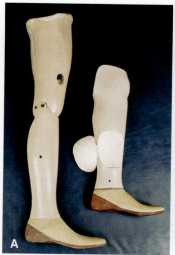
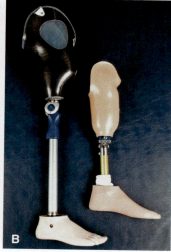

(A) Exoskeletal and (B) endoskeletal prostheses.

LLP Socket Designs: Transtibial and Transfemoral

Transtibial, or below the knee, amputations represent the most common major lower limb amputation level, followed by transfemoral amputations.

🔶 **TABLE 15.10 Lower Limb Prosthetic Transtibial and Transfemoral Socket Designs**

	Description	Advantages	Disadvantages
Transtibial Socket Designs			
Joint and Corset System	• Coronal and sagittal knee stability are maintained by the metal joints that connect the corset to the socket and a posterior check strap • Primary style of prostheses until the PTB prosthesis in the 1950s	• Indicated when someone with a transtibial amputation has severe AP or ML knee instability • De-weights residual limb via custom leather thigh corset, which serves as an extension to the shank section	• Due to constriction and loading, thigh musculature atrophies over time • Hot, heavy, and bulky • Requires waist belt and fork strap for suspension

(table continues on page 954)

PROSTH

TABLE 15.10 Lower Limb Prosthetic Transtibial and Transfemoral Socket Designs (continued)

	Description	Advantages	Disadvantages
Transtibial Socket Designs			
Patellar Tendon-Bearing (PTB) Sockets	• Loads pressure-tolerant RL regions while relieving pressure-sensitive RL areas (see Figs. 16.6 & 16.7) • Existing wearers may find it difficult to switch to another socket design	• Tolerant tissues can be loaded, allowing less tolerant tissues to be off-loaded • Interface materials can be socks or foam liners	• Fitting is more time intensive than total surface bearing designs • Distal end contact must be maintained to prevent verrucous hyperplasia • Gel type is not made for localized loads created in PTB sockets
Total Surface-Bearing (TSB) or Quasi-Hydrostatic Sockets	• Pressure is evenly distributed across the RL by the addition of a roll on silicone, urethane, or similar gel type liner • Gel liners allow the RL to behave quasi-hydrostatically, distributing the forces across the residual limb	• The introduction of gel liners has facilitated fitting of prosthetic sockets • Bony prominences may still need to be accommodated via loading or reliefs to prevent rotation or optimize fitting • Gel liners available in numerous sizes and thicknesses, with different coverings and additional suspension options	• Gel liners require daily cleaning, can be hot, require hand dexterity for donning, and may last a year or less • Air bubbles between the RL and liner may compromise function • Some wearers are allergic to the materials in the gel liners • Gel liners are costly

	Description	Advantages	Disadvantages
Transfemoral Socket Designs			
Quadrilateral Sockets	• Distal ischium is the primary weight-bearing surface • When viewed from the top, the socket has four sides, each with respective contours to accommodate adjacent anatomy • Contains a narrow anteroposterior dimension and a large medial-lateral dimension • Introduced in the 1950s	• Good design for low activity individuals who spend most of their time sitting • Easier to orient for donning • Less aggressive on the ischial ramal complex than IC designs	• Wide ML dimension does not facilitate natural femoral adduction • High loads on ischium may be hard to tolerate • Ischium "rides" on the socket brim instead of being contained within the socket
Ischial Containment Sockets	• Body weight is directed upon the ischium, soft tissues, and in more aggressive designs on the ischial ramal complex • The ischium is contained within the socket to some degree • Maintains a narrow medial lateral dimension in an attempt to create near-normal femoral adduction • Types of ischial containment socket designs include Narrow ML, CAT CAM, Normal Shape Normal Alignment, Sabolich Sockets, ComfortFlex Sockets, and MAS sockets	• Anatomically based design allows for greater rotational control over quad designs	• IC sockets are more challenging to fit • Some wearers do not want a socket to extend so proximally • May be difficult to don

PROSTH

(table continues on page 956)

TABLE 15.10 Lower Limb Prosthetic Transtibial and Transfemoral Socket Designs (continued)

	Description	Advantages	Disadvantages
Transfemoral Socket Designs			
Sub-Ischial Sockets	• Utilizing a combination of elevated vacuum and RL gel, urethane, or silicone liner, socket trim lines may be lowered so as to not contact or encompass the ischium at all (see Table 16.16)	• Unencumbered hip joint gives wearer excellent range of motion • Suspension is optimized	• Multiple layers of liners and inner and outer sockets make donning complicated • Seal must be maintained • For long and medium-length transfemoral RLs • Requires a pump

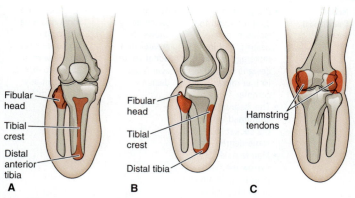

Fibular head
Tibial crest
Distal anterior tibia
A

Fibular head
Tibial crest
Distal tibia
B

Hamstring tendons
C

Pressure tolerant areas are shown as shaded areas for (A) the anterior, (B) lateral, and (C) posterior views of the transtibial residual limb. *Adapted from: Lusardi, MM, and Nielsen, CC: Orthotics and Prosthetics in Rehabilitation. Butterworth-Heinemann, Boston, 2000, with permission.*

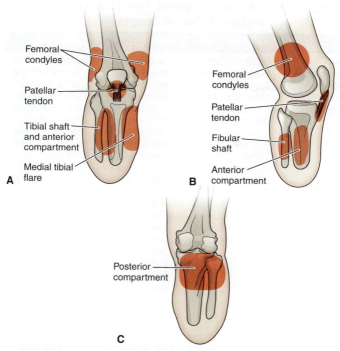

Pressure intolerant areas are shown as shaded areas for (A) the anterior, (B) lateral, and (C) posterior views of the transtibial residual limb. *Adapted from: Lusardi, MM, and Nielsen, CC: Orthotics and Prosthetics in Rehabilitation. Butterworth-Heinemann, Boston, 2000, with permission.*

LLP Socket Designs: Ankle, Knee, and Hip Disarticulations

Knee and ankle disarticulations are similar in that they are performed with the intent of preserving long bones, minimizing surgical trauma by cutting through a joint, and preserving anatomical structures upon which a prosthesis may be suspended. For Syme level amputations (through the ankle), supra malleolar suspension is possible. For knee disarticulation (KD) amputations, prosthetic suspension can be achieved over the femoral condyles. Due to the similarities of these amputation levels, prosthetic socket designs and suspension mechanisms are categorized together. Hip disarticulation and hemipelvectomy amputations are also grouped together in Table 15.11.

PROSTH

⬤▮ **TABLE 15.11** **Lower Limb Prosthetic Transtibial and Transfemoral Socket Designs**

	Description	Advantages	Disadvantages
Knee Disarticulation and Syme Socket Designs	• Disarticulation level amputations have bulbous distal ends that require accommodation to facilitate donning • PTB or TSB (for Syme), quadrilateral or ischial containment (for KD) socket designs are utilized • Distal ends may be partially loaded	• Suspension may be supramalleolar (Syme) or supracondylar (KD) • Amputation is less traumatic through joints than through long bones and muscles remain intact • Disarticulations are preferred for pediatric cases as the possibility for boney overgrowth is eliminated	• Component limitations exist due to the minimal space between the distal end of the RL and the floor (for Syme) and knee center (for KD) • Syme and KD prostheses may lack aesthetic appeal due to bulbous distal ends • In KD, the prosthetic thigh section may be longer and the prosthetic shank section shorter than the ipsilateral side
Hip Disarticulation and Hemipelvectomy (HD/HP) Socket Designs	• Hip disarticulation amputations involve removal of the entire leg through the hip joint; thus weight-bearing must be on the remaining ischium, pelvis, and soft tissues • Very short transfemoral amputations may be treated as HD amputations • Hemipelvectomy amputations involve amputation of some or the entire affected side pelvis and leg thus weight-bearing must be through the remaining skeletal and soft tissues as tolerated	• Suspension is achieved over the sound side iliac crest and is inherent in the socket design • People with HD/HP amputations often ambulate successfully with a prosthesis and some without assistive devices	• Sockets must encompass the affected side and allow for attachment of prosthetic components including a hip, knee and ankle joint, thigh, and shin sections and a prosthetic foot. • The energy cost of ambulation is substantial • Custom sitting socket/cushions are needed for people with hemipelvectomy amputations to facilitate normal spinal alignment and prevent back pain while sitting

LLP Components: Prosthetic Feet

As of 2010, over 180 different designs of prosthetic feet are available in the United States. These components are currently grouped according to coding by the Centers for Medicare & Medicaid Services (CMS) DMEPOS fee schedule. This is relevant because prosthetic feet are appropriate for people with amputations according to their Medicare Functional Classification Levels (see Table 15.2). Efforts are under way to develop functional classifications of prosthetic feet because there is significant variability between feet that are grouped together under the current CMS coding system. For example, all feet classified as SACH do not function in the same way biomechanically. In addition to activity level, other considerations must be addressed when selecting a prosthetic foot such as type of shoes a person with an amputation desires to wear, previous prosthetic wear experience, residual limb length, and the type of terrain for overground ambulation.

⬤ TABLE 15.12 Prosthetic Feet

Prosthetic Foot Groups	Description	Advantages	Disadvantages
SACH (solid ankle cushion heel) (see figure on p. 964)	• Available since the 1950s • Simple, low-maintenance design • Wood, plastic, or composite keel • Compressible foam rubber heels available in different densities • Flexible toe segment	• Inexpensive and durable • Available in different heel heights (0 to 3½ in.) • Good for limited ambulators or when maximum durability and no maintenance are required • Good shock absorption • May be used for post-operative or preparatory prostheses due to light weight and low cost	• Forefoot is rigid • Does not accommodate uneven terrain • May be less energy efficient compared to newer designs • No true inversion/eversion • Not indicated for active community ambulators or athletes
Flexible keel feet (aka elastic keel) (see figure on p. 964)	• Developed in the 1980s • Low maintenance	• Provides a smooth rollover at terminal stance	• Limited push off due to keel flexibility • May feel too "squishy" for some wearers

(table continues on page 960)

TABLE 15.12 Prosthetic Feet (continued)

Prosthetic Foot Groups	Description	Advantages	Disadvantages
	• Resilient keel allows for smooth rollover • Mimics human foot movement without articulations or moving parts • Compressible foam rubber heels available in different densities	• Designs with plantar bands generate a windlass effect to alter stiffness during stance phase similar to the plantar fascia in human feet • Limited inversion/eversion simulated through keel flexibility • May be used for children or preparatory limbs due to smooth rollover	• Athletes or active wearers may prefer foot designs with stiffer, more responsive keels • Not indicated for K1 level ambulators
Single axis feet (see figure on p. 965)	• Rigid keel with molded rubber foot • Articulating joint simulates ankle motion in the sagittal plane • Plantarflexion and dorsiflexion motions are controlled by interchangeable viscoelastic bumpers	• Articulation enables rapid foot flat at loading response, which increases knee stability • Often utilized with transfemoral level amputations, those with weak knee extensors, or very short RLs • Different durometers (hardnesses) of bumpers allow for varying degrees of stiffness depending on the needs of the wearer	• Ankle articulation adds weight • Maintenance is required to lubricate the joint and replace worn bumpers • Foot may become too stiff once bumpers are completely compressed

Prosthetic Foot Groups	Description	Advantages	Disadvantages
Multi-axial feet	• Articulations allow for triplanar motion • Bumpers serve to provide shock absorption and control of motions	• Accommodates to a wide range of terrains • Greater torque forces are absorbed by the foot, reducing forces at the RL/socket interface • Persons with knee instability, poor postural control or vulnerable RLs benefit from reduced stresses on the RL/socket interface • Different durometers of bumpers allow for varying degrees of stiffness depending on the needs of the wearer	• Foot motion provides less static stability than nonarticulating designs • Ankle articulations add weight • Maintenance is required to lubricate the joints and replace worn bumpers • Contraindicated if regular maintenance is unavailable • More expensive than SACH and single axis designs
Dynamic response feet (aka energy storing feet, energy storing and return feet) (see figure on p. 965)	• Keels are often made of single or multiple layers of composites (carbon fiber, Kevlar, etc.) • Energy is stored in the dynamic keel through loading phases of stance and returned to the wearer at terminal stance • Designed to meet performance demands beyond that of walking • Some keel designs include the shank of the prosthesis	• Inherent strength, durability, and lightweight • Appropriate for those wearers involved with high-demand activities • Dynamic push off in terminal stance	• Can be too stiff for those unable to load the foot effectively • High cost • Most effective dynamic response: feet still do not match the propulsion of the human foot/ankle complex • Provide greater energy efficiency at speeds beyond that of normal walking only • Not indicated for K1 or K2 level ambulators

(table continues on page 962)

PROSTH

TABLE 15.12 **Prosthetic Feet** (continued)

Prosthetic Foot Groups	Description	Advantages	Disadvantages
Prosthetic foot manufacturers have now developed prosthetic feet that combine features of the groups outlined above. The rest of this table introduces these combination groups as well as other design features that are important for prosthetic foot selection.			
Single axis ankle/ flexible keel feet	• Combines the articulation of a single axis foot with the flexible keel	• Allows for smooth rollover in terminal stance as well as inherent knee stability • See advantages of single axis feet and flexible keel feet, above	• See disadvantages of single axis feet and flexible keel feet, above
Multi-axial ankle/ dynamic response feet	• Combines multi-axial ankle motions with dynamic response keel properties	• Allows for high activity wearers to reduce forces at the RL/socket interface over uneven terrains	• High cost • See disadvantages of multi-axial feet and dynamic response feet, above
User-adjustable heel heights (see figure on p. 965)	• A button or other mechanism allows the foot to be plantarflexed or dorsiflexed to match different heel height shoes (**Note:** Prosthetic feet are designed to be worn with shoes with predefined heel heights, i.e., ⅜ or ¾ in. If a wearer applies a shoe with a heel height that does not match the heel height of the prosthetic foot, the prosthesis alignment is altered, creating an unstable and potentially unsafe condition.)	• Feet with this feature have the ability to reposition to allow for a variety of shoes with different heel heights and/or walk barefoot • User-adjustable heel height feet may also have flexible or dynamic keels	• High cost • Added weight • User must be able to safely operate the adjustable heel height foot • Not indicated for those with cognitive impairment

Prosthetic Foot Groups	Description	Advantages	Disadvantages
User-adjustable heel durometer	• User can change the heel to be softer or harder depending on needs	• Allows for adaptability of foot to activity and terrain	• May add some maintenance, weight and cost to the foot
Aesthetic appearance	• Prosthetic feet come in different skin shades • Some feet have a split between the first and second toe, some feet have no sculpted toes at all	• If the wearer is interested in shoes that will show the prosthetic foot such as sandals or has shoes that require a strap to be secured between the toes, this must be considered	• These features are not critical to wearers who keep their prosthetic foot in a sock and shoe
Running feet	• Most prosthetic feet are designed to meet biomechanical demands of walking, and are therefore not optimal for running (either sprinting or distance) • Running feet lack a heel	• Running feet for sprinting are designed to be stiff and responsive • Running feet for distance running may be less stiff than those for sprinting	• Running specific feet are not made for walking • Costly
Foot build height	• Some feet designs have keels that extend beyond the malleoli area into the shank	• Symes feet are designed to allow for no leg length discrepancies, yet still allow for dynamic features when possible	• Extended keel feet may not fit under long residual limbs
Micro-processor-controlled foot/ankle	• A battery-powered rechargeable microprocessor actively controls ankle dorsiflexion and plantarflexion	• Mimics human foot/ankle motion in swing phase • Can self-align to different heel heights	• Powered ankle does not provide active push off • Heavy • Very costly

(table continues on page 964)

PROSTH

🔴 **TABLE 15.12 Prosthetic Feet** (continued)

Prosthetic Foot Groups	Description	Advantages	Disadvantages
	• Foot still has a dynamic keel	• Adapts foot/ankle motion to ramps and stair ascent/descent • Will position into dorsiflexion for standing from a chair	• Maintenance • May be noisy to some

Based on: Fergason, J: Prosthetic feet. In Lusardi, MM, and Nielsen, CC (eds): *Orthotics and Prosthetics in Rehabilitation.* Saunders Elsevier, St. Louis, MO, 2007; Michael, JW: Prosthetic suspensions and components. In Smith, D, Michael, J, and Bowker, J (eds.), *Atlas of Amputations and Limb Deficiencies.* American Academy of Orthopaedic Surgeons, Rosemont, IL, 2004.

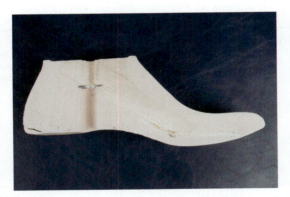

SACH foot cutaway.

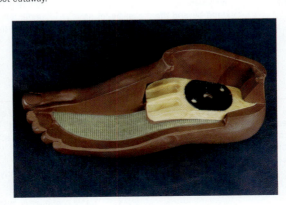

Flexible keel foot cutaway.

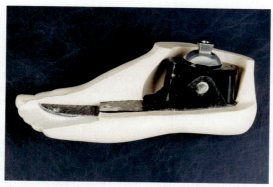

Single axis foot cutaway.

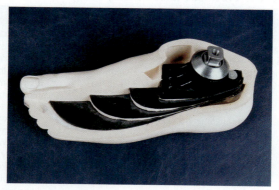

Dynamic response foot cutaway.

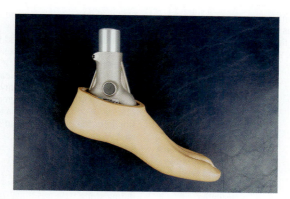

User-adjustable heel height foot.

LLP Components: Prosthetic Knees

Prosthetic knees are designed to simulate the motions and actions of human knees but are limited in that they are passive devices. The following tables introduce prosthetic knees according to primary design options (Table 15.13) and other features (Table 15.14). Primary design options are control of knee axis and knee motion. Regarding knee axis, prosthetic knees are either single axis or polycentric (see figure on pp. 967 and 968). Regarding knee motion control, prosthetic knees have either constant friction or variable friction control. Other features of prosthetic knees include extension assist, manual locks, weight-activated stance control, stance phase knee flexion, and microprocessor control. Prosthetic knees may or may not have these features and they may contain features in a variety of combinations. For example, there are single axis knees with constant friction, extension assist, and manual locks. There are also polycentric knees with constant friction, extension assists, and manual locks.

TABLE 15.13 Prosthetic Knee Primary Design Options

Design Options	Description	Advantages	Disadvantages
Single axis knees (see figure on p. 967)	• Knee mechanism simulates a simple hinge, pivoting about a single axis • Knee stability is affected by alignment, muscular contraction, or built-in microprocessors	• Mechanically simple • Lightweight • Requires minimal maintenance	• Stability may be difficult for those with short RLs or limited hip extension strength to generate a knee extension moment • For individuals with very long TF and knee disarticulations, knee centers may not be symmetrical
Polycentric knees (see figure on p. 967)	• Knee mechanism with multiple articulations and linkages (or bars) • Functional center of knee rotation (instantaneous center of rotation or ICOR) may be located outside of the knee joint • "Four bar" is most common but five, six, and seven bar designs are also available	• Stance stability is inherent in the design • Special designs accommodate long TF RLs and knee disarticulations • Closely simulates the anatomical knee axis through ROM • Facilitates toe clearance during swing	• Increased weight compared to single axis designs • Mechanical complexity equals greater maintenance • Increased cost

PROSTH

Design Options	Description	Advantages	Disadvantages
Constant friction knees	• Friction that modulates the speed that the knee flexes and extends during swing phase is set for one general speed of gait	• Mechanically simple • Indicated for single speed walkers	• Does not accommodate variable speed walking • Contraindicated for high activity wearers (K3 and K4 level ambulators)
Variable friction knees	• Uses fluid dampening to control the rate of knee flexion and extension during swing phase according to the gait of the wearer • Flexion and extension dampening may be set independently • Dampening may be controlled by pneumatic (gas) cylinders, hydraulic (liquid) cylinders, or both	• Allows for high-activity wearers to ambulate at variable cadence without having to wait for the shank/foot/ankle to swing through • Provides a smoother, more natural swing through movement • Pneumatic knees are not affected by ambient temperature • Hydraulic knee units are more robust than pneumatic knee units	• Increased complexity adds cost and maintenance • Increased weight

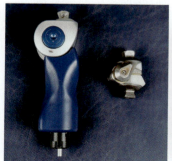 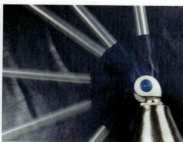

Single axis knees.

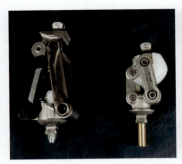
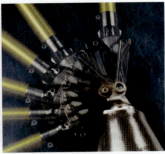

Polycentric knees.

TABLE 15.14 Prosthetic Knee Features

Features	Description	Advantages	Disadvantages
Extension assist	• Elastic mechanism (usually a spring) that facilitates the prosthetic knee into full extension during swing phase • May be adjustable	• Aids knee into extension, thereby enhancing stance phase knee stability	• May cause "terminal impact" upon full extension when resistance to extension is too low or extension assist is too high • May add noise
Manual locks	• Mechanism within the prosthetic knee that locks the knee completely or locks out knee flexion while allowing extension • Usually locks automatically upon full knee extension when wearer is standing, then must be disengaged once wearer is seated • Some models contain control levers on the prosthetic knee, whereas other models route control cables to the proximal aspect of the socket	• For those in need of the greatest stance phase stability • May be used during initial socket fittings to begin building wearer confidence in the prosthesis; only to be replaced after wearer's confidence is demonstrated	• Prosthesis is too long during swing as the knee does not bend, resulting in a compensation such as vaulting, circumduction, or hip hiking • Considered to be the knee design of last resort • Should not be used bilaterally

Features	Description	Advantages	Disadvantages
Weight-activated stance control	• A friction brake engages if weight is loaded onto the prosthetic knee while it is not in terminal extension, which prevents the knee from collapsing • Sensitivity of braking mechanism can be adjusted	• Prevents knee flexion if the knee is partially flexed and loaded due to a stumble or uneven terrain or if the prosthetic foot is "stubbed" on a rug or other obstacle • Best for slow-speed ambulators • Indicated for those with recent amputations, limited strength, and difficulty controlling the prosthesis	• To flex the prosthetic knee, it must be fully unloaded, requiring the wearer to shift all his/her weight onto the sound side to sit or to initiate flexion for swing phase. • Contraindicated bilaterally
Stance phase knee flexion	• A mechanism within the prosthetic knee that allows the knee to flex only slightly at initial contact/loading response (IC/LR) • Mimics normal human knee flexion at IC/LR • Is adjustable to allow for varying degrees of flexion	• Provides a smooth gait and facilitates forward momentum	• Previous wearers may find knee flexion at IC/LR unsettling • Adds cost, mechanical complexity

(table continues on page 970)

PROSTH

🔴 **TABLE 15.14 Prosthetic Knee Features** (continued)

Features	Description	Advantages	Disadvantages
Microprocessor control	• Microprocessors control knee flexion and extension rates during swing, stance, or both • Knee motion control is either pneumatic or hydraulic, yet the control is adjusted instantaneously • Rechargeable batteries	• Algorithms determine the phase of gait and adjust to compensate for next motion • Gait kinematics are closer to normal • Increased energy efficiency • Requires less concentration than using a nonmicroprocessor knee	• Significant expense • Maintenance • Must be electronically charged nightly

LLP Components: Suspension

Suspension of a prosthesis, regardless of the amputation level, is critical. If the suspension is inadequate, the residual limb will move in and out of the prosthesis during gait, which is referred to as *pistoning*. Pistoning of the RL inside a prosthetic socket results in friction, shear, instability, and difficulty of the wearer to control the prosthesis. In some prostheses the means of prosthetic suspension is inherent in the socket design, whereas in other prostheses, suspension is independent of socket design. Furthermore, suspensions are not mutually exclusive, so some prostheses may contain multiple types of suspension. Suspension can be categorized according to the mechanism in which it is achieved: anatomical and atmospheric. In anatomical suspension (see Table 15.15), the prosthesis hangs onto some anatomical prominence such as the iliac crests, the femoral condyles, or the malleoli. In atmospheric suspension (see Table 15.16), a liner and/or a sleeve is utilized to create a condition of negative pressure. Atmospheric suspension utilizes elastomeric gel, silicone, or urethane liners, which are rolled onto the RL. Friction secures the liner to the skin. Many types of attachments are incorporated into the liner to facilitate suspension.

TABLE 15.15 Anatomical Lower Limb Prosthetic Suspension

Suspension Type	Amputation Level	Anatomy Over Which the Prosthesis is Suspended	Description	Advantages	Disadvantages
Window/door designs (see figure on p. 977)	Syme (Ankle disarticulation)	Malleoli	• A window is made to allow for donning • Window may be medial or posterior • Window is covered by a door or panel to provide total contact on the RL	• Medial windows are structurally stronger than posterior windows	• Openings that are too large may adversely affect structural integrity
	Knee disarticulation	Femoral condyles			
Bladder designs	Syme (Ankle disarticulation)	Malleoli	• A silicone bladder is fabricated inside the socket to accommodate bulbous distal end and passage yet still maintain suspension	• Structurally stronger than window/door designs	• The outer appearance is tubular and resembles a "stovepipe" • Difficult to adjust
	Knee disarticulation	Femoral condyles			
Full or partial foam liners	Syme (Ankle disarticulation)	Malleoli	• A soft full- or partial-length foam liner encompasses the RL and is donned first, followed by a sock • Liner/RL are pushed into the prosthesis	• Structurally more sound than window/door designs	• The outer appearance is tubular and resembles a "stovepipe"
	Knee disarticulation	Femoral condyles			

(table continues on page 972)

PROSTH

PROSTH

■ **TABLE 15.15 Anatomical Lower Limb Prosthetic Suspension** (continued)

Suspension Type	Amputation Level	Anatomy Over Which the Prosthesis is Suspended	Description	Advantages	Disadvantages
Supracondylar full foam liner (PTB–SC)	Transtibial	Femoral condyles	• Medial and lateral walls of the PTB prosthesis extend proximal to the tibial tubercle level so that foam wedges can hang the prosthesis onto the condyles	• Provides coronal knee stability • Indicated for short RLs to enhance lever arm to control coronal forces	• High trim lines may be obtrusive • Prosthesis hangs on the femoral condyles
Supracondylar suprapatellar full foam liner (PTB–SCSP)	Transtibial	Femoral condyles & patella	• Similar to the PTB–SC; however, the anterior socket wall is extended to aid suspension and provide a knee extension stop	• Same as with PTB–SC; however, some degree of sagittal knee stability is also present	• High trim lines may be obtrusive
Cuff strap (see figure on p. 977)	Transtibial	Femoral condyles & patella	• Leather or similar material strap "belts" around the distal thigh	• Simple, economical, and durable suspension	• Requires hand dexterity to don • Contraindicated for fleshy or very muscular thighs
Waist belt and fork strap	Transtibial	Iliac crests	• A belt is worn around the waist connected to an elastic inverted "Y" strap that is secured to the prosthesis	• Used for immediate post-operative as well as joint and corset transtibial prostheses	• Bulky and must be worn over clothes

Suspension Type	Amputation Level	Anatomy Over Which the Prosthesis is Suspended	Description	Advantages	Disadvantages
Silesian belt (see figure on p. 977)	Transfemoral	Iliac crests	• A belt is worn around the waist and attached proximally and laterally to the prosthetic socket • Many varieties exist	• Assists with rotational control • May be made from leather or Dacron fabric	• Bulky and hot
Total elastic suspension (TES) belts (see figure on p. 977)	Transfemoral	Iliac crests	• An elastic belt, usually with Velcro closure, is secured around the prosthetic socket and the waist of the wearer	• Neoprene or other woven material • For low activity ambulators	• Can be hot
Hip Joint and pelvic band (see figure on p. 977)	Transfemoral	Iliac crests	• A belt with an incorporated pelvic band is secured to the prosthetic socket by means of a metal hip joint	• Hip joint simulates gluteus medius control of hip abduction • For those with short TF amputations and/or weak abductors	• Bulky • Heavy

PROSTH

TABLE 15.16 Atmospheric Lower Limb Prosthetic Suspension

Suspension Type	Amputation Level	Description	Advantages	Disadvantages
Knee sleeve	Transtibial or Syme	• Sleeve secured around the proximal aspect of the prosthesis as well as the thigh creating a seal • Suspension is through a combination of friction and negative pressure • May be used in conjunction with foam liner, socks, and/or an elastomeric liner as well	• Many different materials exist • Sleeve can mask (or hide) socket trim lines of a prosthesis	• Knee range of motion may be limited by a knee sleeve • Sleeves are not durable especially if the wearer kneels • May be hot
Suction	Transtibial or Syme	• A combination gel liner and knee sleeve is required • A one-way expulsion valve is incorporated into the socket to allow air to escape but not return	• May secure the prosthesis onto the residual limb more effectively than knee sleeves alone	• Debris may clog valve • Knee range of motion may be limited by a knee sleeve • Sleeves are not durable • May be hot
	Transfemoral	• Traditional TF suction is a skin-to-socket fit. The residual limb is pulled into the socket with the aid of a donning sock. Once the RL is fully seated into the socket, the valve is replaced • TF suction can be attained by using a gel liner as well	• No liners or belts are needed	• Consistent tissue volume is required • Donning requires hand dexterity and balance • New amputations and volume fluctuations (i.e., on dialysis) are contraindicated for TF skin fit suction

Suspension Type	Amputation Level	Description	Advantages	Disadvantages
Elevated vacuum	Transtibial or transfemoral	• A combination gel liner and outer sleeve is required • An electric or mechanical pump draws air from the chamber created between the outside of the liner and the inside of the socket wall. The outer sleeve seals the system	• Is proved to be the most secure suspension system • Helps to maintain RL volume throughout the day	• Pump adds weight, maintenance, and cost • Any compromise to the seal of the system reduces suspension
Pin & shuttle locks (see figure on p. 977)	Transtibial or transfemoral	• A pin is incorporated into the distal end of a gel liner that seats into a shuttle mechanism in the socket upon donning • An external button is pressed to release the pin and allow for doffing	• Mechanical suspension is secure • Auditory "clicking" aids some wearers • Can be used in conjunction with an outer sleeve • Allows for ease of doffing for prolonged sitting such as when driving, during airline flight, or eating	• Weight of the prosthesis is concentrated on the distal end causing a "milking effect" for some wearers • Shuttles require extra length so may not be feasible for long RLs • Pins are hard to seat on flabby TF residual limbs
Seal-in liners (see figure on p. 977)	Transtibial or transfemoral	• These liners have a silicone sealing ring around the outside of the liner that flattens and seals against the socket wall when donned	• Allows for a suction seal without the use of outer sleeves	• Liners are required • Requires a fairly stable volume to maintain fit and suspension

(table continues on page 976)

PROSTH

PROSTH

TABLE 15.16 Atmospheric Lower Limb Prosthetic Suspension (continued)

Suspension Type	Amputation Level	Description	Advantages	Disadvantages
		• An expulsion valve is required to allow air to escape while donning. It must be pushed to allow for doffing		
Lanyard systems (see figure on p. 978)	Transfemoral	• A lanyard, incorporated into the distal end of a gel liner, allows for the wearer to pull his/her RL into the socket. Once the RL is seated, the lanyard is secured to the external surface of the socket via a cleat mechanism	• Overcomes difficulties of donning a pin suspension system • Requires less length than shuttle lock systems, so they may be preferable for wearers with long RLs	• Requires hand dexterity
Liner strapping systems	Transfemoral or knee disarticulation	• Straps are incorporated onto the liners, which are then secured to the lateral aspect of the socket via Velcro or buckles	• These may be secured at the proximal end or the proximal and distal ends of the socket	• Straps on the socket add bulk • Requires hand dexterity

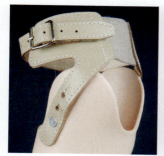

Cuff strap.

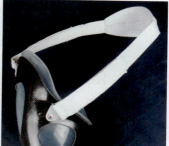

Silesian belt.

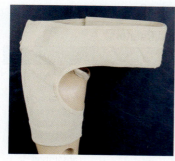

Total elastic suspension (TES) belts.

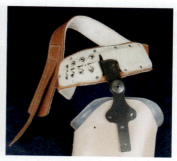

Hip joint and pelvic band.

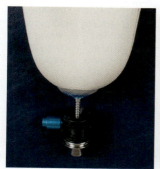

Pin & shuttle locks.

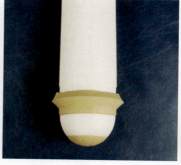

Seal-in liners.

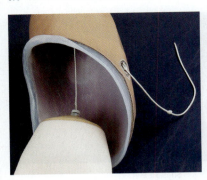

Lanyard systems.

LLP Components: Torque Absorbers and Rotators

TABLE 15.17 Torque Absorbers and Rotators

Component	Description	Advantages	Disadvantages
Torque absorber	• An endoskeletal component that absorbs transverse plane torque • May be adjustable	• Reduces stresses on the residual limb, especially in activities such as golf	• Adds weight, cost, and maintenance • Not necessary if the prosthetic foot provides adequate torque absorption
Rotators (transfemoral & higher level prostheses) Shock-absorbing pylons	• An endoskeletal component mounted proximal to the prosthetic knee that, with the push of a button, allows the user to transversely rotate the distal section of the prosthesis • Pylons, which connect the socket to the foot, have a built-in mechanism to absorb vertical compressive forces	• Allows for easy access to change shoes without removing the prosthesis • Is useful when driving to change position of the distal section of the prosthesis • Reduce impact transferred up to the RL and the rest of the body • May be utilized as a vacuum pump to facilitate elevated vacuum suspension (see Table 15.16) • May absorb torque as well	• Adds weight, cost, and maintenance • Requires the wearer to be cognizant regarding proper usage to be safe • Adds weight, cost, and maintenance • Requires length, so may not be feasible for long transtibial amputations

PROSTH

Upper Limb Prosthetics (ULP)

Loss of upper limb structure(s) will have significant impact on an individual because hands and arms are more apparent than lower limbs. Innumerable tasks are performed with the upper limbs, and prosthetic rehabilitation for upper limb amputees does not restore an individual's function to pre-amputation levels nearly as well as prosthetic rehabilitation does for persons with lower limb amputation. No single prosthesis will replace the multitude of deficits resulting from an upper limb amputation. As such, multiple prostheses; multiple terminal devices; and adaptations to home, recreation, and work environments are warranted if optimal outcomes are to be realized.

ULP Rehabilitation and the Six Prosthetic Options

To optimize the outcome of prosthetic rehabilitation for individuals with upper limb amputations, team rehabilitation must include physical/occupational therapy training throughout the phases of amputation (see Table 15.1), psychological counseling, case management, and prosthetic restorations as well as home, work, and recreational accommodations. It is essential that someone with a recent upper limb amputation be referred to a prosthetist as soon as possible rather than after they are healed and ready for fitting. This will assuage both the amputee and family members'/individual's supporters' concerns by beginning to establish realistic expectations for device designs, components, and prosthetic outcomes as part of a treatment plan of care. Peer visitation is also valuable if the peer is a comparable match with regard to gender, age, outlook, and amputation level.

With regard to prostheses for individuals with upper limb amputations, six options exist (Table 15.18).

TABLE 15.18 Prosthetic Options for Persons With Upper Limb Amputations

No prosthesis	Many upper limb amputees choose not to wear a prosthesis. This may be due to an inability of prosthetic rehabilitation to provide necessary functionality, lack of proper training, limitations of funding, or any number of other reasons. Amputees must know that this may be an acceptable option if they choose to exercise it part or all of the time.
Non-powered prosthesis (aka passive, semi-prehensile, or functional aesthetic)	These devices are functional for balance, carrying, pushing, pulling, and bimanual tasks that do not require active bilateral grasp. They restore an individual's appearance so that the affected limb appears as a whole limb, which facilitates acceptance and social reintegration. They require minimal harnessing and no cabling. They do not offer active prehension.

(table continues on page 980)

PROSTH

TABLE 15.18 Prosthetic Options for Persons With Upper Limb Amputations (continued)

Body-powered prosthesis	Body-powered (BP) devices utilize a harness and cabling system to capture body motions and translate these body motions into operation of mechanical components. BP devices are sturdy, reliable, durable, and economical when compared to externally powered devices.
Externally powered prosthesis	Externally powered (EP) devices utilize batteries to power the motorized arm components. Component control is most often through surface electrodes (myoelectrics) but may also be achieved through force sense resistors (touch pads), switches, or a variety of other input types. EP devices require care and maintenance and should not be used in or near water.
Hybrid prosthesis	A hybrid prosthesis contains some components that are controlled through body power and some that are controlled through external power. They are utilized for amputations at the elbow disarticulation level or proximal when control of multiple components is needed to restore arm motion and hand function.
Activity-specific prosthesis	These devices are designed for a specific work or recreational activity and may or may not include prehensile capabilities. They do not mimic anatomical appearance and are strictly utilitarian in nature.

Upper Limb Amputation Levels

For purposes of classification, amputation levels for the upper limb can be divided into major amputations—those through or proximal to the wrist joint—and minor amputations—those distal to the wrist joint. These terms must be used for classification only, as any amputation is major to the individual who sustained it.

TABLE 15.19 Major Upper Limb Amputation Levels

Interscapular thoracic or forequarter (IST)	Amputation of the entire upper limb as well as the ipsilateral clavicle and scapula
Shoulder disarticulation (SD)	Amputation of the entire upper limb through the shoulder joint
Transhumeral (TH)	Amputation through the humerus further subdivided into long, medium, short, and very short. Very short TH amputations are effectively treated as SDs

PROSTH

Elbow disarticulation (ED)	Amputation through the elbow joint
Transradial (TR)	Amputation through the radius and ulna further subdivided into long, medium, short, and very short
Wrist disarticulation (WD)	Amputation through the wrist joint removing the carpal bones and sometimes modifying the styloid processes

⬤ **TABLE 15.20 Minor Upper Limb Amputation Levels**

Partial hand (PH)	Amputation through any aspect of at least one metacarpal bone, usually with accompanying digit or digits
Metacarpal phalangeal disarticulation (MCP)	Amputation through the metacarpal phalangeal joints of digits 2–5
Thumb amputation	Amputation of all or part of the first digit
Phalangeal amputations	Amputation of all or part of phalanges 2–5

ULP for Minor Level Amputations

A 2002 report indicated that over 90% of upper limb amputations in the United States were at the finger, thumb, or partial hand level. Because 90% of the function of the human arm comes from the digits, even amputation of a finger results in impairment of function. It is common for persons with hand disfigurement to conceal the affected hand rather than draw attention to it. Hence someone with a finger amputation may lose function of the entire hand if the individual persists in concealing it. A misconception of prosthetic rehabilitation for minor level amputations is that the accompanying prostheses and components are only for cosmetic or vanity purposes. In reality, prosthetic fingers and partial hand prostheses provide protection, desensitization, and restoration of anatomical gripping surfaces as well as aesthetic restoration for the wearer.

References:

Dillingham, TR, Pezzin, LE, and MacKenzie, EJ: Limb amputation and limb deficiency: Epidemiology and recent trends in the United States. South Med J 95(8):875–883, 2002.
International Organization for Standardization:, ISO 8548-1:1989: Prosthetics and orthotics—Limb Deficiencies—Part I: Method of describing limb deficiencies present at birth. International Organization for Standardization, Geneva, Switzerland, 1989, pp 1–6.

PROSTH

PROSTH

TABLE 15.21   Minor Upper Limb Amputation Prosthetic Options

Amputation Level	Prosthetic Options	Description	Advantages	Disadvantages
Phalangeal amputations	Custom silicone finger restorations (NP)	• Sculpted and painted to duplicate the missing digit or digits • Suspended through suction onto the remnant finger • If little or no remnant finger exists, prostheses can be "banded" onto other fingers or adhesive may be used • Contraindicated for infants and children	• Restores anatomical gripping surface • Provides protection of sensitive distal ends • Aids desensitization • Restores hand aesthetic appearance	• Costly • Remnant finger sensation is diminished due to silicone coverage
	M-fingers or X-fingers (BP)	• Linkages or cables capture MCP flexion or wrist flexion to activate fingers • Not available for infants or children	• Finger motion is restored	• Limited power • Limited aesthetics
Thumb amputation (with some remnant thumb remaining)	Custom silicone thumb restoration (NP)	• Sculpted and painted to duplicate the missing thumb • Suspended through suction onto the remnant thumb • Contraindicated for infants and children	• All of the advantages/disadvantages of custom silicone fingers • Restores thumb length	• May not be rigid enough for strong grasp

Amputation Level	Prosthetic Options	Description	Advantages	Disadvantages
	Custom silicone partial hand restoration (NP)	• If no remnant thumb exists for suspension, a partial hand restoration is needed • Remaining fingers protrude through apertures allowing for full sensation and ROM • Sculpted and painted to simulate anatomy	• All of the advantages/disadvantages of custom silicone fingers • Restores thumb length • Wires can be added for thumb rigidity	• May not be sufficiently rigid for strong grasp • May be hot as the hand is sheathed in thin silicone
Thumb amputation (complete)	Opposition post (NP)	• Rigid post or thumb is strapped around the wrist to provide opposition to fingers	• Aids in grasp • Heavy duty	• Post is only in one location • Not aesthetic
	Powered thumbs (EP) (i.e., i-limb digits)	• Powered thumb flexes to provide active grasp • Myoelectric or touch-pad controlled • Thumb can be passively abducted • Not available for children	• Active prehension is restored • Aesthetic covering is available	• Not heavy duty • Cannot get wet • Very expensive, requires maintenance

(table continues on page 984)

PROSTH

TABLE 15.21 Minor Upper Limb Amputation Prosthetic Options (continued)

Amputation Level	Prosthetic Options	Description	Advantages	Disadvantages
Metacarpal phalangeal disarticulation (MCP) and partial hand amputations	Custom silicone partial hand restoration (NP)	• Sculpted and painted to simulate missing anatomy • Fingers are positionable due to wires embedded in the silicone • Thumb or unaffected digits protrude through apertures allowing for full sensation and ROM • Rarely utilized in children	• Restores anatomical gripping surface • Provides protection of suture lines • Aids desensitization • Restores hand aesthetic appearance	• Costly • Palm sensation is diminished due to silicone coverage • Not for heavy duty applications
	Powered fingers (EP) (i.e., ProDigits or Transcarpal Hand)	• Powered digits flex to provide active grasp • Myoelectric or touch-pad controlled • Not available for children	• Active prehension is restored • Aesthetic covering is available	• Not heavy duty • Cannot get wet • Very expensive, requires maintenance
	"Prosthosis" (AS) (i.e., N-Abler)	• Wrist hand orthosis with a palmar mounting into which tools or recreational terminal devices can be inserted and quickly exchanged • Not available for children	• Restores power grasp • Facilitates bimanual activities	• Leverage and movement is achieved through forearm, elbow, and shoulder movements • Wrist motion is locked out

NP = nonpowered, BP = body powered, EP = externally powered, AS = activity specific.

ULP for Major Level Amputations

Major ULP: Structure

Major upper limb prostheses are either exoskeletal or endoskeletal in basic structure. Exoskeletal upper limb prostheses are most common.

TABLE 15.22 Major Upper Limb Prosthetic Structure

Prosthetic Structure	Description	Advantages	Disadvantages
Exoskeletal	• Strength and aesthetics of the prosthesis are created by a laminated external shell, allowing for installation of external cabling/harnessing components • Inside of the prosthesis is hollow, allowing space for batteries, wiring and controllers	• Highly durable and low maintenance	• Hard outer surface may lack aesthetic appeal
Endoskeletal	• Strength is from internal pylons that connect the socket to the elbow/wrist/terminal device • Aesthetics are established through a shaped foam cover that is then covered by hosiery, off-the-shelf, or custom-made gloves	• Soft feel of the prosthesis • Realism of the outer skins • Cabling/wiring can run through pylons • Elbow lock can be operated by depressing a lever or button	• Durability of the outer foam cover and skins is limited • Light- to moderate-duty applications

Major ULP: Harnessing

Harnesses serve the roles of securing the prosthesis to the body, thereby providing stability and suspension. They also serve in the capacity as the anchor for the cabling systems, which capture body motions and translate these motions to component operation. Self-suspending prostheses that do not need to capture body motions for component operation can avoid harnessing altogether.

PROSTH

■ **TABLE 15.23 Major ULP Harnessing**

Amputation Level	Harness Type	Description	Advantages	Disadvantages
Wrist disarticulation and transradial amputations	Figure of eight	• Used when both suspension and terminal device activation are required from the harness • Axilla loop anchors harness around contralateral shoulder • Anterior suspensor strap bifurcates to an inverted "Y" strap, which attaches to a triceps cuff and hinges (see Table 15.31) • Control strap attaches to cabling for TD operation • Straps are either sewn together or connected by a metal ring or plastic harness anchor	• Glenohumeral flexion, uni-scapular and/or bi-scapular protraction generate excursion (movement of a cable) to activate the terminal device • Wearer can experience feedback through the harness to have some sense of TD position	• Contralateral axilla pressure may not be tolerated or may cause damage over time to the sound side if excessive force is required for TD activation • Harnessing may feel binding • Bulky compared to figure of nine
	Figure of nine	• Used when only cable activation is required of the harness as suspension is achieved through some other means • Axilla loop anchors harness around contralateral shoulder • Control strap attaches to cabling for TD operation • No anterior strap or triceps cuff	• Glenohumeral flexion, uni-scapular, and/or bi-scapular protraction generate excursion to activate the terminal device • Harnessing is less encumbering than figure of eight	

Amputation Level	Harness Type	Description	Advantages	Disadvantages
	Shoulder saddle	• Used when both suspension and cable activation are required from the harness and the prosthesis will be used to manage heavy loads • A shoulder saddle made of plastic or leather "rides" on the ipsilateral shoulder • Chest strap secures the saddle in place • Anterior strap provides suspension through triceps cuff • Control strap attaches to cabling for TD operation	• Transfers load from the prosthesis through the triceps cuff/hinges to the saddle • Glenohumeral flexion, uni-scapular, and/or bi-scapular protraction generate excursion to activate the terminal device • Eliminates the axilla loop, thereby reducing pressure on the sound side arm	• May be bulky
Elbow disarticulation and transhumeral amputations	Figure of eight	• Same as figure of eight above; however, the anterior strap attaches to an elbow lock cable that locks/unlocks the elbow in different angles of flexion/extension • Lateral suspension strap secures the socket to the RL • "Z" strap or cross back strap are variations	• Glenohumeral flexion, uni-scapular, and/or bi-scapular protraction generate excursion to activate the terminal device • A combination of shoulder abduction, depression, and extension is needed to lock/unlock the elbow	• Control motions and operation take time to master

(table continues on page 988)

PROSTH

PROSTH

■ TABLE 15.23 **Major ULP Harnessing** (continued)

Amputation Level	Harness Type	Description	Advantages	Disadvantages
		• Control strap attaches to cabling that generates elbow flexion (when the elbow is unlocked) and terminal device operation (when the elbow is locked)		
	Shoulder saddle	• Same as with shoulder saddle above; however, the anterior strap provides activation of the elbow lock • Control strap attaches to cabling, which generates elbow flexion (when the elbow is unlocked) and terminal device operation (when the elbow is locked)	• Same advantages as the figure of eight; however, a shoulder saddle allows for higher loads to be distributed onto the upper shoulder, alleviating pressure from the contralateral shoulder • No axilla loop	• May be bulky
	Chest strap	• Used when only suspension is required of the harness or as an auxiliary suspension • Chest strap crosses from the prosthesis around the torso and buckles anteriorly	• Provides a simple and effective suspension • Eliminates the axilla strap	• Contraindicated for women

Amputation Level	Harness Type	Description	Advantages	Disadvantages
Interscapulo-thoracic and shoulder disarticulation amputations	Chest strap	• Used to secure the socket to the torso • May be made of Dacron webbing, leather, or Spenco vulcanized rubber or a similar elastic material	• Provides a simple and effective suspension • Eliminates the axilla strap • Some designs can be used for women	

Major ULP: Cabling

Cabling in UL Prosthetics serves the role to transfer excursion generated from a body motion from the point of origin to some other location. In most cases cabling allows the user to directly operate terminal devices, elbow units, or locks. Concomitantly, cable excursion (i.e., linear displacement of the cable) may also be utilized by the amputee to activate switches for control of externally powered components. Cabling generally consists of housing, housing retainers to anchor housing to the prosthesis, and the cable itself, which may be constructed of braided steel, nylon, or Spectra®, an ultra-high-molecular-weight polyethylene.

TABLE 15.24 Major ULP Cabling

Cable Type	Amputation Level	Description	Advantages
Single control or Bowden cable	WD or TR	• A single cable runs from the control strap, is anchored either on the triceps cuff (for figure of eight) or directly to the posterior aspect of the socket (for figure of nine), and proceeds to the terminal device	• Works on hooks, prehensors, or hands; voluntary opening (VO) or voluntary closing (VC) • Efficient and effective
	ED, TH, SD, or IST	• Utilized when a cable is needed to control only one component or action, i.e., elbow lock, terminal device, elbow flexion/extension, or shoulder lock	• Different motions can control different components • Each cable must be attached to a separate strap on the harness
Dual control or fair lead cable	Very short TR	• A single cable has a split or two-part housing, which allows excursion on the cable to flex the elbow (when the elbow is not locked) or operate the terminal device (when the elbow is locked).	• Provides elbow flexion power and terminal device operation • Requires a split socket design (see Table 15.34) • For use only with RL-activated locking hinges (see Table 15.31)

Cable Type	Amputation Level	Description	Advantages
	ED and TH	• Same as dual control for very short TR above • Elbow lock is achieved by a separate cable activation on external locking hinges (see Table 16.31) or a locking elbow	• Provides elbow flexion power and TD operation • Elbow lock can be operated through body motions or pulled manually by the sound side hand

Major ULP: Body-Powered Terminal Device Operation Strategies—VO versus VC

For body-powered ULP, terminal devices (TDs) are designed to be operated in one of two strategies: voluntary opening (VO) or voluntary closing (VC).

🔴 **TABLE 15.25 Body-Powered Terminal Device Operation Strategies**

Operation Strategy	Description	Advantages	Disadvantages
Voluntary opening (VO) "pull to open"	• Terminal device is closed at rest • Excursion on the cable opens the terminal device • Rubber bands or springs close the device • Used on hooks, prehensors, or hands	• Items once grasped will remain in the TD as long as the force required to maintain the item in the TD does not exceed the pinch force generated by the springs or rubber bands • The wearer can relax the cable and items will stay in the TD • Pinch force is determined by the springs or rubber bands	• To increase pinch force, increased numbers of rubber bands are required that must be overpowered every time the TD is opened. This may result in irritation or shoulder injury over time • Feedback from the harness to the wearer relates to force needed to open the TD, not the pinch force created by the TD

(table continues on page 992)

PROSTH

🔴 **TABLE 15.25** **Body-Powered Terminal Device Operation Strategies** (continued)

Operation Strategy	Description	Advantages	Disadvantages
Voluntary closing (VC) "pull to close"	• Terminal device is open at rest • Excursion on the cable closes the terminal device • Rubber bands or springs open the device • Used on hooks, prehensors, or hands	• TD pinch force can be finely controlled through cable excursion and feedback through the harness to the wearer • Pinch force is only limited by the amount of power the wearer can generate through the harness/cable	• Wearer must either keep tension through the cable, lock the cable in place, or utilize a TD with a back locking feature to maintain pinch force on items once grasped

Major ULP: Externally Powered Prosthesis Control Inputs

Control of the powered components in externally powered prostheses comes from surface myoelectrodes, push switches, linear pull switches, and/or touch pads. Proportional control means that the speed a component operates is proportional to the input signal being generated. This is similar to a dimmer control for a light. Digital control means that once an input signal is generated, a motor is turned on at one speed. This is similar to an on/off light switch.

🔴 **TABLE 15.26** **Externally Powered Prostheses Control Inputs**

Input Type	Description	Advantages	Disadvantages
Myoelectrode	• Surface electrode(s) is mounted into the prosthetic socket, allowing for electromyographic (EMG) signals to be captured • Signals are processed and used to control externally powered components	• Anatomical muscle activity "controls" components (i.e., wrist flexor muscle EMG signals may control TD closing while wrist extensor EMG signals trigger TD opening)	• May not be feasible on scarred, burned, or grafted skin • Moisture or sweat can damage the myoelectrode • Myoelectrodes must be properly shielded to prevent inadvertent operation

Input Type	Description	Advantages	Disadvantages
	• Antagonistic muscle groups provide the best control of componentry • The current control option of choice when available	• Electrodes may be remote from their amplifier or the amplifier may be built into the socket	
Push switches	• Depressing a button commands a motor to operate in one direction or allows the wearer to select between components • Switches can be single position or dual position • Operation is usually by the chin or by bumping the switch against the body	• Usually installed on the socket • Indicated when high level (short TH, SD, or IST) externally powered prostheses require control of multiple components (i.e., TD, wrist rotator, elbow flexion/ extension, elbow lock, and/or shoulder lock)	• Too much gadgetry can lead to wearer frustration
Pull switches	• Pull on a small cable generates an electrical signal that can be used to control componentry • Small amount of excursion (0–1 in.) and a limited amount of force are required • Can be digital (on/off) or proportional (similar to a dimmer switch)	• Usually installed on the socket • Indicated when high-level, externally powered prostheses require control of multiple components (i.e., TD, wrist rotator, elbow flexion/ extension, elbow lock, and/or shoulder lock)	• Too much gadgetry can lead to wearer frustration

(table continues on page 994)

PROSTH

TABLE 15.26 Externally Powered Prostheses Control Inputs (continued)

Input Type	Description	Advantages	Disadvantages
		• Body motion translates to component operation, yielding some measure of feedback	
Touch Pads or frorce sense resistors (FSRs)	• Flat, thin pressure-sensitive pads generate proportional signals when pressed	• Available in a variety of sizes and shapes • Economical when compared to myoelectrodes	• Not as durable as myoelectrodes • Must be used on a flat surface

Major ULP: Componentry

Terminal devices (TDs) represent the distal components of upper limb prostheses. The attachment features of the TDs to the prosthesis allow for installation and removal, thus making them interchangeable to serve different functional uses. It is not unusual for a wearer to have more than one TD or to have more than one prosthesis with a variety of different TDs. TDs can be categorized according to their role in allowing the wearer the ability to grasp: non-prehensile, semi-prehensile, and active prehensile. Non-prehensile and semi-prehensile TDs are utilized on non-powered and activity-specific prostheses. Active prehensile TDs are utilized on body powered, externally powered, or hybrid powered prostheses (see Table 15.18). TDs are classified as hooks, prehensors, hands, or activity specific (i.e., recreational TDs, tools, or utensils). Hooks generally possess a hook shape, whereas prehensors open and close in a manner similar to that of a thumb and finger pinch. Body-powered active prehensile TDs utilize either voluntary opening or voluntary closing operation strategies.

Major ULP: Terminal Devices for Infants and Children

TABLE 15.27 Terminal Devices for Infants and Children With Major Upper Limb Amputations

TD Category	Terminal Device Classification and Operation	Description	Advantages	Disadvantages	Examples
Non-prehensile infant	Baby mitts or crawling TDs	• Mitts look like mittens • Crawling TDs are rubber with a stylized hand • Hands come in different colors	• Durable, lightweight • Designed to promote crawling and bimanual activities	• May or may not have aesthetic appearance • No ability to grasp	Baby mitt Infant 2 Infant crawling hands
Semi-prehensile infant	Hands with stock gloves	• Have wires or elastic properties that allow for lightweight items to be placed into a stylized hand • Gloves come in assorted colors	• Facilitates bimanual activities • Provides light duty holding to allow for item manipulation from unaffected side • No cabling required	• Grasp is limited	Alpha hand Child Passive hand Cosmetic hands
Non-prehensile child	Foam-filled hands/gloves	• PVC gloves are filled with soft or rigid foam, adhered to a prosthetic socket, and then covered with a PVC or silicone glove (TR and WD levels)	• Lightweight and low cost • Gloves come in many colors	• PVC gloves stain and become rigid over time • Fingers are not positionable	Child hard PVC hand

(table continues on page 996)

PROSTH

PROSTH

TABLE 15.27 Terminal Devices for Infants and Children With Major Upper Limb Amputations (continued)

TD Category	Terminal Device Classification and Operation	Description	Advantages	Disadvantages	Examples
	Sports and recreation TDs	• Utilitarian TDs designed specifically for a sport, hobby, or recreational activity	• Good for the purpose they are designed for • Interchangeable	• Do not look like hands	TRS Sports TDs Texas Assistive Devices TDs
Semi-prehensile child	Hand with or without stock gloves	• Have wires or elastic properties that allow for lightweight items to be placed into the hand • Gloves come in assorted colors	• Facilitates bimanual activities • Provides light-duty holding • No cabling required • Fingers may be positionable	• Grasp is limited • Gloves may stain and need replacement	Child passive hand TRS L'il EZ hand System hands
Active prehensile child Body powered (children develop ability to control a BP system around age 5 yr)	Hand VO	• Thumb and/or fingers move • Mechanical hand requires a glove for covering • CAPP hand does not require a glove but comes in different colors	• Grasp is controlled by springs or elastic bands • Stylized appearance aids in acceptability of the TD • Opening is voluntary • Closing is automatic	• Gloves may stain and need replacement • Fine-tip pinch is difficult • Visually obstructive • Heavy compared to hooks	CAPP hand Dorrance mechanical hand System hands RSL Steeper VO hand

TD Category	Terminal Device Classification and Operation	Description	Advantages	Disadvantages	Examples
	Hand VC	• Only the thumb moves • Comes in different colors	• Aesthetic hand appearance and active function enhance acceptance • Grasp is controlled by the wearer	• Fine-tip pinch is difficult with hand TDs	TRS Lite Touch hand RSL Steeper VC hand
	BP hooks VO	• May have plastisol coating in Caucasian or brown colors	• Grasp is controlled by the rubber bands • Fine-tip pinch is available but pinch force is determined by rubber bands	• Hooks can be ominous for children or adults	Hosmer hooks Otto Bock hooks
	BP prehensors VO	• Allows for fine-tip pinch • Has two different colored covers	• Grasp is controlled by springs • Variable surface aids prehension	• Does not have a hand-like appearance	CAPP TD
	BP prehensors VC	• Allows for fine-tip pinch • Comes in three different colors	• Grasp controlled by the wearer • Finger- and thumb-like appearance • Lightweight	• Does not have a hand-like appearance	TRS ADEPT

(table continues on page 998)

PROSTH

PROSTH

TABLE 15.27 Terminal Devices for Infants and Children With Major Upper Limb Amputations (continued)

TD Category	Terminal Device Classification and Operation	Description	Advantages	Disadvantages	Examples
Active prehensile child Externally powered	Electric hands	• Require a battery, controller, and user input for operation • Require gloves for covering • Three jaw chuck is primary grasp pattern • Can be used on toddlers at 15 mo	• Grip force is generated by motors • "Cookie crusher" operation lets the child provide a hand open signal and after a brief delay the hand closes	• Gloves may stain and require replacement • Expensive • Requires maintenance • Heavy	Child Myo hand Electrohand 2000 RSL Scamp hand VASI hands

Major ULP: Terminal Devices for Adults

TABLE 15.28 Terminal Devices for Adults With Major Upper Limb Amputations

Category	Terminal Device Classification and Operation	Description	Advantages	Disadvantages	Examples (not a comprehensive list)
Non-prehensile adult	Foam-filled hands/gloves	• PVC gloves are filled with soft or rigid foam, adhered to a prosthetic socket, and then covered with a PVC or silicone glove (TR and WD levels)	• Lightweight and low cost • Gloves come in assorted colors	• PVC gloves become rigid over time • Fingers are not positionable	Cosmetic or foam-filled hands
	Sports, hobby, and recreation TDs	• Utilitarian TDs designed specifically for a sport, hobby, or recreational activity	• Good for the purpose they are designed for • Interchangeable	• Do not look like hands	TRS sports TDs TX assistive devices TDs
Semi-prehensile adult	Hands with stock gloves	• Have wires that allow for finger positioning • Stock gloves come in assorted colors • Gloves can be silicone or PVC	• Functional for bimanual activities • Provides light-duty holding • No cabling required	• Grasp is limited • PVC gloves may stain and become rigid over time	Cosmetic hands System hands

(table continues on page 1000)

PROSTH

PROSTH

TABLE 15.28 Terminal Devices for Adults With Major Upper Limb Amputations (continued)

Category	Terminal Device Classification and Operation	Description	Advantages	Disadvantages	Examples (not a comprehensive list)
	Custom hands with hand painted gloves	• Molds are obtained of the unaffected hands and an opposite side hand is sculpted to match • Outer silicone skin is hand-painted to match the skin of the wearer • Have wires that allow for finger positioning and for lightweight items to be placed into the hand	• Highest level of aesthetic restoration • Functional for bimanual activities • Provides light-duty holding • No cabling required • Stain resistant	• Grasp is limited • Custom hands/gloves are expensive	ArTech Life Like LIVINGSKIN Otto Bock Silicone Pillet
Active prehensile adult Body powered	Hand VO	• Thumb and fingers open with cable pull • Has three jaw chuck grasp • Most require a glove	• Grip force is controlled by springs	• PVC gloves stain • Fine-tip pinch is difficult with hand TDs • Mechanical hand is visually obstructive • Mechanical VO hands are heavy compared to hooks	Robin Aids hands Hosmer hands Becker hands Otto Bock hands

Category	Terminal Device Classification and Operation	Description	Advantages	Disadvantages	Examples (not a comprehensive list)
	Hand VC	• Thumb, fingers, or a combination close with cable pull to control grasp • Lite Touch hand comes in different colors and has sculpted fingers; others require gloves	• Aesthetic hand appearance and active function enhance acceptance • Grasp is controlled by the wearer • Fine-tip pinch is difficult with hand TDs	• Mechanical hand is visually obstructive • Mechanical VC hands are heavy compared to hooks	TRS Lite Touch hand RSL Steeper VC hand
	Hooks VO	• Split hooks come in a variety of shapes, materials, and styles • Cable pull opens tines or fingers	• Grasp is controlled by the rubber bands • Fine-tip pinch is available but pinch force is determined by rubber bands	• Hooks can be ominous for children or adults	Hosmer hooks Otto Bock hooks
	Prehensors VC	• Allows for fine-tip pinch • Comes in difference colors • Cable pull closes fingers	• Grasp controlled by the wearer • Finger- and thumb-like appearance • Lightweight and rugged	• Not hand shaped	TRS grip prehensors

(table continues on page 1002)

PROSTH

TABLE 15.28 Terminal Devices for Adults With Major Upper Limb Amputations (continued)

Category	Terminal Device Classification and Operation	Description	Advantages	Disadvantages	Examples (not a comprehensive list)
Active prehensile adult Externally powered	Standard electric hands	• Require a battery, controller, and user input for operation • Motors generate opening/closing • Externally powered hands require gloves for covering • Some have faster speeds or sensors in the digits to detect grasp force • Three jaw chuck is primary grasp pattern	• Grip force is generated by motors • Programmable modes of operation	• Gloves may stain and require replacement • Expensive and requires maintenance • Heavy compared to non-externally powered TDs • Grip pressure is focused at the tips of the thumb and first two fingers • Fourth and fifth digits are passive	Otto Bock System hands RSL Steeper Electric hands Motion Control hands Centri Adult hands
	Compliant electric hands	• Same as standard electric hands above; however, multiple grasp patterns exist • Individual digits have separate motors • Thumb can passively abduct	• Reduces body compensation by offering different grip patterns • Grasp pressure is distributed across the entire surface of the hand • Aesthetic movement of the hand appears normal	• More expensive than standard electric hands	Touch Bionics iLIMB hand & iLIMB pulse RSL Steeper BeBionic hand

Category	Terminal Device Classification and Operation	Description	Advantages	Disadvantages	Examples (not a comprehensive list)
		• Digits close around objects and stop when they reach resistance			Motion control ETD
	Powered hooks	• Motors drive split hooks • One tine or finger moves • Require a battery, controller, and user input for operation • Motors generate opening/closing	• Allows for those accustomed to a body powered hook to control a hook externally thereby alleviates stresses on the upper torso • Water resistant	• Hooks can be ominous for children or adults • Expensive and requires maintenance	
	Powered prehensors	• Same as powered hook except both tines of the TD open	• Very strong pinch force • Wide opening	• Hooks can be ominous for children or adults • Expensive and requires maintenance	Greiffer MC Gripper

Major ULP: Wrist Units

Wrist units serve the primary purpose of securing the terminal device to the forearm section or socket of the upper limb prosthesis. In addition, wrist units may provide wrist flexion/extension, allow for simulated pronation/supination, and/or include quick disconnect features to allow for ease of TD exchange. Body-powered prosthetic wrist unit types (Table 15.29) and externally powered wrist unit types (Table 15.30) are described below.

TABLE 15.29 Body-Powered Prosthetic Wrist Units

Wrist Type	Description	Advantages	Disadvantages
Economy wrists	• Basic wrist unit in round or oval shape • TD is screwed into the wrist unit • Friction on pronation/supination is variable	• Simple, low-cost wrist • Optional straps for heavy-duty applications • Available in aluminum, stainless steel, and titanium	• No wrist flexion/extension
Flexion wrists	• Enables terminal device flexion/extension to different angles • Indicated for those with bilateral amputations or a strong need to reach midline • Flexion/extension position may be locked or may be controlled by friction • Pronation/supination may be constant friction or through a ratcheting mechanism • Comes in round or oval shape, adult and child sizes	• Facilitates bimanual mid-line activities • Varieties exist for body-powered hooks, prehensors, or hands as well as externally powered hook, prehensors, or hands • Flexion/extension is achieved through passive motion or by unlocking the wrist and activation by the cable • Externally powered wrist flexion units do not exist in the United States	• Adds weight, cost, and maintenance • Requires length at distal end so may not fit in long TR- or WD-level amputations

Wrist Type	Description	Advantages	Disadvantages
Quick disconnect wrists	• TDs are readily interchangeable by installing an insert that matches with the wrist unit • TDs pronation/supination as well as removal are facilitated by depressing a lever or push button for BP systems • For EP systems, TD removal is facilitated by rotating the TD > one full rotation. Pronation/supination in EP systems can either be powered or achieved through passive motion or a ratcheting mechanism	• Rapid TD exchange facilitates utilization of multiple TDs including hooks, prehensors, hands, sports TDs, and tools • An insert is required for each TD • If BP hook and BP hand are utilized, an adapter is needed for the cabling • Available in aluminum, stainless steel, and titanium	• Adds weight and cost • Requires length at distal end so may not fit in long TR- or WD-level amputations
Five-function wrist	• Incorporates spring-loaded pro/supination, flexion/extension, and a quick disconnect feature • Indicated for those with bilateral amputations who can master operation	• Body powered only • Requires extra skill with cabling and position locks	• Requires length at distal end so may not fit in long TR- or WD-level amputations • Added complexity for operation • Extra weight

🟠 **TABLE 15.30 Externally Powered Prosthetic Wrist Units**

Wrist Type	Description	Advantages	Disadvantages
Flexion/extension wrists	• Enables terminal device to be flexed or extended to different angles • May be locked in positions or controlled by friction	• Facilitates bimanual mid-line activities • TD position can be readily changed for functional task	• Adds weight, cost, and maintenance • Requires length at distal end so may not fit in long TR- or WD-level amputations

(table continues on page 1006)

PROSTH

🔴 **TABLE 15.30 Externally Powered Prosthetic Wrist Units** (continued)

Wrist Type	Description	Advantages	Disadvantages
Universal motion wrists	• Wrist motion is simulated through a "ball and socket" friction-controlled joint	• TD position can be readily optimized for functional task	• Friction may be overpowered by weight of TD and held object
Quick disconnect wrists	• TD removal is facilitated by rotating the TD >one full rotation. • Pronation/supination in EP systems can either be powered or achieved through passive motion or a ratcheting mechanism	• Rapid TD exchange facilitates utilization of multiple TDs including hooks, prehensors, hands, sports TDs, and tools	• Adds weight and cost • Requires length at distal end so may not fit in long TR- or WD-level amputations
Wrist rotators	• Provides motor-driven pronation/supination • Controlled by a variety of inputs	• TD position can be readily optimized for functional task	• Requires length at distal end so may not fit in long TR- or WD-level amputations • Added complexity for operation • Extra weight and cost

Major ULP: Transradial and Wrist Disarticulation Hinges

Transradial (TR) and wrist disarticulation (WD) hinges are utilized to facilitate suspension, provide rotational control, and, in some instances, lock/unlock an elbow to allow for flexion/extension.

TABLE 15.31 Transradial and Wrist Disarticulation Prosthetic Hinges

Hinge Type	Indicated for	Description	Advantages	Disadvantages
Flexible hinges	WD, medium, and long TR with natural pro/supination	• ½ in. Dacron, leather, or flexible metal straps extend from the socket/forearm to the triceps cuff/harness	• Allows for suspension to be transferred to the harness while still allowing for natural pro/supination	• No rotational stability
Rigid hinges	WD, long, medium, and short TR with limited pro/supination Wearers that need strong rotational control	• Metal hinge joints connect the socket/forearm to the triceps cuff/harness • May be single axis or polycentric joints	• Allows for suspension to be transferred to the harness • Maximal rotational stability • Heavy duty applications	• Natural pro/supination is restricted • Pro/supination must be achieved through TD rotation in the wrist unit
Step-up hinges	Very short TR with good strength but limited ROM	• Through utilization of a split socket, when the RL flexes, the forearm section flexes twice as much	• Allows wearers with limited elbow flexion ROM to position the forearm to reach their face • Rotational control is inherent	• Split socket looks unnatural • Requires good strength
Residual limb locking hinges	Very short TR with limited strength and limited ROM	• Once the elbow is flexed to position the forearm into the desired position, when the RL flexes, the hinges lock the elbow to maintain the forearm in place • A split socket is required	• Rotational control is inherent • Requires a dual control cable to operate the TD as well as to flex the elbow	• Split socket looks unnatural • Flexing/extending the elbow lock the prosthetic elbow joints in place, which is counterintuitive

PROSTH

Major ULP: Elbows

Elbow units serve the purpose of securing the humeral section of a prosthesis to the forearm section. They provide the motions of humeral internal/external rotation as well as elbow flexion/extension. For a terminal device to be stable and steady in space, prosthetic elbows must have some method of locking and unlocking as well.

TABLE 15.32 Prosthetic Elbows for Transhumeral and Higher Level Amputations

Elbow Type	Lock/ Unlock	Description	Advantages	Disadvantages	Examples (not a comprehensive List)
Friction elbow	This design does not lock	• Elbow is positioned by sound side and maintains position via friction • Used with non-prehensile or semi-prehensile TDs	• Lightweight and light duty • Available in standard, medium, and small	• Elbow does not lock • Exoskeletal design only	Hosmer friction elbow RSL Steeper friction elbow
Endoskeletal locking elbow	Push button Lever operation Cable pull	• Elbow is positioned by sound side • Lock/unlock can be operated by sound side or through body motions • Can be used with all non-EP TDs	• Endoskeletal design allows for foam cover and aesthetic appearance	• Sound side is required to flex/extend	Hosmer elbows Otto Bock modular arm RSL Steeper modular arm

Elbow Type	Lock/Unlock	Description	Advantages	Disadvantages	Examples (not a comprehensive List)
Exoskeletal locking elbows Body powered flexion/Extension	Cable pull Push button	• Elbow flexion/extension is determined by single or dual control cable operation • Lock/unlock is operated through body motions or sound side • Can be used with all non-EP TDs	• Rugged design • Available in standard, medium, and small • Forearm lift assists or forearm balancers facilitate ease of elbow flexion	• Operation requires training and practice to master • Live lift is limited with anything in the TD	Hosmer elbows RSL Steeper mechanical elbows Ergo arm
	Electric lock	• Elbow flexion/extension is determined by single or dual control cable operation • Lock/unlock is operated electronically • Can be used with all TDs	• Electric lock can be operated by a switch, touch pad, or myoelectrode	• Requires battery and alternate input • Not to be used around water • Increased cost and maintenance	RSL Steeper Electric elbows Ergo arm electric plus
Exoskeletal locking elbows External powered flexion/extension	Electric lock	• Elbow flexion/extension are controlled by external power • Lock/unlock is operated electronically • Used with EP TDs	• Fully electronic system minimizes necessary body motions for control and operation	• Increased cost, weight, and maintenance • Not to be used around water	Motion Control Utah Arms LTI Boston Arms Otto Bock Dynamic Arm

Major ULP: Socket Design and Suspension

Wrist Disarticulation and Elbow Disarticulation Amputations

Socket design for the WD and elbow disarticulation (ED) levels of amputation must consider RL length, suspension, available pronation/supination (WD) or internal/external humeral rotation (ED) and anticipated loads. As the challenges and socket styles of WD and ED are similar, they are grouped together in Table 15.33.

● **TABLE 15.33 Wrist Disarticulation and Elbow Disarticulation Prosthetics: Socket Design and Suspension**

Suspension Type	Suspension Is Achieved	Description	Advantages	Disadvantages
Windows/doors	Over styloids for WD Over humeral epicondyles for ED Auxiliary via harness	• A window is made to allow for donning • Window is covered by a door or panel to provide total contact on the RL	• Bulbous distal ends are accommodated • Suspension is inherent in the socket for light- to moderate-duty loads if tolerable • Rotational control is maintained	• Aesthetic finishing is difficult
Bladder designs	Same as above	• A silicone bladder is fabricated inside the socket to accommodate bulbous distal end passage yet still maintain suspension	• Same as above • Structurally more sound than window/door designs	• The outer appearance is tubular • Difficult to adjust

Suspension Type	Suspension Is Achieved	Description	Advantages	Disadvantages
Full or partial foam liners	Same as above	• A soft full or partial length foam liner encompasses the RL, is covered by a sock, and then the liner/RL are pushed into the prosthesis	• Structurally more sound than window/door designs • Foam is modifiable	• The outer appearance is tubular
Gel liners	Through friction on the skin Via straps, lanyard, or seal-in (see Table 16.16)	• Gel liners reduce shear and pressure on skin and are indicated for scars/burned/grafted tissue • Liners have various means to aid in suspension	• External power is an option using custom liners with openings for electrodes or liners with snap electrodes	• Pins/shuttles are contraindicated due to length limitations • Liners may be hot and require daily washing
Suction	Inner liner with expulsion valve	• Air is evacuated from between the skin/inner liner • Valve seals the system	• Skin fit facilitates electrode contact	• Requires a mature RL with a consistent volume
Special Considerations for WD & ED Prostheses				
WD		• Leaving the full forearm intact allows for near normal pronation/supination, a strong lever arm, and intact muscles • Styloids may or may not be shaved • Space for wrist and TDs is limited; as a result, the overall length of the prosthesis may be longer than the sound side • Special TD mounting options for WD exist to minimize the build height of the components If adequate suspension for a WD can be achieved suprastyloid, a figure of nine harness can be used for BP TD operation; no harness is needed for externally powered operation or semi-prehensile or non-prehensile TDs		

(table continues on page 1012)

(table continues on page 1012)

PROSTH

PROSTH

TABLE 15.33 **Wrist Disarticulation and Elbow Disarticulation Prosthetics: Socket Design and Suspension** (continued)

Suspension Type	Suspension Is Achieved	Description	Advantages	Disadvantages
Special Considerations for WD & ED Prostheses				
ED		• Leaving the full humerus intact allows for near normal humeral internal/external rotations, a strong lever arm, and intact muscles • Epicondyles may or may not be shaved • Space for an elbow is limited; as a result, the overall length of the humeral section may be longer than the sound side if an elbow unit is utilized Outside locking hinge joints are required to prevent humeral length discrepancies; however, they are bulky and require cable activation		

Transradial and Wrist Disarticulation Prosthetics: Relationship Between RL Length and Pronation/Supination

For TR or WD amputations, socket type, suspension, and other componentry are determined by the amount of pronation/supination that can be effectively captured by the socket and translated to prosthesis operation. The figure below details the amount of pronation/supination that remains as the amputation level moves from WD to very short TR amputation.

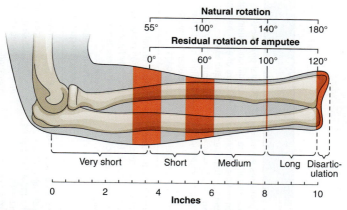

Below-elbow (transradial) amputation and wrist disarticulation.

Transradial Socket Designs

TABLE 15.34 Transradial Socket Designs

Amputation Level	Socket Style	Suspension Is Achieved	Description	Advantages	Disadvantages
Long and mid-length TR	Conventional	Via figure of eight harness, triceps cuff, and flexible hinges	• Socket trim lines extend to or are just distal to the olecranon and the epicondyles • Distal end has flattened volar and dorsal areas, resulting in a "screwdriver" shape • Worn with socks or gel liners	• Natural pronation/supination is maintained • Figure of eight harness is required for moderate-duty loads • Shoulder saddle harness used for heavy-duty loads	
	Suction		• Same trim lines as above • Inner socket contains a valve to allow for air to be expelled from the socket upon donning	• Natural pronation/supination is maintained • BP: Only figure of nine is needed for TD operation • EP: No harnessing, cabling is required	
	Liner assisted		• Gel liner is worn over the RL, which has a Velcro strap or similar to suspend the prosthesis • Pin/shuttle may be used if space permits	• Natural pronation/supination is maintained • BP: Only figure of nine is needed for TD operation • EP: No harnessing, cabling is required	• Liners require daily washing and may be hot

PROSTH

Amputation Level	Socket Style	Suspension Is Achieved	Description	Advantages	Disadvantages
Mid-length and short TR	Conventional	Via figure of eight harness, triceps cuff, and rigid hinges	• Socket trim lines extend to or are just distal to the olecranon and the epicondyles • Rigid hinges stabilize socket on RL preventing rotation • Worn with socks	• Figure of eight harness is required for moderate-duty loads • Shoulder saddle harness used for heavy-duty loads	• Natural pronation/supination is "locked out" by the rigid hinges
	Self-suspending (i.e., Muenster, Northwestern, TRAC, or ACCI)	Humeral epicondyles and triceps tendon	• Socket trim lines extend proximal to and hang onto the epicondyles • For BP: worn with socks or gel liners • For EP: skin fit or gel liner with electrodes	• Elbow flexion/extension ROM is maintained; however, as the RL length decreases, active ROM in the socket decreases • Good for up to moderate-duty loads • BP: Only figure of nine is needed for TD operation • EP: No harnessing, cabling is required	• Natural pronation supination is "locked out" by the socket trim lines • Suspension over epicondyles takes time to be tolerable

(table continues on page 1016)

PROSTH

TABLE 15.34 Transradial Socket Designs (continued)

Amputation Level	Socket Style	Suspension Is Achieved	Description	Advantages	Disadvantages
Very short TR	Split socket	Via figure of eight harness, triceps cuff, and rigid hinges	• Socket trim lines extend to or are just distal to the olecranon and the epicondyles • Rigid hinges stabilize socket on RL, preventing rotation • Socket is separate from the forearm section so that forearm moves separately from the socket • BP only: Worn with socks	• Remaining motions are optimized by using hinges	• Unusual appearance • Challenging fit and fabrication • Short lever arm makes control of prosthesis difficult

Transhumeral, Shoulder Disarticulation, and Interscapulothoracic Socket Designs

High-level upper limb amputations present a challenging scenario because the amputation level moves proximally, the lever arm and remaining anatomy for control of the prosthesis become minimized, while the need for control of multiple components increases.

References

American Medical Association. *Guides to the Evaluation of Permanent Impairment, ed. 5.* American Medical Association, New York, 2001.

PROSTH

TABLE 15.35 Transhumeral, Shoulder Disarticulation, and Interscapulothoracic Socket Designs

Amputation Level	Socket Style	Suspension Is Achieved	Description	Advantages	Disadvantages
Short to long TH	Open shoulder (i.e., Utah Dynamic Socket)	Figure of eight harness	• Socket design is anatomically contoured • Anterior and posterior trim lines extend farther toward midline as the amputation level becomes more proximal	• Durable system with good control, especially with long RLs	• Harness/cabling may be binding and restrict ROM
		Suction	• Same trim lines as above • Inner socket contains a valve to allow for air to be expelled from the socket upon donning	• Harnessing can be reduced because suspension is in the socket	
		Liner assisted	• Gel liner is worn over the RL, which has a Velcro strap or similar to suspend the prosthesis • Pin/shuttle may be used if space permits	• Harnessing can be reduced because suspension is in the socket • Gel liners provide cushion	• Liners need to be washed daily
Humeral neck, SD, and IST	Shoulder cap	Chest straps	• Shoulder cap is used to provide symmetry to the torso as well as to assess patient candidacy for a prosthesis	• Serves as a diagnostic interface to assess candidacy • Restores an aesthetic appearance even without distal components	

Amputation Level	Socket Style	Suspension Is Achieved	Description	Advantages	Disadvantages
			• Plastic or foam buildup designed to match contralateral shoulder	• Can be progressively weighted to simulate the weight of a prosthesis	
Infraclavicular		Chest straps	• Very low profile minimalist sockets provide a secure base for attachment of remaining componentry • Anterioposterior compression on the deltopectoral muscle group and scapula provides stability of the socket on the torso	• Small footprint on the torso reduces discomfort from heat • Can be used with NP, BP, EP, & HP	

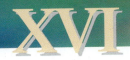

ORTHOTICS

Orthotics Overview

An orthosis is prescribed by a referring health-care provider as part of a treatment plan. When appropriately prescribed and utilized by the wearer correctly, an orthosis applies a series of forces to regions of the body to control motion(s) of the respective segment(s) (i.e., force systems). Essentially, orthoses function as motion control devices and are commonly utilized in concert with other medical or rehabilitation treatments. If one understands this fundamental concept of an orthosis, then patient evaluation and subsequent orthosis prescription formulation, design, and construction as well as optimal fit and function assessments are more clearly targeted. This chapter provides an overview of orthotic management principles and practices with an emphasis on the biomechanical motion(s) that the orthosis is designed to influence.

The fundamentals of orthotic management as part of a treatment plan are founded on a unique combination of normal and abnormal systems anatomy and physiology, which commonly extend beyond the neuromuscular and skeletal systems and include other disciplines of knowledge such as biomechanics, pathomechanics, material science, engineering, normal and abnormal psychology, and other sciences. Integration of this body of knowledge into a treatment plan for rehabilitation requires some basic guiding factors to ensure the orthosis creates optimal fit and functional performance for the wearer. Because biomechanical motion control is a common objective of the majority of orthoses, an important philosophy is to preserve as much natural movement so that the orthosis(es) impose the least constraint to allow the wearer to function to the best of his/her ability. To successfully implement a minimalist strategy of orthotic intervention, other rehabilitation therapies (i.e., physical therapy, occupational therapy) often need to be combined in tandem with orthotic management to optimize the functional outcome for the person who will wear the orthosis(es).

To gain a full appreciation of how orthoses interact with the body segments targeted for biomechanical motion control, a basic understanding of biomechanics, mechanics, force systems, and normal and pathological gait is necessary. Therefore, this chapter also provides a practical review of these fundamental principles that allow orthoses to effectively apply force system(s) to the body. In considering the outcome of the orthosis on the user's efficiency and function, one must be cognizant that an orthosis can only apply a force when the device is worn, and that the manner in which the orthosis is applied determines the device's functional capabilities. In addition, the wearer's "interaction" with the device, such as his/her adaptation, learning, and dose response, are also of considerable importance to the effectiveness of the orthosis as part of the overall treatment plan.

Classification Systems and Nomenclature

The International Standards Organization (ISO) (http://www.iso.org) has created a classification system of orthoses, including terminology and nomenclature (ISO 8540-3:1989 Prosthetics and Orthotics—Vocabulary, Terms relating to external orthoses. Geneva, Switzerland: International Standards Organization; 1989).

ORTHOT

Categories of Orthoses

Orthoses are categorized by the body region(s) incorporated or targeted, except for those designs denoted by (*).

Lower Limb Orthoses
Foot Orthosis (FO)
Ankle Foot Orthosis (AFO)
Knee Orthosis (KO)
Knee Ankle Foot Orthosis (KAFO)
Hip Orthosis (HO)
Hip Knee Ankle Foot Orthosis (HKAFO)
*Reciprocating Gait Orthosis (RGO)

Spinal Orthoses
Cervical Orthosis (CO)
Cervico-thoracic Orthosis (CTO)
Cervico-thoraco-lumbo-sacral Orthosis (CTLSO)
Thoraco-lumbo-sacral Orthosis (TLSO)
Lumbo-sacral Orthosis (LSO)
Sacro-iliac Orthosis (SIO)
Cranial and Facial Orthoses:
*Cranial Orthosis (CO)
*Facial Orthosis (FO)

Upper Limb Orthoses
Finger Orthosis (FO)
Hand Orthosis (HdO)
Wrist Hand Orthosis (WHO)
Wrist Hand Finger Orthosis (WHFO)
Elbow Orthosis (EO)
Elbow Wrist Hand Orthosis (EWHO)
Shoulder Orthosis (SO)

Nomenclature

Over the past several decades, the use of nomenclature and related terminology regarding orthoses has not consistently been utilized by health-care professionals. This section provides appropriate and accurate clarifications.

- An **orthosis** (*noun*) is defined as an externally applied device that is utilized as part of a treatment plan to modify the structural and functional characteristics of the neuromuscular and skeletal systems; the device may impose secondary effects on other systems (i.e., ankle foot orthosis).
- The term **orthoses** (*noun*) refers to the plural form of orthosis and describes more than one orthosis (i.e., bilateral lower limb orthoses).
- The term **orthotic** (*adjective*) is utilized as a descriptor (i.e., orthotic device).
- The term **orthotics** (*noun*) is defined as the science and art involved in treating persons with an orthosis as part of a treatment plan (i.e., the profession of orthotics).

ORTHOT

- An **orthotist** (*noun*) is defined as a person who, having completed an approved course of education and training, is authorized by a credentialing authority to design, measure, manufacture, fit, and alter orthoses as part of a treatment plan.
- **Custom-molded** orthoses are precisely fit to the patient as part of a multiple-step process that usually involves patient assessment, measurement, and creation of a negative impression (i.e., capturing the shape of the external body segment via casting or laser digitizing). From the negative impression, a positive model is created and this model serves as the basis for the custom fabrication process. The final product is an orthosis that fits the patient's particular body segment and addresses the desired biomechanical motion controls.
- **Off-the-shelf/custom-fitted** orthoses (also known as *prefabricated*) are premanufactured products that are commercially available. The off-the-shelf orthosis may be altered by the orthotist to approximate the fit to the patient's body segment to address the desired biomechanical motion controls.
- The term referring to an orthosis as a **splint** is vague and connotes an external device that may hold a body segment and limit natural motion. Because many orthoses serve more than one role beyond a static mechanical constraint, this terminology is unclear and is not recommended. For recommended terminology, see Technical Analysis Form on the following pages.
- Terms referring to function of the orthosis as "**static**" or "**dynamic**" are vague. It is recommended that the rehabilitation specialist avoid using these terms because they are difficult to define. A clearer description of the intended biomechanical motion control by the orthosis can be created by use of key descriptive terms added to the name of the orthosis such as, *solid, articulated, assist, resist, stop, hold, variable,* or *lock* when referring to the desired biomechanical control function (see Technical Analysis Form on the following pages).

TECHNICAL ANALYSIS FORM   **LOWER LIMB**

Name_____ No. _____ Age_____ Sex_____

Date of onset_____ Cause _____

Occupation_____ Present lower-limb equipment _____

Diagnosis _____

_____

_____

Ambulatory ☐   Non-Ambulatory ☐

Major Impairments:

A. Skeletal
  1. Bone and joints: Normal ☐ Abnormal _____
  2. Ligaments: Normal ☐ Abnormal ☐ Knee: AC ☐ PC ☐ MC ☐ LC ☐
                                         Ankle: MC ☐ LC ☐
  3. Extremity Shortening: None ☐ Left ☐ Right ☐

     Amount of discrepency: A.S.S. Heel_____ A.S.S.-MTP_____ MTP-Heel_____

B. Sensation: Normal ☐   Abnormal ☐
  1. Anesthesia ☐   Hypesthesia ☐ Location:_____
     Protective Sensation: Retained ☐   Lost ☐
  2. Pain ☐   Location: _____

C. Skin: Normal ☐ Abnormal _____

D. Vascular: Normal ☐ Abnormal ☐ Left ☐ Right ☐

E. Balance: Normal ☐ Impaired ☐ Support:_____

F. Gait deviations: _____

_____

G. Other Impairments:_____
─────────────────── **LEGEND** ───────────────────

⊕ = Direction of translatory motion

= Abnormal degree of rotary motion 60°

= Fixed position 30° 1 CM.

∿ = Fracture

Volitional Force (V)
N = Normal
G = Good
F = Fair
P = Poor
T = Trace
Z = Zero

Hypertonic Muscle (H)
N = Normal
M = Mild
Mo = Moderate
S = Severe

Proprioception (P)
N = Normal
I = Impaired
A = Absent
D = Local Distention or Enlargement

= Pseudarthrosis

= Absence of Segment

ORTHOT

Technical Analysis Form (for the lower limb). (A) Page 1 contains the summary of major impairments and the legend.

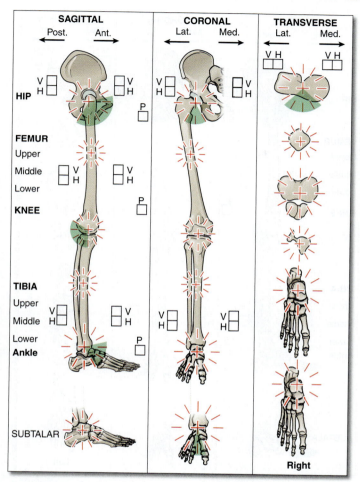

Cont'd from previous page (B) Pages 2 and 3 are the skeletal diagrams in the three cardinal planes.

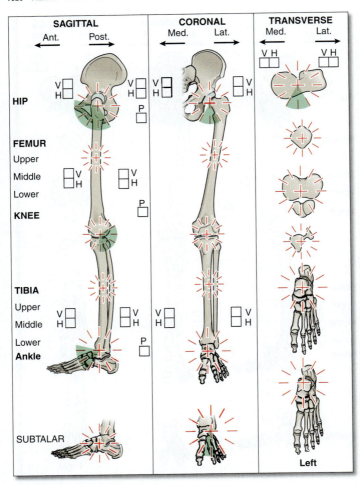

Cont'd from previous page (B)

ORTHOT

Summary of Functional Disability _____

_____

_____

_____

_____

Treatment Objectives:

Prevent/Correct Deformity ☐ Improve Ambulation ☐

Reduce Axial Load ☐ Fracture Treatment ☐

Protect Joint ☐ Other _____

ORTHOTIC RECOMMENDATION

Lower limb		Flex	Ext	ABD	ADD	Rotation		AXIAL LOAD
						Int.	Ext.	
HKAO	Hip							
KAO	Thigh							
	Knee							
AFO	Leg							
	Ankle	Dorsi	Plantar					
	Subtalar					Inver.	Ever.	
FO	Foot Midtarsal							
	Met.-phal.							

Remarks:

_____   _____

Signature   Date

KEY: Use the folowing symbols to indicate desired control of designated function:

F= FREE Free motion

A= ASSIST Application of an external force for the purpose of increasing the range, velocity, or force of motion.

R= RESIST Application of an external force for the purpose of decreasing the velocity or force of motion.

S= STOP Inclusion of the static unit to deter an undesired motion in one direction.

v= Variable A unit that can be adjusted without making a structural change.

H= HOLD Elimination of all motion in prescribed plane (verify position)

L= LOCK Device includes an optional lock.

Cont'd from previous page (C) The last page contains sections for Summary Functional Impairments, Treatment Objectives, and Orthotic Recommendations. *From: Lusardi, MM, and Nielsen, CC: Orthotics and Prosthetics in Rehabilitation, ed. 2. Butterworth-Heinemann, Boston, 2006, pp 22–24.*

Mechanical Principles Related to Orthoses

Although a relatively comprehensive understanding of mechanical principles is necessary for orthotists and bioengineers who design orthoses, rehabilitation specialists need a basic knowledge of mechanics to interpret proper fit and function of an orthosis. This section presents an applied approach to the information and is not intended to be complete. The reader is referred to the medical and engineering literature for further knowledge on the subject.

ORTHOT

Force

- Orthoses are 'force systems' that are applied to the body to control motion of various skeletal segments. A **force** has both direction and magnitude, and the principles guiding their integration into an orthosis determine, in part, their efficiency and effectiveness.
- Usually an orthosis applies several forces that interact and resolve to create the desired orthotic control. This system, known as a *force couple,* contains two equal forces, in opposite directions. A **three-point force couple** is one of the most fundamental mechanical principles incorporated into an orthosis (see the following figures).

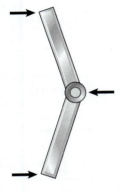

Three-point force couple. A force system that applies two equal forces in opposite directions. The single arrow on the right represents the corrective force and the two opposing arrows represent the counter forces.

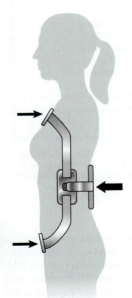

TLSO. A three-point force couple to resist trunk flexion.

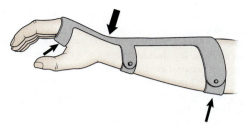

WHO. A three-point force couple to control for wrist flexion.

- Some orthoses have multiple force couples in play. For example, in a KAFO in which both the knee and ankle joints may need to be controlled, multiple force couples are at work in which some of the force application regions may be shared (see the figure below).

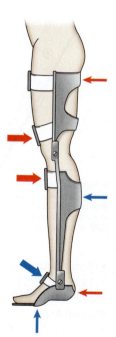

KAFO. Multiple-point force couples in a KAFO. The blue arrows show control of the ankle to resist plantar flexion and the red arrows show the force couple for resisting knee extension.

Gravity

- Gravity pulls the body toward the ground and the opposing reaction force from the body-ground interaction is known as the **ground reaction force (GRF)**. This external force is an important factor because GRFs significantly alter the interface pressures between the orthosis and body segment(s).
- For example, an AFO designed to hold the ankle in the neutral position (i.e., 90°) in a non-weight bearing situation will possess lower interface pressures

than when an individual stands or walks (during the stance phase of gait) due to the external GRFs .

- With a good understanding of the mechanics of gait, GRF can be capitalized to control joint motions. By blocking motion of a joint, the GRF can induce a joint moment at the nearest proximal joint.

- *Example:* A solid AFO may control knee motion during a portion of the stance phase of walking. If the AFO holds the patient's ankle and foot complex in plantar flexion, then the GRF may induce a knee extension moment during the early portion of stance phase, whereas if the AFO holds the patient's ankle and foot complex in dorsiflexion, then a knee flexion moment during the early portion of stance phase may be induced (see the following figure).

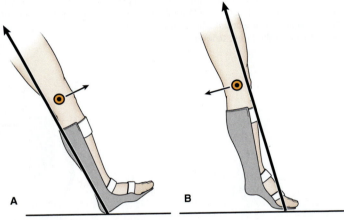

Influence of ground reaction forces (GRF). The influence of GRFs can occur only during the stance phase of gait and if ankle joint motion is blocked. (A) When the foot/ankle is held in dorsiflexion, the GRF is posterior to the knee joint axis and a knee flexion moment is present. (B) When the foot/ankle is held in plantarflexion, the GRF is anterior to the knee joint axis, and a knee extension moment is present.

- Ground reaction force control can only occur during the stance phase of walking unlike three point force couple systems, which provide control during both stance and swing phase.

Moment Arms

- Management of forces in an orthosis may be complicated due to the many interrelated components affecting how the forces are applied to the body. The criteria for orthotic design are founded on basic mechanical principles.

- A **moment arm** is the distance from the respective joint axis to the point where the interface force of the orthosis is applied.

- Orthoses with short moment arms produce higher interface pressures than orthoses with long moment arms (see the following figure).

- *Example*: The length of an orthosis often correlates with the length of its moment arm, due to its corresponding influence on the interface pressure applied by the orthosis.

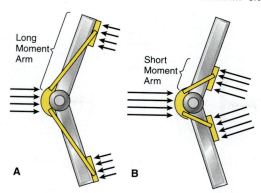

Length criteria for orthoses (*long vs. short*). An orthosis with a short moment arm (i.e., length) will possess higher orthotic interface pressures compared to a device with a longer moment arm.

- Maximizing the length of an orthosis (inherently its moment arm) is generally preferred over shorter orthotic devices. This is an important factor for the capacity of orthoses to provide the necessary forces to control movement while also insuring the wearer's comfort and tolerance.

Pressure and Shear

- Because orthoses interface with the skin and subcutaneous tissues, pressure and shear are extremely important in orthotic design.
- Because **pressure** is defined as force per unit area, the surface area of the force application region by an orthosis could be increased to redistribute a force over larger area or decreased to concentrate the force over a smaller area (see the following figure).

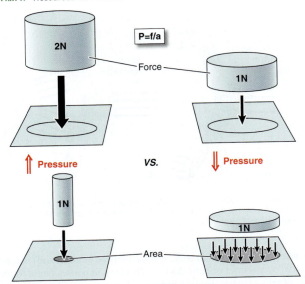

Orthotic interface pressures. Considering the formula, pressure = force × area, pressure can be reduced by decreasing the magnitude of the force or increasing the surface area of the force being applied.

- Decreasing the magnitude of the force may reduce pressure (see figure above).
- In most cases, if a patient is having difficulty tolerating the forces applied by an orthosis, increasing the surface area where the force is applied may be one option to decrease pressure, especially if the amount of force necessary to provide the desired control cannot be changed.
- With pressure, the line of force is perpendicular to the surface and may be easily quantified, whereas with **shear** stress the line of force is parallel with the surface (see figure below). Measurements of shear stresses are more difficult to quantify compared to measurements of pressure.

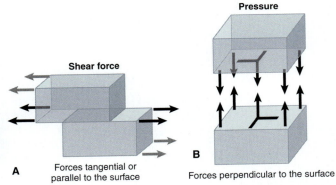

Pressure vs. shear force. The forces that describe pressure are perpendicular to a surface of the structure, whereas with shear the forces are parallel to the surface of the structure.

Shear and Coefficient of Friction

- **Shear** stresses may damage skin and other tissues. To reduce the shear forces in an orthosis, friction between the orthosis and the skin must be decreased.
- Friction may be reduced by introducing a layer of material as a barrier between the orthosis and the skin.
- *Example:* The use of hosiery and socks can reduce friction when one is wearing shoes or an AFO. For a spinal orthosis, a snug-fitting cotton T-shirt without seams may reduce shear stresses to the skin. For an upper limb orthosis, an interface sock may also be used in similar fashion. Stockinet is available in many sizes and is one of the most common materials used to protect the skin from direct contact with an orthosis.
- Another way shear stress can be reduced is to add interface materials that possess mechanical properties with a low friction coefficient value.
- The **coefficient of friction** (symbolized as μ) is the relationship of resistive frictional forces between two surfaces that are pressed together by a normal force. In an orthosis the normal force is the applied force from the device that presses the two surfaces together.
- The coefficient of friction characterizes the roughness between two materials and how those materials slide against each other.
- Coefficient of friction is calculated as: $\mu = F_r/N,$ where μ is the coefficient of friction for the two surfaces, F_r is the resistive force of friction, and N is the normal force pressing the two surfaces together in a perpendicular manner.

Total Contact Fit

- **Total contact fit** may be adopted to increase the surface contact area for force redistribution in an orthosis.
- Often the anatomical surface that an orthosis encompasses is contoured. To optimize the force redistribution over a larger surface area, part of the force system of the orthosis should remain in complete contact with the respective anatomical surface, hence the term *total contact.*
- Conceptually, the shape of the interface of the orthosis should perfectly match the contours and form of the respective anatomical counterpart to be characterized as a total contact fitting device. To achieve this goal, custom-molded orthoses are fabricated from a mold of the patient's body segment that is being treated (see figure on p. 1034).

ORTHOT

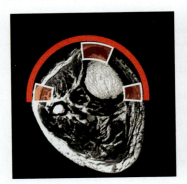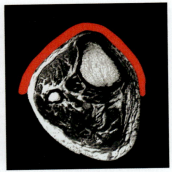

Total contact fit. Custom molded orthoses aim to achieve a total contact fit by having an orthotic interface that is shaped to the patient's anatomy. Theoretically, the goal is to create equal pressure between the orthotic interface and the patient, which may require altering the surface of the orthosis to accommodate for bony prominences.

- In practice, the shape of the interface of the orthosis may not contain the same contours as the shape of the patient's anatomy. Alterations to the shape of the orthosis may be performed by an orthotist to effectively transmit forces via the soft tissue lying superficial to the underlying skeleton (see figure above).
- *Example:* An orthotist may subtly alter the shape of the interface of an orthosis to create a relief for a bony prominence. With only a thin layer of subcutaneous tissue covering a bony prominence, pressures can be concentrated to the area, which may render the region intolerant to pressure and prone to skin breakdown compared to other areas that may contain underlying soft tissue and muscle (which may be pressure tolerant).
- Equalizing interface pressures is another factor associated with total contact principles in orthosis design.

Hydrostatic Pressure
- Uniform compression of soft-tissue in a rigid or semi-rigid cylindrical structure produces internal **hydrostatic pressure.**
- Hydrodynamic principles are used in the orthotic management of long bone fractures to maintain anatomical alignment and to distract fractured segments. As fracture healing progresses, the person wearing the orthosis is encouraged to return to functional tasks (i.e., weight-bearing activities); hence the term *functional fracture bracing* describes this method of treatment.

Intra-Abdominal/Intra-Cavity Pressure
- To lower static loading of the spine, the application of **intra-abdominal pressure** (sometimes known as **intra-cavitary pressure**) via abdominal supports, corsets, and bi-valved rigid shell devices may produce hydrostatic pressure within the abdominal cavity, and decompress intervertebral disc spaces of the lumbar spine.
- Muscle activity of the abdominals may be altered by the use of an orthosis that incorporates intra-abdominal pressure. Because of this, a plan of care that addresses exercise of muscles of the trunk and inferior spine may need

to be included in tandem with the patient's use of the orthosis as part of a treatment plan to address this potential effect.

- Excessive redundant tissue in the abdominal region due to obesity may restrict the effective use of intra-abdominal pressure in the design of spinal orthoses.

Formulating an Orthotic Prescription

Biomechanical Analysis Systems

To improve communication among the prescribing provider, rehabilitation specialists, and the orthotist, and to standardize the approach for orthotic prescription formulation, the American Academy of Orthopaedic Surgeons developed **biomechanical analysis systems** for the lower limb, upper limb, and spine. These systems incorporate the fundamental procedures by which an orthotist assesses and formulates a prescription recommendation for an orthosis as part of a treatment plan. The underlying principle behind the biomechanical analysis systems is to match the person's functional impairment with the biomechanical motion controls incorporated into an orthosis that targets the person's functional goals without disturbing normal function.

Each biomechanical system uses a **Technical Analysis Form** (see figure on pp. 1024–1027) as a guide to document the assessment, which methodically identifies the biomechanical variables and other parameters that are key to formulation of the orthotic prescription recommendation. Although the use of the technical analysis form may not always be practical in the clinical setting, all the elements included in the biomechanical assessment of a patient should be included when formulating a prescription for an orthosis. These systems are now adopted worldwide.

Methods Used in Biomechanical Analysis Systems

A four-step approach is used in biomechanical analysis systems to methodically determine an orthotic prescription. A summary of the Technical Analysis Form procedures follows:

- Describe the Functional Impairments
- Document Details of the Functional Deficits
- Establish Treatment Objectives
- Determine Orthotic Recommendation

Describe the Functional Impairments

An overview of a patient's functional limitations is described in relative detail, followed by a summary statement (see figure on p. 1024). According to McCullough and colleagues, "This summary is intended to be a concise analysis of the factors that are significant to producing functional impairment and for which orthotic biomechanical control is desirable."

Reference:

McCullough, NC III, Fryer, CM, and Glancy J: A new approach to patient analysis for orthotic prescription. Artif Limbs 14:68, 1970.

The categories considered for functional impairment include the following:

- Skeletal
- Sensation
- Skin

- Vascular
- Balance
- Gait Deviations
- Other Impairments

Examples: Summary of Functional Impairment
- *Lower limb example*: a person who displays inability to achieve left ankle and foot clearance during swing phase secondary to inadequate ankle dorsiflexion due to lumbar peripheral neuropathy.
- *Upper limb example*: a person who displays weak grasp of bilateral upper limbs secondary to progressive deformity due to rheumatoid arthritis.
- *Spinal example*: person with L4–L5 compression fractures and co-morbidities of osteoporosis and osteoarthritis.

Document Details of the Functional Deficits
In the Technical Analysis Form, the biomechanical assessment is depicted through figures of the neuromuscular and skeletal systems in each of the three cardinal planes of motion. The figures are intended to visually document the impairments of the body segment(s) (see figure on pp. 1025–1026).

Descriptive Functional Assessments
- Volitional force (i.e., manual muscle testing)
- Range of Motion
- Hypertonic muscle (i.e., rigidity, spasticity)
- Proprioception (i.e., normal, absent, impaired)
- Fractures

Establish Treatment Objectives
Treatment objectives for the three representative body regions (lower limb, upper limb, and spinal) vary considerably. However, examples of possible specific orthotic treatment objectives for each of these regions are listed below. When describing the orthotic treatment objective for a patient, there may be more than one objective applied (i.e., protect joint, fracture treatment, reduce axial load) (see figure on p. 1027).

- **Lower Limb**
  - Prevent/correct deformity
  - Reduce axial load
  - Protect joint
  - Improve ambulation
  - Fracture treatment
  - Other
- **Upper Limb**
  - Prevent/correct deformity
  - Improve function
  - Relieve pain
  - Other
- **Spinal**
  - Spinal alignment
  - Axial unloading
  - Motion control
  - Other

Determine Orthotic Recommendation

Description of Guidelines for an Orthotic Recommendation

- Describe joint(s) that the orthosis encompasses
- Describe motion control in the cardinal plane
- Utilize orthotic motion control mechanisms terminology

The Technical Analysis Form organizes the variables for an orthotic prescription recommendation through the use of a chart that assists in identifying the language in the orthotic prescription recommendation (see figure on p. 1027).

Joint motion control is described by the cardinal plane(s) of motion(s) (i.e., flexion and extension vs. abduction and adduction), using the seven orthotic control terms listed below that describe motion control with regard to function.

■ TABLE 16.1 Terms Used to Describe the Motion Control

Term	Description
Free	Free motion; motion that is unrestricted
Assist	Application of an external force for the purpose of increasing range, velocity, or force of a motion
Resist	Application of an external force for the purpose of decreasing range, velocity, or force of a motion
Stop	Inclusion of a static unit to deter an undesirable motion in one direction
Variable	A unit that can be adjusted without making a structural change
Hold	Elimination of motion in a prescribed plane (verify position)
Lock	The device includes an optional lock

Source: McCullough, NC III, Fryer, CM, and Glancy, J: A new approach to patient analysis for orthotic prescription. *Artif Limbs* 14:68, 1979.

Writing an Orthotic Prescription

A clear and concise prescription for an orthosis establishes the important details of the orthosis design required for the patient to achieve the desired functional outcomes. The following is an outline of the key features of the orthotic prescription:

- Patient name
- Date
- Diagnosis(es) and relevant ICD-9 diagnosis codes
- Body region and side(s) (Right, Left, or Bilateral)
- Descriptor of orthosis (i.e., AFO, WHO, TLSO)
- Describe whether the orthosis is custom molded or off the shelf
- Biomechanical motion control (i.e., free, assist, stop, hold)

ORTHOT

- Relevant reimbursement coding (i.e., HCPCS L-Codes)
- Signature of referring physician (including contact information)

The patient name and date are essential features of the orthotic prescription, particularly to establish the initial date of requested service. It is important to establish a documented reference date, particularly for patients with conditions who may undergo changes in their functional status (i.e., degenerative conditions).

Including diagnosis(es) and relevant ICD-9 diagnosis codes helps to clarify the type of pathological condition of the person to be treated with an orthosis. This information is also important for development of a fee for service because the diagnosis code(s) is/are required documentation.

The body region and side(s) of the orthosis relate important information regarding the targeted body region and the fee for service. The above-mentioned features represent only a starting point in defining the terminology of the orthotic prescription. Additional information is required to describe how the orthosis will address the patient's deficits.

The orthotic descriptor is critical in specifying the extent of the orthotic device to be created for the patient. The descriptor serves as the fundamental design of the orthosis for which biomechanical motion control features will be added.

The desired biomechanical motion control is one of the most important (yet least understood) features of the orthotic prescription. Besides the biomechanical motion controls, the objectives of orthotic treatment (i.e., to relieve pain, to manage deformities, to prevent excessive range of joint motion) must be clarified. Once the objectives of treatment are identified, then the functional requirements of the orthosis are defined (i.e. to prevent, reduce, or stabilize a deformity; to modify the range of motion of a joint).

A **Technical Analysis Form** was developed to assist the rehabilitation specialist in understanding and formulating accurate language that describes the desired biomechanical motion control(s) of the orthosis (see figures on pp. 1024–1027).

Relevant reimbursement coding is formulated as a fee for service involving an orthosis as part of a treatment plan. The fees, descriptors, and accompanying coding appear in a national database (U.S. Department of Health and Human Service Durable Medical Equipment, Prosthetics, Orthotics and Supplies [DMEPOS]), which may be accessed at http://www.cms.hhs.gov/DMEPOSFeeSched/01_overview.asp#TopOfPage).

The coding system is "device focused," whereby coding and fees for services focus on the orthotic device and component parts. There are limited reimbursement codes for other important patient services (i.e., education in care, use, and maintenance; dose response and habituation training; follow-up adjustments).

Orthosis Fit and Function Assessment Guidelines

General Objectives Related to Fit

- **Safety**
  - The orthosis should not harm the user.
  - An orthosis should not produce any irreversible side effects when worn by the patient over a long term or for an extended period of time.

- **Donning and Doffing**
  - Ideally, the patient should be able to don and doff his/her orthosis independently.
  - If a patient requires assistance in donning or doffing, the procedure should be relatively simple for the caregiver.
  - The method of securing the closures of the orthosis should be repeatable and consistent to always ensure a satisfactory fit.
- **Comfort and Skin Tolerance**
  - When an orthosis is removed, any noted discoloration to the patient's skin and soft tissue should dissipate after approximately 10 minutes to ensure that undue pressure or shear is not occurring due to wear or use.
  - Patients should be able to accommodate and tolerate the use of an orthosis well enough to meet the wear schedule of the treatment plan.
  - The orthosis should not create any skin and underlying soft tissue irritations.
  - In orthoses that encompass body segments (i.e., thermoplastic TLSO), heat retention may stress the wearer's thermoregulation capabilities, which may contribute to discomfort and reduced compliance. A common preventive measure is for the patient to use an interface barrier such as fabric stockinet, which acts as a wick to increase air flow while providing an additional benefit of reducing shear forces between the orthosis and the skin.
  - Normal and excessive perspiration that occurs with the use of an orthosis may increase the risk of skin problems related to harboring microorganisms at the skin surface (e.g., bacteria, fungi). A more frequent hygiene regimen may be needed to reduce the potential of trauma related to moist skin problems.
- **Cosmesis**
  - The appearance of the orthosis should be socially acceptable.
  - An orthosis should be as compact as possible and its shape should emulate that of the underlying anatomical shape and contour.
  - The orthosis should not be bulky or cumbersome.
  - The orthosis should not draw undue visual attention.
- **Surface Texture and Finish**
  - The final finish of the orthosis should be smooth with no rough edges and any anchors of the component parts such as rivets should be flush with the surface, particularly on the side that interfaces with the skin and underlying soft tissue.
- **Psychosocial Considerations**
  - Persons wearing orthoses for improved function and mobility should be encouraged to appreciate those benefits to their general well-being so that any psychosocial issues from using an orthosis may be of less concern by comparison.

General Objectives Related to Function

- **Prescription and Treatment Objectives**
  - The orthosis should meet the clinical objectives of the prescription.
  - Confirmation of treatment outcomes should be validated by clinically relevant tests and measures. For example, to confirm that an AFO prescribed

ORTHOT

for the treatment of weak ankle and foot dorsiflexion provides adequate toe clearance during swing phase and controlled plantar flexion during initial stance phase should be performed by observational gait analysis to assess whether the desired outcome is met.

- **Function During Activities of Daily Living**
  - Activities of daily living (ADL) should be maintained at their current level or should improve with the use of an orthosis, as opposed to interfering with functional activities.
  - Confirmation of ADL outcomes should be validated with clinically relevant tests and measures.

Specific Assessments for Lower Limb and Spinal Orthoses

- **Function During Standing**
  - The orthosis should permit double limb stance with no significant impact on normal standing posture. Consideration of the wearer's relative condition may influence what is acceptable standing function (e.g., a user with a moderate knee flexion contracture may not be able to achieve normal terminal knee extension during standing).
  - A balanced stable standing posture for the wearer should be a fundamental functional objective of the orthosis design that aims to maintain normal skeletal alignment of the person's head, trunk, spine, and the limbs.
  - In some instances, standing with the use of an orthosis may require the use of a walking aid (e.g., walker) for safety and stability. However, the healthcare professional must determine that a poorly designed orthosis is not the factor requiring the use of the walking aid.
- **Function During Sitting**
  - A patient should be able to achieve a stable and balanced sitting posture for everyday tasks.
  - The orthosis should not impede the patient's ability to independently stand and sit in an armchair. To achieve this objective, flexion of the trunk, hip, and knee as well as ankle dorsiflexion are required.
  - The minimal alignment requirements of the lower limb for the seated position are that the hip, knee, and ankle be positioned at 90 degrees, respectively.
  - Patients should be able to achieve adequate foot placement and foot/ankle position to rise and sit in an armchair.
- **Function During Walking**
  - Perturbations from an orthosis should be minimized so that an optimal walking pattern can be attained.
  - The biomechanical controls (i.e., assist, resist) incorporated in an orthosis should make a significant improvement to the patient's walking capabilities compared to their respective pathological gait condition with regard to walking speed, step length, and energy expenditure.

Reference

Committee on Prosthetics Research and Development Report of the Seventh Workshop Panel on Lower Extremity Orthosis of the Subcommittee on Design and Development, National Research Council–National Academy of Sciences, March 1970.

ORTHOT

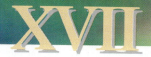
WHEELCHAIR ASSESSMENT AND PRESCRIPTION

Wheelchair selection is best performed by a client-centered team. The *seating clinic* has evolved in present-day rehabilitation facilities and hospitals as a service to both inpatients and outpatients. An individual and his/her family/caregiver can network with a therapist, a qualified rehabilitation technology supplier (RTS), the physician, and other clinicians in a clinic setting dedicated to providing assessments for wheelchair and seating equipment and sometimes other assistive technology devices. The clinic is typically set up with evaluation tools, a mat table, demonstration equipment, samples, equipment catalogs, and other resources. Trial and simulation of demonstration equipment and samples are excellent tools to determine the potential outcome(s) of a prescribed piece of equipment. Proper education in the use of the device is essential and follow-up is arranged for fitting and delivery. People of all ages with various disabilities (e.g., spinal cord injury, spina bifida, cerebral palsy, muscular dystrophy, CVA, traumatic brain injury, multiple sclerosis, amyotrophic lateral sclerosis, post–polio syndrome, burn injuries, osteogenesis imperfecta) can be served.

Goals of a Wheelchair/Seating Assessment

1. *Improved function:* Maximization of the client's learning potential or independence in mobility related activities of daily living (MRADL). Must be specific on letters of medical necessity. How does the equipment improve transfer ability, dressing, toileting, bathing, meal preparation, eating, computer access, driving, work access, and so on?
2. *Comfort:* Improved sitting tolerance (preferred terminology for medical reviewers), documented in hours.
3. *Physiological optimization:* To diminish the progression of deformity, correct deformity, reduce sitting pressures, improve skin integrity, improve sitting balance, normalize muscle tone, decrease influence of abnormal reflex patterns, improve pulmonary hygiene, prevent injury or trauma, and conserve energy.
4. *Cosmetic:* Will the client accept the device(s)? It has to be a mutually agreed-on piece of equipment by all parties involved.
5. *Durability:* Frequent maintenance and repairs are costly and time consuming, and prevent the client from living the benefits of the mobility and seating system.
6. *Financial sensitivity:* Will the equipment meet insurance guidelines? Education is provided in potential insurance coverage and other resources available. A letter of medical necessity is typically generated by the therapist. It should clearly reflect the thought processes behind the evaluation and the recommendations generated. The letter must describe why each feature is needed based on a specific goal. The insurance provider wants to know that each item is the least costly alternative.

Wheelchair Seating and Positioning Assessment

Assessment Elements

- Medical/surgical history
- Home environment: House or apartment; alone or with family/caregivers; accessibility; ramp entry? Narrowest doorway.

- Mode of transportation; ability to drive.
- Community activities and access; school, work.
- Cognitive/visual status.
- ADL status: Dressing, bathing, feeding, grooming, toileting, meal prep.
- Bowel/bladder status.
- Mobility skills: Transfers; gait (functional vs. nonfunctional); manual wheelchair propulsion; power wheelchair propulsion/mode of control; ability to perform weight shifts; hours in wheelchair per day?

Current Equipment. Define the advantages and disadvantages of the current equipment. Determine the need to change to another system. If the equipment works for the client, determine parts of the system that require change. If the client has a changing condition, determine changes that need to accommodate potential deterioration in the future without interfering with the client's current functional capacity.

1. Type of wheelchair and set up, back, and cushion: Age and condition; can it be repaired/modified?
2. Client's posture and stability in system.
3. Check for "bottoming out" on current cushion.
4. Pressure mapping if technology is available.
5. Ability/frequency of weight shifts/pressure relief.
6. Propulsion skills and movement patterns.
7. Transfer technique.
8. Accessibility to home and mode of transportation.

Clinical Criteria/Algorithm Summary. Criteria that serve as the basis for current reimbursement standards for mobility assistive equipment under Medicare and followed by many insurance carriers.

> *Reference:*
> *http://www.cms.hhs.gov/mcd/viewncd.asp?ncd_id=280.3&ncd_version=2&basket=ncd%3A280%2E3%3A2%3AMobility+Assistive+Equipment+%28MAE%29.*

Mat Table Evaluation

Passive ROM Supine. Pelvis, trunk, extremities. Hamstring/flexion test performed to determine influence of hamstrings on pelvic flexibility. Determine the maximum hip flexion angle (may be different left to right) in a gravity-eliminated position before the pelvis begins to rock into a posterior pelvic tilt by placing your hands on the ASIS. The therapists' thigh supports the knee at the angle likely to be placed on the wheelchair footrests (60, 70, 80, 90 degrees or more) (see figure on following page).

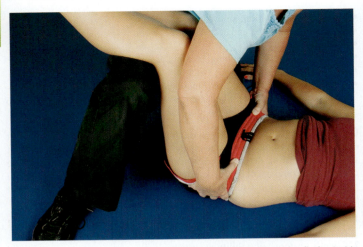

Hand placement for assessment of pelvic and trunk flexibility. Hamstring flexion test to determine flexibility of the hip joints without pelvic rotation. This is done with the knees in the position likely to be supported on the wheelchair footrest.

Spinal/pelvic deformities (noted in supine and then sitting). Note what degree of deformity is fixed vs. flexible.

i. Spinal alignment in sagittal plane: Pelvic tilt. Passively move the pelvis posterior to anterior. Can you create a lumbar curve with anterior tilt of the pelvis? Is there an excessive lordosis? Does the curve flatten in supine position or with movement of the pelvis posteriorly? Upper thoracic area: Does the client's head rest in a neutral position without pillows? If the individual requires multiple pillows, the kyphosis is likely fixed. Note the degree of flexibility of all areas.

ii. Spinal alignment in the frontal plane: Does the spine and/or pelvis neutralize laterally in the gravity-eliminated position? How much effort does it take the therapist to hold the spine in the neutral position? What does correction do to the pelvis? What does correction of the pelvis do to the position of the trunk?

iii. Alignment in the transverse plane: Does your passive motion of the legs correct rotation of the pelvis and/or a windswept deformity? Does this action cause the trunk to rotate?

iv. Muscle tone and abnormal reflex patterns are noted in supine.

Posture and flexibility in sitting. How does gravity contribute to a postural abnormality? Is the postural abnormality caused by a fixed deformity (determined in supine position), high vs. low muscle tone? If abnormal tone is noted in supine, this should be reassessed and noted in sitting. Determine hip-to-back angle. Determine seat angle by altering the position of the thighs with blocks or a lift under the feet.

i. Test the pelvis, hips, knees, trunk/head position, and flexibility in sitting as was done in supine (see figure on p. 1045). The therapist can sit posterior to the client, supporting the pelvis and trunk in the desired posture. Can the client sit in a perfect anatomical position without manual support? Can the client sit comfortably with the knees extended to −70 degrees (common swing-away footrest position)? Rx: Minimal back support such as reg. upholstery; adjustable tension upholstery; 70-degree footrests. Or see the figure below.

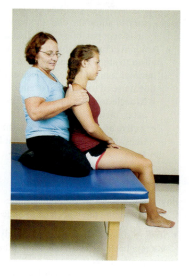

Determine the hip-to-back angle that results in a neutral pelvic tilt (supported) and a position of least resistance. The client may be able to identify the hip-to-back angle that is comfortable for a relaxed but functional posture. Correction of postural abnormalities are done with the therapists' body or hands where needed.

ii. Corrective forces can be applied to the client by using the muscles of the clinician's arms and hands to change both direction and magnitude of the applied force. The therapist's hands then have to translate into a seating system that provides accommodation and/or correction of the postural problems. Picture the seating components that take the place of the clinician's hands.

What corrective forces are needed to allow the client to relax in a seated position without constant effort?

a) *Sagittal plane corrects:* Open the hip-to-back angle to allow the client to relax and sit more symmetrically. Does an open hip-to-back angle accommodate and/or correct a shortened hamstring or a kyphosis? Does an open hip-to-back angle place the client's line of vision more horizontal? Is muscle tone more normal? (Potential Rx: 70-degree footrests with angled back. Adjustable back canes; adjustable back hardware; adjustable tension back upholstery with client positioned between the back canes.) Note the degree of back angle needed. Alternately, accommodate shortened hamstring, placing feet under the mat table. Does this allow the pelvis to reach a more neutral position? Note angle of knee. Rx: 90-degree footrests with more upright back.

b) *Frontal plane corrections:* Does it help to position the *pelvis oblique* (use your hands or a foam pad under one ischium) to correct a scoliosis or improve line of vision? (Potential Rx: Cushion that will accommodate asymmetric pelvic height: Gel cushions, air cushions with bilateral valves; wedges inserted in symmetric cushion, accommodating fixed pelvis, correcting flexible pelvis.) Lateral trunk or pelvic support required? Note degree. (Potential Rx: Lateral trunk support in contoured system vs. modular system vs. custom molded system or combination.)

c) *Transverse plane corrections:* What corrective forces are needed to achieve a horizontal line of vision, face forward position? It may be necessary to allow the client to rotate either at the trunk, pelvis, and/or legs (windswept position). The clinician must decide in the case of a fixed rotational deformity that it is best not to correct one part of the body in an effort to align the head forward or to place the upper body in a position of optimal function (e.g., for communication, enhanced swallowing, functional use of the upper extremities).

- **Muscle tone:** Abnormal reflex patterns are noted throughout the mat assessment.
- **Active muscle control/strength:** Head control; trunk control; extremities.
- **Sensation and skin condition:** Note areas and size of skin breakdown.
- **Pain:** Location and degree.

Simulation

Position the client in simulator frame or sample wheelchair frame of choice. (See determining the wheelchair frame.)

- *Seating simulators:* These are highly adjustable frames with respect to the seat and back surfaces (including tilt and recline) as well as the postural support components.
- *Sample wheelchair:* Higher functioning clients, who do not have significant postural compromise, are not as likely to need to go through the step of using an actual seating simulator.
  - It would be impossible to have every wheelchair frame and seating system to determine a prescription but one can have a select supply of wheelchair frames, seat backs, cushions, and other supplies to simulate the outcome.
  - The equipment supplier and/or local manufacturer's representative can supply other demonstration equipment for trial after the initial evaluation. The equipment can be tried in the client's environment. Sometimes this is a requirement of the third-party funding source.

Body Measurements. Take these measurements either during your sitting mat assessment or in your trial/simulation equipment (see figure on following page).

Patient _____Height (inches): _____Weight (lbs): _____

Body measurements (inches)

  A. Hip width: _____

  B. Thigh length: R_____ L _____

  C. Leg length: R_____ L _____

  D1. Foot length: R_____ L _____

  E. Lower scapula
     height: R_____ L _____

  F. Height to top
     of scapula: R_____ L _____

  G. Shoulder width: _____

  H. Height to top
     of head: _____

  I. Forearm height: R_____ L _____

  J. Chest width: _____

  K. Chest depth: _____

  L. Forearm length: R_____ L _____

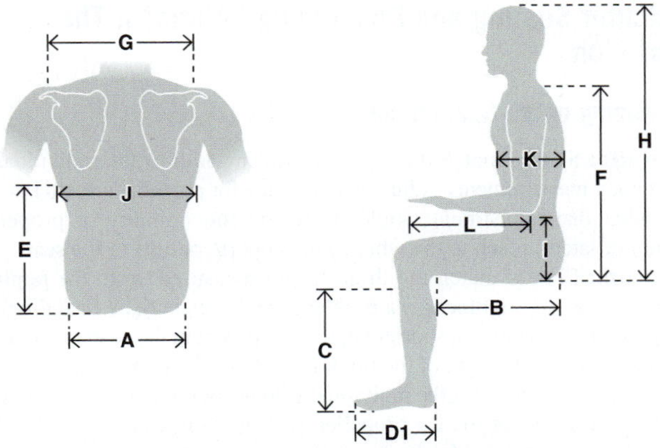

Body measurements taken in sitting. The combination of A and J is sometimes necessary when scoliosis is present. Note client's height and weight for letter of medical necessity.

Angle Measurements. Determined during your mat assessment and simulation and noted in your assessment or final prescription (see figure on the following page).

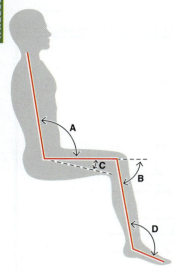

Note angular measurements. (A) Hip-to-back angle. (B) Knee angle (usually measured as the degree of knee flexion from the horizontal). (C) Seat plane angle (usually measured as the height of the rear of the seat compared to the height of the front of the seat). (D) Footrest angle (noted as either a neutral ankle or degree of dorsiflexion vs. plantarflexion).

Wheelchair Seating and Positioning Solutions: The Prescription

Proper Sizing of the Seat Frame

- **Seat width:** Should match the hip or shoulder width of the individual (or widest body measurement). Adjustment is made for potential growth but consider what that adjustment would do to the functionality of propelling (amount of lateral reach to the wheels) or support/comfort of the seat.

- **Seat depth:** Should match the thigh length measured up to the popliteal space. If hamstring tightness is a problem, the knees may be flexed beyond 90 degrees, necessitating a shorter depth or undercut in the seat/cushion. Approximating the full length of the thigh is essential for comfort and pressure relief. The exception is for the individual who is not going to be a permanent wheelchair user or for the leg propeller. At least 2-in. clearance behind the popliteal space is needed for foot propellers.

- **Back height:** The proper back height is determined by personal preference based on injury level, sensory level, balance, functional ability, skill, and chair usage. Generally, the higher the level of injury (as in spinal cord injury), the higher the backrest height that is needed for balance and stability. For optimal propulsion and mobility in a manual wheelchair, the height of the back should be below the inferior angles of the scapula by 0.5 in. Consider the trade-off between comfort (high back support) and increased mobility or functional reach (low back height).

- **Footplate adjustment (lower leg length):** The length of the client's lower leg should match the distance from the top of the cushion to the footplate.

With a few exceptions, the footrest adjustment affects thigh support throughout the distance from the buttocks to the popliteal fossa. A proper adjustment of both the seat depth and footplate height is essential for pressure distribution, comfort, stability, muscle tone management, and safety.

- **Back angle:** This angle is determined during the mat assessment based on flexibility and balance. Accommodates clients who cannot tolerate 90-degree upright sitting due to flexibility restrictions in the hips or hamstrings. Could be used to accommodate a kyphosis or for weakness in trunk musculature/poor sitting balance. Angle adjustment can be achieved by adjusting the wheelchair frame hardware and/or the solid back hardware. (See figures on pp. 1055 and 1062.)

> *From:*
>
> *Quickie Design: The Perfect Fit: An Adjustments Guide to Your Manual Wheelchair. Brochure copywrited by Quickie Designs, Inc., 1990.*

- Recliners allow for full adjustment of the back angle from approximately 90 degrees upright to 160 degrees (varies by model and manufacturer).

Selecting a Seating System.   The therapist's primary responsibility is to have a working knowledge of the principles of human biomechanics, normal and abnormal human growth and development, and neurophysiology. The same principles apply in seating and positioning. Additionally, knowledge of the constantly changing products on the market is advantageous to make the process an interchange of ideas with the client and the supplier. The equipment supplier should have some knowledge of biomechanics, human development, and neurophysiology as well. They should be able to supply all of the wheelchair and seating products on the market and be the primary resource for exploring what the industry has to offer based on the client's needs. The industry has made strides to make the assessment and prescription of complex rehabilitation equipment a specialty area, separate from the durable medical equipment (DME) industry because the provision of seating and mobility equipment serves individuals with the most complex of disabilities, physiological, and functional deficits.

Biomechanics of Seating

Corrective forces must be applied to simply support a midline position or often needed to change both the direction and magnitude of abnormal spinal curves and postures. A therapist's hands can change both direction and magnitude of applied forces. Conversely, a seating system is a static device with limitations in the direction and magnitude of forces that can be applied. This is done in such a manner to improve posture and alignment while compromises are made to maintain or improve function. One cannot expect to correct a deformity or contracture in the seated position that is not correctable in supine.

- **Controlling movement around a joint:** To control a joint, a point of control must be used on both sides of the joint. To do this, three forces must be applied to the body. Two points of control immobilize one side of the joint while a third controls the other side (see figure on following page).

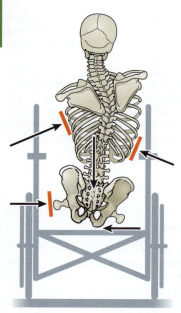

Three-point pressure system for exerting corrective forces in scoliosis. Because the ribs slope inferiorly and because the pads exert pressure through the ribs, which project from the vertebral bodies forming the lateral curvature, placement of the pads should be somewhat inferior to the curve.

From:

Nwaobi, OM: Biomechanics of seating. In Trefler, E (ed): Seating for Children With Cerebral Palsy—A Resource Manual. University of Tennessee Center for the Health Sciences, Memphis, TN, 1984.

- **Pressure distribution:** Pressure is a function of the force and surface area. The greater the surface area, the more widespread will be the force, reducing pressure in any one area. This applies especially in the size and selection of the seat cushion. A contoured seat cushion properly sized will therefore result in reduced seat pressures in any given area over a flat, noncontoured cushion.

- **Shape of forces:** For a controlling force to work effectively, it must be comfortable and promote or enhance function while being aesthetically acceptable to the user. This requires a balance between the shape and size of the seating components. An off-the-shelf, contoured back, for example, may provide more comfort given the increased contact area provided by the lateral support but may not have enough force in any given area for correction of deformity or to improve balance/function in the seat. Angular surfaces (straight lines) tend to hold the body better than do curved surfaces. Surfaces that are curved to match the body contour will allow the body to slip or ride up, whereas angular surfaces tend to distort the soft tissue and provide for more control of unwanted movement. There must therefore be a balance between control and pressure.

- **Firmness:** Firm supports generally hold the posture of the user better than soft supports. The trick is to achieve a balance between the stability offered by a firm surface and the comfort of the user.

- **Balance and base of support:** In a situation in which the base of support remains constant, lowering the center of gravity increases stability. Any change in body structure (e.g., amputation or spinal deformity) will affect the location of the center of gravity. To maintain stability of the body, the center of gravity must remain over the base of support. In cases in which the client has lost a great deal of trunk control, the wheelchair becomes the base of support and the use of an angled back or recliner will be necessary to use gravity to assist with balance and postural control. The combination of back angle and seat angle is important to determining the client's optimal position and angle in space and in relation to the wheelchair frame/base of support.

> *Modified from:*
> Invacare: *Biomechanics of Seating: Avanti Seating and Positioning Products.* Brochure distributed by Invacare Corp., Elyria, OH.

Human Development and Neurophysiological Principles

- **Reducing the influence of primitive reflexes:** The abnormal synergistic movement patterns commonly seen in neurological disorders are the result of the persistence of primitive reflexes. When seating an individual, an attempt is made to position him/her in a reflex-inhibiting posture. For example, a dominant asymmetrical tonic neck reflex (ATNR) makes it difficult for the client to hold his/her trunk and head in midline, prevents use of both hands together, and contributes to a scoliosis. The seating system must therefore provide lateral support at the head and trunk to inhibit the ATNR.
- **Normalizing postural muscle tone:** Individuals who exhibit hypertonia need to be positioned so that postural tone is decreased and normal movement patterns are facilitated. Those who exhibit hypotonia require appropriate support and use of various gravity-assisting positions to compensate for inadequate postural tone.
- **Controlling abnormal movement patterns:** Positioning an individual in a reflex-inhibiting posture that also effectively reduces excessive postural muscle tone will assist in controlling abnormal movement patterns.
- **Promoting normal neuromotor development:** If the above three objectives are achieved, the individual will have a better opportunity to develop his/her motor skills. Maintenance of a symmetrical upright posture will also facilitate the development of righting responses. In this regard, be careful not to provide so much symmetrical support that you inhibit normal activities such as crossing midline, normal weight-bearing through the pelvis and feet, and weight shifting over the base of support either forward or laterally.
- **Prevent the development and/or progression of deformity or correct deformity:** An individual who remains in an unmodified abnormal or asymmetrical posture for a long period of time will almost certainly develop skeletal deformities. A properly fitted seating system may be unable to totally prevent such deformity but it is generally thought that progression of the deformity may be slowed and/or controlled by such a system. Modified seating may also be used to maintain postural alignment following corrective surgical procedures.
- **Functional considerations:**
  - Improved head control: With appropriate trunk, shoulder, and head/neck support if required, an individual will experience increased stability for

communicating more readily, to participate in educational activities more easily, to be more independent in activities of daily living (ADL) such as feeding, and to improve social interaction.

- Improved upper extremity function: By stabilizing the pelvis, trunk, and shoulder girdle if necessary, upper extremity function is improved. The hands are not required for balance or support and are free to perform other activities. The result may be increased independence in ADL; increased ability to use communication devices, computers, or other equipment; and an increased ability to maneuver the wheelchair.

- Ease of nursing care: Improved posture and prevention of deformity will make caring for the severely involved neurologically impaired client easier. Any increase in independence in ADL reduces the burden of care on these individuals. Transfers can be made easier with proper positioning; there is less frequent need for repositioning in the chair; and basic care such as bathing and hygiene is improved.

- Improved cardiorespiratory function: Vital capacity, diaphragmatic excursion, and gas exchange are all improved when an individual is properly positioned in a seating system.

Modified from:

Bergen, AF, Presperin, J, and Tallman, T: Positioning for Function. Valhalla Rehabilitation Publications, 1990.

An introduction to seating and the disabled person. Paper presented at the Third International Seating Symposium–Seating the Disabled. University of Tennessee, Memphis, TN, February 26–28, 1987.

Clinical Standards of Positioning and Pressure Management

- The *pelvis* is the key to postural alignment as it dictates the position of the trunk, head, and extremities. Correction of the client's sitting posture begins with stabilization of the pelvis, which will influence all other parts of the body. The optimal hip angle for any given individual influences pelvic position and is an integral part of stabilizing the pelvis.

- *Flexible deformities* should be corrected and supported within the client's tolerance and ability to function.

- *Fixed deformities* should be accommodated and supported to prevent further progression and to distribute pressure evenly.

- Proximal support and stability will improve distal function.

- Pressure is not the only cause of decubitus ulcers. Consider the client's nutritional status, moisture control, and size and location of sores. (The seating system is often not the cause of an ulcer.) Heat and moisture may be trapped by cushion materials that contour the body.

- Cushion immersion or contouring of bony prominences will reduce peak pressure and improve pressure distribution.

- Cushion materials are a consideration in controlling shear; alternately, they may allow the client to move easier. There needs to be a compromise between stability and function.

- Sitting tolerance must be established and alternative positioning options provided. If a client is unable to perform an independent weight shift, a mechanical weight shift can be provided through manual or power tilt and/or recline.

Seating Products

- **Seats and backs:** Seat cushions and backs are available in planar and contoured designs, either off the shelf or custom measured by the therapist and supplier.
  - **Planar systems:** Flat seats and backs were used more frequently in the past, especially for control of clients with severe extensor thrust. Our bodies are not flat and therefore the industry is making more and more products designed to conform to normal curves. A flat cushion is preferable when the client needs to be able to slide forward and back on the seat or when a sliding board or lateral transfer is performed. Planar systems allow for growth adjustment (see figure below).

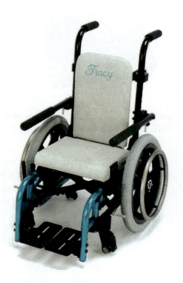

Planar seating system. *Compliments of: Freedom Designs, Inc., http://www. freedomdesigns.com/images/wheel- chair%20Gallery.html.*

  - **Contoured systems:** Off-the-shelf contoured systems are available for those who do not have severe deformities. Minimal to maximal contouring seats and backs are available to facilitate an even distribution of pressure and therefore are usually more comfortable to the user (see figure on the following page). The degree of deformity that must be accommodated dictates whether an off-the-shelf system will work. The therapist might try a contoured system with or without added supports and find that the contact of the system is inadequate with off-the-shelf systems. There is a liquid foam available on the market (foam in place) that would allow the combination of an off-the-shelf product with a custom molding method. Consider that contoured systems do not allow for a significant amount of growth.

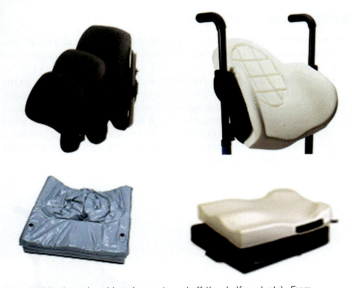

Contoured backs and cushions (precontoured off-the-shelf products). *From: http://www.sunrisemedical.com*.

- **Full custom systems** require the use of a seat simulator that allows the therapist and supplier to make a mold of the client's body contours either mechanically or via computerized tomography. Growth accommodation is even more of an issue with these fully contoured systems (see figure below).

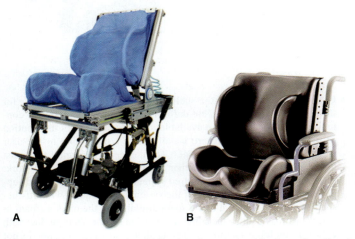

Custom-contoured seating system. (A) Simulator frame and molding bags. *Compliments of: Prairie Seating Corp.* (B) End product made by the manufacturer from a mold (Contour U by Invacare).

- **Back hardware:** If the seat frame of the wheelchair does not allow for back angle adjustment, off-the-shelf and custom systems offer different degrees of back angle adjustment, which is essential to pelvic and trunk stabilization. Most office chairs and standard furniture are designed with a 95-degree or more open hip-to-back angle. Hamstring tightness alone can cause posterior pelvic tilt in the general population. The mat evaluation will allow therapists to determine the angle of choice for any given individual. Some muscular dystrophy clients often assume a more acute hip-to-back angle for functional control of sitting balance with declining muscle power (see figure below).

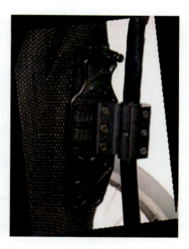

Angle and depth adjustable back hardware by Motion Concepts, Inc.

- **Materials:** Foams, fluids/gels, air floatation, combination foam/air, combination foam/gel, honeycomb. Cushion immersion or contouring of bony prominences will reduce peak pressures. Cushion materials that reduce shear may allow for pelvic movement and compromise stability. Conversely, some clients may be able to function better if they can slide along the surface of the cushion during transfers. Heat and moisture are other considerations. Foams and honeycomb cushions allow for air to circulate. Often the cushion covers will be designed to improve air circulation or wick away moisture. The weight of the cushion can be an important factor when prescribing an ultralight chair. Experience with various products on the market is helpful in making cushion choices.

Modified from:

Levy, B: Clinical uses of seating and positioning products. Paper Presented at MEDTRADE, November 19, 1998.

- **Pressure relief activities:** Clients are expected to move frequently in the wheelchair to maintain skin integrity. It is recommended that weight shifts, forward leaning or side-to-side, be performed every 10 to 20 minutes for duration of at least 3 seconds. The use of manual or power tilt and/or recline systems are said to require at least 45 degrees of tilt or recline to be effective in relief of seat pressure.

- **Pressure mapping:** A pressure measurement system available in most wheel-chair or seating clinics. Multiple-sensor, computerized systems are the most valuable. The input is a map either for a seat, back, or mattress composed of an array of sensors that interfaces with a computer. It is most commonly used in the selection of a seat cushion. It measures the interface pressures between the cushion and the client's buttocks/pelvis. The clinician can determine the ability of potential cushions to distribute pressure. Absolute pressure values are not important but the distribution of pressures on any given surface gives the clinician information on the potential benefits of one cushion over another. It is used to show evidence of asymmetry in sitting and what influence changing the seat-to-back angle or orientation in space may have. In this regard, it is an excellent evaluation and educational tool with which to teach the client weight-shifting techniques (see the following figures).

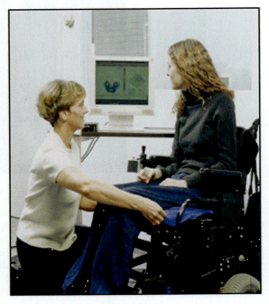

FSA pressure mapping system by Vista Medical.

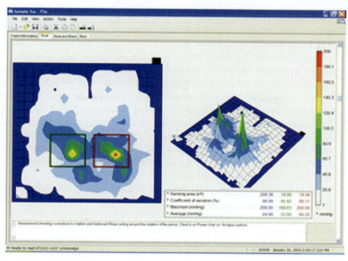

Cont'd from previous page

- **Postural supports**
  - **Adductor pads and thigh supports:** The hips are typically aligned in 0 to 5 degrees of abduction. An adductor pad or thigh support is necessary when the client is apt to abduct excessively, which typically places pressure areas on the outside of the legs. Flip-down or removable hardware is available for side transfers.
  - **Abductor pads or pummels:** Some seats are molded and contoured so that the abduction pummel (or adductor) is built into the cushion. Used to inhibit extensor and adductor muscle tone or posture. They often interfere with the use of a urinal in the chair. Flip-down hardware can assist with toileting and transfers.
  - **Calf pads:** Calf pads, straps, or panels are used to prevent the client's legs from flexing behind the footrests either due to abnormal flexor tone, postural reactions, gravity (as in the case of tilt or recline), and/or poor sensation. This reduces the risk for skin breakdown due to interference of the legs/feet with the footrests, casters, or other parts of the chair.
  - **Foot supports:** Foot or ankle straps or shoe holders are used most often when there is excess flexor or extensor muscle tone and the potential for injury to the feet. This often has to be at the discretion of the client or caregiver, as this should not interfere with functional movement and normal weight-bearing and development. Clients with athetosis often prefer to have their feet stabilized.
  - **Lateral trunk supports:** Curved or flat. Consider placement (where does the pad need to be placed in relation to the seat and back?), size, and hardware. (See figure on p. 1050.)

- **Chest supports and harnesses:** Various types of harnesses and chest pads can provide thoracic support anteriorly. These are used when the client is at risk to pull or fall into flexion at the trunk or hips. Some clients use them only for transport in a van or bus.
- **Upper extremity supports:** Armrests should be of an appropriate height. Adjustable height armrests are typically an option on most wheelchairs. Some arm pads are made with forward-back or medial-lateral adjustments for optimal placement. Accurate adjustment of the arm pads is important for propelling or optimal functional use of the client's upper extremities. Arm pads come in a variety of sizes and materials. The wider arm pads allow for control of arm positioning when the client does not have anti-gravity control. Arm troughs may be necessary for the client with severe hypotonia, quadriplegia, or athetosis.
- **Head supports:** The position of the pelvis and backrest influences head position and therefore should be adjusted before any adjustments or modifications are made to the headrest. An open hip-to-back angle will allow for adequate rest of the head, otherwise the client's head will fall forward. Head supports are made in a large variety of sizes and shape. The hardware associated with the head support is just as critical for accurate head positioning of more severely involved clients, as optimal support is usually multidirectional. Some manufacturers offer headrests with multiple component pads to shape and form the headrest for multidirectional control. A client with a dominant ATNR, for example, will need asymmetrical forces applied to the head to maintain midline and can be achieved with pads and hardware shaped to match the forces determined in your evaluation. Neutral head positioning for clients with neck and head flexion that is associated with or without abnormal muscle tone is difficult to achieve. Placement of an anterior headband across the forehead is sometimes acceptable. A separate cervical collar may be needed to provide support in the chair but can also provide support during transfers. (Note postural supports in figure on p. 1061.)

Considerations for Wheelchair Base Selection

- User's ability: Is the client able to self-propel a manual wheelchair, or is powered mobility the only option?
- Future potential including abilities, growth, weight loss, change in environment, change in caregiver.
- Disease progression.
- Accessibility to the client's home, community, school, or work environment. Access through hallways, clearance under tables and desks.
- Transportation.
- Insurance; cost.

Standard Wheelchair Frames

Typical frames available from a standard DME supplier: The supplier generally sends out what they have in stock. Unless the prescription is specific, you get what happens to be in the supplier's inventory based on the user's height and weight.

1. Standard frames: Likely made of chrome or steel (see figure A below)
   - Typically 18 in. × 16 in. or 16 in. × 16 in. seat dimensions.
   - 20-in. or greater widths are available with varying depths.
   - Available with or without removable or height-adjustable arms and swing-away footrests.
   - Transport wheelchairs (see figure B below): Same dimensions with small, 8 in. or 12 in. rear wheels designed for pushing by a caregiver or in some cases foot propelling. Lightest weight, less durable.
   - Recliners: Semi- or full-reclining wheelchairs (see figure C below).

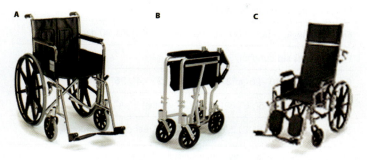

Standard wheelchair frames. *Compliments of: Sunrise Medical.*

2. Lightweight frames: Made of aluminum (similar in appearance to figure on p. 1060 without axle plate).
   - 18 in. × 16 in. or 16 in. × 16 in. with wider widths and depths sometimes available on request (depends on the inventory of the DME provider).
   - Axle adjustment is minimal (1-in. height adjustment; no center of gravity adjustment).

Custom Manual/Ultralight Wheelchair Frames

Custom manual wheelchair frames evolved from the standard options of the 1970s and earlier.

The equipment supplier should be qualified to provide custom, rehabilitation/specialty equipment.

Lightweight and ultralight folding or rigid frames: Generally made of aluminum or titanium. Available in all sizes/dimensions (10-in. to 22-in. widths; 7-in. to 22–in. depths).

TABLE 17.1 **Custom Wheelchair Options**

Options: (++) Folding frames, Rigid frames
Axle adjustability optional std
Back angle adjustable optional std
Quick release axles optional std
Footrest hangers swing-away or rigid mostly rigid*
Elevating/artic. legrests optional no*
Front end angle (knee <) 60; 70; 90 (can be rigid) 70–90 degrees
Push handles std optional
Rear wheel size 20″–26″ in 2″ increments 22″, 24″, 26″
Front caster size 3″, 5″, 6″, 8″ (std or 1/5″ widths) 3″, 4″, 5″ (std or 1.5″ W)
Seat heights Front 15″–21.5″ Rear 14″–21.5″ rear can be lower

++ Sizes and specifications vary from manufacturer and model.
* Some manufacturers offer a rigid chair with swing-away front end.

folding frames: Cross-brace allows the chair to fold in the middle. Folding frames are easier for user or caregiver to load into car from a standing position. Slightly heavier and less mechanically efficient than rigid frames due to the increase in moving parts (see figure at right).

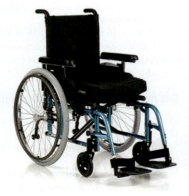

Folding ultralight weight frame (Quickie 2 by Sunrise Medical).

rigid frames: More efficient, generally lighter frames as all the energy that is applied to the wheels goes into propulsion. Usually more compact and have tighter turning radius. Rigid frames are easier for user to load into a car from a sitting position. (The chair is usually brought across the lap of the user and placed either in the front passenger seat or back seat.) Most wheelchairs used for sports are typically rigid but they are also used for everyday mobility and function (see figure at right).

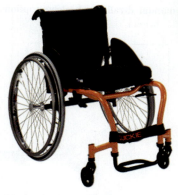

Rigid frame ultralight wheelchair (Quickie GT by Sunrise Medical).

manual tilt-in-space frames: Can be for self-propelling but most often selected for dependent clients who require tilt-in-space feature for pressure-relieving weight shifts, for postural control, or for energy conservation/rest. Although there are exceptions, most tilt-in-space frames do not fold (see figure at right).

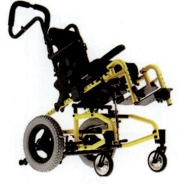

Tilt-in-space frame with planar seating system. *Compliments of Invacare Corp.*

manual ultralight wheelchair options and sizing considerations: (see figure below)

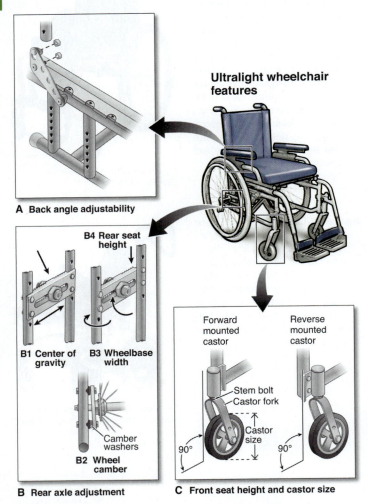

Ultralight wheelchair features

A Back angle adjustability

B4 Rear seat height

B1 Center of gravity **B3 Wheelbase width**

Camber washers

B2 Wheel camber

B Rear axle adjustment

Forward mounted castor

Reverse mounted castor

Stem bolt
Castor fork
Castor size
90° 90°

C Front seat height and castor size

Ultralight wheelchair features and adjustments. (A) Back angle. (B) Rear axle adjustments (B1, center of gravity; B2, wheel camber; B3, wheelbase width; B4, rear seat height). (C) Front seat height and caster size.

optimum pushing position (manual wheelchair): Optimal propulsion is achieved with up to four adjustments: Backrest angle, axle position, seat height and angle (the relationship between front and rear seat height).

- **back angle adjustability:** Not available on all chairs, it is available on most rigid frame models, tilt-in-space chairs, and optional on some folding frame wheelchairs. Back angle adjustment usually allows for angles from 85 degrees to 120 degrees, usually specified by the manufacturer.

- **axle position:** An axle adjustable chair places the wheelchair into an ultra-lightweight category (from reimbursement standards). Center of gravity, wheel camber, wheel base width, and rear seat height are all determined by the axle position:

  - **center of gravity:** More customized frames have anterior adjustability for improving the efficiency of push on the wheel. Center of gravity is determined by a combination of how high a body mass is off the ground and how far weight is distributed from front to back in a chair. Adjustment of the center of gravity is based on the user's balance and skill in varying environments. Moving the center of gravity to the front will lighten the force required to push and turn the chair. The lighter the front end, the less weight there will be on the front caster wheels. By having less weight distributed to the casters, the wheels are less likely to "plow" into the ground, making it easier to stroke the rear wheels and maneuver the chair. (These concepts can apply to the positioning of clients and the performance of power wheelchairs as well.) Conversely, a forward axle position can cause the chair to flip over backward. The further back the axle is, the more stable the chair becomes. As the front end becomes heavier, the more it will pull to the lowest point of any surface wheeled on. The client's shoulder ideally should be vertical to the axle for optimal efficiency.

  - **wheel camber:** Adjustment is made by slanting the tops of the rear wheels toward the frame. It provides for greater side-to-side stability due to the increased angle and width of the wheelbase, quicker turning, and greater access to the top of the hand rims. (It is more natural to push down and out.

  - **wheelbase width:** Axle sleeves can be threaded, allowing for the axle position to be inset or outset in relation to the axle plate. Some of the frames let you adjust the axle sleeves inward or outward in relation to the axle plates. Axle plates may allow the user to mount them on the inside of the frame, which reduces the wheelbase width. This gives the user the option to move the wheels closer or farther away from the hips; proper wheel spacing to maximize pushing efficiency; compensation for camber adjustment; and lateral adjustment for increasing wheelchair stability.

- **rear seat height and rear wheel size:** Allows for the chair to be set higher or lower in the rear. The adjustment of the rear seat height can be used to adjust for mechanical efficiency of propulsion, balance, and transfers. If there is a rear axle plate, the rear seat height is adjusted vertically by moving the axle plate. Used to accommodate the length of the client's arms, relative to trunk length. A 16-in. rear wheel size is typically used to lower frame height for a very short person and/or foot propeller. A 26-in. rear wheel size is usually required for individuals over 6 ft tall and needs more ground clearance under the frame.

- **front seat height:** Front seat height is a consideration for foot propellers, balance, transfer status, and clearance of the user's footrest from the ground. Generally measured from the seating surface in the front of the chair to the floor. Higher front seat heights are usually used when the user is tall and/or has long legs. The size caster, caster fork, and fork stem determine the front seat height. The caster fork generally needs to match the size of the caster. If added height is needed, up to 1.5-in. stem bolts are available. (Always check the caster angle after making any adjustments to the chair's seat height, wheels, casters, or caster forks. It is important for all four wheels of the chair to simultaneously contact the ground for maximum performance. The caster must be aligned to a 90-degree angle with respect to the floor. This will eliminate caster flutter.) A forward-mounted caster compared to a reverse-mounted caster is used when more forward stability is desirable such as with a client with large or edematous legs.

- **caster size/selection:** The wheelchair is more maneuverable and faster to turn with a small caster and small fork size. An 8-in. caster is typically harder to turn than a 3-in. to 6-in. caster. Conversely, the smaller the caster size, the more likely the chair will get hung up on obstacles. A 3-in. caster is most often used by a skilled wheelchair user who can easily "jump" over obstacles by lifting the front end of the chair or doing a "wheely." By contrast, 8-in. casters provide the least amount of clearance from the footplate or foot of the user but provide optimal clearance and maneuvering over obstacles. Five- or 6-in. casters provide a compromise between clearance, height, and maneuverability. Casters are offered in wider widths, sometimes referred to as "soft rolls," adding to the front stability and improved maneuverability over uneven terrain.

- **seat height and angle:** Generally measured from the seating surface to the floor in the front and the rear of the chair. The adjustment of the rear seat height can be used to adjust for mechanical efficiency of propulsion, balance, and transfers. There may be times when it is advantageous to have an angled seat (tilt of frame or "dump") for improved balance and stability.

quick release axles: Allows for more compact travel in a vehicle. Allows client to interchange different sized wheels and/or tire types.

footrest hangers: Optional with different knee angles to accommodate flexibility of client. The length of the chair is shorter with a larger angle to the footrest. Foot propellers who have a low seat to floor height generally require the 60- or 70-degree hangers so that there is clearance between the footrest and floor/ground.

elevating or articulating leg-rests: Allows for elevation of the lower leg from approximately 60 degrees of flexion to 5 degrees of knee extension. Keep in mind that most clients are not flexible enough in the hamstrings to tolerate full elevation. (A shortened hamstring will then often result in posterior tilt of the pelvis.) The degree of elevation often does not approach the level of the heart and therefore does not typically reduce edema in the feet a significant amount. Elevation is more often a comfort measure for someone who cannot tolerate constant positioning of the knee and feet in one position.

front-end angle: Referenced for rigid front frames, accommodates the flexibility of the client's knees and hamstring length. The length on the frame is shorter and has a smaller turning radius when the angle of the front end is 85 or 90 degrees.

From:

Quickie Design: The Perfect Fit: An Adjustments Guide to Your Manual Wheelchair. Brochure copywrited by Quickie Designs, Inc., 1990, including images 4–7.

push handles: Allows caregiver to push the user in the chair. Some individuals in custom frames prefer to keep the frame small and light and prefer or don't require a handle for pushing.

armrests: Available in the full and desk lengths. Styles include L-shaped swing-away, flip back, single and dual post, and height adjustable.

hand rims: Generally made of aluminum, plastic, or other alloy. Available with a plastic coating to improve grip, or with straight or angled projections for improved contact.

clothing guards: Small panel to protect the client's clothing from rain or debris in the wheels. Typically used when client does not use armrests, as the clothing guard is built into many armrest styles.

anti-tip devices: Safety device to prevent the chair from tipping rearward. An anti-tip is almost always ordered on a new frame for safety. Used all the time for amputees whose weight is all carried in the rear of the frame or for those clients who are new to the lighter, more adjustable wheelchair frames.

frame protectors: Used on the footrest hanger or front end of a rigid model to protect the wheelchair frame from scratches and dents. Sometimes can be used to pad the side of the frame to reduce pressure on the lower leg (provides limited protection).

mag wheels: Plastic or composite wheel that is more durable than a spoke wheel but heavier.

spoked wheels: Lighter aluminum wheel but more maintenance involved, as they require truing to maintain spoke tension and the integrity of the wheel.

spoke guards: Plastic wheel protector to reduce bending of a spoke wheel. Often used to protect the client's hands from injury in the spokes, particularly those with decreased coordination.

Spinergy wheels: Spoked wheel made of a carbon fiber material, which is highly durable and resistant to bending and breaking.

grade aides: Device mounted close to the rear wheel and lock to prevent the chair from rolling backward down a hill or incline.

transit options: Added ring-shaped hardware to allow the chair to be hooked to a tie-down strap in a wheelchair-accessible van.

References:
http://www.Sunrisemedical.com; http://www.Invacare.com.

Power Wheelchairs

Power wheelchair options and electronics have evolved and changed over the past 20 years. Belt-driven power wheelchairs were the norm in the 1970s and 1980s. Rear-wheel-drive power wheelchairs were designed in a similar manner to the manual wheelchair, but with large rear wheels and manual braking systems. Recliners were used for quadriplegics. Front-wheel-drive systems came from the European market.

Options include **rear-wheel drive, front-wheel drive,** and **mid-wheel drive** systems (see figure on p. 1066), most of which have direct-drive motors.

WHEELCH

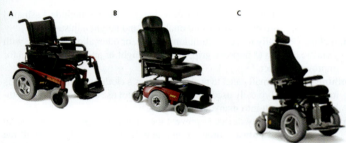

Power wheelchair bases. (A) Rear-wheel drive.(B) Mid- or center-wheel drive (A & B by Invacare Corp.) (C) Front-wheel drive (by Permobil USA).

rear-wheel drive: Generally made with a basic wheelchair type seat frame/rehab seat (part A of figure above).

mid-wheel drive: Accommodates van or captain's seat for clients who do not need customized seating systems and are much more comfortable than with the sling seat and back typical of older, standard wheelchair frames. There are limited size options available on the van type seats (part B of figure above).

front-wheel drive: Usually modular, accepting any type of seat frame (part C of figure above). Performance comparison of rear- vs. mid- vs. front-wheel drive power wheelchairs (see figure on p. 1067).

Modular power wheelchairs (rear, mid, or front wheel) are designed as a separate base from the seating system. A separate power base from the seat allows manufacturers to offer different seating and electronic options for different power bases. It eliminates the need to have a large offering of models by changing the seat options on the chair. The modular system is used for patients with the potential for changing needs whether that is growth, weight loss, progression of disease, or functional improvement. Manufacturer specifications are available on line or through literature provided by a local manufacturer's representative or equipment supplier.

Power seating systems are added to a modular power base for addressing more complex seating needs. Multiple power seat options are available in today's market: tilt, recline, seat elevation, standing, seat to floor, swing-away elevating/articulating leg rests, center-mount elevating/articulating footplates and some custom options (see motionconcepts.com). See Table 17.2 comparison of weight-shifting options.

Power Wheelchairs
Rear v/s Mid v/s Front Wheel Drive

S.I.T.C.O.M.P

Parameters to consider when comparing performance of Rear, Mid, & Front Wheel Drive Power Chairs.

Definitions

Stability	• Front & Rear "Tippy-ness" when driving -- and stopping - on an incline or a decline.
Incline Transition	• The ability of the chair to make the transition from a level surface to an incline, as in maneuvering onto a ramp into a vehicle.
Transfers	• The ability to transfer in & out of the wheelchair without interference from front riggings, front stabilizers, or drive wheels.
Control	• The Driver's confidence the chair will perform in a predictable manner in response to control input. • The Driver's ability to accurately maneuver the chair in all situations & environments.
Obstacle Handling	• The ability of the front most wheel to maneuver over an obstacle.
Maneuverability	• Turning radius, both "Front" and "Full". • Front turning Radius is required to turn a corner into a doorway, and is the distance from the center of the Drive axle, to the farthest point in Front of the chair. • Full turning radius is required to turn the chair 180°, & is the distance from the center of the Drive axle, to the farthest point on the chair.
Positioning	• The ability to position the feet close into the body.

S.I.T.C.O.M.P. Rating Scale

♿ = Average
♿♿ = Above Average
♿♿♿ = Superior

Performance Comparison of Rear - Mid - Front Wheel Drive Power Chairs

	Stability	Incline Transition	Transfers	Control	Obstacle Handling	Maneuverability	Positioning
RWD	♿♿	♿♿	♿♿♿	♿♿♿	♿♿	♿ (♿*)	♿♿
MWD	♿ (♿*)	♿ (♿*)	♿♿	♿♿	♿ (♿*)	♿♿♿	♿♿♿
FWD	♿♿♿	♿♿♿	♿♿	♿♿	♿♿♿	♿♿	♿♿♿

Performance of ALL configurations is greatly affected by Center of Gravity, which must be set (when allowable) for Optimal Chair Performance

(♿*) Denotes significant performance difference dependent on Stabilizer type, or base set-up.

Not One Configuration is clearly better than the other two configurations in all circumstances. An Individual's Clinical & Postural Needs, Preferences, and Environmental Demands need to be matched with the performance capabilities of the Power Wheelchairs considered.

On an overall basis however, FWD out performs MWD and RWD chairs in many performance categories. FWD retains many of the benefits of RWD & MWD, and eliminates many of the disadvantages.

Power Wheelchair Drivers will experience a "Learning Curve" when changing from one configuration to another. The Larger the change, the larger the "Learning Curve.

S.I.T.C.O.M.P. rating scale: Performance comparison of rear-, mid-, and front-wheel drive power wheelchairs developed by Invacare Corp.

WHEELCH

TABLE 17.2 Weight-Shifting Options

	Indications	Functional Use	(-)Considerations	Typical User
Tilt*	Pain or pressure relief Rest Impaired trunk/head control Limited hip extension ROM Increased extensor muscle tone Relief for dysreflexia	Elevation of lower extremities is higher esp. in combination with elevating leg-rests. Front seat ht. raises for ease of transfers or improved balance	Weight capacity may be limited. Overall length of chair increased Should have adjustable hip to back angle to accommodate hip angle and balance	Quadriplegia Spastic quadriplegia Muscular dystrophy ALS MS CP
Recline*	Pain or pressure relief Rest Impaired trunk/head control Limited hip flexion Provides for limited passive ROM of joints (for comfort/pain relief) Relief for dysreflexia	Toileting Pulmonary hygiene can be performed in chair	Shearing forces may cause loss of positioning. Not recommended for increased ms tone Overall length of chair is increased Should have flex/ext limits to accommodate hip ROM (Not to replace ROM program)	Quadriplegia without severe spasticity ALS MS MD with full range of motion *Combination tilt and recline is useful for high quads; end-stage MS; ALS due to severity of impairment

	Indications	Functional Use	(-)Considerations	Typical User
Seat Elevation (Power Only)	Sit to stand transfers are easier. Increases functional reach	Increased independence in all ADLs Improved social interaction/ direct eye contact esp. in work environments	Center of gravity/instability of chair Weight capacity Speed of chair is slowed for safety in elevated position Insurance: Not typically a covered item	Users who live alone or with limited help Employment
Elevating/Articulating Legrests	Pain control and comfort Edema control? Must have knee extension/ hamstring ROM! Limited knee flexion Support of leg braces or casts	Increasing foot clearance off of the ground User cannot use manual leg-rests independently	Limited edema control without tilt or recline. Can cause posterior pelvic tilt when hamstrings tight. Lengthens the chair	Quadriplegia Users with severe edema and poor circulation
Standing	Maintenance of bone density Maintenance of full ROM Improve visceral function User feels less disabled	Improved social interaction/direct eye contact esp. in work environments Increased functional reach	Risk for fractures with existing poor bone density Insurance: Not typically a covered item. Is not used for stand pivot transfers (legs are stabilized)	Newly injured para-plegics or lower level quads. MD
Power Seat to Floor	Need for independent seat to floor transfers	Improved access to play/ school/work environment Improved social interaction with peers	Cannot convert to other power seat features in future Insurance coverage	Pediatrics Dwarfism

Modified from:
Kreutz, D, and Johnson-Taylor, S: Medical and Functional Considerations of Powered Tilt and Recline Systems.

Lower-End Power Wheelchairs

- *Portable power chairs:* Generally smaller power chairs with the capability of coming apart and/or folding. The process of making these units portable so that the chair can be compacted to a car is often time consuming and the pieces are still inherently heavy. It is not conducive to a procedure that one would want to do multiple times a day and in inclement weather. *Examples:* Invacare Nutron, http://www.invacare.com/cgi-bin/imhqprd/inv_catalog/prod_cat.jsp?s=0&catOID=-536887496 and At'm http://www.invacare.com/cgi-bin/imhqprd/inv_catalog/prod_cat.jsp?s=0&catOID=-536887499. Pride Zchair, http://www.pridemobility.com/jazzy/zchair.asp. Accessed February 12, 2010.

- *Add-on power units* (for manual wheelchair frames): These have been popular in the past as an alternative to portable power wheelchairs. The power unit is composed of the motor package, battery unit, and a mounting system that attaches to the manual wheelchair frame. Friction between the power unit and the manual wheelchair tire drive this type of system. Taking the unit on and off the wheelchair frame makes the system less durable. Tires have to be replaced frequently on the friction drive systems.

- *Power-assisted wheels:* The power-assisted wheel is mounted on the wheelchair in place of the manual wheels. The batteries are integrated in the wheel hub. A sensor registers the propelling movement and activates the electrical motors. (See e-motion by frankmobility.com and Xtender by Quickie: http://sunrisemedical.com/products/product_detail.jsp?FOLDER%3C%3Efolder_id=1408474399315797&PRODUCT%3C%3Eprd_id=845524442807833&ASSORTMENT%3C%3East_id=1408474395285139&bmUID=1266179523431.)

- *Power scooters:* Typically narrower units but the length of them makes them less maneuverable for household mobility. Scooters are a basic unit not designed for long-term sitting. Scooters are ideal for the client who can transfer easily in and out of the seat. Not designed for long-term sitting.
  - *Three-wheel units:* Easier to use inside a home. The smaller three-wheel-drive scooters are easiest to break down and transport in a vehicle but only fit smaller individuals (size limits the space between the seat and tiller).
  - *Four-wheel drive:* Less maneuverable indoors but more stable for outdoor use. (Larger three- and four-wheel-drive scooters are available with larger weight capacities but become less and less useful indoors and for transport due to their size and turning radius.)
  - *Fishon seats:* Plastic fold-down shell with foam insert. A more pressure-relieving cushion can be placed in the shell but limited size (only partially addressing pressure distribution needed for pressure relief).
  - *Van or captain's seat:* Similar to bucket seat of a car with or without back-angle adjustment.

Adaptive Switches for Control of Powered Wheelchairs, Communication Devices, and Environmental Controls

- .**Site:** The hands and fingers are the preferred control sites because they are naturally used during manipulation tasks and finer resolution can be achieved.

If the hands or fingers are not an option, the head and mouth are considered next, followed by the foot.

- **Proportional vs. digital control:** A traditional joystick is typically a proportional control in that the client has multidirectional control (360 degrees) over speed and direction of movement. Digital control is nonproportional where individual switches provide on/off control for each direction. Combination systems can be used to provide variable speed control for forward/reverse and on/off directional control.

Proportional Joysticks

- **Traditional joysticks:** Often a single-drive system with a potentiometer or digital speed control. Programmability is limited to speed, acceleration, deceleration, and sometimes sensitivity (turning acceleration).
- **Multi-drive proportional systems:** Generally available with anywhere from two to five drives, each of which is programmed for a different environment such as indoor, outdoor, ramp/van access, etc. Display is typically built in to allow visualization of the drive or control function at hand.
- **Handle shape and size:** A variety of joystick handles and sizes are available for different grasp patterns and strength: T-bars, goal post, balls, mushroom shapes, long extensions, discs, and cups. Handles can be used for mechanical advantage but the "throw" of the joystick then becomes longer.
- **Compact or mini joysticks:** Proportional driver control typically for those with limited hand, finger, chin, foot, or attendant control. Programming parameters can compensate for impaired upper extremity/head/foot control function. Requires a display. Often used with a midline mount for the hand or chin, or recessed in a tray for hand control. Mounting systems must be able to swing away at the chin or mounted on a bib. Mounting can be modified to allow for foot or elbow control.
- **Head controls:** Can be either proportional or digital. Proportional head systems are manufacturer specific such as Magitek (http://www.magitek.com/invacare.pdf). Must have multidirectional/circumferential control of the head.
- **Scanners:** Allows the chair to operate with a single switch. This mode of driving is much less efficient and more time consuming. A client may have as little as a small muscle twitch or eyebrow movement to operate single switch with a scanner but must be highly motivated to do so.

Digital Controls

Digital controls are usually arranged in an array of pads to allow for control of forward, left-right, and reverse directions. Digital systems require the use of an electronic interface and typically a display. A digital system is totally dependent on electronic programming to function safely and from a functional standpoint.

- **Switch types**
  - **Mechanical switches:** Button/plate switches, levers, pneumatic, mercury.
  - **Electronic switches:** Proximity (capacity with range up to 3/8 in.), fiberoptic, infrared, touch pads, sensor (myoelectric), photoelectric, sound activated, piezo electric, ultrasonic.
- **Switch setup**
  - **Single:** Used as a single function for on/off.

- **Array:** Comes in a package to allow for control of multiple directions or functions: Head arrays, sip and puff (intraoral pressure), wafer boards, star board, imbedded in trays.
- **Scanners:** Allows a single switch to operate multiple functions such as a power wheelchair. On-board scanners are used often on various communication devices.
- **Mounting systems:** Swing-away, trays, goosenecks.
- **Manufacturers:** Adaptive Switch Labs, Inc.; Ablenet Inc.; Enabling Devices; Stealth; Tash International Inc.; Whitmeyer Biomechanix.

Programming

- **Power wheelchairs** either have a control module that is built into the joystick box or on higher-end modular systems the control module is typically a box under the chair. Power wheelchairs are typically sent from the manufacturer with a standard program(s) that can be modified with an electronic programmer. (Ask your equipment supplier.) This allows you to match the responses of the chair to coincide with an individual's physical capabilities.
- **Performance adjustments:** Forward speed, turning speed, reverse speed, acceleration (forward/reverse), sensitivity/dampening (turning acceleration), braking adjustment (deceleration).
- **Other adjustments (manufacturer specific):**
  - **Torque:** Amount of power generated by the motor. Higher adjustments are typically used for outdoor performance.
  - **Joystick throw:** The amount of joystick excursion required. A short throw reduces the amount of joystick deflection required for the wheelchair to reach top speed. It is useful when the client has very limited movement because of weakness or contractures.
  - **Momentary vs. latched:** The joystick or switch must be in an activated position for the chair to respond when set in **momentary.** Release of the joystick/switch causes the chair to stop. Most power chairs are set in momentary. In the **latched** setting, once the switch is activated, it can be released and the chair will continue to run until a switch is hit again. Latched mode is often used for sip-and-puff drivers so they do not have to constantly maintain the sip or puff (cruise control)
  - **Stand by/sleep mode:** A timer is set so that the system will remain in a selected mode of operation before automatically turning off. This functions as a safety mechanism so that the user does not inadvertently move the chair when at rest.
  - **RIM control** (developed at the Rehabilitation Institute of Montreal): Allows for one switch to be used for two different directions or functions. For example, a head array is typically made up of three switches with a fourth switch acting as a reset. A single switch is used for both forward and reverse or the turn switches can be programmed to activate a power seat function.
  - **No driving mode:** Allows one particular mode to be used for another function besides driving the chair: power seat functions, communication, environmental controls.

Modified from:

Kreutz, D, and Johnson-Taylor, S: Wheelchair positioning and mobility workshop: A hands on approach, September 17–18, 1993.

Modules and Interfaces

Multifunction control boxes, ACM/ECU (environmental control units), auxiliary interface, COM interface, D-9 ports, wired, and "wireless" are all potential electronic components needed for a system to work with multiple functions. An ECU, for example, allows the electronics of the chair to interface with a communication device or environmental control so that the client can use the same joystick or switch system to operate the alternative device. An ECU is also needed to allow the power seat functions to operate through the joystick as would be required for a client who cannot access more than one switch site. Therapists will consult with their suppliers and manufacturer representatives to understand the function of the electronic boxes to justify the needs for various components.

Modified from:

Lange, M; Assistive Technology Partners, Children's Hospital, Denver, CO: Switch access and assessment. Paper presented at RESNA 2006: Thriving in Challenging Times: The Future of Rehabilitation Engineering and Assistive Technology, June 22–26, 2006.

Communication devices often have to be mounted to the wheelchair for access. A dedicated mounting system that attaches to the seat frame works best in most instances, as the communication device will move with the seating system when tilted or reclined. The mount prevents the device from falling off in the tilted or reclined position and allows the screen to be placed in the client's visual field.

Ventilators are typically mounted to manual reclining wheelchairs under the seat. The older, less expensive, large ventilators require a large tray mounted on the rear of a manual tilting or power wheelchair. In this case, the tray has to be gimbaled, which increases the length of the chair significantly. The newer, brief, case-shaped ventilators take up much less room on the back of the chair and are preferable for portability on most wheelchairs to cut down on the overall size and improve access.

A *power converter* is now available that allows communication devices, ventilators, and other battery-operated equipment to be run by the power wheelchair batteries. In this way, a third battery does not have to be mounted on the wheelchair, taking up even more space on the system.

The Final Prescription

- Typically formatted on the final page of your evaluation form.
- The components of the system should match the goals that are determined throughout the evaluation process.
- A manufacturer's order form is typically used as a reference for the particular options offered on the wheelchair frame.
- Components can come from many manufacturers: Wheelchair base; power seating units; wheels; seat back; seat cushion; headrest; and so on. All the components are listed with the rationale for each component outlined in your letter of medical necessity (see figure on following page).

Body measurements

A. _____

B. R_____ L _____

C. R_____ L _____

D1. _____

D2. _____

E. R_____ L _____

F. _____

G. _____

H. _____

I. R_____ L _____

J. _____

K. _____

L. _____

Overall width of body _____ (when scoliosis present)

Overall depth of body _____ (when kyphosis present)

Equipment specifications

Mobility base _____ Anti-tips _____

Power controls _____ Gel batteries/charger _____

Wheels _____ Wheel locks _____ Wheel lock extensions _____ Spoke guards _____

Tires _____ Plastic coated handrims _____

Casters _____

Back _____
_____

Trunk supports _____

Chest strap/harness _____

Headrest _____

Seat/cushion _____
_____

Thigh/hip guides _____

Pelvic strap _____

Leg/footrest _____

Impact guards _____

Arms _____

Packs/bags/basket _____ Laptray _____ Cane/crutch holder _____ Color _____

Other _____

Please arrange delivert to: _____

Home _____

Emory seating clinic _____

_____ P.T./date

_____

Equipment supplier/RTS

Final prescription document.

Final Fitting and Adjustments

- A follow-up appointment is set up in coordination with the equipment supplier for the delivery of the equipment and final fitting.
- Simple or standard wheelchairs and systems with few adjustments may not have to be coordinated by the team but delivered directly to the client by the equipment supplier. This should be negotiated at the completion of the evaluation.
- The therapist may have to do a brief reevaluation of the client's physical and functional status to confirm the position of the seating system and components. The adjustments are made as a team and feedback is secured from the client, and from postural and functional checkout.
- The client/caregiver is educated in the proper use and function of the system with follow-up arranged as needed.

Sample Custom Wheelchair and Seating System

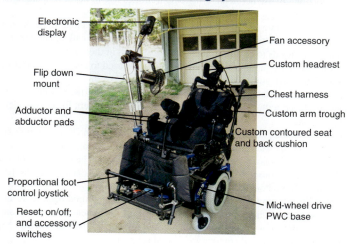

Electronic display — Fan accessory — Custom headrest — Flip down mount — Chest harness — Adductor and abductor pads — Custom arm trough — Custom contoured seat and back cushion — Proportional foot control joystick — Reset; on/off; and accessory switches — Mid-wheel drive PWC base

Client with severe spastic/athetoid cerebral palsy with fixed deformities throughout; scoliosis; pelvic obliquity, windswept deformity, leg length discrepancy; dominated by severe postural extension of the head/neck/trunk, ATNR; resting tremors/dyskinesia; requiring totally customized system with a combination of contoured seating and planar components.

The system was recommended and purchased for a female client with severe spastic/athetoid cerebral palsy with fixed deformities throughout; scoliosis; pelvic obliquity, windswept deformity, leg length discrepancy; dominated by severe postural extension of the head/neck/trunk, ATNR; resting tremors/dyskinesia; requiring totally customized system with a combination of contoured seating and planar components as follows:

Components and Justification

- Wheelchair base: Mid-wheel drive power wheelchair for independent mobility, replacing old dysfunctional equipment; for allowing client to accomplish daily ADL such as feeding via G-tube; computer access; and communication. Movement and upright positioning in a chair contributes to pulmonary hygiene.

- Power tilting seat: For independent weight shifts for rest, postural control, pressure relief, and pulmonary hygiene given the client's severe disability and movement disorder.

- Upgraded/expandable electronics: Allows the chair to be operated with alternative foot control and foot switches, and with programming capability to accommodate the client's unique and special needs.

- Electronic display: Allows the client to know what function is being controlled on the chair. The display screen indicates at any given moment whether the chair is on or off, in what speed, seat function, or communication mode the chair is operating in for accurate control.

- Foot control proportional joystick: Allows the chair to be operated via a foot control, as the client has the most isolated movement in her feet. She is unable to functionally use her head or upper extremities due to her severe athetoid/spastic CP.

- Auxiliary module and four button switches: To allow the client to independently control the tilt, communication device, emergency call signal, and the fan, as she needs to be able to independently do all of these functions for survival and to accomplish simple ADL. The fan is used to control overheating associated with autonomic dysfunction.

- Single actuator interface box: Allows the electronics of the power chair to be interfaced with the electronics of the seating/tilt system for independent operation.

- Custom-molded seat back with aluminum mounting pan: To accommodate and support the client's severely scoliotic spine and to limit extraneous trunk movement associated with her dystonia. The client would be unable to control the joystick without full support of her spine and trunk. The mounting pan contains the custom foam back.

- Lateral trunk supports: Needed in addition to the contoured back to secure the client's trunk laterally due to her severe trunk asymmetry and lack of any balance control in sitting. She has abnormal reflex patterns that will pull her off center without full contour and lateral support.

- Padded customized Dynaform chest harness: To contain the trunk within the contours of the back. Without the chest harness, the client's trunk and chest would hyperextend and cause the remainder of her body to come out of position.

- Custom-molded seat cushion, 4-in. × 8-in. recess for gel insert, and aluminum mounting pan: For full support and control of the pelvis; for pressure relief, as the client has a long history of skin ulcers and hip pain. She would be unable to function or sit for any length of time without a fully contoured and customized seat. The custom foam also has to have a gel insert to provide extra pressure relief on the right as she bears extra weight on the right ischial tuberosity. The contoured foam cushion has to be contained in a mounting pan.

- Padded four-point pelvic belt: To hold the pelvis firmly in the contours of the seat as the client's movement disorder would allow for her to wiggle out of the seat if not fully secured in the pelvic belt.

- Unilateral adductor pad on the right and unilateral abductor on the left with mounting hardware: Holds the legs out of the windswept position; protects the hips from excessive subluxation.
- Custom headrest including an occipital pad, bilateral suboccipital pads, bilateral facial spot pads, gel overlays, and all attaching hardware: The client's abnormal head and neck posturing is a result of a severe ATNR. It is imperative that her neck and head movement be inhibited as much as is possible so that her trunk and extremities maintain as much of a neutral posture as is possible but also accommodates her neck and head deformity because of this lifelong posture. The gel pads inside the headrest components serve to protect the skin on her scalp.
- Custom arm troughs with padded forearms and wrist straps: The client's arms have to be tied down, as she has ballistic arm movements and constant tremors associated with her movement disorder. She would injure herself and others without her arms being completely contained.
- Flip-down mount: To hold accessories in place, including communication device/computer and electric fan.

(Information included in letter of medical necessity to insurance provider(s) in collaboration with certified rehabilitation technology supplier.)

Wheelchair Information and Support Services

WheelchairNet (http://www.wheelchairnet.org; accessed February 12, 2010) is an Internet-based resource initially funded in 1999 by a grant from the National Institute of Disability Research and Rehabilitation (NIDRR) to the University of Pittsburgh. WheelchairNet's purpose is to serve the information needs of anyone interested in wheeled mobility and to create a forum for the free exchange of information regarding wheelchair technology and its successful use. The site has a complete listing of manufacturers of wheelchair and seating products.

Rehabilitation Engineering and Assistive Technology Society of North America (RESNA) is a multidisciplinary and international organization that promotes research and development, education, and advocacy dedicated to promoting the exchange of ideas and information for the provision and advancement of assistive technology. RESNA offers three national certifications:

- *****Assistive Technology Professional (ATP)**
  An assistive technology professional is a service provider who analyzes the needs of individuals with disabilities, assists in the selection of the appropriate equipment, and trains the consumer to properly use the specific equipment. This equipment may include manual and power wheelchairs, alternate computer access, augmentative and alternative communication devices, and other technology to improve the function and quality of life for an individual with a disability.
- **Rehabilitation Engineering Technologist (RET)**
  Service providers who apply engineering principles to the design, modification, customization, and/or fabrication of assistive technology for persons with disabilities.
- **Seating and Mobility Specialist (SMS)**
  An ATP who specializes in the comprehensive seating, positioning, and mobility needs of consumers with disabilities (http://www.resna.org).

National Registry of Rehabilitation Technology Suppliers (http://www.nrrts.com; accessed February 12, 2010) is a professional association supporting individuals/suppliers who provide Complex Rehab wheelchairs and seated positioning systems for people of all ages and diagnoses who have postural or mobility deficits. A rehabilitation technology supplier is credentialed by the organization, Certified Rehabilitation Technology Supplier (CRTS), and is set apart from the durable medical equipment (DME or HME) suppliers who provide no specialized adaptation or services. NRRTS registrants are dedicated to the field of assistive technology and service delivery. An NRRTS professional possesses the experience and knowledge to work with the clinician and client to determine the most appropriate enabling technology for people with disabilities.

National Coalition for Assistive and Rehab Technology (NCART) (http://www.ncart.us/; accessed February 12, 2010) promotes the interests of the Rehab and Assistive Technology industry, ensuring adequate consumer access to appropriate technology and services while creating a stable business environment for providers and manufacturers of rehab and assistive technology. Their vision is to have rehab and assistive technology recognized and accepted as a unique and separate health-care delivery model from DME, then to use this differentiation to effect changes in coding, coverage and payment.

Centers for Medicare & Medicaid Services (CMS) (http://www.cms.gov)

- Medicare Coverage Center (browse by specific topic): Coverage database search
- Durable Medical Equipment (DME) Center (browse by provider type)

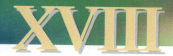

PHYSICAL AGENTS

Interactions Between Drugs and Commonly Used Modalities

TABLE 18.1 Interactions Between Drugs and Commonly Used Physical Modalities

Modality	Desired Therapeutic Effect	Drugs With Complementary/ Synergistic Effects	Drugs With Antagonistic Effects	Other Drug–Modality Interactions
Cryotherapy Cold/ice packs, ice massage, cold baths, vapocoolant sprays	• Decreased pain, edema, and inflammation • Muscle relaxation and decreased spasticity	• Anti-inflammatory steroids (glucocorticoids); non-steroidal anti-inflammatory analgesics (aspirin and similar NSAIDs) • Skeletal muscle relaxants	• Peripheral vasodilators may exacerbate acute local edema. • Nonselective cholinergic agonists may stimulate the neuromuscular junction.	• Some forms of cryotherapy may produce local vasoconstriction that temporarily impedes diffusion of drugs to the site of inflammation.
Thermotherapy Hot packs Paraffin Infrared Fluidotherapy Diathermy Ultrasound	• Decreased muscle/ joint pain and stiffness • Decreased muscle spasms • Increased blood flow to improve tissue healing	• NSAIDs; opioid analgesics; local anesthetics • Skeletal muscle relaxants • Peripheral vasodilators	• Nonselective cholinergic agonists may stimulate the neuromuscular junction. • Systemic vasoconstrictors (e.g., α-1 agonists) may decrease perfusion of peripheral tissues.	
Systemic Heat Large whirlpool Hubbard tank	• Decreased muscle/ joint stiffness in large areas of the body	• Opioid and nonopioid analgesics; skeletal muscle relaxants		• Severe hypotension may occur if systemic hot whirlpool is administered to

Modality	Desired Therapeutic Effect	Drugs With Complementary/ Synergistic Effects	Drugs With Antagonistic Effects	Other Drug–Modality Interactions
				patients taking peripheral vasodilators and some antihypertensive drugs (e.g., α-1 antagonists, nitrates, direct-acting vasodilators, calcium channel blockers).
Ultraviolet radiation	• Increased wound healing	• Various systemic and topical antibiotics		• Antibacterial drugs generally increase cutaneous sensitivity to ultraviolet light (i.e., photosensitivity).
	• Management of skin disorders (acne, rashes)	• Systemic and topical antibiotics and anti-inflammatory steroids (glucocorticoids)	• Many drugs may cause hypersensitivity reactions that result in skin rashes, itching.	• Photosensitivity with anti-bacterial drugs.
Transcutaneous electrical nerve stimulation (TENS)	• Decreased pain	• Opioid and nonopioid analgesics	• Opioid antagonists (naloxone).	
Functional electrical stimulation (FES)	• Increased skeletal muscle strength and endurance		• Skeletal muscle relaxants.	
	• Decreased spasticity and muscle spasms	• Skeletal muscle relaxants	• Nonselective cholinergic agonists may stimulate the neuromuscular junction.	

From Ciccone, CD: *Pharmacology in Rehabilitation*, ed. 3. FA Davis, Philadelphia, 1996, inside front cover, with permission.

Thermal Agents

Thermal agents are modalities that produce a therapeutic transfer of energy to a patient to increase or decrease tissue temperature. **Cryotherapy** is the term used to describe the use of agents that lower tissue temperature, whereas **thermotherapy** is the term used for agents that raise tissue temperature. Temperature changes may be superficial or deep depending on the specific modality used, the body part treated, and the ability of the body to provide thermoregulation.

   Note: Ultrasound and **hydrotherapy** may also be classified as thermal agents; however, because they utilize mechanical forms of energy to produce thermal as well as other therapeutic effects, they are listed as mechanical agents in this section.

Physical Laws

Thermal agents transfer heat by the following five **modes of heat transfer:**

conduction: Heating or cooling that results from the direct energy exchange between materials in direct static contact with each other. The following physical laws apply:

* Energy transfer is always from the material at the higher temperature to the material at the lower temperature.
* The transfer of energy stops when the two materials are at the same temperature.
* The rate at which energy is transferred depends on the temperature difference between the two materials, their thermal conductivity, and their area of contact.

   Examples: hot packs, cold packs, and paraffin.

convection: Heat transfer that occurs as a result of direct contact between a circulating medium and another material of a different temperature. The following physical laws apply:

* Because the thermal agent is in motion and continuously makes contact with the body at the initial temperature of the agent, more heat is transferred in the same time period as in the conduction mode.

   Examples: whirlpools and fluidotherapy.

conversion: Heat transfer that occurs as a result of the conversion of a nonthermal source of energy (e.g., mechanical, electrical, or chemical energy) into heat. The following physical laws apply:

* Unlike conduction or convection modes, heating is not affected by the temperature of the thermal agent.
* The rate of heat transfer depends on the power of the energy source (e.g., the amount of watts for ultrasound, size of the area treated, size of the applicator, efficiency of transmission from applicator to the patient, and the type of tissue being treated.

Example: ultrasound.

radiation: Heat transfer that occurs from a higher to a lower temperature without the need for contact between the two materials or an intervening medium. The following physical laws apply:

• The rate of temperature change depends on the intensity of the radiation, relative size of the radiation source, area being treated, distance, and orientation from the source.

Examples: ultraviolet and solar heat.

evaporation: Heat transfer that occurs as a result of the transformation of a material from a liquid to a gas or vapor.

Examples: vapocoolant spray, or the evaporation of sweat to cool the body.

Cryotherapy

Cryotherapy is the therapeutic application of cold to soft tissue. Cryotherapy exerts its effects by influencing the hemodynamic, neuromuscular, and metabolic processes, such as through direct and indirect vasoconstriction, delayed vasodilation, decreased nerve conduction velocity, increased pain threshold, decreased spasticity, facilitation of muscle contraction, decreased metabolic rate, and decreased inflammation.

TABLE 18.2 Cryotherapy—Indications, Contraindications, and Precautions

Indications
Control inflammation, pain, and edema
Reduce spasticity
Facilitate movement
Control symptoms of multiple sclerosis

Contraindications
Cold hypersensitivity
Cold intolerance
Cryoglobulinemia
Paroxysmal cold hemoglobinuria
Raynaud's disease/phenomenon
Area with regenerating peripheral nerves
Area with circulatory compromise or PVD
Malignancy

Precautions
Over a superficial main branch of a nerve
Over a deep open wound
Hypertension
Poor sensation or poor mentation
Very young or very old person

(table continues on page 1084)

■ **TABLE 18.2 Cryotherapy—Indications, Contraindications, and Precautions** (continued)

Precautions
Over the abdomen of a pregnant patient
History of frostbite

Sources: Cameron, MH (ed): *Physical Agents in Rehabilitation: From Research to Practice*, ed. 3. Saunders, St. Louis, MO, 2009, pp 134–153; Michlovitz, SL, and Nolan, TP: *Modalities for Therapeutic Intervention*, ed. 4. FA Davis, Philadelphia, 2005, pp 44–58.
PVD = peripheral vascular disease.

Cryotherapy Modalities

chemical cold pack: A reusable pack containing silica gel or mixture of saline and gelatin that is stored in a freezer at approximately −5°C (23°F). There are disposable cold packs that are not refrigerated but instead are activated by breaking an inner seal that mixes the chemicals within.

ice pack: A plastic bag filled with ice cubes or crushed ice. Ice packs provide more aggressive cooling than a cold pack at the same temperature (because of its higher specific heat) and therefore more insulation should be used.

ice massage: The stroking of ice on a body part, primarily to anesthetize the skin. The ice is typically frozen in a cylindrical container, such as a paper cup, and held by the lower part of the cup or by a tongue depressor that is frozen into the center of the cup ("lollipop" technique). An ice cube held in a paper towel or gauze is also commonly used.

ice towel: A towel that contains ice shavings or is frozen when wet (rarely used because of its inconvenience and messiness).

controlled cold compression unit: A device that alternately pumps cold water and air into a sleeve that is wrapped around a patient's limb. The water temperature can be set between 10°C and 25°C (50°F and 77°F). Most commonly used directly after orthopedic surgery where it has been reported as more effective than ice or compression alone.

quick icing: A technique developed by Margaret Rood in which the rapid application of ice is used as a stimulus to elicit a desired motor pattern. The effectiveness of its use for patients with flacidity following an upper motor neuron lesion has been questioned.

vapocoolant spray: A method of quickly cooling the skin by the evaporation of a substance sprayed on the skin, for example, ethyl chloride. More recently introduced vapocoolant sprays have appeared on the market that are neither flammable nor volatile in terms of ozone depletion, and are marketed under the trade names Spray and Stretch, Instant Ice, and Pain Ease (Gebauer Company, Cleveland, OH). Generally used as a component for the treatment of trigger points using the spray-and-stretch technique.

References:

Belanger, AY: *Evidence-Based Guide to Therapeutic Physical Agents. Lippincott Williams & Wilkins, Philadelphia, 2002.*

Cameron, MH (ed): *Physical Agents in Rehabilitation: From Research to Practice, ed. 3. Saunders, St. Louis, 2003.*

Thermotherapy

Thermotherapy is the application of heat for therapeutic effects through its influence on hemodynamic, neuromuscular, and metabolic processes.

TABLE 18.3 Thermotherapy—Indications, Contraindications, and Precautions for Thermotherapy

Indications
Control joint pain
Increase soft tissue extensibility
Reduce joint stiffness
Accelerate tissue healing

Contraindications
Recent or potential hemorrhage
Thrombophelebitis
Impaired sensation
Impaired mentation
Malignancy
Over areas treated with topical counterirritants

Precautions
Acute injury or inflammation
Pregnancy (may be applied to limbs)
Impaired circulation or poor thermal regulation
Edema
Cardiac insufficiency
Metal implants, fragments, or jewelry
Over an open wound
Demyelinated nerves

Sources: Cameron, MH (ed): *Physical Agents In Rehabilitation: From Research To Practice*, ed. 3., St. Louis, Saunders, 2009, pp. 134–153, 154–158; Michlovitz, SL, and Nolan, TP: *Modalities for Therapeutic Intervention*, ed. 4. FA Davis, Philadelphia, 2005, pp 44–58.

Thermotherapy Modalities

Heat Packs

Canvas-covered hydrophilic silica gel (bentonite) is immersed in water for at least 2 hours initially (or 30 min to reheat) that is typically between 165°F to 175°F (73.9°C–79.4°C). Hot packs are available in a variety of contours for different body parts. They are applied as a source of conductive moist heat to the body part with layerings of terry cloth toweling between the skin and hot pack.

Paraffin

In most clinical applications, paraffin is applied at temperatures between 113°F to 126°F (45°C–52°C) for lower extremities and 126°F to 135°F (52.2°C–57.2°C) for upper extremities. Paraffin melts rapidly at 130°F (54.4°C) and sterilizes at 200°F (93.9°C). For clinical use, paraffin is usually mixed using the following ratio: 7 parts paraffin:1 part mineral oil, or comes pre-mixed. It is usually applied to distal extremities by dip-wrap method or dip-immersion method but may also be applied by painting the paraffin on the skin for more proximal body parts. May not be used over an open skin lesion. Precaution should be applied when metal is in the area, for example, rings should be covered with gauze to decrease superficial heating.

Fluidotherapy

Small silicon or other solid particles are heated and suspended by circulating air at a temperature range of 115°F to 123°F (46.1°C–50.6°C). Fluidotherapy is used to provide superficial dry convective heating to distal extremities.

Terms Related to the Use of Thermotherapy

reflex heating (consensual heating, remote heating, or the Landis-Gibbons reflex): A technique involving the application of heat to one area of the body that results in an increase in cutaneous circulation and other reactions in another area.

specific absorption rate (SAR): The rate of energy absorbed per unit mass of tissue (expressed in watts per kilogram).

specific heat capacity: The specific heat input required to raise the temperature of 1 g of a substance 1°C.

thermal conductivity: The ability of a substance to conduct heat.

Mechanical Agents

Mechanical agents produce their therapeutic effect through the application of force to the body. Examples of mechanical agents include **ultrasound, hydrotherapy, traction,** and **compression.** Each is described in greater detail below.

Ultrasound

Ultrasound is a physical agent that is used therapeutically for its superficial and deep-heating effects as well as for its non-thermal capabilities to promote wound healing and transdermal drug delivery (**phonophoresis**). Ultrasound is generated from a **transducer head** or **applicator** that is applied in circular motions to the patient's body using a **conductive gel** for **direct contact coupling,** or through immersion, bladder, or gel pad procedures (**indirect coupling**) when direct contact is not tolerable.

Physical Properties

By definition, ultrasound is sound with a frequency greater than 20,000 cycles per second (or hertz (Hz)), the limits of normal human hearing. Therapeutic ultrasound operates at a frequency of 0.7 to 3.3 megahertz (MHz).

The ultrasound wave is produced by the alternating expansion and contraction of a piezoelectric crystal in the sound head when alternating electric current is applied. The resultant **ultrasound beam** acts as a pressure wave (see figure below) on the body's tissue. Ultrasound waves are delivered therapeutically in either a continuous mode (**continuous ultrasound**) or a pulsed mode (**pulsed ultrasound**) where it is characterized by its **duty cycle** (see figure at bottom of page). The strength of the ultrasound wave is determined by the **acoustic power** produced by the ultrasound transducer measured in watts, and is not uniform across its surface (see figure on p. 1088).

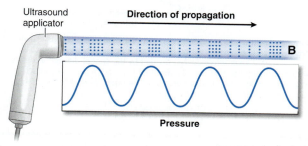

Collimated ultrasound beam (B) produced by the ultrasound applicator. The associated pressure wave is illustrated as periodic areas of increased (condensations) and decreased (rarefactions) molecular concentrations. *Modified from: Michlovitz, SL and Nolan, TP: Modalities for Therapeutic Intervention, ed. 4. FA Davis, Philadelphia, 2012, p. 86, with permission.*

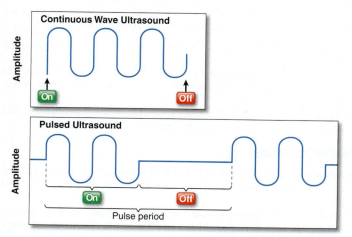

Illustration of continuous-wave (uninterrupted) and pulsed-wave (ON and OFF pulse periods) ultrasound. *Modified from: Michlovitz, SL, et al: Modalities for Therapeutic Intervention, ed. 4. FA Davis, Philadelphia, 2012, p 88, with permission.*

AGENTS

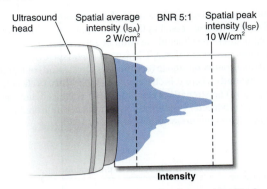

The uneven distribution of acoustic power from the ultrasound head is shown. Power distribution is expressed as the BNR (*beam uniformity ratio*), which is equal to the *spatial peak intensity* (I_{SP}) divided by the *spatial average intensity* (I_{SA}). In the example, the BNR is 5:1. *Modified from: Michlovitz, SL, et al: Modalities for Therapeutic Intervention, ed. 4. FA Davis, Philadelphia, 2012, p 89, with permission.*

Therapeutic Effects

Thermal Effects

Thermal effects are proportional to the absorption of the sound waves by the body tissue. Absorption depends upon the nature of the tissue, its degree of vascularization, and the frequency and intensity of the applied ultrasound. Tissues with high collagen content have a high **absorption coefficient** (e.g., tendons, ligaments, joint capsules, and fascia); tissues with low collagen content have a low absorption coefficient (e.g., water, fat, muscle, and blood).

- Ultrasound heats smaller and deeper tissue areas than most superficial heating agents.
- Penetration is proportional to the ultrasound frequency: 1 MHz ultrasound provides deeper penetration (up to 5 cm) than 3 MHz ultrasound, which penetrates 1 to 2 cm deep.
- Heat absorption is three to four times greater for 3 MHz compared to 1 MHz ultrasound at the same intensity (see figure on p. 1087)

Mechanical Effects

- Intracellular and extracellular ions and fluids subjected to movement, referred to as **microstreaming,** which may alter cell membrane permeability and activity.
- Small gas bubbles present in body fluids undergo compression and expansion (referred to as **cavitation),** which may contribute to diffusional cell membrane changes.

⬤ TABLE 18.4 Indications, Contraindications, and Precautions for Ultrasound

Indications
Continuous ultrasound (superficial and deep tissue heating)
• Muscle spasm
• Contractures
Pulsed or continuous ultrasound (to facilitate tissue healing)
• Acute injury or inflammation of soft tissue
Acute injury or inflammation of peripheral nerve
Open wounds
Fracture

Contraindications
Region of a cardiac pacemaker
During pregnancy near fetus
Eyes
Male or female reproductive organs
Region of active bleeding or infection
Malignant tumors
Region of deep vein thrombosis or thrombophlebitis
Over the heart, stellate, or cervical ganglia
Methylmethacrylate cement or plastic

Precautions
Region of acute inflammation
Epiphyseal plates of growing bones
Fracture
Breast implants

Source: Cameron, MH (ed): *Physical Agents in Rehabilitation: From Research to Practice,* ed. 3. Saunders, St. Louis, MO, 2009, pp. 181–191.

Measurement Terms Related to the Use of Ultrasound

absorption coefficient: A measure of the degree to which a material absorbs ultrasound; expressed in decibels/cm at a specified ultrasound frequency.

beam nonuniformity ratio (BNR): The ratio of the peak intensity of the ultrasound field to the spatial average intensity. The lower the BNR, the more uniform the emitted energy will be.

effective intensity: See *spatial average intensity.*

effective radiating area (ERA): The area of the applicator that emits ultrasound, expressed in square centimeters (cm^2).

enhancement ratio: Ratio of phonophoretic and passive permeability across the skin.

spatial average intensity: The ratio of the ultrasonic power to the effective radiating area (ERA) of the applicator, expressed in watts per square centimeter (W/cm^2). See also *effective radiating area (ERA).*

spatial average, pulse average intensity (SAPA): The average pulse intensity divided by the beam cross-sectional area.

AGENTS

spatial average, temporal average intensity (SATA): The average power output over the pulse repetition period divided by a reference (usually the transducer face area). This is the most quickly determined, most commonly used, and lowest measure of intensity.

spatial average, temporal peak intensity (SATP): The peak intensity over a selected area (most commonly the transducer face) that occurs when the ultrasonic emitting device is "on."

spatial peak, pulse average intensity (SPPA): The pulse-averaged intensity measured at the point in space where the value is maximal.

spatial peak, temporal average intensity (SPTA): The maximal spatial intensity when the sound beam is "on," averaged over the pulse repetition period.

spatial peak, temporal peak intensity (SPTP): The peak intensity at the point in space where the intensity is highest when the sound beam is "on." It is the highest of the measured intensities.

ultrasound absorption coefficient: The spatial average intensity of the ultrasound during the "on" time of the pulse (a measure of the amount of energy delivered to the tissue).

Phonophoresis

Phonophoresis, or *sonophoresis,* refers to the use of ultrasound to enhance transdermal delivery of medication. Current theories propose that ultrasound enhances drug delivery through the skin by increasing the permeability of the stratum corneum through cavitation.

Advantages. Advantages of phonophoresis over oral administration of drugs include higher initial drug concentration at delivery site, avoidance of gastric irritation, and first-pass metabolism by the liver. It allows drug delivery to a larger localized area than injection and avoids the pain, trauma, and infection risk of injection.

Precautions. Drugs delivered by phonophoresis eventually become systemic and therefore contraindications for systemic delivery of the drug also apply to delivery of the drug by phonophoresis. Avoid use of phonophoresis for a drug if that drug is already being administered by another route.

Intervention. Phonophoresis is primarily used to treat tissue inflammation and pain in tendon, bursa, or muscle by transdermal delivery of corticosteroids and NSAIDs. Lower frequency ultrasound (e.g., 20–100 kHz) results in the greatest increase in skin permeability. An example of recommended treatment parameters are pulsed 20% duty cycle, at 0.5 to 0.75 W/cm^2 intensity, for 5 to 10 min.

⬤ TABLE 18.5 Drug Delivery by Phonophoresis

Drug	Solution	Treatment Rationale	Principal Indication(s)
Dexamethasone	0.4% ointment	Synthetic steroidal anti-inflammatory agent	Inflammation

AGENTS

Drug	Solution	Treatment Rationale	Principal Indication(s)
Hydrocortisone	0.5%–1.0% ointment	Anti-inflammatory steroid	Inflammation
Iodine	10% ointment	Iodine is a broad-spectrum antibiotic, hence its use in infections, etc.; the sclerolytic actions of iodine are not fully understood.	Adhesive capsulitis and other soft tissue adhesions; microbial infections
Lidocaine (Xylocaine)	5% ointment	Local anesthetic effects	Soft tissue pain and inflammation (e.g., bursitis, tenosynovitis)
Magnesium sulfate	2% ointment	Muscle relaxant effect may be caused by decreased excitability of the skeletal muscle membrane and decreased transmission at the neuromuscular junction.	Skeletal muscle spasms; myositis
Salicylates	10% trolamine salicylate ointment, or 3% sodium salicylate ointment	Aspirin-like drugs with analgesic and anti-inflammatory effects.	Muscle and joint pain in acute and chronic conditions (e.g., overuse injuries, rheumatoid arthritis)
Zinc oxide	20% ointment	Zinc acts as a general antiseptic; may increase tissue healing.	Skin ulcers, other dermatologic disorders

Adapted from: Ciccone, CD: *Pharmacology in Rehabilitation,* ed. 3. FA Davis, Philadelphia, 1996, p 651 with permission.

References:

Belanger, AY: *Evidence-Based Guide to Therapeutic Physical Agents.* Lippincott Williams & Wilkins, Philadelphia, 2002.

Cameron, MH (ed): *Physical Agents in Rehabilitation: From Research to Practice,* ed. 3. Saunders, St. Louis, MO, 2003.

Gersh, MR: *Electrotherapy in Rehabilitation.* FA Davis, Philadelphia, 1992.

Mitragotri, S, et al: *Determination of threshold energy dose for ultrasound-induced transdermal drug transport. J Control Release 63(1–2):41–52, 2000.*

Mitragotri, S, and Kos, J: *Low frequency sonophoresis: A review. Adv Drug Deliv Rev 56(5):589–601, 2004.*

Hydrotherapy

One of the oldest therapeutic modalities, **hydrotherapy** (water therapy) is the application of water for the treatment of physical or psychological dysfunctions. Hydrotherapy achieves it effects through the following physical properties of water:

Thermal Properties. Water has high specific heat (ability to retain heat) and thermal conductivity (rate at which it can transfer thermal energy). During hydrotherapy, heat can be transferred by *conduction* (if water is stationary) or *convection* (if water is moving). **Note:** Refer to the section Thermal Agents for descriptions of heat transfer by physical agents.

Bouyancy. The upward (anti-gravity) force exerted on a body when it is immersed in water. The bouyancy of water offers a therapeutic medium for decreasing forces on tissue, or assisting weakened muscles to resist gravity. According to *Archimedes' principle,* the force exerted on a body that is immersed in water is equal to the weight of the water displaced by the body. Bouyancy is proportional to the density of the body relative to the density of water (i.e., *specific gravity*). Substances with a specific gravity less than 1.0 float in water (the human body has specific gravity of approximately 0.974).

Resistance. The *viscosity* of water produces a resistance to movement of a body in water that is proportionate to the speed of the body's movement. Strengthening exercises in water are designed to take advantage of this resistance.

Hydrostatic Pressure. A body immersed in water is subjected to pressure by the water. According to *Pascal's law*, the pressure is equal on all surfaces of the body at a given depth and increases proportionately to the depth of the fluid. (Water exerts 0.73 mm Hg pressure per cm of depth). This property is the basis for the joint support, reduction in edema, and cardiac conditioning effects of water immersion.

Water Temperature Classifications
Very Cold: 1°C to 13°C (33°F to 55°F)
Cold: 14°C to 18°C (56°F to 65°F)
Cool: 19°C to 26°C (66°F to 80°F)
Tepid: 27°C to 32°C (81°F to 92°F)
Neutral: 33°C to 35°C (93°F to 96°F)
Warm: 36°C to 37°C (97°F to 99°F)
Hot: 38°C to 40°C (100°F to 104°F)
Very Hot: 41°C to 43°C (105°F to 110°F)

● TABLE 18.6 Hydrotherapy—Indications, Contraindications, and Precautions

Indications
Wound healing (cleansing effect)
Joint disorders (bouyancy effect)
Musculoskeletal diseases (resistance effect)
Peripheral edema (hydrostatic pressure effect)
Aging (all effects)
Pain control (sensory stimulation and bouyancy effect)
Burns (cleansing, bouyancy, and resistive effects)
Wound healing (cleansing effect)

Contraindications
Local immersion hydrotherapy
• Maceration around a wound
• Active bleeding
• Malignancies
• Acute inflammatory conditions
• Tissues devitalized by x-ray therapy
Full body immersion hydrotherapy
• Cardiac instability
• Severe epilepsy
• Acute inflammatory conditions
• Tissues devitalized by x-ray therapy
• Malignancies
• Peripheral vascular disease (PVD)
• Infection conditions
• Bowel Incontinence

Precautions
Local immersion hydrotherapy
• Impaired thermal sensation
• Infection
• Impaired cognition and confusion.
• recent skin grafts
Full body immersion hydrotherapy
• Impaired cognition and confusion
• Ingestion of alcohol
• Extreme limitations in strength, endurance, balance, ROM
• Certain cardiovascular medicines (refer to Table 19.1)
• Urinary incontinence
• Respiratory problems
• Fear of water
• Wound infection
Full body immersion in hot or very warm water
• Pregnancy
• Multiple Sclerosis

Source: Cameron, MH (ed): *Physical Agents In Rehabilitation: From Research to Practice,* ed. 3. Saunders, St. Louis, MO, 2009, pp 252–264.

Hydrotherapy Modalities

contrast bath: A treatment technique to increase superficial blood flow by alternately placing the body part in very hot (105°F–110°F, 40.6°C–43.3°C) and very cold (59°F–68°F, 15°C–20°C) water. Whirlpool tanks are typically used.

Hubbard tank: See *whirlpool*.

moist air cabinet: A cabinet that encompasses approximately one-half of the patient's body, which is either seated or supine. Water is heated to 103°F to 113°F (40°C–45°C), and air is blown past the water, absorbing the moisture and heat and circulating it within the cabinet.

peloid: Mineral mud is heated and applied to the body.

sauna bath: A chamber made of wood in which stones or bricks are heated so that the room air, which is typically kept at low humidity, is raised to approximately 140°F to 176°F (60°C–80°C) or higher. The hot and dry air promotes sweating and subsequent evaporation on the body. This treatment is commonly followed by a cold shower.

Scotch douche: A shower of alternating hot (100°F–110°F, 37.8°C–43.3°C) and cold (80°F–60°F, 26.7°C–15.5°C) water.

sitz bath: A bath in which the pelvic and perineal areas are covered in water. Hot sitz baths require a temperature of 105°F to 115°F (40.5°C–46°C). Cold sitz baths require a temperature of 35°F to 75°F (17°C–24°C).

whirlpool: A modality used for warm, hot, or cold immersion therapy. Stainless steel or plastic tanks contain water that is thermostatically controlled and aerated to produce turbulence. Whirlpool tanks come in various sizes, such as the low boy tank in which the patient can sit, or the Hubbard tank for full-body treatment.

Spinal Traction

This section describes modalities used to apply forces to the cervical or lumbar spine as a means of seperating the joint surfaces or elongation of surrounding tissue.

Physical Effects of Spinal Traction

- Distract joint surfaces
- Stretch soft tissue
- Relax muscles
- Mobilize joints
- Reduce disc protrusion

🔴 TABLE 18.7 **Types of Spinal Traction**

Type	Description	Application
Continuous	Application of relatively small (20 lb) constant force (e.g., several hours each day for 10–14 hr).	To keep the patient immobile, e.g., to enforce strict bed rest. Currently rarely used as an intervention for neck and back pain.
Sustained (static)	Continuous short-period of traction (10–45 min). Can also be applied at much higher force levels (50% body weight) for even shorter periods.	Reduction of disc herniation or bulging, lengthening of soft tissue, relaxation of muscle,* and reduction of pain. Usually chosen for more acute conditions to avoid stretch reflex response and hypersensitivity of soft tissue that may be associated with intermittent traction.
Intermittent	Alternating brief periods of traction force application (hold) and force release (rest). Duration of each may vary 5–60 sec. Ratio of hold/rest is typically 1:1 or 1:2. Total duration of treatment ranges from 10–30 min. Forces are typically less than with static traction.	Reduction of disc herniation or bulging, lengthening of soft tissue, relaxation of muscle,* and reduction of pain. May be better suited for joint mobilization or for patients who cannot tolerate static traction.

Source: Michlovitz, SL, and Nolan, TP: *Modalities for Therapeutic Intervention,* ed. 4. Philadelphia, FA Davis, 2005, pp 166, 170–171.
*Note: The choice of static or intermittent traction for lumbar paraspinal muscle relaxation may depend solely on patient tolerance.

🔴 TABLE 18.8 **Methods of Traction Delivery**

Method	Description	Purpose
Bed traction	Continuous application of relatively low traction force using weights and pulleys for long periods (several hours to most of a day) while the patient is in bed.	To help maintain immobilization during an acute phase of neck or back pain; however, it is currently rarely used.
Mechanical traction	Traction forces are applied to the patient by an electrical or mechanical device (e.g., traction table)	Used to distract joint surfaces, reduce protrusions of disc material, stretch soft tissue, relax muscles,

(table continues on page 1096)

AGENTS

● **TABLE 18.8 Methods of Traction Delivery** (continued)

Method	Description	Purpose
	that can be programmed for force, duration, and duty cycle. Duration typically limited to 10–30 min. Available as electrical mechanical traction units or as inexpensive over-the-door cervical traction devices for in-home use.	and mobilize joints. Electrical devices have the advantage of being able to deliver higher, well-controlled, replicable forces and offer either static or intermittent delivery of traction and adjustability.
Manual traction	Application of traction force manually by a practitioner.	Most often applied to cervical spine, but may also be applied to lumbar spine via a hooklying position utilizing a belt around thighs and practitioner. Has the advantage of enabling the practitioner to feel patient's reaction to manual traction forces which may be delivered statically for short durations (15–60 sec), or as a sudden thrust.
Positional traction	Application of traction force by the positioning of the body in a way that will alter the relationship of the bony surfaces in the area to be treated. Pillows and bolsters are often used to achieve the desired position. Duration is determined by patient tolerance and response to treatment.	Used to alleviate pressure on an entrapped spinal nerve and promote paravertebral muscle relaxation.
Gravity-assisted traction	Traction to the lumbar spine by the use of a chest harness on a table that can be tilted to a vertical position, allowing the lower half of the body to hang free and provide a distraction force to lumbar spine. Amount of force adjusted by the degree of tilt to the table.	Treatment of lumbar disc herniation; paravertebral muscle relaxation.

Method	Description	Purpose
Inversion traction	Traction forces applied to lumbar spine via gravity by having the patient hang in an inverted position using straps or boots. Duration is usually 5–15 min.	Same use as gravity-assisted traction; added precautions for patients who may be apprehensive, fragile, or not tolerate the cardiovascular demands (increase in blood pressure) of inversion. More commonly used when introduced in the late 1980s to mid-1990s; less commonly used today.
Autotraction	Traction forces applied to lumbar spine using a combination of mechanical table traction and self-applied forces by holding or pulling on overhead bars.	Requires a special adjustable traction bench which has grown out of favor due to cost and difficulty for some patients to use.

Source: Michlovitz, SL, and Nolan, TP: *Modalities for Therapeutic Intervention*, ed 4. FA Davis, 2005, Philadelphia, pp 166, 170–171.

■ TABLE 18.9 Traction—Indications, Contraindications, and Precautions

Indications
Radiculopathy from herniated or bulging disc
Narrowing of the intervertebral foramen
Osteophytes encroachment
Ligament encroachment
Spondylolisthesis
Degenerated zygapophyseal joints

Contraindications
Systemic diseases affecting the integrity of the spine; e.g., rheumatoid arthritis
Fracture, subluxation, or dislocation of the spine following trauma
Spinal hypermobility or instability
Hiatal or abdominal hernia
Spinal cord compression
Pregnancy (lumbar traction only)
Vertebral artery occlusion (cervical traction only)
Aortic aneurysm
Temperomandibular joint pain or dysfunction (use of halter for cervical traction)
Uncontrolled hypertension (inversion traction only)
Non-musculoskeletal causes of neck or back pain

(table continues on page 1098)

AGENTS

● **TABLE 18.9 Traction—Indications, Contraindications, and Precautions** (continued)

Precautions
Acute neck and back pain
Claustrophobia
Mental disorientation or confusion
Children or frail, elderly patients
History of surgery to the spine
Hyperactivity or restlessness
Obesity
Respiratory problems (particularly with lumbar traction)
Cardiovascular problems
History of domestic violence (especially in cervical region)

Sources: Michlovitz, SL, and Nolan, TP: *Modalities for Therapeutic Intervention,* ed. 4. FA Davis, Philadelphia, 2005, pp 166, 169–170; Cameron, MH: *Physical Agents in Rehabilitation: From Research to Practice,* ed. 3. Saunders, St. Louis, MO, 2009, pp 288–297.

● **TABLE 18.10 Recommended Parameters for the Application of Spinal Traction**

Phases or Goals of Treatment	Force	Hold/Relax Times (seconds)	Total Traction Time (minutes)
Lumbar Spinal Traction Initial acute phase	13–20 kg (29–44 lb)	Static	5–10
Joint distraction	22.5 kg (50 lb; 50% of body weight)	15/15	20–30
Decrease muscle spasm	25% of body weight	5/5	20–30
Disc problem or stretch soft tissue	25% of body weight	60/20	20–30
Cervical Spinal Traction Initial acute phase	3 to 4 kg (7–9 lb)	Static	5–10
Joint distraction	9 to 13 kg (20–29 lb); 7%	15/15	20–30
Decrease muscle spasm	5 to 7 kg (11–15 lb)	5/5	20–30
Disc problem or stretch of soft tissue	5 to 7 kg (11–15 lb)	60/20	20–30

Source: Cameron, MH: *Physical Agents in Rehabilitation: From Research to Practice,* ed. 3. Saunders, St. Louis, MO, 2009, pp 301, 304.

Mechanical Compression

Mechanical compression is defined as the therapeutic application of external mechanical pressure that is used most commonly for control or reduction of edema. It is often applied intermittently through a pump device (intermittent pneumatic compression [IPC] or sequential pump) or through compression bandaging, compression garments, or Velcro closure devices.

Physical Properties of External Compression

- Increase circulation by increasing hydrostatic extravascular pressure (interstitial space outside the blood and lymphatic vessels). Increased extravascular pressure limits the outflow and pooling of fluid from the vessels, thereby keeping it in circulation.
- Intermittent compression may "milk" fluids from distal to proximal vessels, thereby improving circulation more than static compression
- Sequential compression can create a wave of compression from distal to proximal that may provide even more effective milking than single-chamber, intermittent compression.
- Static compression garments and bandages may provide a form to limit the shape and size of new tissue formation.
- Most compression devices have a secondary effect of increasing superficial tissue temperature by the insulation provided by the garment, sleeve, or stocking. This may explain possible wound-healing benefits from compression.

TABLE 18.11   IPC—Indications, Contraindications, and Precautions

Indications
Edema
Traumatic edema
Venous stasis ulcers
Stump reduction in amputated limbs
Prevention of deep vein thrombosis (DVT)
Wound healing
Arterial insufficiency
Lymphedema

Contraindications
Acute pulmonary edema
Congestive heart failure
Acute DVT, thrombophlebitis, or pulmonary embolism
Obstructed lymphatic or venous return
Severe peripheral arterial disease
Severe hypoproteinemia (<2g/dL)

(table continues on page 1100)

TABLE 18.11 IPC—Indications, Contraindications, and Precautions (continued)

Contraindications
Acute trauma or fracture
Acute local dermatologic infections
Arterial revascularization

Precautions
Impaired sensation or mentation
Uncontrolled hypertension
Cancer
Stroke or cerebrovascular insufficiency
Over superficial peripheral nerves

Source: Michlovitz, SL, and Nolan, TP: *Modalities for Therapeutic Intervention,* ed. 4. FA Davis, Philadelphia, 2005, pp 174–175; Cameron, MH: *Physical Agents in Rehabilitation: From Research to Practice,* ed. 3. Saunders, 2009, St. Louis, MO, pp 325–328.

Reference:

Belanger, AY: Evidence-Based Guide to Therapeutic Physical Agents. Lippincott Williams & Wilkins, Philadelphia, 2002.

TABLE 18.12 Treatment Guidelines for IPC Recommended by the Jobst Institute

Indications	Pressure (mm Hg)	Recommended Treatment Periods	Inflation Time (on)	Deflation Time (off)
Post-mastectomy lymphedema	30–50	Two treatments per day for 3 hr	80–100 sec	25–30 sec
Edema of lower extremities	30–60	Two treatments per day for 3 hr	80–100 sec	25–30 sec
Peripheral edema and venous stasis ulceration	85	One treatment period of 2.5 hr, three times per week	80–100 sec	30 sec
Stump reduction	30–60	Three treatment periods per day for 4 hr	40–60 sec	10–15 sec
Hand edema	30–50	Two treatment periods a day of 30 min to 1 hr each	Extended position: 5–10 min	Flexed position: 5–10 min

From: Michlovitz, SL, and Nolan, TP: *Modalities for Therapeutic Intervention,* ed. 4. FA Davis, Philadelphia, 2005, pp 203, with permission.

Electromagnetic Agents

Electric currents are used widely in health care for diagnosis, treatment, surgery, and communication. The recent integration of digital technology into electrotherapeutic devices has revolutionized the use of these agents and increased their versatility in rehabilitation practice. The fundamental principles of electromagnetic radiation and its application in practice are unchanged despite these advances.

Note: The use of electromagnetic agents for wound care is presented primarily in Section VIII, Integumentary.

Physical Laws

Electromagnetic agents are components of the **electromagnetic spectrum.** The therapeutic effects of electromagnetic radiation are determined primarily by their frequency and wavelength characteristics. The intensity of the electromagnetic source reaching the body is determined primarily by the amplitude or intensity of its waveform as well as the proximity and orientation of the source to the surface of the body.

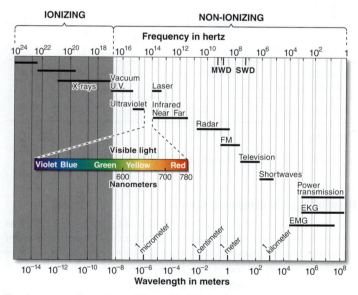

The electromagnetic spectrum. *Source: IES Lighting Handbook: The Standard Lighting Guide, ed. 5. Illuminating Engineering Society, New York, 1972.*

AGENTS

● TABLE 18.13 Wavelength and Frequency of Electromagnetic Agents

Radiation	Wavelength (range in nm)*	Frequency (upper limit in Hz)
Electric power	0.5×10^{15}	60
Long-wave diathermy	300×10^9–30×10^9	10^6
Short-wave diathermy	30×10^9–3×10^9	10^7
Microwave	1×10^9–1.5×10^9	3×10^8
Long (far) infrared	15,000–1,500	2.0×10^{13}
Short (near) infrared	1,500–800	2.0×10^{14}
Laser	10,600–193 (nm)	1×10^{16} (upper limit in Hz)
Visible light	800–400	3.75×10^{14}
Long (near) ultraviolet—UVA	400–280	7.5×10^{14}
Long (near) ultraviolet—UVB	315–280	9.0×10^{14}
Short (far) ultraviolet—UVC	280–230	1.03×10^{15}
Roentgen (x-rays)	120–0.14	5.9×10^{15}
Gamma 0	14–0.01	2.14×10^{18}

*Nanometer (nm) is equal to 10 angstrom (Å) or 10^{-7} cm.

Intensity of Electromagnetic Agents

- **inverse square law:** The intensity of the electromagnetic radiation received (RR) varies inversely with the square of the distance (D) from the source of the radiation. The following formula predicts the radiation received from a single source; it is not applicable to reflected radiation:

$$RR = \text{Radiation source} / D^2$$

- **cosine law:** Maximal radiation is applied when the source of radiation is at a right angle to the patient. The applied radiation is directly proportional to the cosine of the angle formed by the patient's body with the source of radiation.

Electrotherapy

Physical Principles of Electricity

An **electric current** is a flow of charged particles (electrons or ions). Electric charge is determined by the net sum of protons (+) and electrons (−). When like charged particles are in proximity they repel each other; opposite charges attract. The force is proportional to the magnitude of the charge and the distance between them (according to **Coulomb's law**). These attractive and repulsive forces create an **electric field.** Substances that allow the movement of charged particles are called **conductors;** those that limit movement are called **insulators.** The electric force that is capable of moving a charged particle through a conductor between two regions is the **potential difference** or **voltage (V,** measured in **volts).** The movement of charged particles in a conductor as a result of an applied voltage is referred to as **current (A,** measured in **amperes).** Charged particles encounter some opposition to movement, referred to as resistance (Ω, measured in ohms). **Ohm's law** states that current in a conductor will vary proportionately to the voltage, and inversely to the resistance.

Physiological Effects of Electricity

The therapeutic application of electrical current to the body requires the placement of at least two electrodes on the body, one negatively charged **(cathode)** and the other positively charged **(anode).** When electric currents pass through biological tissue, chemical, thermal, and physical effects result as summarized below:

- **Electrochemical:** Electrical compounds are formed beneath the electrodes. Chlorides in the skin combine with water to produce hydrochloric acid under the anode **(acid reaction).** Sodium in the skin combines with water to form sodium hydroxide under the cathode **(alkaline reaction).** Extreme acid reaction (only in interventions using DC, such as iontophoresis) may lead to sclerosis (hardening) of tissue and chemical burns. Alkaline reaction may cause liquefication of proteins in skin, resulting in a softening of the tissue.

- **Electrothermal:** The vibration of moving charges combined with friction from the tissue will cause energy to be released in the form of heat. High root mean square (RMS) average current applied for prolonged periods across skin with high impedance may result in burning or blistering of skin. DC currents will encounter high skin impedances whereas AC or pulsed currents typically do not. Pulsed current also has lower RMS and therefore even less of a thermal effect.

- **Electrophysical:** The therapeutic effect of electrical modalities results from the flow of ions in the biological tissue beneath the anode-cathode electrodes (refer to the figure on p. 1105). This is also referred to as the **electrokinetic effect.** The most apparent result of this movement of ions is the depolarization of peripheral nerves, resulting in either motor or sensory responses.

Current Types

There are two basic types of current, **direct current (DC)** and **alternating current (AC).** Basic DC and AC waveforms are not well suited for most electrotherapeutic interventions and are therefore either modulated as described in the figure below and on p. 1105, or delivered as **pulsed current (PC)**, which is described in the figure at the bottom of p. 1105 and the figure on p. 1106.

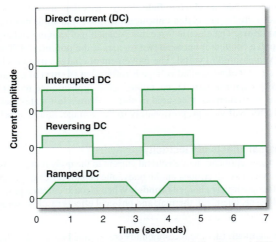

Continuous, interrupted, reversing, and ramped forms of direct current (DC) are illustrated. *Adapted from: Michlovitz, SL, and Nolan, TP: Modalities for Therapeutic Intervention, ed. 4. FA Davis, Philadelphia, 2005, p 99, with permission.*

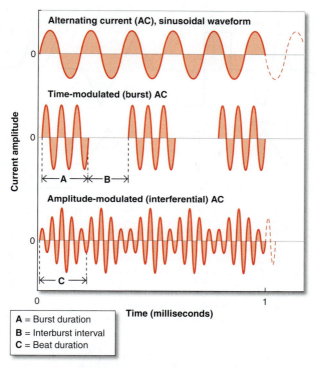

A = Burst duration
B = Interburst interval
C = Beat duration

Continuous, Time-modulated, and Amplitude-modulated forms of Alternating Current (AC) are illustrated. *Adapted from: Michlovitz, SL, and Nolan, TP: Modalities for Therapeutic Intervention, ed. 4. FA Davis, Philadelphia, 2005, p 100, with permission.*

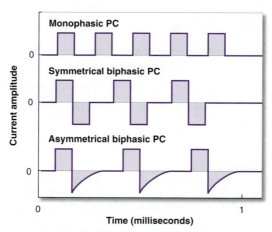

A monophasic, and two types of biphasic, waveforms are illustrated. *Modified from: Michlovitz, SL, and Nolan, TP: Modalities for Therapeutic Intervention, ed. 4. FA Davis, Philadelphia, 2005, p 101, with permission.*

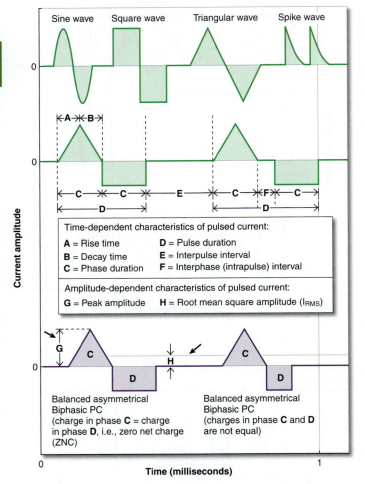

Four common types of pulsed waveforms (*sine wave, square wave, triangular wave,* and *spike wave*) are illustrated (upper diagram) as well as the time-dependent (A–F) and amplitude-dependent (G, H) parameters. *Adapted from: Michlovitz, SL, and Nolan, TP: Modalities for Therapeutic Intervention, ed. 4. FA Davis, Philadelphia, 2005, pp 101–103, with permission.*

Electrical Stimulation

There are several therapeutic forms of electrical stimulation that are included in this section, each with its own terminology. **Neuromuscular electrical stimulation (NMES)** is the application of electric currents to innervated muscle for the purpose of strengthening or improving motor control, decreasing muscle spasticity, or enhancing tissue extensibility. When applied to create or enhance the performance of a functional activity, such as in patients with neurological disorders, it is referred to as **functional electrical stimulation (FES).** Different electrical waveforms are utilized for therapeutic activation of denervated muscle, which is more accurately referred to as **electrical muscle stimulation (EMS).** Electrical activation of sensory fibers for the purpose of providing analgesia is referred to as **transcutaneous electrical nerve stimulation (TENS).**

The use of electrical stimulation for wound healing is covered in Section VII, Integumentary.

Neuromuscular Electrical Stimulation (NMES)
Responses to Nerve and Muscle Stimulation
There are three types of responses to electrical stimulation: *sensory, motor,* and *noxious.*

- **Sensory-level stimulation:** Often elicits a "pins-and-needles" sensation; occurs as a result of excitation of sensory nerve fibers that are located in or near the skin in the vicinity of the electrodes.
- **Motor-level stimulation:** Production of a muscle contraction in the intact nervous systems when the activation threshold of alpha motoneuron axons in peripheral nerves innervating the skeletal muscle is reached.
- **Noxious-level stimulation:** Activation of A-delta and C nerve fibers, which carry signals associated with painful stimuli, occurs with increasing amplitude of stimulation. Strong muscle contractions may also occur.

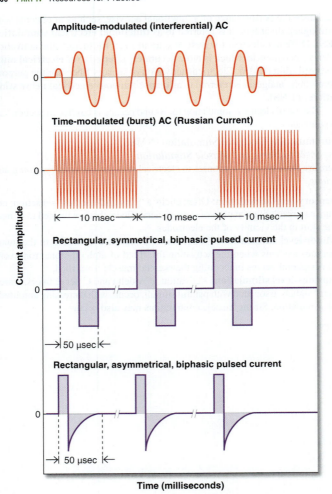

Examples of currents used with commercially available stimulators designed for neuromuscular electrical stimulation. *From Robinson, AJ, and Snyder-Mackler, L (eds): Clinical Electrophysiology: Electrotherapy and Electrophysiologic Testing, ed. 2. Williams & Wilkins, Baltimore, 1995, p 64, with permission.*

TABLE 18.14 NMES Parameters Typically Used for Muscle Strengthening

Waveform	Symmetrical or asymmetrical biphasic pulsed current, burst-modulated alternating current (ex: Russian current)
Pulse duration	200–600 μsec

Frequency	20–100 pps (bursts per second)
Amplitude	To obtain strong muscle contraction (maximum tolerated or current necessary to achieve ≥50% of MVC)
Ramp-up time	1–5 sec
Ramp-down time	1–2 sec
Duty cycle	1:3 to 1:5 with on times up to 10 sec and off time up to 50 sec
Treatment time and duration	At least 10 contractions or up to 1 hr/day 3–5 times/wk 4–8 wk
Carrier frequency*	1,000–2,500 Hz
Burst duration*	2–10 msec
Relative duty cycle*	10%–50%

MVC = Maximal Voluntary Contraction
* Specific to burst-modulated AC (BMAC)
Adapted from: Michlovitz, SL, et al: *Modalities for Therapeutic Intervention,* ed. 5. FA Davis, Philadelphia, 2012, p 288, with permission.

● TABLE 18.15 NMES Parameters Typically Used for Enhancing Tissue Extensibility

Waveform	Symmetrical or asymmetrical biphasic PC
Pulse duration	200–300 μsec
Frequency	12–33 pps
Amplitude	To obtain 3+/5 contraction
Ramp-up time	3 sec (for comfort)
Ramp-down time	1–2 sec
Duty cycle	1:1 (typically 10 sec on, 10 sec off)
Treatment time and duration	15 min–6 hr per day, 1–4 times/day, 2 wk–6 mo

Adapted from: Michlovitz, SL, and Nolan, TP: *Modalities for Therapeutic Intervention,* ed. 4. FA Davis, Philadelphia, 2005, p. 254, with permission.

AGENTS

TABLE 18.16   NMES Parameters Typically Used for Decreasing Muscle Spasticity

Waveform	Symmetrical or asymmetrical biphasic PC, or medium-frequency burst AC (Russian current)
Pulse duration	250–500 μsec
Frequency	20–60 pps
Amplitude	To obtain a contraction (at least a grade 3+/5)
Ramp-up time	2–3 sec
Ramp-down time	2–3 sec
Duty cycle	Variable (1:1, 3:4, 10:7) but typically larger ratio than for muscle strengthening
Treatment time and duration	10–45 min per day. Treatment typically needs to continue for effect to remain, unless recovery of movement is occurring.

Adapted from: Michlovitz, SL, and Nolan, TP: *Modalities for Therapeutic Intervention,* ed. 4. FA Davis, Philadelphia, 2005, p. 255, with permission.

Functional Electrical Stimulation (FES)

TABLE 18.17   FES Parameters Typically Used for Shoulder Subluxation

Waveform	Symmetrical or asymmetrical biphasic PC
Pulse duration	200–350 μsec
Frequency	30–40 pps
Amplitude	To achieve effect without abduction or shoulder elevation
Ramp-up time	3 sec
Ramp-down time	3 sec
Duty cycle	Range 1:5 to 15:1. Typically start with a 1:5, 1:3, or 1:1, but goal is to quickly increase on time and decrease off time as muscle endurance improves. On times up to 30 sec can be used if tolerated by muscles.
Treatment time and duration	30 min–6 hr (start low and increase as endurance improves), 5–7 days per wk, 4–6 wk

Adapted from: Michlovitz, SL, and Nolan, TP: *Modalities for Therapeutic Intervention,* ed. 4. FA Davis, Philadelphia, 2005, p. 259, with permission.

🔴 TABLE 18.18 FES Parameters Typically Used for Hand Function

Waveform	Symmetrical or asymmetrical biphasic PC
Pulse duration	200–350 µsec
Frequency	30–40 pps
Amplitude	To achieve desired movement for function. Keep as low as is feasible.
Ramp-up time	Relatively short to achieve effect
Ramp-down time	Relatively short to achieve effect
Duty cycle	N/A. Stimulation is timed with demand of functional activity.
Treatment time and duration	Determined by muscle fatigue

Adapted from: Michlovitz, SL, and Nolan, TP: *Modalities for Therapeutic Intervention,* ed. 4. FA Davis, Philadelphia, 2005, p. 261, with permission.

🔴 TABLE 18.19 FES Parameters Typically Used for Dorsiflexion Assist

Waveform	Symmetrical or asymmetrical biphasic PC
Pulse duration	200–350 µsec
Frequency	30–40 pps
Amplitude	To achieve grade 3+/5 contraction
Ramp-up time	0 sec
Ramp-down time	0 sec
Duty cycle	N/A. Stimulation is timed with demand of functional activity.
Treatment time and duration	Determined by muscle fatigue

Adapted from: Michlovitz, SL, and Nolan, TP: *Modalities for Therapeutic Intervention,* ed. 4. FA Davis, Philadelphia, 2005, p. 263, with permission.

FES for Urinary Incontinence

AGENTS

● **TABLE 18.20 FES Parameters for Reducing Urinary Incontinence**

Parameter	Setting
Waveform	Symmetrical or asymmetrical biphasic PC or interferential medium frequency
Pulse duration	300–1,000 μs
Frequency	Urge incontinence: 5–20 pps (12 pps common) Stress incontinence: 20–50 pps (50 pps common)
Ramp-up time	2 sec
Ramp-down time	2 sec
Duty cycle	1:3, 1:2, 1:1 (typically 5 sec "on" time)
Treatment time	15–30 min
Duration	1–3 times/day, 4–12 wk

Adapted from: Michlovitz, SL, and Nolan, TP: *Modalities for Therapeutic Intervention,* ed. 4. FA Davis, Philadelphia, 2005, p 264, 2005, with permission.

Electrical Muscle Stimulation

● **TABLE 18.21 EMS Parameters Typically Used for Stimulating Denervated Muscle**

Waveform	Monophasic
Pulse duration	1–450 ms (long)
Frequency	1–500 pps
Amplitude	To obtain contraction but low to prevent burns
Ramp-up time	Not identified
Ramp-down time	Not identified
Duty cycle	Highly variable 30 min–8 hr per day
Treatment time and duration	5–7 days per wk 4 days–4 yr

Adapted from: Michlovitz, SL, et al: *Modalities for Therapeutic Intervention,* ed. 5. FA Davis, Philadelphia, 2012, p 296 with permission.

Iontophoresis

Iontophoresis is the parenteral delivery of medicinal ions using a direct (DC) electrical current. Current devices in use are battery operated and portable with commercially available reservoir electrodes. Ionized forms of the medication must be placed in the electrode receptacle of the same polarity as the medication for it to be "repelled" into the tissue. The exact pathway by which the ions travel is not known.

TABLE 18.22 Optimal Current Variables for Iontophoresis

Type	DC
Amplitude	1.0–4.0 mA
Duration	20–40 min
Total current dosage	40–80 mA/min
Optimal current density at delivery electrode	0.1 – 0.5 mA/cm

Adapted from: Robinson, AJ, and Snyder-Mackler, L (eds): *Clinical Electrophysiology: Electrotherapy and Electrophysiologic Testing,* ed. 2. Williams & Wilkins, Baltimore, 1995, p 339, with permission.

TABLE 18.23 Indications and Drugs Used for Iontophoresis Interventions

Drug	Indication	Solution	Polarity of Delivery Electrode	Effect
Dexamethasone	Inflammation	4 mg/mL in aqueous solution	Negative	Anti-inflammatory
Acetic acid	Calcific tendonitis, myositis ossificans	2%–5% aqueous solution	Negative	Believed to increase solubility of calcium deposits
Iodine	Adhesive capsulitis and other soft tissue adhesions	5%–10% solution or ointment	Negative	Sclerolytic effects
Lidocaine	Soft tissue pain and inflammation	4%–5% solution or ointment	Positive	Local anesthetic effects

(table continues on page 1114)

● TABLE 18.23 Indications and Drugs Used for Iontophoresis Interventions (continued)

Drug	Indication	Solution	Polarity of Delivery Electrode	Effect
Salicylates	Muscle and joint pain	10% tro- lamine salicylate ointment or 2%–3% sodium salicylate solution	Negative	Analgesic and anti- inflammatory
Hyaluronidase	Local subacute or chronic edema	Reconstitute with 0.9% sodium chloride to provide a 150 mg/mL solution	Positive	Dispersion of local edema
Calcium chloride	Skeletal muscle spasms	2% aqueous solution	Positive	Decreased excitability of periph- eral nerves and skele- tal muscle
Magnesium sulfate	Skeletal mus- cle spasms, myositis	2% aqueous solution or ointment	Positive	Muscle relaxant
Zinc oxide	Skin ulcers	20% ointment	Positive	Acts as a general antiseptic and may increase tissue healing
Tap water	Hyperhidrosis	N/A	Alternat- ing polarity	Decreased sweating of palms, feet, or axillae

From Michlovitz, SL, et al: *Modalities for Therapeutic Intervention,* ed. 5. FA Davis, Philadelphia, 2012, p 270 with permission.
Source: Ciccone, CD: *Pharmacology in Rehabilitation,* ed 3. FA Davis, Philadelphia, 2002, p 651.

Transcutaneous Electrical Nerve Stimulation (TENS)

TENS for pain control, also referred to as **electroanalgesia,** was first popularized in the 1960s following the gate-control theory that electrical stimulation may modulate the sensation of pain by interference with its transmission from the spinal cord. This mechanism led to **conventional TENS,** which is applied for relatively long periods as needed to "close the gate" on pain sensation. A second short-term TENS application, referred to as **acupuncture-like TENS,** stimulates motor or A-delta nociceptor fibers that may elicit the release of endorphins or enkephalins. The recommended parameter settings for these uses of TENS are summarized. **Note: Accommodation,** or the decrease in therapeutic response over time, can be minimized by modulating the pulse duration or pulse frequency, or a combination of both.

■ **TABLE 18.24 Recommended Parameter Settings for TENS**

Technique	Target	Waveform	Pulse Frequency	Pulse Duration	Amplitude	Mechanism	Duration
Conventional TENS	Sensory	Monophasic or biphasic PC	100–150 pps	Short: 50–100 μs	To produce tingling sensation	Gating at the spinal cord	Worn as needed for pain control
Acupuncture-like TENS	Motor	Biphasic	2–10 pps	Long: 200–300 μs	To produce muscle twitching	Endorphin and enkephalon release	20–45 min

Sources: Michlovitz, SL, and Nolan,TP: *Modalities for Therapeutic Intervention*, ed. 4. FA Davis, Philadelphia, 2005, p 112; Cameron, MH, ed: *Physical Agents in Rehabilitation: From Research to Practice*, ed. 3. Saunders, St. Louis, 2009, p 219.

TABLE 18.25 Electrical Stimulation—Contraindications and Precautions

Contraindications
Demand cardiac pacemaker
Unstable cardiac arrhythmias
Over carotid sinus
Venous thrombosis, arterial thrombosis, or thrombophlebitis is present
Pregnancy (abdomen or lower back)
Demand cardiac pacemaker

Precautions
Cardiac disease
Impaired mentation
Areas with impaired sensation
Malignant tumors
Open wounds or skin irritation
Bony prominences

Laser and Light

Laser is an acronym for *l*ight *a*mplification by *s*timulated *e*mission *r*adiation. In the field of rehabilitation medicine lasers are categorized as either "hot" lasers for their thermal properties, or "cold" lasers, which produce their effect through radiant energy imparted into the tissue, referred to as **photobiostimulation.**

Physical Principals

Laser is a special form of electromagnetic energy that is within the visible or infrared region of the electromagnetic spectrum (see figure on p. 1101). Lasers have three physical properties that distinguish them from incandescent and fluorescent light sources: *coherence, monochromaticity,* and a *collimated beam.* Laser light can be transmitted into the tissue without alteration of its characteristic properties (*direct penetration*) or with alteration due to the hyperscopic absorption properties of the tissue (*indirect penetration*).Originally, these devices used gas-filled tubes in which electrical stimulation of the gases would cause emission of radiation at a specific wavelength. Current devices use **photodiodes** instead of glass tubes .

Types of Lasers Used in Physical Therapy

Lasers can be classified as **high-power** or **low-power.** Only low-power lasers (i.e., "cold" laser light with average power less than 60 mW) are available for physical therapy treatments. The power of most laser diodes used for therapy is between 5 and 500 mW and these devices are classified as **Class IIIb** lasers according to the Food and Drug Administration (FDA) and the IEC 60825-1 (International Electrotechnical Commission) standard for safety. Cold lasers for **low-level laser therapy (LLLT)** include the following agents:

HeNe Laser. Electrical stimulation of helium and neon gases causes the emission of radiation at a wavelength of 632.8 nm (within the red band of visible light). The light is amplified and directed to the tip of a handheld fiber optic wand that applies the laser beam in a pulsed or continuous mode to the tissue to be stimulated. Penetration of this laser light is to a depth of 0.8 mm (direct) or 10 mm to 15 mm (indirect).

GaAs Laser. The gallium arsenide laser is the first "semiconductor" laser and is produced in a diode composed of a thin coating of zinc on gallium arsenide, which allows electric current to pass in only one direction. The reaction at the gallium arsenide–zinc junction produces laser light at a wavelength of 910 nm (within the infrared or invisible spectrum). The energy is delivered in the pulsed mode and has a reported depth of tissue penetration of 5 cm (indirect).

GaAlAs Laser. Similar to the GaAs laser, the gallium aluminum arsenide laser (830 nm) was approved by the U.S. Food and Drug Administration (FDA) in early 2002 for the treatment of carpal tunnel syndrome and designated a Class II medical device.

TABLE 18.26 Laser Classification

Class	Power	Effects
1 1M	< 0.5 mW	No hazard No hazard because the beam has a large diameter or is divergent.
2	< 1 mW	Safe for momentary viewing; will provoke a blink relex.
3A	< 5 mW	Commonly used for laser pointers. Poses an eye hazard with prolonged exposure.
3B	< 500 mW	Used for therapy. Can cause permanent eye injury with brief exposure. Direct viewing of the beam should be avoided. Viewing of the diffuse beam reflected from the skin is safe. Can cause minor skin burns with prolonged exposure.
4	> 500 mW	Surgical and industrial cutting lasers. Can cause permanent eye injury before you can react. Can cause serious skin burns. Can burn clothing. Use with extreme caution.

From Cameron, MH (ed): *Physical Agents in Rehabilitation: From Research to Practice,* ed. 3. Saunders, St. Louis, MO, 2009, p 353, with permission.

FDA Classification of Low-Power Lasers

Although their use in medicine is expanding, low-power lasers (cold lasers) until recently had all been classified by the FDA as Class III medical devices for approved experimental use. Therefore, practitioners must ordinarily obtain an investigational device exemption from the FDA (FDA regulation 812.2[b]) prior to use.

 TABLE 18.27 Laser: Indications, Contraindications, and Precautions

Indications
Soft tissue healing Bone healing Pain management for musculoskeletal conditions Lymphedema Neuropathy

Contraindications
Pregnant women Enclosed fontanelles of children Cancerous lesions Cornea (note: operator and patient should wear filter goggles) Thyroid and other endocrine glands Hemorrhaging lesions Within 4–6 mo following radiotherapy

Precautions
Epilepsy Fever Areas of decreased sensation Infected tissue Application to gonads, epiphyseal plates of children, sympathetic ganglia, vagus nerve, mediastinum, and low back or abdomen of pregnant women

Source: Cameron, MH (ed): *Physical Agents in Rehabilitation: From Research to Practice*, ed. 3. Saunders, St. Louis, MO, 2009, pp 355–359

Ultraviolet

Ultraviolet (UV) is a form of electromagnetic energy invisible to the human eye that has been traditionally used for treatment of skin conditions such as psoriasis, acne vulgaris, or open skin wounds.

⬤ TABLE 18.28 Types of Ultraviolet and their Properties

Types	Wavelength	Description	Effects
UVA (long-range)	420–320 nm	Derived from a hot quartz mercury lamp requires warm-up and cool-down periods; more difficult to adjust output	Produces flourescence; greatest penetration in tissue (several mm); used alone or in conjunction with oral or topical agents (phototherapy) to treat skin disorders
UVB (middle-range)	320–290 nm	Derived from a hot quartz mercury lamps; requires warm-up and cool-down periods; more difficult to adjust output	Produces the most skin erethema; absorbed by superficial layers of skin; most effective for psoriasis treatment, particularly with narrowband UVB (311–313 nm)
UVC (short-range)	290–185 nm	Derived from a cold quartz mercury lamp; has safety advantages and easier to use than hot quartz (requires warm-up and cool-down periods; more difficult to adjust output)	Bacteriacidal; absorbed by superficial layers of skin; most effective for wound healing
PUVA	A variation of UVA	Psoralen ingested, followed by UVA	Intensifies effectiveness of psoralen for treating scleroderma, psoriasis, and other skin disorders; produces equivalent erythema to UVB when combined with sensitizing drugs

Sources: Cameron, MH (ed): *Physical Agents In Rehabilitation: From Research to Practice,* ed. 3. Saunders, St. Louis, MO, 2009, 370–375; and Michlovitz, SL, and Nolan, TP: *Modalities for Therapeutic Intervention,* ed. 4. FA Davis, Philadelphia, 2005, 233–237.

Erythemal Doses
Definitions of Erythemal Doses
Two systems of classifying erythemal doses have been used. In one classification, the level where erythema, or reddening of the skin, first appears after UV exposure is called the *minimal erythemal dose* (MED). In the other system, the first level is called *first-degree erythema.* When the term MED is used, there

will be three degrees of erythemal doses. When the minimum level of erythema is called *first-degree erythema,* there will be four degrees of erythemal doses.

suberythemal dose (SED): Ultraviolet exposure insufficient to cause reddening.

minimal erythemal dose (MED) (also called *first-degree*): Slight reddening of skin, without desquamation; possible slight itching sensation.

first-degree erythemal (1D or E1) (also called *second-degree*): More reddening than occurs with an MED and slight desquamation (peeling); itching and burning as with sunburn.

second-degree erythemal (2D or E2) (also called *third-degree*): Marked reddening with considerable itching, burning, and desquamation (peeling) of epidermis, some edema; similar to severe sunburn.

third-degree erythemal (3D or E3) (also called *fourth-degree*): Intense reaction with edema, swelling, blister formation.

TABLE 18.29 Characteristics of Erythemal Doses

Dose	Characteristic Effect	Appears	Disappears
SED	No visible reaction		
MED	Slight reddening	4–6 hr	24 hr
1D (2.5 × MED)	Mild sunburn	4–6 hr	48 hr
2D (5.0 × MED)	Severe sunburn	2 hr	Several days
3D (10.0 × MED)	Edema and blistering	2 hr	Several days

TABLE 18.30 Ultraviolet—Contraindications and Precautions

Contraindications
Irradiation of eyes (**Note:** Therapist and patient wear polarizing goggles)
Skin cancer
Pulmonary TB
Within 3 mo of receiving radiation therapy
Lupus erythematosus
Decreased hepatic or renal function
Fever

Precautions
Exposure to areas of skin rarely exposed to light
Acute eczema
Hyperthyroidism
Pregnancy
Photosensitivity; use of photosensing medications
Exposure to areas of skin rarely exposed to light

Sources: Cameron, MH (ed): *Physical Agents in Rehabilitation: From Research to Practice,* ed. 3. Saunders, St. Louis, MO, 2009, pp 370–375;
Michlovitz, SL, and Nolan, TP: *Modalities for Therapeutic Intervention,* ed. 4. FA Davis, Philadelphia, 2005, 233–237

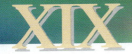
PHARMACOLOGY

This section provides generalized information on pharmacology and also describes drugs categorized by their common mode of action, rather than by clinical application. Information on pharmacology for specific clinical applications can be found in other sections of the *Handbook* that are organized according to area of rehabilitation practice.

Pharmacology material in this *Handbook* is predominantly derived from Ciccone, CD: *Pharmacology in Rehabilitation,* ed. 4. FA Davis, Philadelphia, 2007, with permission. Readers interested in understanding pharmacology and its relationship to rehabilitation are urged to examine this text. The authors wish to thank Dr. Ciccone for the use of his material and for his assistance.

General Principles

TABLE 19.1 Common Drug Suffixes

Drug Class	Suffix	Common Examples	Primary Indication or Desired Effect
Angiotensin-converting enzyme (ACE) inhibitors	-pril	Captopril, enalapril, lisinopril	Antihypertensive, congestive heart failure
Azole antifungals	-azole	Fluconazole, miconazole	Fungal infections
Barbiturates	-barbital	Phenobarbital, secobarbital	Sedative-hypnotic, antiseizure, anesthetic
Benzodiazepines	-epam or -olam	Diazepam, temazepam, alprazolam, triazolam	Sedative-hypnotic, antianxiety, antiseizure, anesthetic
Beta blockers	-olol	Metoprolol, propranolol	Antihypertensive, antianginal, antiarrhythmic, congestive heart failure
Bronchodilators (adrenergic)	-erol	Albuterol, pirbuterol	Bronchodilation
Bronchodilators (anticholinergic)	-tropium	Ipratropium, tiotropium	Bronchodilation
Bronchodilators (xanthine derivatives)	-phylline	Theophylline, aminophylline	Bronchodilation

(table continues on page 1124)

PHARM

🔲 TABLE 19.1 **Common Drug Suffixes** (continued)

Drug Class	Suffix	Common Examples	Primary Indication or Desired Effect
Calcium channel blockers (dihydropyridine group)	-ipine	Nifedipine, nicardipine	Antihypertensive, antianginal
Cyclooxygenase (COX)-2 inhibitors	-coxib	Celecoxib	Analgesic, nonsteroidal anti-inflammatory
Glucocorticoids	-sone or -olone*	Cortisone, dexa-methasone, prednisone, prednisolone, triamcinolone	Anti-inflammatory, immunosuppres-sants
Histamine H_2-receptor blockers	-idine	Cimetidine, ranitidine	Gastric ulcers
HIV protease inhibitors	-avir	Ritonavir, saquinavir	HIV infection
HMG-CoA reductase inhibitors (statins)	-statin	Pravastatin, simvastatin	Hyperlipidemia
Local anesthetics	-caine	Lidocaine, bupivicaine	Local anesthetic, antiarrhythmics
Low molecular weight heparins	-parin	Dalteparin, enoxaparin	Anticoagulants
Oral antidiabetics (sulfonylurea group)	-amide	Chlorpropamide, tolbutamide	Antidiabetic (type 2 diabetes mellitus)
Penicillin antibiotics	-cillin	Penicillin, ampicillin, amoxicillin	Bacterial infections
Proton pump inhibitors	-prazole	Omeprazole, lansoprazole	Gastric ulcers
Tetracycline antibiotics	-cycline	Tetracycline, doxycycline	Bacterial infections

Drug Class	Suffix	Common Examples	Primary Indication or Desired Effect
Various other antibacterials	-micin or -mycin†	Streptomycin, gentamicin, erythromycin	Bacterial infections

From: Ciccone, CD: *Pharmacology in Rehabilitation,* ed. 4. FA Davis, Philadelphia, 2007, back cover, with permission.
*Some anabolic steroids also end with -olone, e.g., nandrolone, oxymetholone.
†Some antibiotics ending with -mycin or -rubicin are used as antineoplastics.

TABLE 19.2 Routes of Drug Administration

Route	Advantages	Disadvantages	Examples
Enteral			
Oral	Easy, safe, convenient	Limited or erratic absorption of some drugs; chance of first-pass inactivation in liver.	Analgesics, sedative-hypnotics, many others
Sublingual	Rapid onset; not subject to first-pass inactivation	Drug must be easily absorbed from oral mucosa.	Nitroglycerin
Rectal	Alternative to oral route; local effect on rectal tissues	Poor or incomplete absorption; chance of rectal irritation.	Laxatives, suppository forms of other drugs
Parenteral			
Inhalation	Rapid onset; direct application for respiratory disorders; large surface area for systemic absorption	Chance of tissue irritation; patient compliance sometimes a problem.	General anesthetics, anti-asthmatic agents
Injection	Provides more direct administration to target tissues; rapid onset	Chance of infection if sterility is not maintained.	Insulin, antibiotics, anticancer drugs, narcotic analgesics

(table continues on page 1126)

PHARM

● TABLE 19.2 **Routes of Drug Administration** (continued)

Route	Advantages	Disadvantages	Examples
Parenteral			
Topical	Local effects on surface of skin	Effective in treating outer layers of skin only.	Antibiotic ointments, creams used to treat minor skin irritation and injury
Transdermal	Introduces drug into body without breaking the skin	Drug must be able to pass through dermal layers intact.	Nitroglycerin, motion sickness medications, drugs used with phonophoresis and iontophoresis

From Ciccone, CD: *Pharmacology in Rehabilitation,* ed. 4. FA Davis, Philadelphia, 2007, p 14, with permission.

● TABLE 19.3 **Newer Techniques for Drug Delivery**

Technique	Purpose	Advantages	Examples
Controlled-release preparations	To permit a slower and more prolonged absorption of the drug from the GI tract and other routes of administration.	Decreases # doses needed per day; prevents large fluctuations of plasma drug levels; sustains plasma levels through the night.	Timed-release, sustained-release, extended release, or prolonged-action preparations for cardiovascular meds, narcotic analgesics, and anti-Parkinson's meds that contain L-dopa.
Implanted drug delivery systems			
Programmable	Allows a small, measured dose of the drug to be released periodically from a reservoir implanted in the body. Release is electronically programmed from either within or outside of the body	Same as above, and allows for adjustment of delivery rate.	Reservoir placed under the skin in the abdomen for delivery of insulin or a reservoir is connected to the subarachnoid space or epidural space for delivery of analgesics, anesthetics, or muscle relaxants to spinal cord.

Purpose	Advantages	Examples
Reservoir incorporated into a gel or matrix where the drug is released biodegradably or nonbiodegradably.	Lower cost and easier maintenance than programmable drug delivery systems.	Administration of contraception hormones such as progesterone (Norplant)

Ciccone, CD: *Pharmacology in Rehabilitation,* ed. 4. FA Davis, Philadelphia, 2007, pp 23–24, with permission.

Anesthesia

Anesthetics are categorized as *general* or *local,* depending on whether or not the patient remains conscious when the anesthetic is administered. These categories are described below, beginning with preoperative medications that are used to sedate the patient prior to the administration of general anesthesia.

General Anesthetics

TABLE 19.4 Preoperative Premedication: Drugs and Doses Used

Classification	Preoperative Indication	Drug	Method of Administration*
Barbiturates	Decrease anxiety; facilitate induction of anesthesia	Amobarbital	Oral: 200 mg 1 to 2 hr before surgery
		Butabarbital	Oral: 50–100 mg 60 to 90 minutes before surgery
		Pentobarbital	Oral: 100 mg IM: 150–200 mg
		Phenobarbital	IM: 130–200 mg 60 to 90 min before surgery
		Secobarbital	Oral: 200–300 mg 1 to 2 hr before surgery
Opioids[†]	Provide analgesic, antianxiety, and sedative effects	Butorphanol	IV: 2 mg 60–90 minutes before surgery
		Meperidine	IM: 1–2.2 mg/kg body weight (100 mg maximum) 30 to 90 minutes before surgery

(table continues on page 1128)

PHARM

● **TABLE 19.4 Preoperative Premedication: Drugs a**
Used (continued)

Classification	Preoperative Indication	Drug	Method of Administration
Benzodiazepines	Decrease anxiety and tension: provide sedation and amnesia	Chlordiazepoxide	IM: 50–100 mg before surgery
		Diazepam	IM or IV: 5–10 mg prior to surgery
		Lorazepam	IM: 0.05 mg/kg body weight (4 mg maximum) 2 hr before surgery IV: 0.044–0.05 mg/kg bodyweight (4 mg maximum) 15 to 20 min before surgery
Antihistamines	Provide sedative–hypnotic effects	Diphenhydramine	Oral: 50 mg 20 to 30 minutes before surgery
		Hydroxyzine	Oral: 50–100 mg
Anticholinergics	Prevent excessive salivation and respiratory tract secretions	Atropine	Oral: 2 mg IM: 0.2–0.6 mg 30 to 60 min before surgery
		Glycopyrrolate	IM: 0.0044 mg/kg body weight 30 to 60 min before induction of anesthesia
		Scopolamine	IM: 0.2–0.6 mg 30 to 60 min before induction of anesthesia

From: Ciccone, CD: *Pharmacology in Rehabilitation,* ed. 4. FA Davis, Philadelphia, 2007, p 142, with permission.
*Typical adult doses. IV, intravenous; IM, intramuscular.
†Virtually all opioids can be used as a preoperative medication. Selection of a specific type and dose can be individualized based on the needs of each patient.

TABLE 19.5 **Neuromuscular Junction Blockers: Nondepolarizing and Depolarizing Forms**

Drug	Time of Onset*(min)	Clinical Duration (min)	Relative Duration
Nondepolarizing Blockers			
Atracurium (Tracrium)†	2–4	30–60	Intermediate
Doxacurium (Nuromax)	4–6	90–20	Long
Mivacurium (Mivacron)	2–4	12–18	Short
Pancuronium (Pavulon)	4–6	120–180	Long
Pipecuronium (Arduan)	2–4	80–100	Long
Rocuronium - (Zemuron)	1–2	30–60	Intermediate
Vecuronium (Norcuron)	2–4	60–90	Intermediate
Depolarizing Blockers			
Succinylcholine (Anectine, others)	1–1.5	5–8	Ultrashort

Adapted from: Ciccone, CD: *Pharmacology in Rehabilitation,* ed. 4. FA Davis, Philadelphia, 2007, p 143, with permission.
*Reflects usual adult intravenous dosage.
†Trade name in parentheses.

Local Anesthetics

TABLE 19.6 **Clinical Use of Local Anesthetics by Method of Administration**

Administration	Description	Use
Topical	Applied to surface of skin, mucous membranes, cornea, and other regions. Can be made from a single agent or combination of agents	• Symptomatic relief of minor surface irritations and injury. • Reduce pain prior to minor surgical procedures.

(table continues on page 1130)

◗ TABLE 19.6 Clinical Use of Local Anesthetics by Method of Administration

Administration	Description	Use
	(e.g., lidocaine and prilocaine).	• Improve motor function in patients with muscle hypertonicity (e.g., 20% benzocaine spray).
Transdermal	Applied to surface of skin with the intent that the drug will be absorbed into underlying tissue. • May be enhanced by the use of electric current (iontophoresis; see Section XVIII) or ultrasound (phonophoresis; see Section XVIII).	• Provides localized delivery of drug before treating painful subcutaneous soft tissues following musculoskeletal injury. Iontophoresis provides a noninvasive alternative to subcutaneous injection of local anesthetic prior to certain dermatological surgical procedures.
	• May be administered via a transdermal patch (e.g., 5% lidocaine patch).	• Treat localized pain in musculoskeletal conditions (e.g., osteoarthritis, low back pain, myofascial pain) and various types of neuropathic pain (e.g., postherpetic neuralgia, diabetic neuropathy).
Infiltration anesthesia	Drug is injected directly into the selected tissue, allowing it to diffuse to sensory nerve endings within the tissue.	To saturate a skin area, such as a skin laceration, prior to suturing or other minor surgical repair.
Peripheral nerve block	Noncontinuous • *Minor:* Drug is injected close to a single nerve trunk (e.g., ulnar, median) so that transmission along the peripheral nerve is interrupted.	• Common in dental procedures or for surgical procedures of the hand, foot, shoulder, etc.

Administration	Description	Use
	• *Major:* Several peripheral nerves or a nerve plexus (e.g., brachial, lumbosacral) is blocked.	• Used to anesthetize larger areas of the upper and lower extremity for more extensive surgery.
	Continuous • A small catheter is left implanted near the nerve(s) so that small dosages of the drug can be administered continuously for extended periods.	• To control post-surgical pain. (**Note:** Prolonged administration can produce localized muscle pain and weakness through necrosis).
Central neural block	Anesthetic is injected within the spaces surrounding the spinal cord. Can be done at any level of cord, but usually administered at the L3–4 or L4–5 vertebral interspace (see figure on p. 1133). • *Epidural Nerve Blockade:* Injection of drug into the epidural space (i.e., between bony vertebral column and the dura mater). Variation performed as "caudal block" by injecting drug into lumbar epidural space via the sacral hiatus (see figure on p. 1133). • *Spinal Nerve Blockade (Intrathecal Anesthesia):* Injection of drug within the subarachnoid space (i.e., between the arachnoid membrane and the pia mater).	Central neural blockade is used whenever analgesia is needed in a large region, e.g., used frequently during obstetric procedures (including caesarean delivery). Can also be used as an alternative to general anesthesia during lumbar spine surgery, hip or knee arthroplasty, or to administer anesthetics or narcotic analgesics for relief of acute and chronic pain (e.g., with the use of an indwelling catheter).
Sympathetic block	One approach is to inject the local anesthetic into the area surrounding the sympathetic	For the selective interruption of sympathetic efferent discharge rather than to provide

(table continues on page 1132)

PHARM

● TABLE 19.6 Clinical Use of Local Anesthetics by Method of Administration (continued)

Administration	Description	Use
	chain ganglion that innervates the affected limb. Alternately, the anesthetic can be administered subcutaneously to the affected limb using regional intravenous block techniques.	analgesia. Especially useful in cases of complex regional pain syndrome (CRPS); also known as reflex sympathetic dystrophy syndrome (RSDS).
Intravenous regional block (Bier block)	Drug injected into a peripheral vein located in a selected limb. The local vasculature carries the anesthetic to the nerves in the extremity. A tourniquet is also applied proximally on the limb to localize the drug temporarily within the extremity, and to prevent drug from reaching the systemic circulation where it could be toxic.	Produces anesthesia of an upper or lower limb. Primarily for anesthetizing the forearm-hand or distal leg-ankle-foot for short periods to allow surgical procedures or to treat conditions such as complex regional pain syndrome (CRPS), also known as reflex sympathetic dystrophy syndrome (RSDS).

Adapted from: Ciccone, CD: *Pharmacology in Rehabilitation,* ed. 4. FA Davis, Philadelphia, 2007, pp 150–154, with permission.

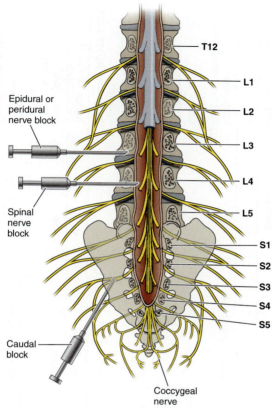

PHARM

Sites of epidural and spinal administration of a local anesthetic. Caudal block represents epidural administration via the sacral hiatus. *Adapted from: Clark, JB, Queener, SF, and Karb, VB: Pharmacological Basis of Nursing Practice, ed. 4. Mosby, St. Louis, MO, 1993 p 688.*

PHARM

TABLE 19.7 Common Local Anesthetics

Generic Name	Trade Name(s)	Onset of Action	Duration of Action	Principle Use(s)
Articane	Septocaine	Rapid	Intermediate	Peripheral nerve block
Banzocaine	Americaine, others	—	—	Topical
Bupivacaine	Marcaine, Sensorcaine	Slow to Intermediate	Long	Infiltration; Peripheral nerve block; Epidural; Spinal; Sympathetic block
Butamben	Butesin Picrate	—	—	Topical
Chloroprocaine	Nesacaine	Rapid	Short	Infiltration; Peripheral nerve block; Epidural; Intravenous regional block
Dibucaine	Nupercainal	—	—	Topical
Etidocaine	Duranest	Rapid	Long	Infiltration; Peripheral nerve block; Epidural
Levobupivacaine	Chirocaine	Slow to Intermediate	Short to Long	Infiltration; Peripheral nerve block; Epidural
Lidocaine	Xylocaine	Rapid	Intermediate	Infiltration;

PHARM

Generic Name	Trade Name(s)	Onset of Action	Duration of Action	Principle Use(s)
				Peripheral nerve block; Epidural; Spinal; Transdermal; Topical; Sympathetic block; Intravenous regional block
Mepivacaine	Carbocaine, Polocaine	Intermediate to Rapid	Intermediate	Infiltration; Peripheral nerve block; Epidural; Intravenous regional block
Pramoxine	Prax, Tronolane	—	—	Topical
Prilocaine	Citanest	Rapid	Intermediate	Infiltration; Peripheral nerve block
Procaine	Novocain	Intermediate	Short	Infiltration; Peripheral nerve block; Spinal
Tetracaine	Pontocaine	Rapid	Intermediate to Long	Topical; Spinal

From: Ciccone, CD: *Pharmacology in Rehabilitation*, ed. 4. FA Davis, Philadelphia, 2007, pp 151–152, with permission.
Source: USP DI, ed. 25. Copyright 2005. Thomson MICROMEDEX. Permission granted.
*Values for onset and duration of action refer to use during injection. Relative durations of action are as follows: short = 30–60 min; intermediate = 1–3 hr; and long = 3–10 hr of action.

PHARM

TABLE 19.8 Relative Size and Susceptibility to Block of Types of Nerve Fibers

Fiber Type*	Function	Diameter (μm)	Myelination	Conduction Velocity (m/s)	Sensitivity to Block
Type A Alpha	Proprioception, motor	12–20	Heavy	70–120	+
Beta	Touch, pressure	5–12	Heavy	30–70	++
Gamma	Muscle spindles	3–6	Heavy	15–30	++
Delta	Pain, temperature	2–5	Heavy	12–30	+++
Type B	Preganglionic, autonomic	<3	Light	3–15	++++
Type C Dorsal Root	Pain	0.4–1.2	None	0.5–2.3	++++
Sympathetic	Postganglioric	0.3–1.3	None	0.7–2.3	++++

From: Ciccone, CD: *Pharmacology in Rehabilitation*, ed. 4. FA Davis, Philadelphia, 2007, p 156, with permission.
*Fiber types are classified according to the system established by Gasser and Erlanger: *Am J Physiol*; 88:581, 1929. Reproduced with permission from Katzung BG. *Basic and Clinical Pharmacology*, ed.9. Lange Medical Books/ McGraw Hill; New York, 2004.

Opioid Analgesics

Opioid analgesics are a group of agents that are used to relieve moderate to severe pain. They exert their effects by binding to specific neuronal receptors that are located primarily in the central nervous system.

Common Analgesics

TABLE 19.9 Opioid Analgesics

Drug	Route of Administration*	Onset of Action (min)	Time to Peak Effect (min)	Duration of Action (hr)
Strong Agonists				
Fentanyl (Sublimaze)	IM	7–15	20–30	1–2
	IV	1–2	3–5	0.5–1
Hydromorphone (Hydrostat, Dilaudid)	Oral	30	90–120	4
	IM	15	30–60	4–5
	IV	10–15	15–30	2–3
	Sub-Q	15	30–90	4
Levorphanol (Levo-Dromoran)	Oral	10–60	90–120	4–5
	IM	—	60	4–5
	IV	—	Within 20	4–5
	Sub-Q	—	60–90	4–5
Meperidine (Demerol)	Oral	15	60–90	2–4
	IM	10–15	30–50	2–4
	IV	1	5–7	2–4
	Sub-Q	10–15	30–50	2–4
Methadone (Dolophine, Methadose)	Oral	30–60	90–120	4–6
	IM	10–20	60–120	4–5
	IV	—	15–30	3–4
Morphine (many trade names)	Oral	—	60–120	4–5
	IM	10–30	30–60	4–5
	IV	—	20	4–5
	Sub-Q	10–30	50–90	4–5
	Epidural	15–60	—	Up to 24
	Intrathecal	15–60	—	Up to 24
	Rectal	20–60	—	—
Oxymorphone (Numorphan)	IM	10–15	30–90	3–6
	IV	5–10	15–30	3–4
	Sub-Q	10–20	—	3–6
	Rectal	15–30	120	3–6

(table continues on page 1138)

TABLE 19.9 Opioid Analgesics (continued)

Drug	Route of Administration*	Onset of Action (min)	Time to Peak Effect (min)	Duration of Action (hr)
Mild-to-Moderate Agonists				
Codeine (generic)	Oral	30–45	60–120	4
	IM	10–30	30–60	4
	Sub-Q	10–30	—	4
Hydrocodone (Hycodan)	Oral	10–30	30–60	4–6
Oxycodone (OxyContin, Roxicodone)	Oral	—	60	3–4
Propoxyphene (Darvon)	Oral	15–60	120	4–6
Mixed Agonist–Antagonist				
Butorphanol (Stadol)	IM	10–30	30–60	3–4
	IV	2–3	30	2–4
Nalbuphine (Nubain)	IM	Within 15	60	3–6
	IV	2–3	30	3–4
	Sub-Q	Within 15	—	3–6
Pentazocine (Talwin)	Qral	15–30	60–90	3
	IM	15–20	30–60	2–3
	IV	2–3	15–30	2–3
	Sub-Q	15–20	30–60	2–3

From: Ciccone, CD: *Pharmacology in Rehabilitation,* ed. 4. FA Davis, Philadelphia, 2007, pp 186–187, with permission.
*IM = intramuscular; IV = intravenous; Sub-Q = subcutaneous.

Patient-Controlled Analgesia (PCA)

Description. A method of analgesia administration that enables the patient to self-administer small doses of a drug (usually an opioid) at relatively frequent intervals to provide optimal pain relief. The delivery is typically administered intravenously or into the spinal canal by a pump that is controlled by the patient.

Use. PCA is typically used to manage acute pain following surgery or to treat patients with cancer and other conditions associated with chronic pain.

Advantage. The primary advantage of PCA over more traditional dosing regimens is the reduction of side effects.

Disadvantages. Problems associated with PCA can include operator errors (misprogramming PCA device, improperly loading syringe or cartridge), patient errors (misunderstanding device or therapy), and mechanical problems (failure to deliver on demand; defective vials, syringes, connectors, or alarms).

Terminology Describing PCA Dosing Strategies and Parameters

loading dose: A single large dose is given initially to establish anesthesia by bringing the level of analgesic to the therapeutic window.

demand dose: The amount of drug that is self-administered by the patient each time he/she activates the PCA pump. See Table 19.10.

locked (or lockout) interval: The minimum amount of time allowed between each demand dose. The PCA pump will not deliver the next dose until the lockout interval has expired. See Table 19.10.

1- and 4-hour limits: Some PCA systems can be set to limit the total amount of drug given in a 1- and 4-hour period.

background infusion rate: In some patients, a small amount of the analgesic is infused continuously to maintain a low, background level of analgesia. Demand doses are superimposed when the patient feels an increase in pain. Particularly beneficial when patient is asleep or is unable to activate the pump.

successful vs. total demands: The PCA pump keeps track of activation demands by the patient that actually results in drug delivery ("successful demands") vs. those that do not (e.g., when the demand is made during the lockout period). The ratio of successful to total demands can be used to adjust the parameters of the demand dose.

Adapted from:

Ciccone, CD: *Pharmacology in Rehabilitation*, ed. 4. FA Davis, Philadelphia, 2007, pp 238–239, with permission.

TABLE 19.10 Parameters for Intravenous PCA Using Opioid Medications

Drug (Concentration)	Demand Dose	Lockout Interval (min)
Alfentanil (0.1 mg/mL)	0.1–0.2 mg	5–8
Buprenorphine (0.03 mg/mL)	0.03–0.1 mg	8–20
Fentanyl (10 µg/mL)	10-20 µg	3–10
Hydomorphone (0.2 mg/mL)	0.05–0.25 mg	5–10
Meperidine (10 mg/mL)	5–25 mg	5–10
Methadone (1 mg/mL)	0.5–2.5 mg	8–20
Morrphine (1 mg/mL)	0.5–2.5 mg	5–10

(table continues on page 1140)

TABLE 19.10 Parameters for Intravenous PCA Using Opioid Medications (continued)

Drug (Concentration)	Demand Dose	Lockout Interval (min)
Nalbuphine (1 mg/mL)	1–5 mg	5–15
Oxymorphone (0.25 mg/mL)	0.2–0.4 mg	8–10
Pentazocine (10 mg/mL)	5-30 mg	5–15
Sufentanil (0.2 µg/mL)	0.2–0.5 µg	3–10

From: Ciccone, CD: *Pharmacology in Rehabilitation*, ed. 4. FA Davis, Philadelphia, 2007, p 239, with permission.
Source: Ready, p. 2328, with permission.

TABLE 19.11 Administrative Routes During PCA and Their Advantages

Administrative Route	Description	Advantages/Disadvantages
Patient-controlled intravenous analgesia (PCIA)	Administration of drugs by inserting a needle into a peripheral vein and then connecting the needle to a catheter or IV line that is connected to the PCA pump. For long-term administration, the catheter can be implanted surgically in a large central vein or connected to an **access port** implanted subcutaneously.	Provides the simplest and most common method of PCA administration. As with any invasive method, there is an increased risk of infection, reduction of patient mobility, and increased need for management.
Patient-controlled epidural analgesia (PCEA)	Administration of drugs directly into the epidural space at a specific spinal cord level or into the subarachnoid space (referred to as **intrathecal administration**). For short-term use, the catheter is inserted through the skin and taped to the back; for long-term use it is often tunneled subcutaneously through the abdomen.	Provides more effective analgesia than other parenteral methods with a smaller amount of drug and reduced side effects. More difficult than simple intravenous delivery using a peripheral vein. Shares the same disadvantages as other invasive methods, as described above.

Administrative Route	Description	Advantages/Disadvantages
Patient-controlled transdermal analgesia (PCTA)	A more recent variant of PCA providing drug delivery through iontophoresis via a medicated patch that is adhered to the patient's skin. The patch is impregnated with an opioid and the patient can self-administer small doses by pushing a button on the patch.	Easy to apply and enables the patient to be more mobile w/o an IV line. Can provide pain control comparable to PCIA techniques. As a noninvasive technique, there is less risk of infection, greater patient mobility, and less need for management.
Patient-controlled regional analgesia (PCRA)	Self-administered drug delivery directly into a specific anatomical site (e.g., peripheral joint, nerve, or wound). A small catheter attached to a PCA pump is inserted into the affected site.	Versatile method that can be used alone or in combination with other methods to provide self-administered delivery of drug for localized pain control. Shares the same risks and disadvantages as other invasive methods described above.

Based on: Ciccone, CD: *Pharmacology in Rehabilitation,* ed. 4. FA Davis, Philadelphia, 2007, pp 240–242, with permission.

PHARM

PHARM

■ TABLE 19.12 Basic Features of Some Common PCA Pumps

Feature	Abbott AMP II	Abbott LifeCare 4100 PCA Plus II	Baxter 6060	Baxter PCA II
Ambulatory use	Yes	No	Yes	No
Size (inches)	6.75 × 4.0 × 2.3	8.25 × 13.4 × 6.0	4.7 × 3.9 × 2.3	13.0 × 6.3 × 2.8
Weight (lb)	1.3	15	1.0	4.2
Power souce	Wall plug in AC; 2 × 9-volt alkaline battery; NiCd rechargeable battery pack	Wall plug in AC; one 8-volt sealed lead-acid battery	2 × 9-volt alkaline or lithium batteries; external lead-acid battery pack	Four D-cell alkaline batteries; AC power kit with two rechargeable NiCd batteries
Comments	Meets all basic requirements for performance, safety, and ease of use.	Performs adequately, but has a number of drawbacks in its ease of use and safety features.	Meets most requirements; has a mix of minor advantages and disadvantages; ease of use is only fair.	Meets most requirements and offers some advantages, but also has some drawbacks, most notably in its data logs and alarms.

From: Ciccone, CD: *Pharmacology in Rehabilitation*, ed. 4. FA Davis, Philadelphia, 2007, p 243, with permission.
Source: Adapted from Patient-controlled analgesic infusion pumps. *Hemth Devices.* 2001; 30:168, 169, 182 with permission.

Controlled Substances

In 1970, federal legislation was enacted to help control the abuse of legal and illegal drugs. The Comprehensive Drug Abuse Prevention and Control Act (or Controlled Substances Act (21 U.S.C. §801; http://www.deadiversion.usdoj.gov/ 21cfr/21usc/801.htm) placed drugs into specific categories, or "schedules," according to their potential for abuse. Since then, approximately 160 substances have been added, removed, or transferred from one schedule to another. Descriptions of these schedules for controlled substances can be found in the Code of Federal Regulations Section 1308—Schedules of Controlled Substances (http://www.deadiversion.usdoj.gov/21cfr/cfr/1308/1308_11.htm). A summary description of the schedule categories follows:

Schedule I

These drugs are regarded as having the highest potential for abuse, and the legal use of agents in this category is restricted to approved research studies or therapeutic use in a very limited number of patients (e.g., use of marijuana as an antiemetic). Examples of Schedule I drugs include heroin, lysergic acid diethylamide (LSD), psilocybin, mescaline, peyote, marijuana, tetrahydrocannabinols, and several other hallucinogens.

Schedule II

Drugs in this category are approved for specific therapeutic purposes but still have a high potential for abuse and possible addiction. Examples include opioids such as morphine and meperidine, barbiturates such as pentobarbital and secobarbital, and drugs containing amphetamines.

Schedule III

Although these drugs have a lower abuse potential than those in Schedules I and II, there is still the possibility of developing mild to moderate physical dependence or strong psychologic dependence, or both. Drugs in Schedule III include certain anabolic steroids, and opioids (e.g., codeine, hydrocodone) that are combined in a limited dosage with other nonopioid drugs. Other drugs in this category are certain barbiturates and amphetamines that are not included in Schedule II.

Schedule IV

Drugs in Schedule IV include narcotics, depressants (e.g., barbital, chloral hydrate, phenobarbital), and stimulants.

Schedule V

Drugs in Schedule V include narcotic drugs containing non-narcotic active medicinal ingredients, and certain depressants and stimulants.

Drug Abuse and Withdrawal

⬤ **TABLE 19.13 Signs of Drug Interactions, Overdose, and Withdrawal**

Drug	Acute Intoxication[a] and Overdose	Withdrawal Syndrome
CNS stimulants: Cocaine, amphetamine, dextroamphetamine, methylphenidate, phenmetrazine, phenylpropanolamine, STP[b], MDMA[c], Bromo-DMA[d], diethylpropion, most amphetamine-like antiobesity drugs	*Vital signs:* temperature elevated; heart rate increased; respirations shallow; BP elevated. *Mental status:* sensorium hyperacute or confused; paranoid ideation; hallucinations; delirium; impulsivity; agitation; hyperactivity; sterotypy. *Physical exam:* pupils dilated and reactive; tendon reflexes hyperactive; cardiac dysrhythmias; dry mouth; sweating; tremors; convulsions; coma; stroke.	Muscular aches; abdominal pain; chills, tremors, voracious hunger; anxiety; prolonged sleep; lack of energy; profound depression, sometimes suicidal; exhaustion
Opioids: heroin, morphine; codeine, meperidine, methadone, hydromorphone, opium, pentazocine, propoxyphene, fentanyl, sufentanil	*Vital signs:* temperature decreased; respiration depressed; BP decreased, sometimes shock. Mental status: euphoria; stupor. *Physical exam:* pupils constricted (may be dilated with meperidine or extreme hypoxia); reflexes diminished to absent; pulmonary edema; constipation; convulsions with propoxyphene or meperidine; cardiac dysrhythmias with propoxyphene; coma.	Pupils dilated; pulse rapid; gooseflesh; lacrimation; abdominal cramps; muscle jerks; "flu" syndrome; vomiting; diarrhea; tremulousness; yawning; anxiety
CNS depressants: barbiturates, benzodiazepines, glutethimide, meprobamate, methaqualone, ethchlorvynol, chloral hydrate, methyprylon, paraldehyde	*Vital signs:* respiration depressed; BP decreased, sometimes shock. Mental status: drowsiness or coma; confusion; delirium. *Physical exam:* pupils dilated with glutethimide or in severe poisoning; tendon reflexes depressed; ataxia; slurred speech; nystagmus; convulsions or hyperirritability with methaqualone; signs of anticholinergic poisoning with glutethimide; cardiac dysrhythmias with chloral hydrate.	Tremulousness; insomnia; sweating; fever; clonic blink reflex; anxiety; cardiovascular collapse; agitation; delirium; hallucinations; disorientation; convulsions; shock

PHARM

Drug	Acute Intoxication[a] and Overdose	Withdrawal Syndrome
Hallucinogens: LSD[e], psilocybin, mescaline, PCP	*Vital signs:* temperature elevated; heart rate increased; BP elevated. *Mental status:* euphoria; anxiety or panic; paranoia; sensorium often clear; affect inappropriate; illusions; time and visual distortions; visual hallucinations; depersonalization; with PCP hypertensive encephalopathy. *Physical exam:* pupils dilated (normal or small with PCP); tendon reflexes hyperactive; with PCP cyclic coma or extreme hyperactivity, drooling, blank stare, mutism, amnesia, analgesia, nystagmus (sometimes vertical), gait ataxia, muscle rigidity, impulsive or violent behavior; violent, scatological, pressured speech.	None
Cannabis group: marijuana, hashish, THC, hash oil, sinsemilla	*Vital signs:* heart rate increased; BP decreased on standing. *Mental status:* anorexia, then increased appetite; euphoria; anxiety; sensorium often clear; dreamy, fantasy state; time/space distortions; hallucinations may be rare. *Physical exam:* pupils unchanged; conjunctiva injected; tachycardia, ataxia, and pallor in children.	Nonspecific symptoms including anorexia, nausea, insomnia, restlessness, irritability, anxiety, depression
Anticholinergics: atropine, belladonna, henbane, scopolamine, trihexyphenidyl, benztropine mesylate, procyclidine, propantheline bromide; jimson weed seed	*Vital signs:* temperature elevated; heart rate increased; possibly decreased BP. *Mental status:* drowsiness or coma; sensorium clouded; amnesia; disorientation; visual hallucinations; body image alterations; confusion; with propantheline restlessness, excitement. *Physical exam:* pupils dilated and fixed;	Gastrointestinal and musculoskeletal symptoms

(table continues on page 1146)

🔵 **TABLE 19.13 Signs of Drug Interactions, Overdose, and Withdrawal** (continued)

Drug	Acute Intoxication[a] and Overdose	Withdrawal Syndrome
	decreased bowel sounds; flushed, dry skin and mucous membranes; violent behavior, convulsions; with propantheline circulatory failure, respiratory failure, paralysis, coma.	

Reprinted with permission from the *Medical Letter,* vol 29, September 11, 1987.
BP = blood pressure.
[a]Mixed intoxications produce complex combinations of signs and symptoms.
[b]STP (2,5-dimethoxy-4-methylamphetamine)
[c]MDMA (3,4-methylenedioxymethamphetamine)
[d]Bromo-DMA (4-bromo-2,5-dimethoxyamphetamine)
[e]LSD = D-lysergic acid diethylamide
[f]PCP (phencyclidine)
[g]THC (γ-9-tetrahydrocannabinol)

Autonomic Pharmacology

The use of therapeutic drugs to alter autonomic function is one of the major areas of pharmacology. Autonomic agents are categorized as either *cholinergic* or *adrenergic,* depending on whether the neurotransmitters involved in autonomic discharge affect either cholinergic or adrenergic receptors.

Cholinergic Drugs

🔵 **TABLE 19.14 Cholinergic Stimulants: Direct-Acting and Indirect-Acting Forms**

Generic Name	Trade Name(s)	Primary Clinical Use(s)*
Direct-Acting (Cholinergic Agonists)		
Bethanechol	Duvoid, Urabeth, Urecholine	Post-operative gastrointestinal and urinary atony
Carbachol	Isopto Carbachol, Carbastat, Miostat	Glaucoma
Pilocarpine	Pilocar, Adsorbo-carpine, many others	Glaucoma

Generic Name	Trade Name(s)	Primary Clinical Use(s)*
Indirect-Acting (Cholinesterase Inhibitors)		
Ambenonium	Mytelase	Myasthenia gravis
Demecarium	Humorsol	Glaucoma
Donepezil	Aricept	Dementia of the Alzheimer type
Echothiophate	Phospholine Iodide	Glaucoma
Edrophonium	Enlon, Reversol, Tensiolon	Myasthenia gravis, reversal of neuromuscular blocking drugs
Galantamine	Reminyl	Dementia of the Alzheimer type
Isoflurophate	Diflupyl	Glaucoma
Neostigmine	Prostigmin	Post-operative gastrointestinal and urinary atony, myasthenia gravis, reversal of neuromuscular blocking drugs
Physostigmine	Antilirium, Eserine, Isopto Eserine	Glaucoma, reversal of CNS toxicity caused by anticholinergic drugs
Pyridostigmine	Mestinon	Myasthenia gravis, reversal of neuromuscular blocking drugs
Rivastigmine	Exelon	Dementia of the Alzheimer's type
Tacrine	Cognex	Dementia of the Alzheimer's type

From Ciccone, CD: *Pharmacology in Rehabilitation,* ed. 4. FA Davis, Philadelphia, 2007, p 265, with permission.

CNS = central nervous system.

*Agents used to treat glaucoma and other visual disturbances are administered topically, that is, directly to the eye. Agents used for other problems are given systemically by oral administration or injection.

🟠 TABLE 19.15 Common Anticholinergic Drugs*

Generic Name	Trade Name(s)	Primary Clinical Use(s)*
Anisotropine	Generic	Peptic ulcer
Atropine	Generic	Peptic ulcer, irritable bowel syndrome, preoperative antisecretory agent, cardiac arrhythmias (e.g., sinus bradycardia, postmyocardial infarction, asystole), reversal of neuromuscular blockade, antidote to cholinesterase inhibitor poisoning
Belladonna	Generic	Peptic ulcer, irritable bowel syndrome, dysmenorrhea, nocturnal enuresis
Clidinium	Quarzan	Peptic ulcer, irritable bowel syndrome
Cyclopentolate	Pentolate, Cyclogyl, others	Induces mydriasis for ophthalmologic procedures
Dicyclomine	Bentyle, others	Irritable bowel syndrome
Glycopyrrolate	Robinul	Peptic ulcer, preoperative antisecretory agent, antidiarrheal, reversal of neuromuscular blockade
Homatropine	Homapin	Peptic ulcer, irritable bowel syndrome
Hyoscyamine	Cystospaz, Levsin, others	Peptic ulcer, irritable bowel syndrome, urinary bladder hypermotility, preoperative antisecretory agent
Ipratropium	Atrovent, others	Bronchodilator
Mepenzolate	Cantil	Peptic ulcer
Methantheline	Banthine	Peptic ulcer
Oxybutynin	Ditropan	Neurogenic or overactive bladder
Propantheline	Pro-Banthine	Peptic ulcer, irritable bowel syndrome, urinary incontinence

Generic Name	Trade Name(s)	Primary Clinical Use(s)*
Scopolamine	Transderm Scop, others	Motion sickness, preoperative antisecretory agent, postoperative nausea and vomiting, antivertigo
Tiotropium	Spiriva	Bronchodilator
Tolterodine	Detrol	Overactive bladder

From Ciccone, CD: *Pharmacology in Rehabilitation,* ed. 4. FA Davis, Philadelphia, 2007, p 269, with permission.
*Clinical uses listed for a specific agent reflect the agent's approved indication(s). Actual clinical use, however, may be limited because anticholinergics have often been replaced by agents that are more effective and better tolerated.

Adrenergic Drugs

Adrenergic drugs primarily influence activity in the sympathetic nervous system through their effect on adrenergic synapses. Norepinephrine usually functions as the neurotransmitter between sympathetic postganglionic neurons and peripheral tissues. Most of the adrenergic agonist drugs are therefore used to augment sympathetic responses, whereas the adrenergic antagonists are used to attenuate sympathetic-induced activity.

● TABLE 19.16 Adrenergic Agonists*

Type	Action	General Indication
Alpha Agonists		
Alpha-1-selective agonists	These agents activate the alpha-1 receptors located primarily on vascular smooth muscle; thus producing vasoconstriction.	Used to increase blood pressure (by increasing peripheral vascular resistance) and treat acute hypotension from shock or following surgery. Also used to treat nasal congestion and decrease heart rate.
Alpha-2-selective agonists	As an anti-hypertension agent, these drugs stimulate alpha-2 receptors located in the brain and brainstem, exerting an inhibitory effect on sympathetic discharge from the vasomotor center. As an anti-spasticity agent, these drugs activate alpha-2 receptors in the	Used primarily in the treatment of hypertension and spasticity.

(table continues on page 1150)

◗ TABLE 19.16 Adrenergic Agonists*

Type	Action	General Indication
	spinal cord where they produce inhibition of interneuron activity, resulting in reduced excitability of motoneurons supplied by the interneurons.	
Beta Agonists Beta-1-selective agonists	These agents activate beta-1 receptors located primarily on the myocardium, resulting in increased heart rate and increased force of myocardial contraction.	Used primarily to increase cardiac output in emergency situations such as cardiovascular shock or in the event of complications in cardiac surgery. Also used for short-term treatment of certain heart diseases, including heart failure. See Section V for information on specific beta-1-selective agonist drugs.
Beta-2-selective agonists	These agents bind to and activate beta-2 receptors on bronchial smooth muscle, resulting in relaxation of the bronchioles. These agents can also bind to and activate beta-2 receptors on uterine muscle, resulting in relaxation of the uterus.	Most are administered to treat the bronchospasm associated with respiratory ailments such as asthma, bronchitis, and emphysema. Also used to inhibit premature uterine contractions during pregnancy, thus preventing premature labor and delivery.
Mixed Alpha- and Beta-Agonist Activity	Multiple receptor drugs that can affect a number of adrenoceptive sub-types. Some (e.g., epinephrine) are able to stimulate all four adrenergic receptor sub-types, whereas others (e.g., norepinephrine) have different degrees of affinity to alpha- and beta-receptors.	Clinical uses are varied and depend upon which combination of receptors these agonists have an affinity for.

Adapted from: Ciccone, CD: *Pharmacology in Rehabilitation,* ed. 4. FA Davis, Philadelphia, 2007, pp 274–279, with permission.
*Refer to Section VI, Cardiovascular, for specific information on adrenergic drugs used to treat cardiopulmonary clinical conditions.

■ TABLE 19.17 Adrenergic Antagonists*

Type	Action	General Indication
Alpha antagonists		
Alpha-1-selective antagonists	These agents reduce peripheral vascular tone by blocking the alpha-1 receptors located on vascular smooth muscle, causing peripheral vasodilation. A primary adverse effect associated with alpha antagonists is **reflex tachycardia**, to compensate for the decrease in BP, and **orthostatic hypotension** due to the decrease in peripheral vascular tone.	Used primarily to treat hypertension by means of decreasing peripheral vascular resistance. Other uses include reversal of HBP following autonomic crisis, improving circulation in patients with vascular insufficiency or Raynaud's phenomenon, and relaxing smooth muscles to promote normal urinary flow during micturition in patients with benign prostatic hyperplasia (BPH).
Alpha-2-selective antagonists	These antagonists would increase peripheral vascular tone by increasing central sympathetic drive, and therefore are considered counterproductive to the primary use of alpha antagonists.	None.
Beta Antagonists		
Beta-1-selective antagonists	These agents are typically used to block the beta-1 receptors located on the heart, thereby reducing the rate and force of myocardial contractions.	Frequently used to decrease cardiac workload in conditions such as hypertension and angina pectoris. Also used to limit extent of myocardial damage following a heart attack and improve cardiac function in certain types of heart failure and cardiac dysrhythmias.
Beta-2-selective antagonists	Because beta-2 receptors are found primarily on bronchial smooth muscles, beta-2 selective blockers are not clinically useful because they would facilitate bronchoconstriction.	None.

(table continues on page 1152)

PHARM

◖ TABLE 19.17 **Adrenergic Antagonists*** (continued)

Type	Action	General Indication
Beta-nonselective antagonists	Beta antagonists that have relatively equal affinity for cardiac beta-1 and beta-2 receptors.	Even if the beta antagonist is nonselective, the beta-1 blockade is considered clinically beneficial for treating hypertension, angina pectoris, arrhythmias, prevent infarction.

Adapted from: Ciccone, CD: *Pharmacology in Rehabilitation,* ed. 4. FA Davis, Philadelphia, 2007, pp 279–284, with permission.
BP = blood pressure; HBP = high blood pressure

Endocrine Pharmacology

This section provides information on the classes of drugs that are intended to maintain internal homeostasis through the regulation and control of hormones produced by the endocrine glands. These glands, their secretory hormones, and therapeutic use are summarized below.

Endocrine Glands

◖ TABLE 19.18 **Hypothalamic and Pituitary Hormones**

Hypothalamic Hormones and Releasing Factors	Effect
Growth hormone–releasing hormone (GHRH)	↑ GH release
Growth hormone–inhibitory hormone (GHIH)	↓ GH release
Gonadotropin–releasing hormone (GnRH)	↑ LH and FSH release
Thyrotropin–releasing hormone (TRH)	↑ TSH release
Corticotropin–releasing hormone (CRH)	↑ ACTH release
Prolactin–inhibitory factor (PIF)	↓ Pr release

Pituitary Hormones	Principal Effects
Anterior Lobe	
Growth hormone (GH)	↑ tissue growth and development
Luteinizing hormone (LH)	Female: ↑ ovulation; ↑ estrogen and progesterone synthesis from corpus luteum Male: ↑ testosterone synthesis
Follicle-stimulating hormone (FSH)	Female: ↑ follicular development and estrogen synthesis Male: enhance spermatogenesis

Pituitary Hormones	Principal Effects
Thyroid-stimulating hormone (TSH)	↑ synthesis of thyroid hormones (T_3, T_4)
Adrenocorticotropic hormone (ACTH)	↑ adrenal steroid synthesis (e.g., cortisol)
Prolactin (Pr)	Initiates lactation
Posterior Lobe Antidiuretic hormone (ADH)	↑ renal reabsorption of water
Oxytocin	↑ uterine contraction; ↑ milk ejection during lactation

Adapted from: Ciccone, CD: *Pharmacology in Rehabilitation,* ed. 4. FA Davis, Philadelphia, 2007, p 404, with permission.

TABLE 19.19 Other Primary Endocrine Glands

Gland	Hormone(s)	Principal Effects
Thyroid	Thyroxine (T_4), Triiodothyronine (T_3)	Increase cellular metabolism; facilitate normal growth and development
Parathyroids	Parathormone (PTH)	Increase blood calcium
Pancreas	Glucagon Insulin	Increase blood glucose Decrease blood glucose; increase carbohydrate protein, and fat storage
Adrenal cortex	Glucocorticoids Mineralocorticoids	Regulate glucose metabolism; enhance response to stress Regulate fluid and electrolyte levels
Adrenal medulla	Epinephrine, Norepinephrine	Vascular and metabolic effects that facilitate increased physical activity
Testes	Testosterone	Spermatogenesis; male sexual characteristics
Ovaries	Estrogens, Progesterone	Female reproductive cycle and sexual characteristics

Adapted from: Ciccone, CD: *Pharmacology in Rehabilitation,* ed. 4. FA Davis, Philadelphia, 2007, p 404, with permission.

Glucocorticoids

▌ TABLE 19.20 Therapeutic Glucocorticoids

Generic Name	Common Trade Name(s)	Type of Preparation Available					
		Systemic	Topical	Inhalation	Ophthalmic	Otic	Nasal
Alclometasone	Aclovate		X				
Amcinonide	Cyclocort		X				
Beclomethasone	Beclovent, Vanceril, others		X	X			X
Betamethasone	Celestone, Diprosone, others	X	X		X	X	
Budesonide	Pulmicort Turbohaler, Rhinocort			X			X
Clobetasol	Dermovate, Temovate		X				
Clocortolone	Cloderm		X				
Cortisone	Cortone	X					
Desonide	DesOwen, Tridesilon		X				
Desoximetasone	Topicort		X				
Dexamethasone	Decadron, Dexasone, others	X	X		X	X	X

PHARM

Generic Name	Common Trade Name(s)	Type of Preparation Available					
		Systemic	Topical	Inhalation	Ophthalmic	Otic	Nasal
Diflorasone	Florone, Maxiflor		X				
Flunisolide	AeroBid, Nasalide			X			X
Fluocinolone	Flurosyn, Synalar, others		X				
Fluocinonide	Lidex, others		X				
Fluorometholone	FML, S.O.P., Fluor-Op, others				X		
Flurandrenolide	Cordran		X				
Fluticasone	Cultivate, Flonase		X				X
Halcinonide	Halog		X				
Halobetasol	Ultravate		X				
Hydrocortisone	Cortaid, Dermacort, Hydrocortone, many others	X	X		X		
Medrysone	HMS Liquifilm				X		

(table continues on page 1156)

PHARM

■ TABLE 19.20 **Therapeutic Glucocorticoids** (continued)

Generic Name	Common Trade Name(s)	Type of Preparation Available						
		Systemic	Topical	Inhalation	Ophthalmic	Otic	Nasal
Methylprednisolone	Medrol, others	X					
Mometasone	Elocon, Nasonex		X				X
Prednicarbate	Dermatop		X				
Prednisolone	Pediaped, Prelone, others	X			X		
Prednisone	Deltasone, Meticorten, others	X					
Triamcinolone	Azmacort, Aristocort, Nasacort, others	X	X	X			X

From Ciccone, CD: *Pharmacology in Rehabilitation*, ed. 4. FA Davis, Philadelphia, 2007, pp 422–423, with permission.

TABLE 19.21 Nonendocrine Disorders Treated With Glucocorticoids

General Indication	Principal Desired Effect of Glucocorticoids	Examples of Specific Disorders
Allergic disorders	Decreased inflammation	Anaphylactic reactions, drug-induced allergic reactions, severe hay fever, serum sickness
Collagen disorders	Immunosuppression	Acute rheumatic carditis, dermatomyositis, systemic lupus erythematosus
Dermatologic disorders	Decreased inflammation	Alopecia areata, dermatitis (various forms), keloids, lichens, mycosis fungoides, pemphigus, psoriasis
Gastrointestinal disorders	Decreased inflammation	Crohn disease, ulcerative colitis
Hematological disorders	Immunosuppression	Autoimmune hemolytic anemia, congenital hypoplastic anemia, erythroblastopenia, thrombocytopenia
Nonrheumatic inflammation	Decreased inflammation	Bursitis, tenosynovitis
Neoplastic disease	Antilymphocytic effects	Leukemias, lymphomas, nasal polyps, cystic tumors
Neurological disease	Decreased inflammation and immunosuppression	Tuberculous meningitis, multiple sclerosis, myasthenia gravis
Neurotrauma	Decreased edema,* inhibit free radical-induced neuronal damage	Brain surgery, closed head injury, certain brain tumors, spinal cord injury
Ophthalmic disorders	Decreased inflammation	Chorioretinitis, conjunctivitis, herpes zoster ophthalmicus, iridocyclitis, keratitis, optic neuritis
Organ transplant	Immunosuppression	Transplantation of liver, kidney, heart, and others
Renal diseases	Decreased inflammation	Nephrotic syndrome, membranous glomerulonephritis

(table continues on page 1158)

PHARM

● TABLE 19.21 Nonendocrine Disorders Treated With Glucocorticoids (continued)

General Indication	Principal Desired Effect of Glucocorticoids	Examples of Specific Disorders
Respiratory disorders	Decreased inflammation	Bronchial asthma, berylliosis, aspiration pneumonitis, symptomatic sarcoidosis, pulmonary tuberculosis
Rheumatic disorders	Decreased inflammation and immunosuppression	Ankylosing spondylitis, psoriatic arthritis, rheumatoid arthritis, gouty arthritis, osteoarthritis

From: Ciccone, CD: *Pharmacology in Rehabilitation,* ed. 4. FA Davis, Philadelphia, 2007, p 424, with permission.
*Efficacy of glucocorticoid use in decreasing cerebral edema has not been conclusively proved.

Adrenocorticosteroids

Steroid hormones, also referred to as **adrenal steroids,** are produced by the adrenal cortex. There are two primary types of adrenal steroids, glucocorticoids and mineralocorticoids, as well as small amounts of sex hormones produced by the adrenal cortex. These hormones exert a number of diverse physiological effects, which are summarized below. Adrenal steroids and their synthetic analogues can be administered pharmacologically to mimic the effects of their endogenous counterparts, frequently as a means of replacement therapy for various hormonal deficiencies. Some of these uses are summarized below and some can be found in other sections of the *Handbook* where clinically based therapeutics involving these agents are presented.

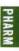

TABLE 19.22 Primary Types of Adrenocorticosteroids and Their Characteristics

Type	Function	Mechanism of Action	Physiological Effect	Clinical Use
Glucocorticoids • *Cortisol* • *Corticosterone*	Primarily involved in the control of glucose metabolism and the body's ability to deal with stress.	Effect cells in a manner that is characteristic of steroid hormones in general. It alters protein synthesis in responsive cells through a direct effect on the cell's nucleus by modulating the transcription of DNA into messenger RNA (mRNA).	Affects the metabolism of glucose, fat, and protein. Maintains blood glucose and liver glycogen levels to provide energy substrates for increased activity. Also reduces the effects of inflammation, allergic reactions, and a variety of other processes.	Available as systemic, topical, inhalation, ophthalmic, otic, or nasal types of preparation.*
Mineralocorticoids (principally *aldosterone* in humans)	Primarily involved in maintaining fluid and electrolyte balance in the body.	Works on the kidneys to increase sodium and water reabsorption and potassium excretion. It is produced in response to low plasma sodium levels, increased *angiotensin II*, and increased plasma potassium levels.	Binds to specific receptors in epithelial cells that line the distal tube of the nephron. They increase sodium reabsorption by affecting sodium channels and sodium pumps. Excessive production can have detrimental effects on the heart and vasculature.	*Aldosterone agonists* are used as replacement therapy for patients with Addison disease, or other forms of adrenal hypofunction. *Aldosterone antagonists* are used primarily as diuretics in treating hypertension and heart failure.

Adapted from: Ciccone, CD: *Pharmacology in Rehabilitation*, ed. 4. FA Davis, Philadelphia, 2007, pp 415–421, with permission.

*Refer to Table 29-1 in Ciccone, CD: *Pharmacology in Rehabilitation*, ed. 4. FA Davis, Philadelphia, 2007, pp 422, 423.

Glossary of Pharmacological Terms

affinity: The mutual attraction between a drug and a specific receptor site.

agonist: A drug that binds to a receptor causing a change in cell activity.

antagonist: A drug that binds to a receptor but does not cause a change in cell activity.

antimetabolite: A general term for drugs (e.g., anti-infectious and anti-neoplastic agents) that impair function in harmful cells by replacing normal metabolic substrates in those cells.

antineoplastic: A drug that prevents or reduces the growth and proliferation of cancerous cells.

antipyresis: The process of reducing fever. Drugs with this ability are known as *antipyretics*.

antitussive: A drug that reduces coughing.

bioavailability: The degree to which a drug reaches the systemic circulation following administration.

blocker: See *antagonist*.

blood-brain barrier: The cerebral capillary walls that restrict the passage of some drugs into the brain.

cathartic: A drug that causes rapid evacuation of the bowels.

ceiling effect: The plateau region of a drug's dose-response curve where no further increase in response occurs as a drug dose is progressively increased.

clearance: The removal of a drug from the bloodstream by either metabolism or excretion.

demand dose: Amount of drug administered when a patient activates a drug delivery system.

desensitization: A brief and transient decrease in the responsiveness of cellular receptors to drug effects.

diuretic: A drug that increases the production and elimination of urine.

dosage: The amount of medication that is appropriate for treating a given condition or illness.

dose: The amount of medication that is administered at one time.

dose-response relationship: The relationship between the drug dose and the drug concentration at the cellular level.

down-regulation: A prolonged decrease in the number and/or sensitivity of drug receptors, such as occurs following overstimulation of the receptor.

emetic: A drug that elicits or facilitates vomiting.

enteral administration: Administration of drugs by way of the alimentary canal (digestive tract).

expectorant: A drug that facilitates the production and removal of mucous secretions from the respiratory tract.

first-pass effect: The process by which drugs absorbed from the stomach and small intestine must first pass through the liver (for hepatic metabolism) before reaching the systemic circulation.

generic name: Typically a shortened version of a drug's chemical name that is not protected by a trademark.

half-life: The time required to eliminate 50% of a drug from the body.

hypnotic: A drug that initiates or maintains relatively normal sleep.

intrathecal: Typically refers to injection of a drug into the subarachnoid space surrounding the spinal cord.

loading dose: Amount of drug initially administered to rapidly achieve a therapeutic level in the body.

maximal efficacy: See *ceiling effect.*

median effective dose (ED$_{50}$): The drug dose that produces a specific therapeutic response in 50% of the patients tested.

median lethal dose (LD$_{50}$): The drug dose that causes death in 50% of the experimental animals tested.

median toxic dose (TD$_{50}$): The drug dose that produces a specific toxic response in 50% of the patients tested.

mucolytic: A drug that facilitates the clearance of mucous secretions from the respiratory tract through coughing by decreasing the viscosity and increasing the fluidity of these secretions.

neuroleptic: A term frequently used to describe antipsychotic drugs.

ototoxicity: The harmful side effect of some drugs that impairs hearing and balance functions mediated by the ear.

over-the-counter (OTC) drugs: Nonprescription drugs that can be purchased directly by the consumer.

parenteral administration: Administration of drugs by routes other than via the digestive tract (e.g., by injection, transdermally, topically).

pharmacological dose: The administration of a drug in an amount that exceeds the quantity of the same, or similar, compound produced by the body. This increased dose is used to amplify the beneficial effects normally produced by the endogenous compound.

physiological dose: The administration of a drug in an amount that is roughly equivalent to the quantity normally produced within the body. This dose is typically used to replace an endogenous substance that is no longer produced by the body.

potency: A measure of the ability of a drug to produce a response for a given dose. A more potent drug will produce a given response at a lower dose.

sedative: A drug that produces a calming effect and serves to pacify the patient.

side effect: Any effect produced by a drug that occurs in addition to the principal therapeutic response.

supersensitivity: An increased response to drugs and endogenous compounds caused by an increase in the number and/or sensitivity of receptors for that drug.

therapeutic index (TI): A measure of the relative safety of a particular drug. It is the ratio of the median toxic dose divided by the median effective dose.

therapeutic window: The optimal range of drug concentrations in the body that will promote beneficial effects with minimal side effects.

tolerance: The acquired phenomenon produced by prolonged administration of some drugs that requires larger doses of the drug over time to achieve a given effect.

trade name: The proprietary name given to a drug by the pharmaceutical company that is protected by a trademark and used for marketing.

volume of distribution (V$_d$): A measure used to estimate the distribution of a drug within the body relative to the total amount of fluid in the body. It is the ratio of the amount of drug administered divided by the plasma concentration of the drug.

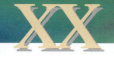
TRANSLATIONS: USEFUL EXPRESSIONS

English

Hello. I want to help you. I do not speak (English) but will use this book to ask you some questions. I will not be able to understand your spoken answers. Please respond by shaking your head or raising one finger to indicate "no"; nod your head or raise two fingers to indicate "yes."

TABLE 20.1 Introduction

Language	Phonetic
SPANISH	Sah-loo'dohs. Ki-air'oh ah-joodar' loh. Joh noh ah' bloh es'pan-yohl, pair'oh voy ah oo-sawr'es'tay lee'broh pahr'ah ah-sair' lay ahlgoo 'nahs pray-goon'tahs. Noh voy ah poh-dair'en-tendair' soos res-poo-es'tahs; pore es-soh ah'gah el fahvohr 'day kohn-tes-tahr', nay-gahn'doh kohn lah kahbay 'thah oh lay-vahntahn 'doh oon day'doh pahr'ah een-dee-kahr'noh ee ah-feer-manh'doh kohn lah kah-bay'thah oh lay-vahn-tahn'doh dohs day'dohs pahr'a een-dee-kahr'see.
KOREAN	Ahn-young-ha-sey-yo. Juh-noon-hahn-gook-mahl-run moht-ha-ji-mahn ee check-un sah-young-heh-suh myut-kah-ji-jeel-moon-url ha-keh-soom-nee-dah. Juh-nun dahng-sheen-ee dep-dahp-url ah-luh doot-jee moht-hahm-nee-da. "Ah-ne-yo" nuhn sohn-ka-lahk hahn-keh-lul do sey-yo. Jew-kuh-nah muh-rhee-rue yup-poo-roh hoon-doo-roh jew-seh-yo. "Yeah" noon sohn-ka-lahk do-ken-roh do seh-yo. Muh-rhee-url ah-rey we-roh hoon-doo-roh jew-she-yo.
MANDARIN	Hai. Wo Shiang Yau Bang Ju Nee. Wo Bu Huai Shuo Chung Wen. Dan Wo Huai Yung Juh Ben Shu Lai Wen Nee Ji Ge Wen Ti. Ke Shr Wo Ting Bu Dung Nee Shuo De Huei Da. Ching Yau Tau Huo Jiu Yi Chih Shou Chih Biau Shi "Bu Shi." Dian Tau Huo Jiu Liang Chih Shou Chih Biau Shi "Shi."
CANTONESE	Hello, Ngor Sheung Hall Yee Bong Nay. Ngor Mm Sic Gong Kong Tung Wai, Darn Hai Wui Yung Jair Boon She Lai Mun Nay Mun Tai. Ngor Mm Wui Tang Doug Ming Nay Gong Mud Yeah. Ching Nay Ling Tau, Wart Gui Hay Yut Jack Sau Gee Doy Bill "No"; Dim Tau Wart Gui Hay Leung Jack Sau Gee Doy Bill "Yes."

⬤ **TABLE 20.2 Common Physical Therapy Directions**

English	Spanish	Korean	Mandarin	Cantonese
Good morning/ afternoon/	Buenos días/ Buenas tardes/ Buenas	Ahn-young-ha-seh-yo Ahn-young-ha-seh-yo	Tsao An Wu An	Joe Sun (Term does not exist in Cantonese) Substitute: Lay Ho
evening.	noches.	Ahn-young-ha-seh-yo	Wan An	(Term does not exist in Cantonese) Substitute: Lay Ho
I am a physical therapist; my name is . . .	Soy la terapista; me llamo . . .	Juh-nun mool-lee-chi-loh-sah-eep-nee-dah. Neh ee-rhum-un . . .	Wo Shi Wu Li Chih Liau Shi; Wo De Ming Zi Shi . . .	Ngor Hai Mutt Lay Gee Liu See, Ngor Hai . . .
Answer only . . .	Conteste solamente . . .	Deh-dap-mahn hah-sey-yo . . .	Chih Yau Hui Da . . .	Ching Wuu Darp . . .
Yes.	Sí.	Yai	Shi	Hai
No.	No.	Ah-nee-yo	Bu Shi	Mm Hai
Speak slower.	Hable más despacio.	Chun-chun-nee mahl-suhm-ha-say-yo	Shuo Man Yi Dian	Ching Mann Mann Gong . . .
Say it once again.	Repítalo, por favor.	Dah-she hahn-bun mahl-suhm-hey jew-seh-yo	Tsai Shuo Yi Bian	Ching Gong Doh Yut Chee
Please wait; I will be right back.	Espere usted, por favor; re-gresaré pronto.	Jahm-she-mahn key-dah-rhee-she-yo, kohd dohl-ah-oh-keh-sum-rhee-dah	Ching Deng Yi Shia, Wo Ma Shang Huei Lai.	Ching Dung Dung; Ngor Yut Chun Farn Lai

English	Spanish	Korean	Mandarin	Cantonese
Don't be afraid.	No tenga miedo.	Kub-neh-jee mah-sey-yo	Bu Yung Pa	Mm Sai Par/Mm Sai Gang
Try to remember.	Trate de recordar.	Kee-uk-ha-doe-rouk no-roo-ha-she-yo	Shi Juh Shiang Yi Shi-ang	Ching Gay Jui
Pay attention.	Preste attención.	Jew-mohk-ha-she-yo	Ju Yi	Ching Lau Sum
Come to my office.	Venga a mi oficina.	Jeh sah-mu-sheel-ro oh-sey-yo	Dow Wo De Ban Gung Shi	Ching Yup Lai Ngor Office
Show me . . .	Muéstreme . . .	Juh-eh-keh bo-yo-jew-she-yo	Gei Wo Kan . . .	Ching Bay Ngor Tigh Tigh
Right.	Derecha.	Oh-luhn-chok	Yo	Yau Bin
Left.	Izquierda.	When-chok	Tzuo	Jaw Bin
Here.	Aquí.	Yuh-ki	Juh Li	Lay Doh
There.	Allí. OR Allá.	Kuh-ki	Na Li	Goh Doh
Good.	Bien (adv.); Bueno (a) (adj.).	Choi-ah-yo	How	Ho
Bad.	Mal OR Malo (a).	Nah-boob-nee-dah	Bu How	Mm Ho
More or less.	Más o menos.	Koo chung-doh-myun dehm-nee-dah	Char Bu Duo	Char Mm Doh/Dai Koi
That is correct.	Es correcto (a).	Koo-keh mah-soom-nee-dah	Duei	Arm La
Not much.	No mucho.	Byul-loh	Bu Duo	Mm Doh/Mo Mud

(table continues on page 1166)

TRANSLAT

🔴 **TABLE 20.2 Common Physical Therapy Directions** (continued)

English	Spanish	Korean	Mandarin	Cantonese
Never.	Nunca.	Juhn-hyo	Tsung Lai Mei Yo	Mo/May See Gor
Never mind.	Olvídelo.	Sheen-kyung-soo-jee mah-sey-yo	Mei Guan Shi	Mm Gun Yiu
That will do.	Es suficiente.	Koo-kuh-she-muhn dep-nee-dah	Juh Jiou Ke Yi	Gum Doh Hall Yee
You must be very careful.	Tiene que tener mucho cuidado.	Ah-jew jo-sheem heh-yah hahb-nee-dah	Nee Yi Ding Yau Fei Chang Shiau Shin	Lay Yiu Ho Siu Sum
Please listen.	Escuche, por favor.	Dool-uh boh-sey-yo	Ju Yi Ting	Ching Lau Sum Tang Jui
It is important to be safe.	Es importante tener cuidado.	Ahn-jyun-han kuh-she-hahb-nee-dah	An Chiuan Hen Jung Yau	On Chuen Jee Sheung/ On Chuen Dai Yat
Keep very quiet.	No haga ningún ruido. OR Quédese quieto(a).	Jo-young-hee hah-sey-yo	Bow Chi An Jing	Ching Soak Jing
You must not speak.	No tiene que hablar.	Mahl-ha-muhn ahn-dep-nee-dah	Bu Yau Shuo Hua	Ching Soak Jing

TABLE 20.3 Questions Used in History Taking

English	Spanish	Korean	Mandarin	Cantonese
What is your name?	¿Como se llama usted?	Ee-lum-ee moo-us-eeb-nee-kah?	Nee Jiau Shu Mo Min Zi?	Lay Giu Mutt Menn?
How old are you?	¿Cuántos años tiene usted?	Nah-ee-kah muht sahl-eem-nee-kah?	Nee Ji Suei?	Lay Gay Shui?
Do you understand me?	¿Me en-tiende? OR ¿Me com-prende?	Geh mahl-url ee-hey-hah-s he-kehs-soob-nee-kah?	Nee Zhi Dow Wo Shua Shu Mo Ma?	Lay Ming Baht Ngor Gong Mutt Yeah?
What did you say?	¿Qué dijó usted?	Moh-lah-koh hehs-soom-nee-kah?	Nee Shuo Shu Mo?	Lay Gong Mutt Yeah?
Are you married?	¿Está usted casado (a)?	Kyul-hone-hah-suhs-soom-nee-kah?	Nee Jie Huen Le Ma?	Lay Git Fun May?
Do you have children?	¿Tiene usted hijos OR niños?	Jah-nyo-kah ees-soom-nee-kah?	Nee Yo Hai Zi Ma?	Lay Yau Mo Jai Lui?
What are your children's ages?	¿Cuántos años tienen sus niños OR hijos?	Ah-hee-dool-eh nah-ee-nun myut sahl-eeb-nee-kah?	Nee Hai Zi Ji Suei?	Lay Jai Lui Gay Shui?
Do you have any sisters/brothers?	¿Tiene usted hermanas/hermanos?	Jah-meh-nah hyung-jeh-kah ees-soom-nee-kah?	Nee Yo Shiung Di Jie Mei Ma?	Lay Yau Mo Hing Dai Gee Mui?

(table continues on page 1168)

TRANSLAT

TABLE 20.3 Questions Used in History Taking (continued)

English	Spanish	Korean	Mandarin	Cantonese
Is your mother/ father alive?	¿Vive su madre/ padre?	(Mother) Uh-mon-nee kah sahl-ah-kehs-seeb-nee-kah? (Father) Ah-bun-nee kah sahl-ah-kehs-seeb-nee-kah?	Nee De Mu-Chin/ Fu-Chin Hai Huo Juh Ma?	Lay Fu Mo Geen Joy Ma?
Of what did your mother die? And your father?	¿De qué murió su madre? ¿Y su padre?	(Mother) Uh-mon-nee-noon moo-soon byung-oo-loh doh-lah-kah-suhs-nee-kah? (Father) Ah-bun-ghee-noon moo-soon byung-oo-loh doh-lah-kah-suhs-nee-kah?	Nee Mu Chin Shi Tze Mo Guo Shi De? Nee Fu Chin Ne?	Lay Ma Ma Dim Yeung Guo Sai? Lay Ba Ba Dim Yeung Guo Sai?
Where were you born?	¿Dónde nació usted?	Uh-dee-suh teh-uh-nah-suhs-soom-nee-kah?	Nee Tzai Na Chu Sheng De?	Lay Bin Doh Chut Sung?
Can you read?	¿Puede usted leer?	Ghul-url eel-koo-sue ees-soom-nee-kah?	Nee Huei Du Ma?	Lay Ho Yee Duk Ma?
Can you write?	¿Puede usted escribir?	Ghul-url surl sue ees-soom-nee-kah?	Nee Huei Shie Ma?	Lay Ho Yee Sair Gee Ma?
Are you nervous?	¿Está usted nervioso (a)?	Boo-lahn hop-nee-kah?	Jin Jang Ma?	Lay Gun Jeung Ma?

English	Spanish	Korean	Mandarin	Cantonese
Can you remember?	¿Puede usted recordar?	Kee-yok-hahl sue ees-soom-nee-kah?	Nee Ji De Ma?	Lay Gay Doug Ma?
Is it possible?	¿Es posible?	Kah-noong hahn-kah-yo?	Ke Neng Ma?	Hall Mm Hall Yee?
Is it necessary?	¿Es necesario?	Pee-loh-hahn-kah-yo?	Yo Bi Yau Ma?	Yut Ding Ma?
Which side?	¿A qué lado?	Uh-new johk-eeb-nee-kah??	Na Yi Bian?	Bin Been?
Since when?	¿Desde cuándo?	Uhn-jeh-boo-tuh-eeb-nee-kah?	Tsung Shu Mo Shi Ho Kai Shi De?	Yau Gay See Hoi Chee?
How long?	¿Cuánto tiempo?	Uhl-mah'-nah oh-leh?	Duo Jiu Le?	Gay Loi?
How often?	¿Cuántas veces? OR ¿Con cuánta frequencia?	Uhl-mah-nah jah-ju?	Duo Chang Fa Sheng?	Yau Gay Doll Chee?
Why?	¿Por qué?	Whey-yo?	Wei Shu Mo?	Dim Gai?
When?	¿Cuándo?	Un-jey-yo?	Shu Mo Shi Ho?	Gay See?
About how much?	¿Cuánto?	Uh-new jung-doe-eeb-nee-kah?	Da Gai Duo Shau?	Gay Doll?
Do you have any questions?	¿Tiene usted algunas preguntas?	Jeel-moon-ees-soom-nee-kah?	Nee Yo Ren He Wen Ti Ma?	Yau Mo Mun Tai?
Why are you here?	¿Por qué está usted aquí?	Yo-kee whey oh-shut-soom-nee-kah?	Nee Wei Shu Mo Lai?	Dim Gai Lay Yiu Tai Yee Sung?

(table continues on page 1170)

TRANSLAT

🔴 **TABLE 20.3 Questions Used in History Taking** (continued)

English	Spanish	Korean	Mandarin	Cantonese
How do you feel?	¿Cómo está usted? OR ¿Cómo se siente usted?	Kee-boon-ee uh-deh-sheem-nee-kah?	Nee Jiue De Tzen Yang?	Lay Gock Doug Dim?
When did you first become sick?	¿Cuándo se enfermó usted al principio?	Chuh-oom ah-paht-dun keh un-jeh-eem-nee-kah?	Nee Shu Mo Shi Ho Kai Shi Bing?	Lay Gay See Hoi Chee Mm Shu Folk?
How long have you felt like this?	¿Cuánto tiempo se ha sentido así?	Ee-lok-keh noo-keen-gee url-mahn-nah oh-reh-des-soom-nee-kah?	Juh Yang Tz Duo Jiou Le?	Lay Yau Gay Loi Mm Shu Folk?
How did this illness begin?	¿Cómo empezó esta enfermedad?	Byung-ee uh-duk-keh she-jahk-deh-us-soom-nee-kah?	Juh Bing Shi Ru He Kai Shi De?	Lay Behn Hai Dim Yeung Hoi Chee?
What happened?	¿Qué ocurrió? OR ¿Qué pasó?	Moo-soon ee-il-nee-kah?	Fa Sheng Shu Mo Shi?	Yau Mud Yeah Fat Sung?
Did you have an accident?	¿Había un accidente? OR ¿Tuvo un accidente?	Sah-ko-kah nahs-soom-nee-kah?	Nee Tseng Yo Yi Wai Ma?	Lay Gee Chin Yau Mo Yee Oi?
Did it begin gradually?	¿Empezó gradualmente?	Suh-suh-hee she-jahk-deh-us-soom-nee-kah?	Ta Shi Man Man Kai Shi De Ma?	Yau Mo Mann Mann Hoi Chee?
Did you take anything for it?	¿Tomó usted algo para esto?	Koo-kuhs deh-moon-hey uh-duhn chee-rol-url bahd-ahs-soom-nee-kah?	Nee Yo Ru He Chu Li?	Lay Yau Mo Sick Yerk?

English	Spanish	Korean	Mandarin	Cantonese
Do you feel like you are falling?	¿Le parece que se va a caer?	Nuh-muhn-jee-nun kuht chuh-rum noo-kim-neh-kah?	Nee Jiue De Shi-ang Yau Die Dow Ma?	Lay Yau Mo Gock Doug Sheung Dit?
Do you feel dizzy?	¿Tiene usted vértigo?	Uh-jew-loh-sey-yo?	Nee Yo Tow Yun Ma?	Lay Yau Mo Gock Doug Won?
Have you any difficulty in breathing?	¿Tiene dificultad de respirar?	Soom-she-kee-kah uh-lohb-soom-nee-kah?	Nee Huei Hu Shi Kuen Nan Ma?	Lay Yau Mo Foo Cup Kwon Larn?
Have you lost weight?	¿Ha perdido usted peso?	Mohm-moo-keh-kah jew-luhs-soom-nee-kah?	Nee Ti Jung Yo Shia Jiang Ma?	Lay Yau Mo Sau Doh?
Are you warm?	¿Tiene usted calor?	Dupt-soom-nee-kah?	Nee Nuan Ma?	Lay Gock Doug Luen Ma?
Are you cold?	¿Tiene usted frío?	Choop-soom-nee-kah?	Nee Leng Ma?	Lay Gock Doug Dong Ma?
Can you eat?	¿Puede usted comer?	Muk-url sue ees-soom-nee-kah?	Nee Ke Yi Chi Ma?	Lay Sick Yeah Yau Mo Mun Tai?
Do you have a good appetite?	¿Tiene usted buen apetito?	Sheek-yoke-oon cho-soom-nee-kah?	Nee Shi Yu Hau Ma?	Lay Yau Mo Wai Hau?
Are you thirsty?	¿Tiene usted sed?	Mohk-mah-loo-sheem-nee-kah?	Nee Kou Ke Ma?	Lay Gang Hot Ma?
Do you still feel very weak?	¿Se siente muy débil todavía?	Ah-jeek-doh meh-oo yak-ha-dah-koh-noo-kim-nee-kah?	Nee Hai Shi Jiue De Hen Shiu Ruo (Mei Li) Ma?	Lay Yau Mo Gock Doug Hui Yerk?

(table continues on page 1172)

TRANSLAT

TRANSLAT

TABLE 20.3 Questions Used in History Taking (continued)

English	Spanish	Korean	Mandarin	Cantonese
Had you been drinking an alcoholic beverage?	¿Había tomado usted alguna bebida alcohólica?	Sool mah-shuhs-sheem-nee-kah?	Nee Yo He Ren He Yo Jiou Jing De Yin Liau Ma?	Lay Yau Mo Yum Jau?
Do you drink alcohol?	¿Bebe usted alcohol?	Sool mah-sheem-nee-kah?	Nee He Jiou Ma?	Lay Yum Jau Ma?
Do you smoke cigarettes?	¿Fuma usted cigarillos?	Dahm-beh pee-oo-sheem-nee-kah?	Nee Cho Yan Ma?	Lay Sick Yin Ma?
Have you had any surgeries?	¿Ha tenido usted algunas operaciones?	Sue-sool bah-doon juk ees-soom-nee-kah?	Nee Yo Guo Ren Her Show Shoo Ma?	Lay Yau Mo Joe Gaw Sau Shirt?
Does your (body part) feel paralyzed?	¿Se siente (parte del cuerpo) paralizado (a)?	. . . uh mah-bee-kah-eet-dah-koh noo-ghim-nee-kah?	Nee Jiue De ____ Ma Bi Ma?	Lay Yau Mo Gock Doug Sing Sun Mm Yuk Doug?
Are you tired?	¿Está usted cansado (a)?	Pee-kohn-hah-seep-nee-kah?	Nee Jiue De Lai Ma?	Lay Yau Mo Ho Gui?
Have you slept well?	¿Ha dormido bien usted?	Jahl jahs-soom-nee-kah?	Nee Shuei De Hau Ma?	Lay Fun Gow Ho Ma?
In what position do you sleep?	¿En qué posición duerme usted?	Uh-done jah-sey-loh jahb-nee-kah?	Nee Dou Shuei Shi Mo Tz Shi?	Lay Fun Gow Gee Sai Dim Yeung?
How long do you sleep at night?	¿Cuántas horas duerme usted por la noche?	Bahm-eh uhl-mah-nah oh-leh jew-moo-sey-yo?	Nee Wan Shang Shuei Duo Jiou?	Lay Fun Gow Yau Gay Doh Siu See?

English	Spanish	Korean	Mandarin	Cantonese
How many times do you wake up during the night?	¿Cuántas veces se despierta usted durante la noche?	Jahm jah-dah-kah url-mah-nah jah-jew-gheb-nee-kah?	Nee Wan Shang Shing Lai Ji Tsz?	Lay Fun Gow Seng Gay Doh Chee?
How many times do you get up to use the bathroom?	¿Cuántas veces se levanta usted para usar el baño?	Hwa-jang-sheel kah-kee we-hey-soh myut bun ee-loh-nam-nee-kah?	Nee Wan Shang Shing Lai Shang Tse Suo Ji Tsz?	Lay Hay Gay Doh Chee Sun Hui Siu Bin?

TABLE 20.4 Questions Used to Assess Pain

English	Spanish	Korean	Mandarin	Cantonese
Have you any pain?	¿Tiene dolor?	Tyong-jyung-ee Ees-sue-she-yo?	Nee Hui Tung Ma?	Lay Yau Mo Tone?
Where does it hurt?	¿Dónde le duele?	Uh-dee-kah Ah-poo-sheem-nee-kah?	Na Li Tung?	Bin Doh Tone?
Point to where it hurts.	Muéstreme dónde le duele.	Ah-poon koh-surl jeep-puh boh-sey-yo.	Chih Gei Wo Kan Na Li Tung?	Ching Jee Bay Ngor Tai Bin Doh Tone?
When does it hurt?	¿Cuándo le duele?	Un-jeh ah-poo-sheem-nee-kah?	Shu Mo Shi Ho Huei Tung?	Gay See Wui Tone?
Do you have pain here?	¿Le duele aquí?	Yo-kee-eh tyong-jyung-ee ees-soom-nee-kah?	Juh Li Tung Ma?	Lay Doh Tone Mm Tone?

(table continues on page 1174)

TABLE 20.4 Questions Used to Assess Pain (continued)

English	Spanish	Korean	Mandarin	Cantonese
Do you have a pain in your chest?	¿Le duele el pecho?	Kay-soom-eh tyong-jyung-url mah-nee noo-gyut-soom-nee-kah?	Nee Shi-ung Bu Huei Tung Ma?	Hone Hau Yau Mo Tone?
Does it hurt you to breathe?	¿Le duele respirar?	Soom-sheel-deh Ah-poo-sheep-nee-kah?	Hu Shi Huei Tung Ma?	Tau Hay Yau Mo Tone?
Did you feel much pain at the time?	¿Sintió mucho dolor entonces? OR ¿Le dolia mucho?	Khut-den tyung-jyung-url mah-nee noo-gyut-soom-nee-kah?	Na Shi Ho Hen Tung Ma?	Lay Goh See Yau Mo Gock Doug Tone?
Is it better/ worse now?	¿Está mejor/peor ahora?	(Better) Gee-koom-un duh choi-ah-juhs-soom-nee-kah? (Worse) Gee-koom-un duh nah-bah-juhs-soom-nee-kah?	Shian Tzai Jiau Hau/ Jiau Cha Ma?	Yee Ga Ho Mm Ho Dee?
Does it still hurt you?	¿Todavía le duele?	Ahh-jig-toh Ah-pooh-she-yo?	Reng Tan Jiue De Tung Ma?	Yee Ga Ying Yin Yau Mo Tone?
Is your pain a shooting pain?	¿El dolor es un dolor punzante?	Sew-doo-she-ahp-poom-nee-kah?		Tone See Gok Doug Kek Tone Ma?
Is your pain an aching pain?	¿El dolor es un latido doloroso?	Sue-sheem-nee-kah?	Suan Tung Ma?	Tone See Gok Doug John Tone Ma?

English	Spanish	Korean	Mandarin	Cantonese
Is your pain a burning pain?	¿El dolor es un dolor que quema?	Hwak-goon-kuh-leeb-nee-kah?	Shuo Re Tung Ma?	Tone See Gok Doug Chee Seal Sheung Ma?
Is your pain as if one were pricking you with pins?	¿El dolor es como pinchar a uno?	Bah-newl-lo jee-loo-doo-see-ahp-poom-nee-kah?	Hau Shi-ang Yung Jen Chuo De Tung Ma?	Tone See Gok Doug Jump Gut Ma?
Does it feel the same as the other side?	¿Se siente lo mismo al otro lado?	Dah-rhun jyok-kwa kah-jee-new-key-sey-yo?	Han Ling Wai Yi Bian Gan Jiue Yi Yang Ma?	Ling Oi Yat Bin Yat Yeung Tone Ma?
Does your (body part) feel like "pins and needles"?	¿Está (parte del cuerpo) en brazas?	. . . eh bah-nuhl-ro ghe-rue-noon kuht kaht-oon new-ghim-ee ees-soom-nee-kah?	Nee De ____ Gan Jiue Shiang Jen Tsz Yi Yang Ma?	Tone See Gok Doug Jump Gut Ma?

TRANSLAT

TABLE 20.5 Questions Used to Assess Function

English	Spanish	Korean	Mandarin	Cantonese
What are your goals?	¿Cuáles son sus objetivos?	. . . mohk-pyi-kuh moo uht-im-nee-kah?	Nee De Chi Wang Shi Shu Mo?	Lay Hay Mong Dim?
What are you unable to do because of your condition?	¿Cuáles son las cosas que no puede usted hacer a causa de esta condición?	Kun-kang sahng-teh deh-moon-eh hahl sue up-noon kuh-she moo-us-sheem-nee-kah?	Shu Mo Shi Yin Wei Nee Shian Tzai De Juang Kuang Tzuo Bu Dow De?	Lay Yau Mud Yeah Mm Joe Doug?
What would you like to be able to do?	¿Qué quisiera hacer?	Moo-us-sool hahl sue eh-keh deh-kee-url won-hah-sheem-nee-kah?	Shu Mo Shu Nee Shiang Tzuo Dow De?	Lay Hay Mong Joe Mud Yeah?
What could we help you do better?	¿Qué podremos hacer para ayudarle a usted?	Duh nah-ah-ghee-doh-lohk juh-heee-kah moo-uh-sool doh-ah-doo-rhee-kah-yo?	Wo Men Ru He He Ke Yi Bang Ju Nee Tzuo Geng Hau?	Ngor Day Hall Yee Bong Lay Dee Mud Yeah?
Are you able to dress yourself?	¿Puede usted vestirse?	Hyon-jah oht-soon ee-bool sue ees-soob-nee-kah?	Nee Ke Yi Tz Ji Chuan Yi Fu Ma?	Lay Hall Yee Jee Gay Jerk Sarm Ma?
Are you able to bathe yourself?	¿Puede usted ban~arse?	Hyon-jah mohk-yohk-hahl sue ees-soob-nee-kah?	Nee Ke Yi Tz Ji Shi Tzau Ma?	Lay Hall Yee Jee Gay Chung Leung Ma?
Are you able to drink from a glass?	¿Puede usted beber de un vaso?	You-rhee cup-ee-roh mool-ool mah-sheel sue ees-soom-nee-kah?	Nee Ke Yi Tz Ji Na Bei Tz He Ma?	Lay Hall Yee Jee Gay Yum Shui Ma?

English	Spanish	Korean	Mandarin	Cantonese
Are you able to feed yourself?	¿Puede usted comer por sí solo/sola?	Hyon-jah-suh oom-sheek-un muhk-url-sue ees-soom-nee-kah?	Nee Ke Yi Tz Ji Chi Dung Shi Ma?	Lay Hall Yee Jee Gay Sick Yeah Ma?
Are you able to use the toilet?	¿Puede usted irse al baño?	Hwa-jyang-sheel-un sah-young-hahl sue ees-soom-nee-kah?	Nee Ke Yi Tz Ji Shang Tse Suo Ma?	Lay Hall Yee Jee Gay Hui Sai Sau Gahn Ma?
Are you able to use the telephone?	¿Puede usted usar el teléfono?	Jhun-hwa-rhur sah-young-hahl sue ees-soob-nee-kah?	Nee Ke Yi Tz Ji Da Dian Hua Ma?	Lay Hall Yee Jee Gay Da Dean Wa Ma?
Does anyone help you?	¿Hay alguien que le ayuda?	Dah-rhun sah-lahm-ee doh-hwa joob-nee-kah?	Yo Ren He Ren Bang Nee Ma?	Yau Mo Yon Bong Lay?
Whom do you live with: Mother/father? Husband/wife?	¿Vive usted con: Su madre/padre? Su esposo/esposa?	Noo-koo-wah-koo kah-chee saab-nee-kah? : (Mother/Father)? Uh-mohn-nee/Ab-buh-ghee? (Husband/Wife)? Nahm-pyon/Ah-ney?	Nee Gen Shei Ju? Mu Chin/Fu Chin? Shian Sheng/Tai Tai?	Lay Tung Bin Goh Yah Chai Juu? Fu Mo? Tai Tai/Jeung Fu?
Children?	Sus niños?	Ah-ee-nun-yo?	Hai Zi?	Yee Lui?
Alone?	Por sí solo/sola?	Hwon-jah eeb-nee-kah?	Zi Ji?	Jee Gay?

(table continues on page 1178)

TRANSLAT

TABLE 20.5 Questions Used to Assess Function (continued)

English	Spanish	Korean	Mandarin	Cantonese
Aunt/uncle?	Su tía/tío?	Ee-moh/Sahm-chyon?	A Yi/Bo Shu?	Yee? Sook?
Grandmother/ grandfather?	Su abuela/abuelo?	Hahl-mohn-nee/ Ha-la-buh-ghee?	Tzu Fu/Tzu Mu?	Joe Fu Mo?
Friend(s)?	Su amiga(o)/ amigas (amigos)?	Cheen-koo (dool)?	Peng Yo?	Pung Yau?
Where do you live?	¿Dónde vive usted?	Uh-dee-eh-suh sahl-ko ees-soom-nee-kah?	Nee Ju Na Li?	Lay Ju Bin Doh?
Do you have to go up/down stairs?	¿Tiene usted que pasearse en las escaleras o arriba o abajo?	Keh-dahn-un oh-roo neh-il-soo ees-soom-nee-kah?	Nee Shi Yau Shang Shia Lo Tea Ma?	Lay Yiu Sheung Lock Lau Tai Ma?
Do you have stairs in your house?	¿Hay escaleras en casa?	Jeeb ahn-eh keh-dahn-ee ees-soom-nee-kah?	Nee Jia Li Yo Lo Ti Ma?	Yau Mo Lau Tai Hai Uk Loi?
Do you have stairs outside?	¿Hay escaleras afuera?	Jeeb bahk-eh keh-dahn-ee ees-soom-nee-kah?	Nee Jia Wai Mian Yo Jie Ti Ma?	Yau Mo Lau Tai Hai Uk Oi?
Is there a handrail?	¿Hay pasamano?	Nahn-kang-ee ees-soom-nee-kah?	Yo Fu Shou Ma?	Yau Mo Fu Sau?

TRANSLAT

English	Spanish	Korean	Mandarin	Cantonese
Do you have an elevator?	¿Hay ascensor?	Elevator-kah ees-soom-nee-kah?	Nee Jia Yo Dian Ti Ma?	Yau Mo Dean Tai?
Do you use a walker?	¿Usa usted un walker?	Wohk-kuh-url sah-yong-hah-sheep-nee-kah?	Nee Yo Yong Ju Shing Chi Ma?	Lay Yung Hang Low Hay Ma?
Do you use a cane?	¿Usa usted un bastón?	Kee-pahng-ee-url sah-yong-hah-sheep-nee-kah?	Nee Yo Yong Guai Jang Ma?	Lay Yung Gwai Jeung Ma?
Do you use crutches?	¿Usa usted muletas?	Mohk-bahl-url sah-yong-hah-sheep-nee-kah?	Nee Yo Yong Yi Shia Guai Jang Ma?	Lay Yung Gwai Jeung Ma?
Do you use a brace?	¿Usa usted una abrazadera?	Boh-joh-kee-url sah-yong-hah-sheep-nee-kah?	Nee Yo Young Jr Jia Ma?	Lay Yung Gee Ga Ma?
Do you play any sports?	¿Juega usted a los deportes?	Ooon-dong ha-nuhn-kut ees-soom-nee-kah?	Nee Yo Tzuo Shu Mo Yun Dung Ma?	Lay Yau Mo Joe Won Dhone?

TABLE 20.6 Questions Used to Assess Work

English	Spanish	Korean	Mandarin	Cantonese
Are you working?	¿Trabaja usted?	Eel-hah-ko ees-soom-nee-kah?	Nee Gung Tzuo Ma?	Lay Yau Mo Gung Jock?
What work do you do?	¿Cuál es su ocupación?	Moo-soon ee-rhun Hah-sheep-nee-kah?	Nee Tzuo Shu Mo Gung Tzuo?	Lay Joe Mud Yeah Gung Jock?
Is it heavy physical work?	¿Es un tra-bajo corpo-ral pesado?	Mohm-un mahn-ee sue-nun ee-im-nee-kah?	Shi Lau Li De Gung Tzuo Ma?	Lay Joe Choad Chung Gung Jock Ma?
What work have you done?	¿Qué trabajo ha hecho?	Moo-soon ee-er heh boh-shush-soob-nee-kah?	Nee Tzuo Guo Na Shie Shi Ching?	Lay Joe Mud Yeah Gung Jock?

TABLE 20.7 Expressions Related to Medications

English	Spanish	Korean	Mandarin	Cantonese
Are you taking any medications?	¿Toma usted medicina?	Yahk muhk-nun kuhs ees-soob-nee-kah?	Nee Yo Chi Yao Ma?	Lay Yau Mo Sick Yerk?
What medications do you take?	¿Cuáles son las medicinas que toma?	Moo-soon yah-khun muhk-soob-nee-kah?	Nee Yung Na Shie Yao?	Mud Yeah Yerk?
Have you taken the medicine?	¿Ha tomado usted la medicina?	Yahk-un muhk-uhs-soob-nee-kah?	Nee Tseng Yung Yao Ma?	Lay Yau Mo Sick Yerk?
Bring in your pill bottle.	Traiga consigo la botella de pildoras.	Yahk-byung-un-kah-jyo oh-sey-yo.	Dai Nee De Yao Guan Lai.	Ching Dai Mai Yerk Jun Lai.
Bring in a list of the names of the medications you are taking.	Traiga consigo una lista de las medici-nas que toma.	Ghee-koom muhk-koh eet-nun yahk-kurl mohk-lohk-url kah-jyo oh-sey-yo.	Dai Nee Suo Yo Tzai Chi De Yao De Ming Dan Lai.	Ching Dai Mai Lay Sick Saul Yau Yerk Lai.

TABLE 20.8 Terms Used to Describe Diseases and Medical Conditions

English	Spanish	Korean	Mandarin	Cantonese
What diseases/ medical problems have you had?	¿Cuáles son las enfermedades o problemas que usted ha tenido?	Uh-duhn Gheel-byong-ee-nah yah-keh deh-heh mon-jeh-kah ee-suhs-soup-nee-kah?	Nee Tseng Yo Guo Shi Mo Ji Bing?	Lay Yau Mud Yeah Behn?
Arthritis.	Artritis.	Kahn-juhl-yum	Guan Jie Yan	Fung Sub.
Bleeding.	Flujo de sangre.	Chool-hyurl	Chu Shie	Chut Huet.
Burn.	Quemadura.	Hwa-sahng	Shau Shang	Siu Shueng.
Cancer.	Cáncer.	Ahm	Ai Jeng	Arm Behn.
Chickenpox.	Varicela.	Soo-doo	Shuei Do	Shui Dull.
Diabetes.	Diabetes.	Dahng-nyo-byung	Tang Neeau Bing	Tong Liu.
Diphtheria.	Difteria.	"Diptheria"	Bai Ho	Bart Hou.
Ear infections.	Dolores de oído.	Ee-yohm	Jung Er Yan	Yee Fat Yim.
Fracture.	Fracturas.	kohl-juhl	Gu Juh	Tun Gwat.
German measles.	Rubéola.	poong-jean	De Guo Ma Jen	Doug Gawk Ma Chun.
Gonorrhea.	Gonorrea.	Eem-jeel	Lin Bing	Lum Behn.
Head injury.	Daño de cabeza.	Doo-boo sohn-sahng	Tow Bu Shou Shang	Tau John Sheung.
Headaches.	Dolores de cabeza.	Doo-tyong	Tow Tung	Tau Tone.
Heart disease.	Enfermedad del corazón.	Sheem-jyang-byung	Shin Tzang Bing	Sum Jong Behn.

(table continues on page 1182)

TRANSLAT

TABLE 20.8 Terms Used to Describe Diseases and Medical Conditions (continued)

English	Spanish	Korean	Mandarin	Cantonese
High blood pressure.	Tensíon sanguinea elevada.	koh-hurl-ahp	Gau Shie Ya	Go Huet Art.
High fevers.	Fiebres elevadas.	koh-yurl	Gau Shau	Fat Go Siu.
HIV.	HIV.	"HIV"	Ai Zi Bing Du	Oi Gee Behn.
Influenza.	Gripe (influenza).	Dohk-kahm	Liu Shing Shing Gan Mau	Gum Moh.
Measles.	Sarampión.	Hyong-yuk	Ma Jen	Ma Chun.
Mental disease.	Enfermedad mental.	Jhung-sheen-jeel-hwan	Jing Shen Bin	Jing Sun Behn.
Mumps.	Paperas.	You-heng-sung ee-hah-sun-yum	Sai Shian Yan	Jar Soy.
Nervous disease.	Enfermedad nerviosa.	Sheen-kyung-jeel-hwan	Shen Jing Ji Bing	Sun Ging Hai Tone Behn.
Pleurisy.	Pleuresía.	Nook-mahk-yum	Shiung Mo Yan	Hone Mock Yim.
Pneumonia.	Pulmonía.	Peh-um	Fei Yan	Fai Yim.
Polio.	Poliomielitis. OR Parálisis infantíl.	So-ah-mah-bee	Shiau Er Ma Bi	Siu Yee Ma Bay.
Rheumatic fever.	Fiebre reumática.	Rue-mah-tee-juhm yurl	Feng Shi Shing Re	Fung Sub Behn.
Rheumatoid arthritis.	Artritis reumatoidea	Rue-mah-tee-sue-sung kwan-churl-yum	Lei Feng Shi Shing Guan Jie Yan	Fung Sub Sing Guan Jit Yim.
Scarlet fever.	Escarlatina.	sung-hyong-url	Shing Hung Re	Sing Hung Yeat.

English	Spanish	Korean	Mandarin	Cantonese
Seizures.	Ataques.	kahn-jeel byong	Dian Jian	Chau Gun.
Smallpox.	Viruela.	chun-youn-do	Tian Hua	Shui Dull.
Sprain.	Torcedura.	Yum-jah	Neou Shang	Lau Sheung.
Stroke.	Ataque fulminante.	Nweh-jorl-joong	Jung Feng	Jung Fung.
Syphilis.	Sífilis.	Meh-dohk	Mei Du	Mui Duk.
Tuberculosis.	Tuberculosis.	Kurl-heck	Fei Jia Her	Fai Low.
Typhoid fever.	Fiebre tifoidea.	Jahng-tee-boo-sue	Shang Han Jeng	Sheung Hong.
Ulcer.	Úlcera.	Kweh-yang	Ru Chuang	Kwui Yeung.

🔴 **TABLE 20.9 Examination: General Instructions**

English	Spanish	Korean	Mandarin	Cantonese
Please.	Por favor	Jeh-bahl	Ching	Ching.
Thank you.	Gracias.	Kahm-sah-hahb-nee-dah	Shie Shie	Doh Jieh.
You are welcome.	De nada.	Chun-mahn-eh-im-nee-dah.	Bu Ker Chi	Mm Sai Hart Hay.
Please remove your	Por favor quítese.	. . . url chee-woh-jew-sey-yo	Ching Tuo Diau Nee De	Ching Chui Hui Lay
Dress.	El vestido.	Ohd	Yi Fu	Sarm
Pants.	Los pantalones.	bah-jee	Ku Zi	Fu
Shirt.	La camisa.	shue-sue	Chen Shan	Shirt Sarm
Shoes.	Los zapatos.	Sheem-bahl	Shie Zi	Hai

(table continues on page 1184)

TRANSLAT

⬤ **TABLE 20.9 Examination: General Instructions** (continued)

English	Spanish	Korean	Mandarin	Cantonese
Socks.	Las calcetines.	Yang-mahl	Wa Zi	Mud
Let me see . . .	Déjeme ver . . .	. . . url juh-eh-keh boh-yo jew-she-yo	Rang Wo Kan	Dung Ngor Tai Tai . . .
Let me feel your pulse.	Déjeme tomarle el pulso.	Mehk-bahk-un jee-puh boh-kehs-soob-nee-dah	Rang Wo Mo Yi Shia Nee De Mai Bo	Dung Ngor Learn Mug Bok.
Show me your right/left (body part).	Muéstreme (parte del cuerpo) derecho (a)/ izquierdo (a).	(Right) Oh-luhn-chohk . . . url boh-yo jew-sey-yo. (Left) When-chohk . . . url boh-yo jew-sey-yo.	Gei Wo Kan Nee Der yo/tzuo Bian	Bay Ngor Tai Tai Lay Yau/ Jaw Bin.
Look straight ahead.	Mire usted hacia delante.	Jong-myun-url boh-she-yo.	Kan Chian Mian	Mong Chin Min.
You are not going to fall.	Usted no se va a caer.	Nuhm-muh-gee-gee ahn-arl-kub-nee-dah.	Nee Bu Huei Dow	Lay Mm Wui Dit Dai.
This will not hurt.	Ésto no le va a doler.	Ah-poo-gee ahn-arl-kub-nee-dah.	Juh Ger Bu Huei Tong	Lay Dee Mm Tone.
Tell me when it starts to hurt.	Dígame cuándo empieza a doler.	Ah-poo-ki she-jahk-hahl deh mahl-soom hah-sey-yo.	Kai Shi Tong Der Shi Ho Gau Sue Wo	Tone See Wah Bay Ngor Gee.
You are okay.	Usted está bien.	Kehn-chahn-soob-nee-dah.	Nee Hen Hau	Lay OK.
Don't cry.	No llore.	Ool-jee mah-sey-yo.	Bu Yau Ku	Mm Sai Harm.

English	Spanish	Korean	Mandarin	Cantonese
Don't worry.	No se preocupe.	Yum-yo-ha-gee mah-sey-yo.	Bu Yung Dan Shin	Mm Sai Darm Sum.
Sit up.	Siéntese.	Eel-uh-nah ahn-jew-she-yo.	Tzuo Hau	Chore Jick.
Sit down.	Siéntese.	Ahn-jew-seh-yo.	Tzuo Shia	Chore Dight.
Stand.	Levántese.	Suh she-yo.	Jan Chi Lai	Kay Hay Sun.
Walk.	Ande.	Kuh-rhoo-she-yo.	Tzou Lu	Harn La.
Roll over.	Vuelva.	Doh-rah Noo-oo-sey-yo.	Fan Shen	June Sun.
Lie on your stomach on the table (face down).	Acuéstese en la mesa con boca abajo.	Table-eh urhl-kur-url deh-koh noo-oo-sey-yo.	Par Juh Par Tzai Chuang Shang	Fun She-ung Toy (Min Heung Ha).
Lie on your back on the table (face up).	Acuéstese en la mesa con boca arriba.	Table-eh urhl-ku-url we-loh-ha-ko noo-oo-sey-yo.	Town Juh Tang Tzai Chuang Shang	Fun Sheung Toy (Min Heung Sheung).
Lie on your side.	Acuéstese de lado.	Yoh-poo-loh noo-oo-seh-yo.	Tse Town	Fun Yat Bean.
Lie on your other side.	Acuéstese al otro lado.	Dah-rhum chohk yoh-poo-loh noo-oo-she-yo.	Tse Town Ling Wai Yi Bian	Fun Ling Yat Bean.
Squat.	Agáchese usted.	Oong-kuh-rhee-koh ahn-jah boh-sey-yo.	Duen	Mau Dight.
Kneel.	Arrodíllese usted.	Moo-rhoop-url ggor-ruh-boh-sey-yo.	Guei	Guai.

(table continues on page 1186)

TRANSLAT

⬤ TABLE 20.9 Examination: General Instructions (continued)

English	Spanish	Korean	Mandarin	Cantonese
Raise.	Levante.	Durl-uh-boh-she-yo.	Tai Gau	Hay Sun.
Lower.	Baje.	Neh-rhee-sey-yo.	Fang Di	Fong Dight.
This way.	Por aca.	Ee-rho-keh.	Juh Bian	Lee Bean.
Again.	Otra vez.	Dah-she	Tzai Yi Tsz	Joy Lai.
Hold it.	Sosténgalo.	Do-roo-she-yo.	Na Juh	Jar Ju.
Push against me.	Empuje contra mí.	Juh-url me-ro boh-sey-yo.	Tuei Wo	Heung Ngor Tui.
Push down with your hands to lift your body.	Empuje con las manos para levantar el cuerpo.	Sohn-oo-rho me-loh-suh mohm-url durl-uh boh-she-yo.	Shou Wang Shia Ya Ba Shen Ti Tai Chi Lai	Tui Hay Lay Sun.
Push as hard as you can.	Empuje con la fuerza que sea posible.	Heem kuht-mee-ro boh-sey-yo.	Jin Chi-uan Li Tuei	Dai Lik Tui.
Is that the best you can do?	¿Es lo mejor que puede usted hacer?	Koo-kuh-she hahrl sue ees-nun-jung-doh-eeb-nee-kah?	Juh Shi Nee Tzuei Hau De Juang Kuang Ma?	Hai Mm Hai Lay Lung Joe Doug Jui Ho?
Relax.	Cálmese.	Heem kuht beh-sey-yo.	Fun Song	Fong Zone.
Slowly.	Lentamente.	Chun-chun-ee	Mann Mann Der	Mann Mann.
Not so fast.	No tan rápido.	Nuh-moo bah-luh-jee ahn-keh.	Bu Yung Juh Yang Kuai	Mm Ho Gum Fai.
Rest.	Descánse.	She-she-yo.	Shiou Shi	Yau Sik.
Stay there.	Quédese allí.	Kuh-kee-suh Keh-she-yo.	Ting Tzai Na	Lau Hai Lay Doh.

English	Spanish	Korean	Mandarin	Cantonese
Move your (body part) like this.	Mueve su (parte del cuerpo) así.	Ee-loh-keh . . . uhl oom-jeek-ee-she-yo.	Shiang Juh Yang Yi Dung Nee Der Shen Ti Bu Wei	Gun Ngor Yuk Don Lay Dic (Bo Fun).
Now with your other (body part).	Ahora con el otro/la otra (parte del cuerpo).	Ee-jeh Dah-rhun chohk . . . uhl.	Shian Tzai Yi Dung Shen Ti Bu Wei	Ling Yat Bean (Bo Fun).

TRANSLAT

● **TABLE 20.10 Expressions Used When Examining the Face and Neck**

English	Spanish	Korean	Mandarin	Cantonese
Lift your head.	Levante la cabeza.	Koh-keh durl-uh boh-sey-yo.	Tow Tai Chi Lai	Occ Go Tau.
Open your mouth.	Abra la boca.	Eeb-burl url-ruh-boh-sey-yo.	Da Kai Tzuei	Da Hoi Hau.
Close your mouth.	Cierre la boca.	Eeb-burl dah-murl-uh boh-sey-yo.	Tzuei Her Chi Lai	Hub My Hau.
Open your eyes.	Abra los ojos.	Noon-uhl duh boh-seh-yo.	Da Kai Yan Jing	Da Hoi Ngan.
Close your eyes.	Cierre los ojos.	Noon-uhl kahm-ah boh-seh-yo.	Yan Jing Her Chi Lai	Hub My Ngan.
Wrinkle your nose.	Arruga la nariz.	Koh-url jing-koo-roh boh-sey-yo.	Jou Yi Shia Bi Tz	Yuk Bay.
Smile.	Sonréase.	Oo-soo-sey-yo.	Shia	Seal.
Bend your head toward your chest.	Incline la cabeza hacia el pecho.	Kah-soom choh-koo-loh muh-rhee-url sook-kyo boh-sey-yo.	Tow Shi-ang Chian Wan	Tau Heung Hone Shui Dight.

(table continues on page 1188)

⬤ **TABLE 20.10 Expressions Used When Examining the Face and Neck** (continued)

English	Spanish	Korean	Mandarin	Cantonese
Bend your head backward.	Incline la cabeza hacia atrás.	Muh-rhee-url twee-roh jek-kuh-boh-sey-yo.	Tow Shi-ang Ho Yang	Tau Heung Hau.
Turn your head to look behind you.	Vuelva la cabeza para mirar atrás.	Muh-rhee-url dwe-roh boh-sey-yo.	Juan Tow Kan Nee Ho Tow	Ling Tau Heung Hau Mong.
Bend your neck so that your ear moves toward your shoulder.	Incline la cabeza para que su oído se mueva hacia el hombro.	Kwe-kah-uh-keh-eh dah-do-lohk mohk-uhl yo-poo-roh oom-jeek-yuh boh-sey-yo.	Tow Tse Wan Rang Er Duo Tie Dow Jian Bang	Jug Tau, Jeung Yee Tip Heung Bok Tau.

⬤ **TABLE 20.11 Expressions Used When Examining Hearing**

English	Spanish	Korean	Mandarin	Cantonese
Do you have ringing in the ears?	¿Le pitan los oídos?	Kwe-eh-suh ool-rhee-nun-soh-rhee-kah nahb-nee-kah?	Nee Yo Er Ming Ma?	Lay Yee Tang Gin Ling Sing Ma?
Do you have discharge from the ears?	¿Sale flúido de los oídos?	Kew-eh-suh boon-bee-moo-lee nah-oob-nee-kah?	Nee Er Duo Yo Fen Mi Wu Ma?	Lay Yee Yau Lau Lone Ma?
Do you have difficulty hearing?	¿Tiene dificultad para oír?	Jahl ahn durl-leeb-nee-kah?	Nee Ting Yo Kuen Nan Ma?	Lay Tang Yau Mo Mun Tai?
Do you wear a hearing aid?	¿Lleva usted auxilio para oír?	Boh-chong-url sah-yong-ha-koh ees-soob-nee-kah?	Nee Yo Dai Ju Ting Chi Ma?	Lay Yau Mo Dai Jor Ting Hay?

🔴 TABLE 20.12 Expressions Used When Examining Vision

English	Spanish	Korean	Mandarin	Cantonese
Look up.	Mire usted hacia el cielo.	We-ro boh-sey-yo.	Shiang Shang Kan	Mong Sheung Min.
Look down.	Mire usted hacia el suelo.	Ah-reh-roo boh-sey-yo.	Shiang Shia Kan	Mong Ha Min.
Look toward your nose.	Mire usted hacia la nariz.	Koh-url boh-sey-yo.	Kan Nee De Bi Zi	Mong Lay Goh Bay.
Look at me.	Míreme.	Juh-url boh-seh-yo.	Kan Wo	Mong Ju Ngor.
Can you see what is on the wall?	¿Puede usted ver lo que está en la pared?	Byuk-eh eet-nun kuh-she boh-eeb-nee-kah?	Nee Kan De Dow Chiang Shang De Dung Shi Ma?	Lay Tight Doe Cheung Sheung Yau Mud Yeah?
Can you see it now?	¿Puede usted verlo ahora?	Eee-jeh-bo-eeb-nee-kah?	Shian Tzai Dan De Dow Ma?	Lay Yee Ga Tight Doe May?
What is it?	¿Qué es ésto?	Koo-kuh-she moo-us-eeb-nee-kah?	Shi Shu Mo Dung Shi	Hai Mud Yeah?
Tell me what number it is.	Dígame qué número es.	Moo-soon soos-jah-een-jee mahl-heh jew-sey-yo.	Gau Su Wo Shi Shu Mo Shu Zi	Gong Ngor Gee Hai Gay Hol Number?
Tell me what letter it is.	Dígame qué letra es.	Moo-soon kuhl-jah-een-jee mahl-heh jew-sey-yo.	Gau Su Wo Shu Shu Mo Zi	Gong Ngor Gee Hai Mud Yeah Gee Mo?
Can you see clearly?	¿Puede ver claramente?	Jahl bo-eeb-nee-kah?	Nee Dan De Ching Chu Ma?	Lay Tight Doug Ching Chor Ma?

(table continues on page 1190)

TRANSLAT

⬤ **TABLE 20.12 Expressions Used When Examining Vision (continued)**

English	Spanish	Korean	Mandarin	Cantonese
Can you see better at a distance?	¿Puede usted ver mejor a la distancia?	Muhl-lee-suh duh jahl bo-eeb-nee-kah?	Yo Yi Dian Jiu Li Shi Bu Shi Dan De Bi Jiau Ching Chu?	Lay Yuen Dee Tight Doug Ching Chor Ma?
Do your eyes water?	¿Derraman lágrimas los ojos?	Noon-mool-ee nahb-nee-kah?	Nee De Yan Jing Yo Shuei Ma?	Lay Yau Mo Ngan Shui?
Can you open your eyes?	¿Puede usted abrir los ojos?	Noon-url dur sue ees-soob-nee-kah?	Nee Yan Jing Da De Kai Ma?	Lay Ho Yee Da Hoi Sheung Ngan Ma?
Did anything get into your eye?	¿Hay algo en el ojo?	Noon-eh moo-uhs-she dew-uh kahs-soob-nee-kah?	Yo Dung Shi Tzai Nee De Yan Jing Ma?	Yau Mo Yeah Yup Jor Ngan?
Do you some-times see things double?	¿Ve usted las cosas doble algunas veces?	Kah-koom mool-cheh-kah do keh-roh bo-eeb-nee-kah?	Nee Huei Yo Shi Ho Kan Dow Liang Ge Ying Zi Ma?	Lay Yau Mo Tight Doe Chung Deep?
Do you wear glasses?	¿Lleva usted anteojos?	Ahn-kyong-url sah-young-ha-sheep-nee-kah?	Nee Dai Yan Jing Ma?	Lay Yau Mo Dai Ngan Gang?
Has your vision changed?	¿Ha cambi-ado la visión?	She-luh-kee byun-hehs-soob-nee-kah?	Nee De Shi Li Yo Gai Bian Ma?	Lay Tight Yeah Yau Mo Bean Far?
Do your eyes hurt?	¿Le duelen los ojos?	Noon-ee dah-kahb-soob-nee-kah?	Nee Yan Jing Tung Ma?	Lay Yau Mo Ngan Tone?

TABLE 20.13 Expressions Used When Examining the Upper Extremity

English	Spanish	Korean	Mandarin	Cantonese
Raise your arm.	Levante el brazo.	Pahl-url dool-uh bo-sey-yo.	Shou Tai Gau	Dai Go Sau.
Move your arm out to the side.	Mueve el brazo arriba al lado.	Pahl-url bah-kaht joh-koo-loh byul-uh bo-sey-yo.	Shou Shi-ang Tse Mian Tai Gau	Sau Jeung Hoi Learn Bean.
Move your arm back to your side.	Mueve el brazo a su lado.	Pahl-url mohm joh-koo-loh boo-chuh bo-sey-yo.	Shou Fang Huei Liang Bian	Sau Jeung Fong Hai Juck Bean.
Bend your elbow.	Doble el codo.	Pahl-koom-jee-url koob-hyo bo-sey-yo.	Shou Jou Wan Chi Lai	Wut Hay Sau Jarn.
Straighten your elbow.	Enderece el codo.	Pahl-koom-jee-url pyo bo-sey-yo.	Shou Jou Shen Jr	Yung Lick Wut Hay Sau Jarn.
Turn your hand over.	Revuelva la mano.	Sohn-url dole-roh bo-sey-yo.	Shou Fan Guo Lai	Farn Sau.
Bend your fingers.	Doble los dedos.	Sohn-kah-lahk-url koo-boo-ruh bo-sey-yo.	Wan Shou Jr Tow	Wut Hay Sau Gee.
Straighten your fingers.	Enderece los dedos.	Sohn-kah-lahk-url jook pyo bo-sey-yo.	Shou Jr Tow Sheng Jr	Yung Lick Wut Hay Sau Gee.
Bend your wrist (flexion).	Doble la mun~eca.	Sohn-mohk-url koo-boo-luh bo-sey-yo.	Shou Wan Wan Chi Lai	Wut Hay Sau Woon.
Lift your wrist (extension).	Levante la mun~eca.	Sohn-mohk-url chut-chuh bo-sey-yo.	Shou Wan Shiang Ho Wan	Sing Hay Sau Woon.
Pull your shoulders back.	Mueve los hombros hacia atrás.	Uh-keh-url dwe-roh chut-chuh dang-kyo bo-sey-yo.	Jian Bang Wang Ho	Bok Tau Lie Hau.

(table continues on page 1192)

TRANSLAT

TABLE 20.13 Expressions Used When Examining the Upper Extremity (continued)

English	Spanish	Korean	Mandarin	Cantonese
Circle your shoulder.	Haga círculo con el hombro.	Uh-keh-url dole-roh bo-sey-yo.	Jian Bang Rau Chiuan Chiuan	Bok Tau Da Hoon.
Let me see your hand.	Muéstreme la mano.	Sohn-url bo-yo jew-sey-yo.	Rang Wo Kan Nee De Shou	Bay Ngor Tight Lay Sau.
Squeeze my hand.	Apriete mi mano.	Jeh sohn-url gwok jahb-ah bo-sey-yo.	Yung Li Wo Jin Wo De Shou	Jar Ju Ngor Sau.
Take this from me.	Tome éste.	Ee-guh Gah-joo-geh Suh-yo	Tsung Wo Shou Jung Na Tzou	Lor Lay Gor.
When did you notice weakness in your arms?	¿Cuándo notó usted la debilidad de los brazos?	Uhn-jeh pahl-reh heem-ee up-nun kuhs-surl arl-ahs-soob-nee-kah?	Nee Shu Mo Shi Ho Kai Shi Jiue De Shou Mai Yo Li?	Gay See Lay Gee Doh Lay Sau Mo Lick?
Had you been sleeping on your arm?	¿Había usted dormido encima del brazo?	Pahl-url beh-koh jahs-soob-nee-kah?	Nee Yi Jr Ya Shou Bi Shuei Ma?	Lay Yau Mo Fun Gow Jart Ju Sau?
Can you move your arm at all?	¿Puede usted mover el brazo?	Pahl-url joh-koom-ee-lah-doh oom-jeek-eel soo ees-soob-nee-kah?	Nee De Shou Ke Yi Dung Ma?	Lay Hall Yee Yuk Lay Sau Jarn Ma?

TABLE 20.14 Expressions Used When Examining the Lower Extremity

English	Spanish	Korean	Mandarin	Cantonese
Bend your hip.	Doble la cadera.	Dah-rhee-rur koob-hyo bo-sey-yo.	Da Tuei Wan Chi Lai	Wan Dai Sun.
Lift your leg.	Levante la pierna.	Dah-rhee-rur dool-uh bo-sey-yo.	Ba Jiau Tai Gau	Dai Go Gert.
Bend your knee.	Doble la rodilla.	Moo-doop-url koob-hyo bo-sey-yo.	Shi Gai Wan Chi Lai	Kuk Sud Tau.
Straighten your knee.	Enderece la rodilla.	Moo-doop-url pyo bo-sey-yo.	Shi Gai Shen Jr	Sun Jik Sud Tau.
Roll your leg in.	Mueva la pierna hacia el interior.	Dah-rhee-rur ahn-oo-roh dole-roh bo-sey-yo.	Jiau Shi-ang Nei Juan	June Lay Jack Gert Heung Yup.
Roll your leg out.	Mueva la pierna hacia el exterior.	Dah-rhee-rur bahk-koo-roh dole-roh bo-sey-yo.	Jiau Shi-ang Wai Juan	June Lay Jack Gert Heung Chut.
Lift your foot	Levante el pie.	Bahl-url orl-luh bo-sey-yo.	Ba Jiau Ban Tai Chi Lai	Dai Hay Jack Gert.
Push your foot down.	Empuje el pie para abajo.	Bahl-url ah-rhey johk-koo-roh mee-ruh bo-sey-yo.	Jiau Ban Fang Shia Chiu	Fong Dight Jack Gert.
Lift your toes.	Levante los dedos de pie.	Bahl-kah-lahk-url dur-uh bo-sey-yo.	Jiau Jr Tow Tai Chi Lai	Dai Go Gert Gee.
Bend your toes.	Doble los dedos de pie.	Bahl-kah-lahk-url koo-boo-luh bo-sey-yo.	Wan Jiau Jr Tow	Wut Hay Gert Gee.
Pull your foot in.	Mueva el pie para adentro.	Bahl-url ahn johk-koo-roh dahng-kyo bo-sey-yo.	Jiau La Jin Lai	Lie Jack Gert Yup Lai.
Pull your foot out.	Mueva el pie para afuera.	Bahl-url bah-kaht johk-koo-roh dahng-kyo bo-sey-yo.	Jiau Shen Chu Chiu	Lie Jack Gert Chut Hui.

TRANSLAT

TABLE 20.15 Expressions Used When Examining the Back

English	Spanish	Korean	Mandarin	Cantonese
Bend forward.	Doble hacia adelante.	Mohm-url ahp-poo-roh koo-boo-ruh bo-sey-yo.	Shiang Chian Wan	Heung Chin Wan Sun.
Bend backward.	Doble hacia atrás	Mohm-url dwe-roh koo-boo-ruh bo-sey-yo.	Shiang Ho Wan	Heung Hau Wan Sun.
Bend sideways.	Doble al lado.	Mohm-url up-poo-roh koo-boo-ruh bo-sey-yo.	Shiang Liang Bian Wan	Heung Pong Bean Wan Sun.
Keep your knees straight/bent.	Mantenga las rodillas directas/dobladas.	Moo-roop-url jook pyo-koh key-sey-yo/koo-boo-rhee-koh keh-sey-yo.	Shi Gai Shen Jr/Wan	Sun Jik Sud Tau/Wan Kuk Sud Tau.
Lift this way.	Levante así.	Ee luhk-keh ohl-luh bo-sey-yo.	Shiang Jr Yang Tai Chi Lai	Lik Hay.
Keep things close to your body.	Mantenga cosas cerca del cuerpo.	Mur-kuhn-url mohm-eh kah-kahb-keh hah-sey-yo.	Dung Shi Na Kau Jin Nee De Shen Ti	Lor My Sun Bean.

TABLE 20.16 Expressions Used When Examining the Respiratory System

English	Spanish	Korean	Mandarin	Cantonese
Cough.	Tosa	Kee-cheem-ha-sey-yo.	Ke Sou	Cud.
Cough again.	Tosa otra vez.	Dah-she kee-cheem-ha-sey-yo.	Tzai Ke Sou	Joy Cud.
Open your mouth.	Abra la boca.	Eeb-url purl-luh bo-sey-yo.	Jang Kai Tzuei	Da Hoi Hau.

English	Spanish	Korean	Mandarin	Cantonese
Does it hurt you to open your mouth?	¿Le duele abrir la boca?	Eeb-url byul-rhee deh tong-joong-ee ees-soom-nee-kah?	Jang Kai Tzuei Huei Tung Ma?	Lay Da Hoi Hau See Yau Mo Tone?
When did you first start coughing?	¿Cuándo empezó usted toser?	Chu-oom kee-cheem-url she-jahk-hahn kuh-she un-jeh-eeb-nee-kah?	Nee Shu Mo Shi Ho Kai Shi Ke De?	Lay Gay See Hoi Chee Cud?
Do you cough a lot?	¿Tose mucho?	Kee-cheem-url mahn-hee hahb-nee-kah?	Nee Jing Chang Ke Ma?	Lay Yau Mo Cud Ho Doh?
I will now listen to your lungs.	Ahora voy a es-cuchar los pul-mones.	Chung-jeen-url hah-kehs-soom-nee-dah.	Wo Shian Tzai Yau Ting Ting Nee De Fei	Ngor Yee Ga Tang Lay Gor Fai.
Take a deep breath.	Respire profundamente	Soom-url kee-pee dur-rhee she-sey-yo.	Shen Hu Shi	Tau Dai Hay.
Exhale.	Espire.	Soom-url neh she-sey-yo.	Tu Chi	Foo Hay.
Do you cough up fluid?	¿Cuando tosa, es-puta flema?	Kah-leh-kah nah-ohb-nee-kah?	Nee Yo Ke Chu Yi Ti Ma?	Lay Yau Mo Yeah Cud Chut Lai?
What is the color of what you cough up?	¿De qué color es la flema?	Kah-leh-kah moo-soon sehk eeb-nee-kah?	Nee Ke Chu Lai De Dung Shi Shr Shu Mo Yan Se?	Lay Cud Chut Lai Hai Mud Ngan Sik?

(table continues on page 1196)

TRANSLAT

🟠 **TABLE 20.16 Expressions Used When Examining the Respiratory System** (continued)

English	Spanish	Korean	Mandarin	Cantonese
Does your tongue feel swollen?	¿Siente usted hinchada la lengua?	Hyuh-kah boo-uhs-soob-nee-kah?	Nee De Shu Tow Jung Ma?	Lay Till Lay Yau Mo Jung?
Do you have a sore throat?	¿Le duele la garganta?	Moh-kee ah-poob-nee-kah?	Nee De Ho Lung Tung Ma?	Lay Yau Mo Hau Lone Tone?
Does it hurt to swallow?	¿Le duele tragar?	Sahm-kil deeh ah-poob-nee-kah?	Tuen De Shi Ho Tung Ma?	Lay Tun Yeah See Yau Mo Tone?

🟠 **TABLE 20.17 Expressions Used When Examining the Gastrointestinal System**

English	Spanish	Korean	Mandarin	Cantonese
Do you have stomach cramps?	¿Tiene usted calambres en el estómago?	We kyong-rhun-ee ees-soob-nee-kah?	Nee Yo Wei Jiau Tung Ma?	Lay Yau Mo Wai Chau Gun?
Do you have pain in your stomach?	¿Le duele el estómago?	We-eh tong-joong-ee ees-soob-nee-kah?	Nee Yo Wei Tung Ma?	Lay Yau Mo Wai Tone?
Are you nauseated?	¿Está mareado (a)?	Meh-soo-kuh-oom-url noo-keeb-nee-kah?	Nee Yo Fan Wei Ma?	Lay Yau Mo Jok Moon?
Does eating make you vomit?	¿Cuando come, tiene que vomitar?	Muh-koo-myun toh-hahb-nee-kah?	Chi Dung Shi Rang Nee Tu Ma?	Lay Sic Yeah See Yau Mo Ngau Toll?
Have you vomited?	¿Ha usted vomitado?	Toh-hahn juhk-kee ees-soob-nee-kah?	Nee Yo Tu Ma?	Lay Yau Mo Ngau Toe?

English	Spanish	Korean	Mandarin	Cantonese
Do you still vomit?	¿Vomita todavía?	Ah-jeek-doh toh-hahb-nee-kah?	Nee Hai Tzai Tu Ma?	Lay Yau Mo Ying Yin Ngau Toe?
Is it of a dark or bright red color?	¿Es de color rojo oscuro o claro?	Koo-kuhs-she bahl-koon bar-kahn seh-im-nee-kah uh-doo-oon bar-kahn-sehk-eeb-nee-kah?	Shi An Se De Hai Shi Shian Hung Se?	Hug Sic Yik Wart Sin Hung Sic?
Are any of your limbs swollen?	¿Están hincha-dos alguno miembros?	Pahl dah-rhee-kah boo-uhs-soob-nee-kah?	Nee De Si Juh Yo Jung Ma?	Lay Sau Gert Yau Mo Jung?
How long have they been swollen like this?	¿Desde cuándo estan hin-chados así?	Ee-luhk-keh boo-un-jee are-mah-nah deh-uhs-soob-nee-kah?	Shiang Juh Yang Jung Yo Duo Jiou Le?	Lay Yau Mo See Guo Gum Yeung Jung?
Were they ever swollen before?	¿Han estado hinchados alguna vez antes?	Jun-eh-doh boo-us-dun johk-kee ees-soob-nee-kah?	Yi Chian Tseng Jing Juh Yang Jung Ma?	Yee Chin Yau Mo Jung?
How long has your tongue been that color?	¿Cuánto tiempo hace que la lengua está de ese color?	Hyuh-kah ee-rhun sey-kee-den-jee are-mah-nah oh-reh-deh-us-soob-nee-kah?	Nee De Shu Tow Shiang Juh Ge Yan Se Yo Duo Jiou Le?	Lay Till Lay Yau Gay Loi Hai Gum Ngan Sic?
How are your stools?	¿Cómo son las defeca-ciones?	Byun-un uh-duh-soom-nee-kah?	Nee De Da Bian Tzen Mo Yang?	Lay Dai Bean Dim Yeung?

(table continues on page 1198)

● **TABLE 20.17 Expressions Used When Examining the Gastrointestinal System** (continued)

English	Spanish	Korean	Mandarin	Cantonese
Are they regular?	¿Son regulares?	Byun-un qu-cheek-juhk-koo-roh bohb-nee-kah?	Guei Liu Ma?	Jing Sheung Ma?
Have you noticed their color?	¿Se ha fijado usted en el color?	Sehk-kahr-url boh-ahs-soob-nee-kah?	Nee Ju Yi Guo Shi Shu Mo Yan Se?	Lay Yau Mo Lau Yee Ngan Sic?
Are you constipated?	¿Está usted es-treñado?	Byun-bee-kah ees-soob-nee-kah?	Nee Yo Bian Mi Ma	Lay Yau Mo Bean Bay?
Do you have diarrhea?	¿Tiene diarrea?	Sur-sah-roo hahb-nee-kah?	Nee Yo La Du Tz Fu Shie? Ma?	Lay Yau Mo Toe Shair?
Do you pass any blood?	¿Hay sangre en las defeca-ciones?	Pee-kah nah-om-nee-kah?	Nee Da Bian Yo Shie Ma?	Lay Yau Mo Pai Huet?
Have you any difficulty urinating?	¿Tiene usted dificultad en orinar?	Soh-byun-boh-nun-keh uh-lub-soob-nee-kah?	Nee Shiau Bian Yo Kuen Nan Ma?	Lay Siu Bean Yau Mo Kwon Larn?
Do you urinate involuntarily?	¿Orina usted sin querer?	Jah-sheem-doh moh-roo-keh soh-byun-ee nah-ohb-nee-kah?	Nee Yo Neeau Shi Jin Ma?	Lay Yau Mo Yun Mm Doe Siu Bean?

● TABLE 20.18 Expressions Used When Examining the Central Nervous System

English	Spanish	Korean	Mandarin	Cantonese
How does your head feel?	¿Cómo e siente la cabeza?	Muh-rhee-kah uh-duh-tah-koh noo-kee-sheeb-nee-kah?	Nee De Tow Jiue De Tzen Mo Yang?	Lay Gor Tau Gawk Doug Dim?
Do you have a good memory?	¿Tiene usted buena memoria?	Kee-uk-yoh-kee joh-oob-shim-nee-kah?	Nee Ji Yi Li Hau Ma?	Lay Gay Doug Yeah Ma?
Do you have any pain in the head?	¿Le duele usted la cabeza?	Muh-rhee-eh tong-joong-ee ees-soob-nee-kah?	Nee Tow Na Li Huei Tung Ma?	Lay Tau Yau Mo Tone?
Did you fall?	¿Se cayó usted?	Num-uh-juhs-soob-nee-kah?	Nee Tseng Die Dow Ma?	Lay Yau Mo Dit Chun?
How did you fall?	¿Cómo se cayó?	Uh-duh-keh num-uh-juhs-soob-nee-kah?	Nee Tze Mo Die Dow De?	Lay Dim Yeung Dit Chun?
Did you faint?	¿Se desmayó?	Kee-jurl-hehs-soob-nee-kah?	Nee Tseng Yun Shiuan Ma?	Lay Yau Mo Tau Won?
Have you ever had fainting spells?	¿Se desmayó usted alguna vez?	Kee-jurl-hahn juhk-kee ees-soob-nee-kah?	Nee Tseng Huen Dow Ma?	Lay Yau Mo Tau Ngan Fa?
Do you get headaches?	¿Tiene usted dolores de cabeza?	Doo-tong-ee ees-soob-nee-kah?	Nee Tow Tung Ma?	Lay Yau Mo Tau Tone?

(table continues on page 1200)

TRANSLAT

● **TABLE 20.18 Expressions Used When Examining the Central Nervous System** (continued)

English	Spanish	Korean	Mandarin	Cantonese
Did you become unconscious?	¿Estuvo inconsciente?	Ui-sheek-url ee-lus-soob-nee-kah?	Nee Yin Tsz Sang Shi Jer Jiue Ma?	Lay Yau Mo Mm Ching Sing?
Do people have difficulty understanding you?	¿Tiene la gente dificultad de entenderle?	Sah-lahm-durl-ee dahng-sheen mahl-url ah-rah dood-kee uh-ruh-woh hahb-nee-kah?	Bie Ren Yo Kuen Nan Liau Jie Nee Ma?	Kay Ta Yun Yau Mo Tang Mm Ming Lay?
Do you have difficulty understanding what people say to you?	¿Tiene usted dificultad de entender lo que le dice la gente?	Sah-lam-durl-nee moo-soon mahl-url hah-noon-jee ee-heh-hah-kee-kah uh-rub-soob-nee-kah?	Nee Yo Kuen Nan Liau Jie Bie Ren Duei Nee Shuo De Hua Ma?	Lay Tang Kay Ta Yun Gong Yeah Yau Mo Kwun Larn?
What is the date?	¿Cuál es la fecha de hoy?	Myut chil-eeb-nee-kah?	Jin Tian Shu Mo Ri Zi?	Gum Yat Lai Bai Gay?
What month is it?	¿En qué mes estamos?	Myut warl-eeb-nee-kah?	Jin Tian Ji Yue?	Gum Gor Yuet Gay Yuet?
What day is it?	¿Qué día es hoy?	Moo-soon yoh-eel-eeb-nee-kah?	Jin Tian Ji Hau?	Gum Yat Gay Ho?
What year is it?	¿En qué año estamos?	Myut nyun-doh-eeb-nee-kah?	Jin Neean Ji Neean?	Gum Lean Gay Lean?

English	Spanish	Korean	Mandarin	Cantonese
What do you use this for?	¿Para qué se usa esto?	Ee-kuhs-sun moo-us hahr deh soob-nee-kah?	Juh Ge Shi Yung Lai Tzuo Shu Mo De?	Lay Go Yung Lai Joe Mud Yeah?
Follow the moving pencil with your eyes.	Siga el movimiento del lápiz con los ojos.	Yun-peel-url noon-oo-roh dah-lah-hwa bo-sey-yo.	Yan Jing Gen Juh Chian Bi Dung	Ngar Jing Gun Ju Yoon Bud Mong?
Copy this.	Copie esto.	Ee-kuhs-sur behk-kyo soo-she-yo.	Mo Fang Juh Ge	Jill Joe.
Tell me when you see it.	Dígame cuando lo vea.	Koo-kuhs-she bo-eel deh mahr-soom-heh joo-sey-yo.	Dang Nee Kan Dow Shu Gau Su Wo	Dong Lay Tai Doe Gong Bay Ngor Gee.
Do not move your head.	No mueva la cabeza.	Muh-rhee-roo oom-jee-kee-jee mah-sey-yo.	Tow Bu Yau Dung	Mm Ho June Tau.
Draw a circle.	Dibuje un círculo.	Won-url koo-ruh bo-sey-yo.	Hua Yi Ge Yuan	Wart Yuen Hoon.
Draw a triangle.	Dibuje un triángulo.	Sahm-kahk-hyong-url koo-ruh bo-sey-yo.	Hua Yi Ge San Jiau Shing	Wart Sarm Gok.
Draw a cross.	Dibuje una cruz.	Sheeb-jah-kah-rur koo-yuh bo-sey-yo.	Hua Yi Ge Shi Zi	Wart Sub Gee.

(table continues on page 1202)

TABLE 20.18 Expressions Used When Examining the Central Nervous System (continued)

English	Spanish	Korean	Mandarin	Cantonese
Draw a house.	Dibuje una casa.	Jeeb-url koo-roh bo-sey-yo.	Hua Yi Ge Fang Zi	Wart Yat Gan Uk.
Pick the one that is different.	Escoja el(la) que es diferente.	Dah-run kuht hah-nah-rur jeep-puh bo-sey-yo.	Ba Bu Tung De Jau Chu Lai	Shoon Jark Mm Tone Gor Goh.
Pick the one that is the same.	Escoja el(la) que es igual.	Dohk-kaht-oon kuh-sur keep-uh bo-sey-yo.	Ba Yi Yang De Jau Chu Lai	Shoon Jark Yat Yeung Gor Goh.
Connect these dots.	Conecte estos puntos.	Ee juhm-duhl-url yun-kurl-hashe-yo.	Ba Juh Shie Dian Lian Chi Lai	Jeung Dim Lean My.
Draw a person.	Dibuje una persona.	Sah-lahm-url koo-ruh bo-sey-yo.	Hua Yi Ge Ren	Wart Yat Gor Yan.
Put this . . .	Ponga esto . . .	Ee-kuhs-surl . . . eh noh-oo-sey-yo.	Ba Juh Ge Fang Tzai . . .	Fong Lay Gor Hai . . .
Under.	Debajo.	Ah-reh	Shia Mian	Dai Har.
Behind.	Detrás.	Dwe-eh	Hau Mian	Hau Bean.
In front.	Enfrente.	Ahp-eh	Chian Mian	Chin Min.

TABLE 20.19 **Expressions Used for Sensory Testing**

English	Spanish	Korean	Mandarin	Cantonese
Close your eyes.	Cierre los ojos.	Noon-url kah-moo-sey-yo.	Yan Jing Bi Chi Lai	Hop My Sheung Ngan.
Point to where I touch you.	Apunte adonde yo le toco a usted.	Neh-kah dahng-sheen-url mahn-jee-noon koh-she uh-deen-jee kah-rhee-kuh bo-sey-yo.	Wo Peng Nee Na Li Nee Jiou Juh Na Li	Gee Chut Ngor Dim Lay Day Fong.
Say "yes" when I touch you.	Dígame "sí" cuando yo le toco a usted.	Jeh-kah mahn-jeel-deh "yeh" rah-go mahl-heh joo-sey-yo.	Dang Wo Peng Nee Nee Jiou Shuo Yo	Gong "Yes" Dong Ngor Dim Lay.
Tell me if you feel:	Dígame si se siente:	Noo-kee-myun mahl-heh-joo-sey-yo:	Ru Guo Nee Jiue De __ Jiou Gau Su Wo	Gong Ngor Gee Lay Gawk Doug:
Hot or cold.	Calor o frío.	Do-cup-dah doh-nun cha-cup-dah.	Re Huo Leng	Yeet Wart Larn.
Sharp or dull.	Punteagudo o sin punta.	Byo-juh-ha-dah doh-nun moo-dee-dah.	Jian Huo Duen	Jim Wart Dun.
Tell me what is in your hand without looking:	Dígame lo que tiene en la mano sin mirar:	Po-jee mahl-koh sohn on-eh een-nun kuh-she moo-uh-sheen-jee mahl-hey-bo-sey-yo:	Bu Yau Kan Gau Su Wo Nee Shou Shang Yo Shu Mo	Mm Ho Mong Lay Sheung Yau, Gong Ngor Gee Yau Mud Yeah:
Coin.	Moneda.	Dong-jun	Chian Bi	Un.

(table continues on page 1204)

TABLE 20.19 Expressions Used for Sensory Testing (continued)

English	Spanish	Korean	Mandarin	Cantonese
Cotton.	Algodón.	Sohm.	Mian Hua	Min Fa.
Key.	Llave.	Url-sey.	Yau Shi	Sor See.
Pencil.	Lápiz.	Um-peel.	Bi	Yuen Bud.
Safety pin.	Imperdible.	Ahn-jun-pin	Bie Jen	Cul Jump.

TABLE 20.20 Patient Instructions

English	Spanish	Korean	Mandarin	Cantonese
Follow these instructions.	Siga usted estas instrucciones.	Ee jee-she-do-url dah-rah-ha-sey-yo.	Tzuen Shou Juh Shie Chi Shi	Gun Gee See.
Do exactly as I tell you.	Haga exacta-mente lo que le digo.	Jeh-kah mahl-hah-noon deh-roh jung-hwak-hah-keh dah-rah ha-sey-yo.	Chiue Shi Tzuo Wo Gau Su Nee De	Gun Ngor Jill Joe.
Do like this.	Hágalo así.	Ee-rohk-keh ha-sey-yo.	Shiang Juh Yang Tzuo	Jill Joe.
I will demonstrate.	Demostraré.	Jeh-kah she-bum-url boh-ee-kehs-soom-ne e-dah.	Wo Huei Shi Fan	Ngor See Farn.
Watch how I do the exercise.	Mire cómo hago yo el ejercicio.	Jeh-kah uht-duk-keh ha-noon-jee bo-sey-yo.	Kan Wo Tzen Mo Tzuo Juh Yun Dung	Tight Ngor Joe Won Dhone.

English	Spanish	Korean	Mandarin	Cantonese
Do this at home.	Hágalo en casa.	Jeeb-eh-suh ee-kuhs-surl ha-sey-yo.	Huei Jia Tzuo Juh Shie	Joy Ga Joe.
Do it ___ times each day.	Hágalo ___ veces cada día.	May-il . . . bun sheek ha-sey-yo.	Mei Tian Tzuo ___ Ci	Mui Yat Joe ___ Chee.
Let me do the movement for you.	Permítame hacer el movimiento para usted.	Jeh-kah oom-jee-kyo poh-kehs-soom-nee-dah.	Ren Wo Bang Nee Tzuo Juh Dung Tzuo	Ngor Bong Lay Joe Dhone Jok.
It is nothing serious.	No es nada grave.	Juhn-hyuh sheem-kahk-hah-jee ahn-soom-nee-dah.	Juh Bu Yan Jung	Mm Gun Yiu.
You will get better.	Usted se mejorará.	Duh cho-ah-jeel cum-nee-dah.	Nee Huei Jian Jian Hau	Lay Wui Ho Farn.
Soak your (body part) in hot/cold water.	Tiene que em-paparse el/la (parte del cuerpo) en agua caliente/fría.	. . . url doo-kuh-oon/cha-kah-oon mool-eh dahm-koo-sey-yo.	Jiang Nee De___ Jin Tzai Re/Leng Shuei Jung	Jum Lay Sun Tight Joy Yit/Larn Sui Chung.
Do it for ___ minutes.	Hágalo por ___ minutos.	. . . boon dong-ahn koo-ruhk-keh ha-sey-yo.	Tzuo ___ Fan Jung	Joe ___ Fun Chung.
I will use electricity.	Usaré la electricidad.	Juhn-kee-rur sah-young-ha hl cum-nee-dah.	Wo Yau Shi Yung Dian Liau	Ngor Wui Yung Din.

(table continues on page 1206)

TRANSLAT

TABLE 20.20 Patient Instructions (continued)

English	Spanish	Korean	Mandarin	Cantonese
You will feel a tingling sensation.	Se sentirá la sensasión de brasas.	Dah-koom-kuh-rhee-nun noo-kim-ee ee-surl cum-nee-dah.	Nee Huei Jiue De Tsz Tsz De	Lay Wui Gok Doug Yau Siu Siu Hun.
Tell me if it hurts too much.	Dígame si le duele demasiado.	Nuh-moo ahp-poo-myun mahl-soom-hah-sey-yo.	Ru Guo Tung Yau Gau Su Wo	Yu Guo Tai Tone Ching Wa Ngor Gee.
Apply bandage to . . .	Ponga un vendaje a . . .	. . . eh poong-deh-rur kah-moo-sey-yo.	Ba Beng Dai Bang Tzai . . .	Tip Gau Bo Hai . . .
Apply ointment.	Ponga ungüento.	Yun-ko-rur pah-roo-sey-yo.	Tu Yau Gau	Char Yerk Go.
Heat.	Calor.	Url.	Re	Yeet.
Cold.	Frío.	Neng.	Leng	Larn.
Ultrasound.	Ultrasonido.	Choh-oom-pah.	Chau Yin Po	Chiu Sing Ball.
Use a ___ pound weight.	Use una pesa de ___ libra(s).	. . . pound-doo-rur sah-young-hah-sey-yo.	Yung ___ Bang De Jung Liang	Yung ___ Bong Lik.
Repeat this exercise ___ times without stopping	Repita este ejercicio ___ veces sin parar.	Mohm-choo-jee mahl-koh ee oon-dong-url . . . bun pahn-bohk hah-sey-yo.	Chung Fu Tzuo Juh Dung Tzuo ___ Tsz Bu Yau Ting	Bud Ting Day Chung Fook Joe ___ Chee.

English	Spanish	Korean	Mandarin	Cantonese
Take a break between exercises	Pause entre los ejercicios.	Oon-dong-hah-nun joon-kah-eh shoo-sheek-url chee-hah-sey-yo.	Liang Tsz Dung Tzuo Jian Shiou Shi Yi Shia	Ting Yat Jun Joy Joe.
Do these exercises ___ times a day every day.	Haga usted estos ejercicios ___ veces por día, cada día.	Ee oon-dong-url hah-roo-eh . . . bun meh-il hah-sey-yo.	Mei Tian Tzuo Juh Shie Yung Dung ___ Tsz	Mui Yat Joe Won Dhone ___ Chee.
Stop the exercise if your pain increases.	Si crece la pena, páre de hacer el ejercicio.	Tong-joong-ee joong-kah-hah-myun oon-dong-url mum-choo-sey-yo.	Ru Guo Jiue De Tung Jiou Ting Juh Yung Dung	Yu Guo Lay Ho Tone, Ching Ting Joe Won Dhone.
Sit with your back straight.	Siéntese con la espalda erecta.	Doong-url jook pyu-koh ahn-joo-sey-yo.	Tzuo Jeng Bei Ting Jer	Chor Jig.
Place your heel on the ground first.	Ponga primero el talón en el piso.	Dee-koom-cheel-rur mun-juh pah-dahk-eh daht-keh hah-sey-yo.	Shian Ba Jiau Gen Fang Tzai Di Shang	Fong Gerk Jarn Seen.
Place your foot flat on the ground.	Ponga el pie de plano en el piso.	Pahl-bah-dahk-url mun-juh dang-eh daht-keh hah-sey-yo.	Ba Jeng Ge Jiau Ban Ping Fang Tzai Di Shang	Fong Ping Gerk Barn Seen.

(table continues on page 1208)

TRANSLAT

🔴 **TABLE 20.20** **Patient Instructions** (continued)

English	Spanish	Korean	Mandarin	Cantonese
Take a step with your right/left leg.	Camine primero con la pierna derecha/ izquierda.	Oh-roo-johk/ when-johk dah-rhee-roh neh dee-dee-sey-yo.	Yo/Tzuo Jiau Tzou Yi Bu	Yung Lay Yau/Jor Gerk Harn Yat Bo.
Your next appointment is on ___.	Su próxima cita es el ___.	Dah-oom yahk-soh she-kahn-oon . . . im-nee-dah.	Nee Shia Yi Tsz Jer Liau De Shi Jian Shi __	Lay Ha Chee Yu Yerk See Gan Hai ___.

🔴 **TABLE 20.21** **Anatomical Names**

English	Spanish	Korean	Mandarin	Cantonese
Head.	La cabeza.	Muh-rhee	Tow	Tau.
Forehead.	La frente.	Ee-mah	Er Tow	Arc Tau.
Neck.	El cuello.	Mohk	Jing; Or Bo Zi	Gang.
Face.	La cara.	Url-koo	Lian	Min.
Ear.	El oído.	Kwe	Er	Yee.
Nose.	La nariz.	Koh	Bi Zi	Bay.
Mouth.	La boca.	Eep	Tzuei	Hau/Jui.
Eyes	Los ojos.	Noon	Yan	Ngan.
Chest.	El pecho.	Ka-soom	Shiung	Hone.
Back.	La espalda.	Doong	Bei	Bui.
Spine.	La espina dorsa.	Doong-byuk	Ji Juei	Jack Jui.
Abdomen.	El abdomen.	Peh	Du Zi	Toll.
Arm.	El brazo.	Pahl	Shou Bei	Sau Bay.

English	Spanish	Korean	Mandarin	Cantonese
Shoulder.	El hombro.	Ut-keh	Jian Bang	Bog Tau.
Elbow.	El codo.	Pah-koom-chee	Shou Joe	Sau Jarn.
Wrist.	La muñeca.	Sohn-mohk	Shou Wan	Sau Woon.
Hand.	La mano.	Sohn	Shou	Sau.
Fingers.	Los dedos.	Sohn-kah-rahk	Shou Zhi	Sau Gee.
Thumb.	El dedo grande.	Um-jee-soohn-kah-rahk	Da Mu Zhi	Sau Gee-Gung.
Leg.	La pierna.	Dah-rhee	Tuei	Gerk.
Hip.	La cadera.	Huh-rhee	Kuan	Poon.
Buttocks.	Las nalgas.	Ung-dung-ee	Pi Gu	Pay Goo.
Knee.	La rodilla.	Moo-roop	Shi Gai	Sut Tau.
Ankle.	El tobillo.	Pahl-mohk	Jiau Huai	Gerk Ngan.
Foot.	El pie.	Pahl	Jiau	Gerk Bahn.
Heel.	El talón	Pahl dee-koom-chee	Jiau Gen	Gerk Jarn.
Toes.	Los dedos de pie.	Pahl-kah-rahk	Jiau Chih Tow	Gerk Gee.
Side.	El lado.	Yup	Pang Bian	Bean.
Top of . . .	Encima de; el pico.	. . . ui we	Tzuei Shang Mian	Dang.
Bottom of . . .	Al fondo de; el fondo.	. . . ui pah-dahk	Tzuei Shia Mian	Dight.

TABLE 20.22 Numbers and Time of Day

English	Spanish	Korean	Mandarin	Cantonese
One.	Uno.	Hah-nah	Yi	Yat.
Two.	Dos.	Dool	Er	Yee.
Three.	Tres.	Set	San	Sarm.
Four.	Cuatro.	Net	Sz	Say.
Five.	Cinco.	Dah-suht	Wu	Mm.
Six.	Seis.	Uh-suht	Liou	Luk.
Seven.	Siete.	Il-kohp	Chi	Chut.
Eight.	Ocho.	Uh-durl	Ba	Bhat.
Nine.	Nueve.	Ah-hope	Jiou	Gau.
Ten.	Diez.	Url	Shih	Sub.
Twenty.	Veinte.	Soo-murl	Er Shih	Yee Sub.
Thirty.	Treinta.	Suh-roon	San Shih	Sarm Sub.
Forty.	Cuarenta.	Mah-hoon	Sz Shih	Say Sub.
Fifty.	Cincuenta	.Sheen	Wu Shih	Mm Sub.
Sixty.	Sesenta.	Yeh-soon	Liou Shih	Luk Sub.
Seventy.	Setenta.	Il-hoon	Chi Shih	Chut Sub.
Eighty.	Ochenta.	Uh-doon	Ba Shih	Bhat Sub.
Ninety.	Noventa.	Ah-hoon	Jiou Shih	Gau Sub.
One hundred.	Cien (by itself); ciento (a, os, as) (otherwise).	Behk	Yi Bai	Yat Bark.
At 10:00.	A las diez.	Oh-juhn url-she-eh.	Shih Dian	Sub Dim.
At 2:30.	A las dos y media.	Doo-she sahm-sheep poon-eh.	Liang Dian Ban	Leung Dim Boon.

English	Spanish	Korean	Mandarin	Cantonese
Early in the morning.	Temprano por la mañana.	Ah-chim il-jeek.	Yi Da Tzau	Dai Ching Joe.
In the daytime.	Durante el día.	Naht-she-kahn eh.	Bai Tian	Yat Gan.
At noon.	A mediodía.	Jung-oh-eh.	Jung Wu	Jung Mm.
At bedtime.	Al acostarse.	Jahm-jahl deh.	Shuei Chian	Shui Min See.
At night.	Por la noche.	Pahm-eh.	Wan Shang	Yeah Mann.
Before meals.	Antes de comer.	Sheek-sah juhn.	Fan Chian	Farn Chin.
After meals.	Después de comer.	Sheek-sah hoo.	Fan Ho	Farn Hull.
Today.	Hoy.	Oh-nurl.	Jin Tian	Gum Yat.
Tomorrow.	Ma~nana.	Neh-il.	Min Tian	Ming Yat.
Every day.	Todos los días; OR cada día.	Meh-il.	Mei Tian	Mui Yat.
Every hour.	Cada hora.	Meh-she-kahn-mah-dah.	Mei Shiau Shih	Mui Siu See.

🔴 TABLE 20.23 Seasons

English	Spanish	Korean	Mandarin	Cantonese
Summer.	El verano.	Yuh-room.	Shia Tian	Har Teen.
Autumn.	El otoño.	Kah-url.	Chiou Tian	Chow Teen.
Winter.	El invierno.	Kuh-url.	Dung Tian	Dong Teen.
Spring.	La primavera.	Pohm.	Chuen Tian	Chun Teen.

TABLE 20.24 Months

English	Spanish	Korean	Mandarin	Cantonese
January.	enero.	Il-wor.	Yi Yue	Yat Yuet.
February.	febrero.	Ee-wor.	Er Yue	Yee Yuet.
March.	marzo.	Sahm-wor.	San Yue	Sarm Yuet.
April.	abril.	Sah-wor.	Sz Yue	Say Yuet.
May.	mayo.	Oh-wor.	Wu Yue	Mm Yuet.
June.	junio.	Yoo-wor	Liou Yue	Look Yuet.
July.	julio.	Chil-wor.	Chi Yue	Chud Yuet.
August.	agosto.	Pahl-wor.	Ba Yue	Baht Yuet.
September.	septiembre.	Koo-wor.	Jiou Yue	Gow Yuet.
October.	octubre.	Sheep-wor.	Shih Yue	Sub Yuet.
November.	noviembre.	Sheep-il-wor.	Shih Yi Yue	Sub Yat Yuet.
December.	diciembre.	Sheep-ee-wor.	Shih Er Yue	Sub Yee Yuet.

TABLE 20.25 Days of the Week

English	Spanish	Korean	Mandarin	Cantonese
Sunday.	domingo.	Il-yoh-il	Sing Chi Tian	Sing Kay Yut.
Monday.	lunes.	War-yo-il.	Sing Chi Yi	Sing Kay Yat.
Tuesday.	martes.	Hwa-yo-il	Sing Chi Er	Sing Kay Yee.
Wednesday.	miércoles.	Soo-yo-il	Sing Chi San	Sing Kay Sarm.
Thursday.	jueves.	Mohk-yo-il	Sing Chi Sz	Sing Kay Say.
Friday.	viernes.	Koom-yo-il	Sing Chi Wu	Sing Kay Mm.
Saturday.	sábado.	Toh-yo-il.	Sing Chi Liou	Sing Kay Look.

TABLE 20.26 Colors

English	Spanish	Korean	Mandarin	Cantonese
Black.	Negro (a, os, as).	Cum-jung.	Hei	Hug Sig.
Blue.	Azul.	Pah-rang.	Lan	Nam Sig.
Green.	Verde.	Choh-ruhk.	Lyu	Look Sig.
Pink.	Rosado (a, os, as).	Poon-hong.	Fen Hung	Fun Hung Sig.
Red.	Rojo (a, os, as).	Bahl-kang.	Hung	Hung Sig.
White.	Blanco (a, os, as).	Heen-sehk.	Bai	Baht Sig.
Yellow.	Amarillo (a, os, as).	Noh-rahng.	Huang	Wong Sig.

TRANSLAT

REFERENCE TABLES, CONVERSION CHARTS, AND FIRST AID

SI Units

🔴 TABLE A.1 SI Base Units

Quantity	Name	Symbol
Length	Meter	m
Mass	Kilogram	kg
Time	Second	s
Electric current	Ampere	A
Temperature	Kelvin	K
Luminous intensity	Candela	Cd
Amount of a substance	mole	mol

🔴 TABLE A.2 Some SI-Derived Units

Quantity	Name of Derived Unit	Symbol
Area	Square meter	m^2
Volume	Cubic meter	m^3
Speed, velocity	Meter per second	m/s
Acceleration	Meter per second squared	m/s^2
Mass density	Kilogram per cubic meter	kg/m^3
Concentration of	Mole per cubic meter	mol/m^3 a substance
Specific volume	Cubic meter per kilogram	m^3/kg
Luminescence	Candela per square meter	cd/m^3

🔴 TABLE A.3 SI-Derived Units With Special Names

Quantity	Name	Symbol	Expressed in Terms of Other Unit
Frequency	Hertz	Hz	s^1
Force	Newton	N	$kg{\bullet}m{\bullet}s^{-2}$ or $kg{\bullet}m/s^2$
Pressure	Pascal	Pa	$N{\bullet}m^{-2}$ or N/m^2
Energy, work, amount of heat	Joule	J	$kg{\bullet}m^2{\bullet}s^{-2}$ or $N{\bullet}m$
Power	Watt	W	$J{\bullet}s$ or J/s
Quantity of electricity	Coulomb	C	$A{\bullet}s$
Electromotive force	Volt	V	W/A
Capacitance	Farad	F	C/v
Electrical resistance	Ohm	Ω	V/a
Conductance	Siemens	S	A/V
Inductance	Henry	H	Wø/A
Illuminance	Lux	lx	ln/m^2
Absorbed (radiation)	Gray	Gy	J/kg dose
Dose equivalent	Sievert	Sv	J/kg (radiation)
Activity (radiation)	Becquerel	Bq	s^{-1}

Temperature Conversions

To Convert Centigrade to Fahrenheit

Degrees Fahrenheit = (Degrees Centigrade × 9/5) + 32

To Convert Fahrenheit to Centrigrade

Degrees Centigrade = (Degrees Fahrenheit – 32) × 5/9

To Convert Centigrade to Absolute (Kelvin)

Degrees Kelvin = Degrees Centigrade – 273

To Convert Absolute (Kelvin) to Centigrade

Degrees Centigrade = Degrees Kelvin + 273

TABLE A.4 Common Equivalent Temperatures

Fahrenheit	Centigrade
–19.4	12.04
32	0
98.6	37
100	37.7
212	100
0	–17.8

TABLE A.5 Metric Prefixes and Multiples Used in SI

Quantity	Multiples/ Submultiples	Prefix	Symbol
1,000,000,000,000	10^{12}	tera	T
1,000,000,000	10^9	giga	G
1,000,000	10^6	mega	M
1,000	10^3	kilo	K
100	10^2	hecto	H
10	10^1	deka	Da
0.1	10^{-1}	deci	D
0.01	10^{-2}	centi	C
0.001	10^{-3}	milli	M
0.000 001	10^{-6}	micro	μ
0.000 000 001	10^{-9}	nano	N
0.000 000 000 01	10^{-12}	pico	P
0.000 000 000 000 001	10^{-15}	femto	F
0.000 000 000 000 000 001	10^{-18}	atto	A

English-to-Metric Conversions

To convert an English measurement to a metric measurement, multiply by the factor shown. To convert a metric measurement into an English measurement, divide by the factor shown in the tables.

Area

To obtain square meters, multiply:

Sq inches	×	6.4516^{-4}
Sq feet	×	0.092903
Sq yards	×	0.8361274
Sq miles	×	2,589,988
Acres	×	4,046.856
Sq millimeters	×	1.0^{-6}
Sq centimeters	×	1.0^{-4}
Sq meters	×	1.0
Sq kilometers	×	1,000,000
Hectares	×	10,000

Length

To obtain meters, multiply:

Inches	×	0.0254
Feet	×	0.3048
Statute miles	×	1,609.344
Nautical miles	×	1,852
Millimeters	×	0.001
Centimeters	×	0.01
Meters	×	1.0
Kilometers	×	1,000

Pressure

To obtain pascals (N/m^2), multiply:

Inches Hg at 0°C	×	3,386.389
Feet H_2O 4°C	×	2,988,98
Pounds per sq inch	×	6,894.757
Pounds per sq foot	×	47.88026
Short tons per sq foot	×	95,760.52
Atmospheres at 760 mm Hg	×	101,325
Centimeters Hg at 0°C	×	1,333.22
Meters H2O at 4°C	×	9,806.38
Kilograms per sq centimeters	×	98,066.5
Pascals (N/m^2)	×	1.0

Speed and Velocity

To obtain meters per seconds, multiply:

Inches per minute	×	4.2333^{-4}
Feet per second	×	0.3048
Feet per minute	×	0.00508
Miles per second	×	1,609.344
Miles per hour	×	0.44704
Knots	×	0.5144444
Centimeters per minute	×	1.6667^{-4}
Meters per second	×	1.0
Meters per minute	×	0.0166667
Kilometers per hour	×	0.2777778

Volume and Capacity

To obtain cubic meters, multiply:

Cubic inches	×	1.6387^{-5}
Cubic feet	×	0.0283168
Cubic yards	×	0.7645549
Ounces	×	2.9574^{-5}
Quarts	×	9.4634^{-4}
U.S. gallons	×	0.0037854
Imperial gallons	×	0.0045461
Cubic centimeters	×	1.0^{-6}
Cubic meters	×	1.0
Liters	×	0.001

Weight, Mass, and Force

To obtain kilograms, multiply:

Grains	×	6.4799^{-5}
Ounces (avdp)	×	0.0283495
Pounds (avdp)	×	0.4535924
Short tons	×	907.1847
Long tons	×	1,016.047
Milligrams	×	1.0^{-6}
Grams	×	0.001
Metric tons	×	1,000,000
Newtons	×	0.1019716

To obtain newtons, multiply:

Grains	×	6.3546^{-4}
Ounces (avdp)	×	0.2780139
Pounds (avdp)	×	4.448222
Short tons	×	8,896.443
Tons	×	9,964.016
Milligrams	×	9.8067^{-6}
Grams	×	0.0098067

Kilograms	×	9.80665
Metric tons	×	9,806.65
Newtons	×	1.0

Work, Energy, and Power

To obtain joules (watt-sec), multiply:

Foot-pounds	×	1.355818
Btu (IT)	×	1,055.056
Btu (mean)	×	1,055.87
Btu (TC)	×	1,054.350
Meter-kilograms	×	9.80665
Kilocalories (IT)	×	4,186.8
Kilocalories (mean)	×	4,190.02
Kilocalories (TC)	×	4,184.0
Joules (watt-second)	×	1.0
Watt-hours	×	3,600

To obtain watts, multiply:

Foot-pounds per second	×	1.355818
Foot-pounds per minute	×	0.0225970
Btu (IT) per hour	×	0.2930711
Btu (TC) per minute	×	17.57250
Horsepower (550 fpps)	×	745.6999
Horsepower (electric)	×	746
Horsepower (metric)	×	735.4988
Kilocalories (TC) per second	×	4,184
Watts	×	1.0
Kilowatts	×	1,000

pH Nomenclature and Values

The pH scale is simply a series of numbers stating where a given solution would stand in a series of solutions arranged according to acidity or alkalinity. At one extreme (high pH) lies a highly alkaline solution, which may be made by dissolving 4 g of sodium hydroxide in water to make a liter of solution; at the other extreme (low pH) is an acid solution containing 3.65 g of hydrogen chloride per liter of water. Halfway between lies purified water, which is neutral. All other solutions can be arranged on this scale, and their acidity or alkalinity can be stated by giving numbers that indicate their relative positions. If the pH of a certain solution is 5.3, it falls between gastric juice and urine on the above scale, is moderately acid, and will turn litmus red.

Tenth-normal HCl	−1.00
Gastric juice	1.4
Urine*	6.0
Water	7.00 (neutral)
Blood	7.35–7.45
Bile*	7.5

Pancreatic juice	8.5
Tenth-normal	13.00 NaOH

For the acid mixture solutions of pH values of –1.00 to 6.0, litmus paper will turn red. For the alkaline mixture solutions of pH values of 7.35 to 13.00, litmus paper will turn blue.

*These body fluid values vary widely in pH; typical values have been used for simplicity.

Symbols

m	Minim
℈	Scruple
ˆ	Dram
f	Fluidram
J	Ounce
fJ	Fluidounce
O	Pint
lb	Pound
[Rx]	Recipe (L. take)
M	Misce (L. mix)
ā ā	Of each
A,Å	angstrom unit
C-1, C-2, etc.	Complement
c, c⁻	cum (L. with)
Δ	Change; heat
E0	Electroaffinity
F1	First filial generation
F_2	Second filial generation
mμ	Millimicron, nanometer
μg	Microgram
mEq	Milliequivalent
mg	Milligram
mg%	Milligrams percent; milligrams per 100 ml
Q_{O2}	Oxygen consumption
m-	Meta-
o-	Ortho-
p-	Para-
p⁻	After
P_{O2}	Partial pressure of oxygen
P_{CO2}	Partial pressure of carbon dioxide
s⁻	Without
s⁻ s⁻	[L. semis] One-half
μm	Micrometer
μ	Micron (former term for micro-meter)
μμ	Micromicron
+	Plus; excess; acid reaction; positive
−	Minus; deficiency; alkaline reaction; negative
±	Plus or minus; either positive or negative; indefinite

Symbol	Meaning
#	Number; following a number, pounds
÷	Divided by
×	Multiplied by; magnification
/	Divided by
=	Equals
≈	Approximately equal
>	Greater than; from which is derived
<	Less than; derived from
≮	Not less than
≯	Not greater than
≤	Equal to or less than
≥	Equal to or greater than
≠	Not equal to
√	Root; square root; radical
2√	Square root
3√	Cube root
∞	Infinity
:	Ratio; "is to"
::	Equality between ratios; "as"
∴	Therefore
°	Degree
%	Percent
π	3.1416—ratio of circumference of a circle to its diameter
elaM,♂	Male
o,♀	Female
s	Denotes a reversible reaction
n	Subscripted n indicates the number of the molecules can vary from two or greater

Abbreviations Used in Prescription Writing and Notes (in alphabetical order)

A		ante	before
a	before	aq	water
abs feb	while the fever is absent	aq ferv	hot water
		aq frig	cold water
ac	before meals	aq tep	tepid water
ad lib	as desired	**B**	
ADL	activities of daily living	b	bath
		bal	bath
adv	against	bib	drink
aeg	the patient	bid	twice a day
alt	alternate	bin	twice a night
alt die	alternate days	bis	twice
alt hor	every other hour	bol	pill
alt noc	every other night	BR	bedrest
AMA	against medical advice	BRP	bathroom privileges

C

c, c̄	with
C/O	complains of
cc	chief complaint
CCW	counterclockwise
cf	compare, refer to
cib	food
CM	tomorrow morning
cms	to be taken tomorrow morning
CN	tomorrow night
cns	to be taken tomorrow night
cont	continue
CV	tomorrow evening
CW	clockwise

D

d	day
D	dose, duration, give, let it be given, right
D/C	discharge
da	give
dc, D/C	discontinue
de d in d	from day to day
decr	decrease
decub	lying down
det	let it be given
dieb alt	on alternate days
dieb tert	every third day
dil	dilute
DISC	discontinue
disch	discharge
div	divide
DP	with proper direction
dur dolor	while the pain lasts

E

ead	the same
EMP	as directed
et	and
eval	evaluation

F

feb dur	while the fever lasts
FLD	fluid
freq	frequent

G

GRAD	gradually, by degrees

H

Hd	at bedtime
HOB	head of bed
hor decub	at bedtime
hor interm	at intermediate hours
hor som	at bedtime
hor un spatio	at the end of an hour
hs	at bedtime

I

id	the same
in d	daily
Incr	increase

L

L	left
LIQ	liquid
loc dol	to the painful spot
lt	left

M

M&R	measure and record
mit	send
mor dict	as directed
mor sol	in the usual way
mp	as directed

N

NB	note well
NBM	nothing by mouth
noc	night
noct	at night
non rep	do not repeat
NOS	not otherwise specified
NPO	nothing by mouth
NPO/HS	nothing by mouth at bedtime
NR	do not repead

O

Occ	occasional
OD	once daily
om	every morning
om quar hor	every quarter of an hour
omn bih	every two hours
omn hor	every hour
omn noct	every night
on	every night
OOB	out of bed

P

P	after, position
par aff	the part affected
PC, p.c.	after meals
per	by, for each, through
PO	postoperative
PO, po	by mouth
POD	postoperative day
pp	postpartum, post-prandial
prn	as the occasion
pta	prior to admission

Q

q	each, every
q2h	every two hours
q3h	every three hours
q4h	every four hours
qam	every morning
qd	every day
qh	every hour
qhs	every bedtime
qid	four times a day
ql	as much as desired
qm	every morning
qn	every night
qns	quantity not sufficient
qod	every other day
qoh	every other hour
qp	at will
qqh	every four hours
qqhor	every hour
quotid	daily
qv	as much as you like

R

R	right
REP	let it be repeated
RO/R/O	rule out
ROM	range of motion
ROS	review of systems
Rot	rotate
RT	right
RX, Rx	prescription, take, treatment

S

s,s̄	without
S	label, left, sign, without
S/P	status post
si op sit	if it is necessary
simul	at the same time
SOS	if it is necessary, when necessary
stat	immediately
std	let it stand

T

Tab	tablet
tds	take three times a day
tid	three times a day
TLC	tender loving care
TO	telephone order

U, V, W

UNK	unknown
ut dict	as directed
VIZ	namely
VO, vo, V/O	verbal order
WNL	within normal limits

Manual Alphabet

Braille Alphabet and Numbers

A	B	C	D	E	F	G	H	I
○	○ ○	○ ○	○ ○	○ ○	○ ○	○ ○	○ ○	○ ○

J	K	L	M	N	O	P	Q	R

S	T	U	V	W	X	Y	Z	1

2	3	4	5	6	7	8	9	0

Body Mass Index

Body mass index (BMI) is a statistical estimator of body fat based on height and weight. The BMI is used to screen for weight categories that may lead to health problems. BMI is defined as the individual's body weight (kg) divided by the square of his/her height (m). The formula universally used in medicine produces a unit of measure of kg/m^2.

$$BMI = weight\ (kg)\ /\ [height\ (m)]^2$$

or,

$$BMI = weight\ (lb)\ /\ [height\ (in.)]^2 \times 703$$

BMI values are age-independent and the same for both sexes. However, BMI does not directly measure body fat. As a result, some people, such as athletes, may have a BMI that identifies them as overweight even though they do not have excess body fat.

For a Web-based calculator of BMI refer to the Centers for Disease Control and Prevention (CDC) website: http://www.cdc.gov/healthyweight/assessing/bmi/adult_bmi/english_bmi_calculator/bmi_calculator.html

BMI for Children and Teens 2 to 20 Years

Although the BMI number is calculated the same way for children and adults, the criteria used to interpret the meaning of the BMI number for children (and teens) are different from those used for adults.

For children and teens, BMI age- and sex-specific percentiles are used because the amount of body fat changes with age, and differs for girls and boys.

The CDC BMI-for-age growth charts take into account these differences and allow translation of a BMI number into a percentile for a child's sex and age (see figures below and on p. 1228).

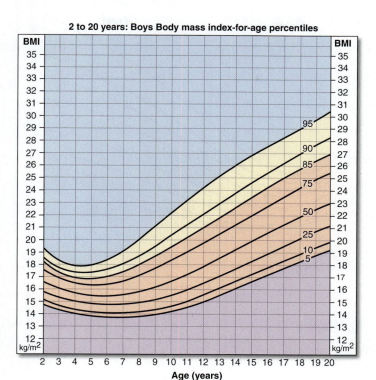

2 to 20 years: Boys Body mass index-for-age percentiles

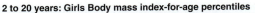

2 to 20 years: Girls Body mass index-for-age percentiles

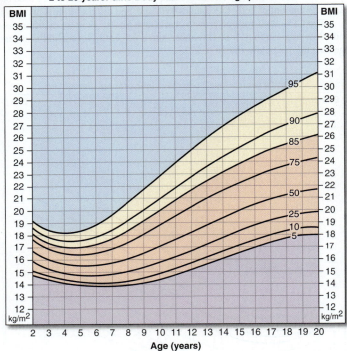

Adapted from

The Center for Disease Control and Prevention (CDC) website: http://www.cdc.gov/growthcharts/

Weight Classifications for Adults

The current international classification of body weight categories for adults, established by the World Health Organization (WHO), is based on the BMI.

TABLE A.6 WHO International Classifications for Adult Weight

Classification	BMI(kg/m²) Principal Cut-Off Points	Additional Cut-Off Points
Underweight	**<18.50**	**<18.50**
Severe thinness	<16.00	<16.00
Moderate thinness	16.00–16.99	16.00–16.99
Mild thinness	17.00–18.49	17.00–18.49
Normal range	**18.50–24.99**	**18.50–22.99**
		23.00–24.99
Overweight	**≥25.00**	**≥25.00**
Pre-obese	25.00–29.99	25.00–27.49
		27.50–29.99
Obese	**≥30.00**	**≥30.00**
Obese class I	30.00–34.99	30.00–32.49
		32.50–34.99
Obese class II	35.00–39.99	35.00–37.49
		37.50–39.99
Obese class III	≥40.00	≥40.00

From: World Health Organization (WHO). http://apps.who.int/bmi/index.jsp?introPage=intro_3.html

For more information:

Obesity: preventing and managing the global epidemic. Report of a WHO Consultation. WHO Technical Report Series 894. Geneva, Switzerland: World Health Organization, 2000. http://whqlibdoc.who.int/trs/WHO_TRS_894.pdf

Weight Classifications for Children and Teens

The CDC and the American Academy of Pediatrics (AAP) recommend the use of BMI to screen for overweight and obesity in children beginning at 2 years of age. However, BMI is not a diagnostic tool; that is, a child may have a high BMI for age and sex, but to determine if excess fat is a problem, a health-care provider would need to perform further assessments. These assessments might include skinfold thickness measurements and evaluations of diet, physical activity, family history, and other appropriate health screenings.

To establish the weight status category, use the following percentile ranges for the calculated BMI-for-age percentile (from the charts in the figures on pages 1227–1228):

Weight Status Category	Percentile Range
Underweight	Less than the 5th percentile
Healthy weight	5th percentile to less than the 85th percentile
Overweight	85th to less than the 95th percentile
Obese	Equal to or greater than the 95th percentile

For more information:

Consult the Centers for Disease Control and Prevention (CDC) website:
http://www.cdc.gov/healthyweight/assessing/bmi/

Cardiopulmonary Resuscitation (CPR)

The following is an overview of cardiopulmonary resuscitation (CPR). The information in this section is based on the American Heart Association's 2010 Guidelines for Basic Life Support for Healthcare Providers and the International Liaison Committee on Resuscitation (ILCOR) Consensus on CPR and Emergency Cardiovascular Care (ECC) Science With Treatment Recommendations. This overview does not qualify an individual to perform CPR in a professional capacity and does not substitute for an official training course. This information should serve as a guide for those who have completed CPR training and are certified.

The main purpose of CPR is to provide oxygenated blood to the brain and the heart and create a return of spontaneous circulation (ROSC) in an unresponsive victim. Brain damage begins after 4 to 6 minutes and irreversible brain damage occurs after about 10 minutes. Once the brain cells die, biological death will occur. CPR by itself is unlikely to create a ROSC and hence the need for early activation of the Emergency Response System (call 911) and use of an automatic external defibrillator (AED). An AED is a simple device to use, which analyzes a victim's heart rhythm and prompts the rescuer to deliver a "shock" when necessary, allowing the victim's heart to return to a normal electrical rhythm and work effectively to support a pulse.

Clincial death occurs when breathing and heartbeat stop. This is often caused by a sudden cardiac arrest (SCA). An SCA may be caused by an arrhythmia, such as ventricular fibrillation (VF), in which the heart's electrical signals become chaotic and ineffective and the victim loses conciousness. Cardiac arrests also result from brain damage, choking, drowning, drug abuse, electrocution, traumatic injury, congenital heart disease, sudden infant death syndrome (SIDS), and more. Clinical death may be reversible through CPR and other treatments.

The 2010 guidelines have been changed from the ABC sequence (Airway, Breathing, Chest Compression) to the CAB sequence (Chest Compressions, Airway, Breathing) to ensure higher quality CPR by focusing on uninterrupted compressions, pushing hard and fast, and early defibrillation. However, the ABC sequence may still be used for arrests of an asphyxial nature and for neonates, as the etiology is often respiratory. The "look, listen, and feel" step for breathing has been removed and there is a de-emphasis on checking for a pulse. Performing CPR as a team and with effective communication will also result in more effective CPR, allowing multiple steps to be completed simultaneously. Compression-only CPR is effective and is taught to lay rescuers, although whenever possible ventilations should be delivered as well, particularly for pediatric victims.

The reader is encouraged to check with the American Heart Association (http://heart.org/) for any updated recommendations. (Note: the recommendations in this section were accessed from the AHA website on July 1, 2011.)

⬤ TABLE A.7 Components of CPR—Adult*

*Defined as the onset of puberty or older in appearance.
Signs of puberty include chest or underarm hair in males and any breast development in females.

Assess the Victim	Ensure that the scene is safe for the rescuer and the victim. If necessary, consider moving the victim.
Check for Response and Breathing	Tap the victim's shoulder and shout, "Are you all right?"
	Simultaneously check the victim's breathing in ≤ 10 seconds.
	If there is no response from victim, or the victim is not breathing or not breathing normally (agonal gasps), shout for help.
	The emergency response system must be activated immediately (call 911) and an automated external defibrillator (AED) retrieved, if available. If alone, first perform these steps and then return to the victim and proceed. If bystanders are available, the rescuer should designate them to activate the emergency response system (call 911) and retrieve an AED, if available, while the rescuer continues with CPR.
	If the victim is definitely breathing adequately and has no suspected spinal injury, place in the recovery position on the left side and reassess every 2 minutes.

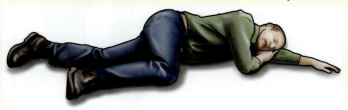

Recovery position.

If the victim suffered an asphyxial arrest, first provide 5 cycles of CPR (ABC sequence preferred). If bystanders have not already done so, activate the emergency response system and retrieve an AED, if available, and then return to continue CPR.

(table continues on page 1232)

● TABLE A.7 Components of CPR—Adult* (continued)

Pulse Check	Check the victim's carotid artery at the side of the neck in the groove between the trachea and muscles. If in ≤ 10 seconds no pulse is present or the rescuer is unsure if a pulse is present, immediately perform 5 cycles of compressions and breaths (CAB sequence). If in ≤ 10 seconds a pulse is definitely present, provide rescue breaths by delivering 1 breath every 5–6 seconds (1–12 breaths/minute). Reassess pulse every 2 minutes.
Compression Depth	≥ 2 inches (5 cm)
Compression Rate	≥ 100/minute
Compression Techniques	Position the victim face up on a firm, flat surface. Position yourself at the victim's side and expose the chest. If you suspect the victim has a spinal injury, try to keep the head, neck, and torso of the victim in a line while rolling the victim to a faceup position. Place the heel of one hand on the center of the victim's chest on the lower half of the sternum or breastbone, midline between the nipples. Place the heel of the other hand on top of the first hand. Alternatively, with the second hand grab the wrist of the first hand.

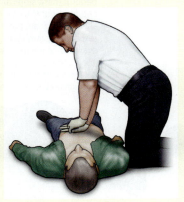

Location of hand position for chest compressions in CPR.

Push hard and fast on the chest.
Keep arms straight and locked, positioning shoulders directly over hands.
Push straight down in a smooth and rhythmic fashion.
Allow for full chest recoil between compressions.

Count number of compressions out loud.
Minimize interruptions between compressions to ≤ 10 seconds.
Ensure fingers are not compressing chest, only heel of hand.

Compression: Ventilation Ratio	30:2 (universal ratio for ≥ 1 rescuers) → 30 compressions in ≤ 18 seconds The universal ratio should be repeated continuously, or in steps of 5 cycles when an AED is present. If a second rescuer is available, switch roles every 5 cycles, or about 2 minutes, taking ≤ 5 seconds and minimizing interruptions. This should be done while the AED, if available, is analyzing the victim. The second rescuer should be positioned by the victim's head and maintain an open airway, deliver breaths, and monitor the primary rescuer for effective compressions.
Opening the Airway	Head Tilt–Chin Lift Technique Lift the jaw by placing fingers under the bony part of the lower jaw near the chin, without using the thumb. With the other hand, push with your palm on the victim's forehead to tilt the head back. Make sure not to close the victim's mouth completely.

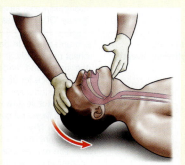

Head tilt–chin lift technique: Open airway by raising jaw and tilting head backward from chest. This forces epiglottis and tongue away from airway.

Jaw Thrust Technique
This technique should be used when there is a suspected head or neck injury. It typically requires at least 2 rescuers to perform. If this technique does not open the airway, switch to the Head Tilt–Chin Lift Technique.

(table continues on page 1234)

TABLE A.7 **Components of CPR—Adult*** (continued)

The jaw is lifted without tilting the head. Place one hand on each side of the victim's head, resting elbows on the surface on which the victim is lying. Place fingers under the angles of the victim's lower jaw and lift with both hands, displacing the jaw forward. If the lips close, push the lower lip with the thumb to open the lips.

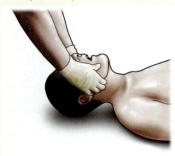

Jaw thrust technique.

If available, insert an airway adjunct, such as an nasopharyngeal airway (NPA) or an oropharyngeal airway (OPA), unless otherwise contraindicated.

Ventilation: Delivering Breaths	Each breath should be 1 second long and make the chest rise visibly. If breaths do not enter, reposition the airway and reattempt. If breaths still do not enter, check for an obstruction and continue with compressions. Avoid excessive ventilation.
	Ensure effective airway device seals against the victim's face and connect supplementary oxygen if available. Mouth-to-mouth may also be performed by pinching the nose closed.
	Note: The routine use of cricoid pressure (Sellick's maneuver) is no longer recommended.
	With an advanced airway (endotracheal intubation, laryngeal mask airway, supraglottic airway) in place, maintain a compression rate ≥ 100/minute and deliver 1 breath every 6–8 seconds (8–10 breaths/min). Do not pause or attempt to synchronize compressions while delivering ventilations.
AED	Use the AED as soon as it becomes available.
	See Table A.9
	If the victim was down for ≥ 4–5 minutes or the arrest is asphyxia related, consider first providing 1–2 minutes of CPR before using the AED.

* Standard safety precautions and personal protective equipment should always be used.

TABLE A.8 Steps of Pediatric CPR—Child and

	Child	Infant
	Defined as 1 year of age to puberty. Signs of puberty include chest or underarm hair in males and any breast development in females.	Defined as younger than 1 year of age (12 months), excluding newly born infants in the delivery room.
...im	Ensure the scene is safe for the rescuer and the victim. If necessary, consider moving the victim.	
...ck for Response and Breathing	Tap the victim's shoulder and shout, "Are you all right?" Simultaneously check the victim's breathing in ≤ 10 seconds.	Tap the bottom of the foot to illicit response. Simultaneously check the victim's breathing in ≤ 10 seconds.
	If there is no response from victim or the victim is not breathing or not breathing normally (agonal gasps), shout for help. • If the rescuer did not witness the arrest and is alone, or the victim suffered an asphyxia arrest, immediately provide 5 cycles of CPR. Then leave the victim to activate the emergency response system (call 911) and retrieve an automated external defibrillator (AED), if available, and return to continue CPR. • If the rescuer witnessed the sudden arrest and is alone, first activate the emergency response system (call 911) and retrieve an AED, if available, and then return to the victim and begin CPR. • If bystanders are available, the rescuer should designate them to activate the emergency response system (call 911) and retrieve an AED, if available, while the rescuer continues with CPR.	
	If the victim is definitely breathing adequately, place in the recovery position on left side, unless the child is small or there is suspected spinal injury (see figure on p. 1231). Reassess every 2 minutes.	Do not place infants in the recovery position, as this may block the airway. Continuously assess the infant's breathing.

(table continues on page 1236)

■ **TABLE A.8 Components of Pediatric CPR—Child Infant** (continued)

	Child	Infant
Pulse Check	Check the victim's carotid artery at the side of the neck in the groove between trachea and muscles, or the femoral artery in the inner thigh, midway between the hipbone and the pubic bone and just below the crease where the leg meets the abdomen.	Check brachial on the inside upper arm, between the elbow and shoulder. Press gently with the index and middle fingers.
	If in ≤ 10 seconds no pulse is present, the rescuer is unsure if a pulse is present, or pulse is ≤ 60 beats/minute with signs of poor perfusion despite adequate oxygenation and ventilation, immediately perform 5 cycles of compressions and breaths (CAB-sequence). If in ≤ 10 seconds a pulse is definitely present and adequate, provide rescue breaths by delivering 1 breath every 3 seconds. Reassess pulse every 2 minutes.	
Compression Depth	≥ ⅓ anterior-posterior depth of chest	
	≈ 2 inches/5 cm	≈ 1.5 inches/4 cm
Compression Rate	≥ 100 per minute	
Compression Techniques	Position the victim faceup on a firm, flat surface. Position yourself at the victim's side and expose the chest. If you suspect the victim has a spinal injury, try to keep the head, neck, and torso of the victim in a line while rolling the victim to a faceup position.	
	Place the heel of one hand on the center of the victim's chest on the lower half of the sternum or breastbone, midline between the nipples. Optionally, place the heel of the other hand on top of the first hand, as in adult CPR (refer to figure on p. 1232).	**1 rescuer:** 2 fingers (see figure below at left on p. 1237). **2 rescuers:** 2 thumb-encircling hands technique, or alternatively 2 fingers (see figure below at right on p. 1237).

Child	Infant

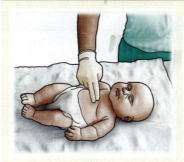

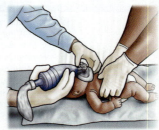

Two-finger chest compressions for infants.

Two thumb-encircling hands chest compressions for infants.

Keep arms straight and locked, positioning shoulders directly over hands. *Ensure fingers are not compressing chest, only heel of hand.*	For each scenario, press on the lower half of the breastbone in the center of the chest, just bellow the nipple line, with the tips of your fingers. Do not press on the bottom of the breastbone.

Push hard and fast on the chest.
Push straight down, in a smooth and rhythmic fashion.
Allow for full chest recoil between compressions.
Count number of compressions out loud.
Minimize interruptions between compressions to ≤ 10 seconds.

Compression: Ventilation Ratio	**1 Rescuer:** (universal ratio) 30:2 ➜ 30 compressions in ≤ 18 seconds **2 Rescuers:** 15:2 ➜ 15 compressions in ≤ 9 seconds The compression:ventilation ratio should be repeated continuously, or in steps of 5 cycles when an AED is present. If a second rescuer is available, switch roles every 5 cycles, or about 2 minutes, taking ≤ 5 seconds and minimizing interruptions. This should be done while the AED, if available, is analyzing the victim. The second rescuer should be positioned by the victim's head and maintain an open airway, deliver breaths, and monitor the primary rescuer for effective compressions.
Open the Airway	Open the airway using the head tilt–chin lift technique, as in adult CPR (see figure on p. 1233). Do not hyperextend the neck.

(table continues on page 1238)

TABLE A.8 Components of Pediatric CPR—Child and Infant (continued)

	Child	Infant
		For infants, place the head and neck in the neutral or sniffing position, so that the external ear canal is level with the top of the infant's shoulder. Hyperextending the neck can cause the airway to become blocked. If spinal injury suspected, use the jaw thrust technique, as in adult CPR (see figure on p. 1234). Note: Children's and infants' airways are more difficult to open and may require a few attempts to open and maintain an airway. If available, insert an airway adjunct, such as an NPA or OPA, unless otherwise contraindicated.
Ventilation: Delivering Breaths		Each breath should be 1 second long and make the chest rise visibly. If breaths do not enter, reposition the airway and reattempt. If breaths still do not enter, check for an obstruction and continue with compressions. Avoid excessive ventilation. Ensure effective airway device seals against the victim's face and connect supplementary oxygen if available. Mouth-to-mouth may also be performed, by pinching the nose closed. For infants, mouth-to-mouth may be performed by also surrounding the nose. Note: The routine use of cricoid pressure (Sellick's maneuver) is no longer recommended. With an advanced airway (endotracheal intubation, laryngeal mask airway, supraglottic airway) in place, maintain a compression rate ≥ 100/minute and deliver 1 breath every 6–8 seconds (8–10 breaths/min). Do not pause or attempt to synchronize compressions while delivering ventilations.
AED		If a witnessed event, use the AED immediately. If the event was u-witnessed or asphyxia related, consider first providing 1–2 minutes of CPR before using the AED.

⬤ TABLE A.9 Steps for Using an Automatic External Defibrillator (AED) for Adults, Children, and Infants*

Indications	Verify the victim is unresponsive, is not breathing, and has no pulse. Use the AED as soon as it becomes available. If the arrest is asphyxia related, or the adult victim was down for ≥ 4–5 minutes, or an unwitnessed pediatric event, consider providing 1–2 minutes of CPR first before using the AED.
Attachment and Placement	The first step in using an AED is to power the device on. Attach adhesive pads to the victim while CPR is in progress. If a second rescuer is not available, pause CPR if already initiated. Remove the backing from the pads. Place one adhesive pad on the victim's bare, upper-right chest, directly below the collarbone. The second pad is placed to the side of the left nipple (midaxillary), with the top edge of the pad a few inches below the armpit. Proper location of each pad is indicated by an image on the pad. 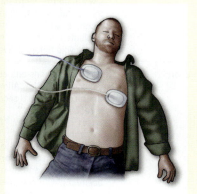 Automated external defibrillator (AED) electrode pad placement. Attach cables to AED device if not already connected. Note: Pediatric pads should be used on children ages 1 to 8 and should never be used on an adult. If no pediatric pads are available for pediatric victims, adult pads can be used. For infants, a manual defibrillator is preferred. If not available, an AED with pediatric pads is acceptable, and if necessary adult

(table continues on page 1240)

TABLE A.9 Steps for Using an Automatic External Defibrillator (AED) for Adults, Children, and Infants* (continued)

	pads may still be used. Ensure the pads do not touch or overlap. For pediatrics, one pad can be placed on the chest (anterior) and the other on the back (posterior). Note: If the AED instructs to "check electrodes," press down firmly on the pad. If the AED continues to prompt and the victim is excessively hairy, quickly remove the pads and then replace pads, optimally with a new pair if available. Consider using a razor to shave the area. Notes: • Remove any transdermal medication patches and quickly wipe the area clean, if it won't delay shock delivery, before attaching the AED pad. • Move or wipe down the victim if in standing water or excessively wet or sweaty. If the victim is lying on snow or in a small puddle, the AED may still be used. • If victim has an internal pacemaker/defibrillator, avoid placing the pads directly over the device. Follow the normal steps for operating an AED unless the implanted defibrillator is delivering shocks to the victim, in which case allow 30–60 seconds for the implanted defibrillator to complete the shock treatment cycle before delivering a shock from the AED.
Operation	Stop compressions and ensure no one is touching or moving the victim. Allow the AED to analyze the victim for about 5–15 seconds and determine if shock is required. If shock is advised say, "I'm going to shock. I'm clear. Everybody clear." Perform a visual check to ensure that no one is touching the victim or equipment. Deliver a shock, and then resume CPR immediately beginning with compressions. If no shock is advised, resume CPR immediately beginning with compressions. Minimize interruptions between last compressions and shock delivery or resumption of compressions. Note: The shock may produce a sudden contraction of the victim's muscles.
Continue CPR and Reanalyze	After every 5 cycles, or about 2 minutes, the AED will automatically instruct the discontinuation of CPR and reanalyze. At this point, rescuers can switch roles. After determining if a shock needs to be delivered, resume CPR beginning with compressions.
Continued Care	Continue CPR and leave the AED attached and on until advanced care providers assume responsibility and take over continued care, or CPR is terminated.

If the victim shows obvious signs of life, stop CPR, turn off the AED, and leave the pads attached to the victim. Continue to monitor the victim.

*If possible, become familiar with the AED that you may need to use in an emergency prior to using it.
Most AEDs have similar operating procedures and will provide voice prompts and step-by-step instructions, to be used by untrained rescuers.

Airway Obstructions and Relieving Choking

Mild Airway Obstruction. If a victim has a mild airway obstruction, the airway will be only partially blocked. The victim will still have good air exchange, will be able to cough forcefully, and may wheeze between coughs.

- Encourage the victim to continue spontaneous coughing and breathing efforts.
- Do not interfere with the efforts.
- Monitor the condition, as a mild airway obstruction may become severe.
- Activate the emergency response system if the obstruction is not relieved.

Severe Airway Obstruction. If a victim has a severe airway obstruction, he or she usually expresses the universal choking sign, in which the person grabs his throat or neck with one or both hands (see figure below). The victim will be unable to speak, breathe, or cough effectively, indicating that the person is not getting enough air to sustain life. She may make high-pitched noises while inhaling and will have increased respiratopry difficulty. His lips or skin may become blue (cyanotic) and younger children won't be able to cough, breathe, or make any sounds. Always ask the victim if she is choking. If the victim nods yes and cannot talk, attempt to relieve the obstruction.

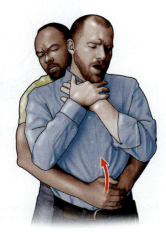

Abdominal thrust hand positioning for a standing adult or child who is choking. Note: The victim is displaying the universal choking sign.

- **Adult & Child:** For a conscious standing adult victim, abdominal thrusts* (Heimlich maneuver) should be performed:
  - Stand behind victim with a strong stance and wrap your arms around the victim.
  - Place the fist of one hand against the abdomen—midline slightly above the navel and well below the breastbone.
  - Grab the fist with the other hand and press into the victim's abdomen with a quick and forceful upward and inward thrust (J motion).
  - Continue thrusts with separate and distinct movements until the object is expelled from the airway or until the victim loses consciousness.
  - If the victim is pregnant or obese, chest thrusts can be used instead. If the victim is a child, the rescuer can kneel behind him.
- **Infant:** For a conscious choking infant, the Heimlich maneuver is not recommended.
  - Bare the infant's chest and hold the infant facedown with the head lower than the trunk, resting on your forearm (see figure below).
  - Support the infant's head and jaw with your hand, resting your arm on your thigh or lap. Avoid compressing the soft tissues of the infant's throat.
  - Deliver up to five backslaps forcefully in the middle of the back between the shoulder blades with the heel of the hand.
  - Then, place the free arm on the infant's back, supporting the back of the head with your hand, and turn the infant as a unit. Support the infant on your forearm and thigh, keeping the head lower than the trunk.
  - Provide up to five chest thrusts at a rate of about one per second, in the same location and manner as two-finger chest compressions.
  - Repeat this sequence of backslaps and chest thrusts until the object dislodges or the infant become unconscious.

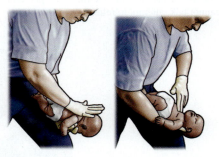

Hand position for backslaps and chest thrusts for a choking infant.

---

*Abdominal thrusts may cause medical complications. If abdominal thrusts were performed, the victim should be examined by a health-care provider to rule out any complications.

- **Unconscious Adult, Child, & Infant:** If the victim becomes unresponsive, the following procedures should be followed:
  - Safely position the victim on the floor.
  - Check the airway to remove any visible objects and immediately begin CPR with compressions. Do not check for a pulse.
  - Each time the victim's airway is opened, any visible objects should be removed before providing ventilations. Perform finger sweep only if the object is visible.
  - After breaths are delivered, continue with compressions, even if the breaths did not enter.
  - After five cycles, activate the emergency response system if someone has not already done so.
  - Once the obstruction is cleared and breaths enter, continue with CPR until the victim regains consciousness or until advanced care providers assume responsibility.

For more information:

2010 American Heart Association Guidelines for Cardiopulmonary Resuscitation and Emergency Cardiovascular Care Science. Circulation 2010;122;S639. doi:10.1161/CIR.0b013e3181fdf7aa

2010 International Consensus on Cardiopulmonary Resuscitation and Emergency Cardiovascular Care Science With Treatment Recommendations. Circulation. 2010;122:S249, doi:10.1161/CIR.0b013e3181fdf77e

Resource

American Heart Association
http://heart.org/
1-877-AHA-4CPR
International Liaison Committee on Resuscitation (ILCOR)
http://www.ilcor.org/en/home/

Index

Note: *f* denotes figure; *t*, table, and *tt*, several tables over a page range.